MW00380590

A PRACTICE OF CARDIAC PACING

Second Revised and Enlarged Edition

A PRACTICE OF CARDIAC PACING

Second Revised and Enlarged Edition

by

Seymour Furman, MD, FACC

Attending Cardiothoracic Surgeon
Montefiore Medical Center
Professor of Surgery
Professor of Medicine
Albert Einstein College of Medicine of Yeshiva University
Bronx, New York

David L. Hayes, MD

Consultant, Division of Cardiovascular Diseases
and Internal Medicine
Director, Cardiac Pacing Services
Mayo Clinic and Mayo Foundation
Assistant Professor of Medicine
Mayo Medical School
Rochester, Minnesota

David R. Holmes, Jr., MD

Consultant, Division of Cardiovascular Diseases
and Internal Medicine
Mayo Clinic and Mayo Foundation
Professor of Medicine
Mayo Medical School
Rochester, Minnesota

Futura Publishing Company, Inc
Mount Kisco, New York
1989

Library of Congress Cataloging-in-Publication Data

Furman, Seymour.
    A practice of cardiac pacing / by Seymour Furman, David L.
Hayes, David R. Holmes, Jr.—2nd rev. and enl. ed.
        p.   cm.
    Includes index.
    ISBN 0-87993-350-X
    1. Cardiac pacing.   I. Hayes, David L.   II. Holmes, David R.,
1945– . III. Title.
        [DNLM: 1. Cardiac Pacing, Artificial—methods.   2. Pacemaker,
Artificial.   WG 168 F986p]
RC684.P3F867   1989
617.4'12059—dc20
DNLM/DLC
for Library of Congress   89-7687
                                CIP

Copyright 1989
Futura Publishing Company, Inc.

Published by:
Futura Publishing Company, Inc.
P.O. Box 330, Bedford Ridge Road
Mount Kisco, New York 10549

L.C. No.:89-7687
ISBN No.: 0-87993-350-X

Printed in the United States of America

FOREWORD

There is a wealth of literature that includes articles and monographs concerning cardiac pacing in English and in other languages. Books published during the early 1960s had one or several authors and developed a specific point of view; later books commonly were the proceedings of various world or regional symposia or were multi-authored edited texts. The need for multiple authors is a reflection of the diversity and the vitality of the field and the comprehension that even an experienced worker cannot know more than a modest portion. Still, we felt that there was room for a more personal volume that would reflect the attitudes and approaches of a small group rather than of the diversity of large numbers. Something is lost by limiting approaches and perceptions, but a great deal is gained by a personal approach from two large practices of cardiac pacing, i.e., Montefiore Medical Center and the Mayo Clinic. We hope that this book will be a readable, accessible tutorial, responsive to the needs of the less experienced worker and valuable to the more experienced, in addition to being a significant contribution to the cardiac pacemaker literature.

The volume is extensively illustrated and diagrams the operation of cardiac pacemakers. The bibliography focuses on those references that seem most necessary rather than attempting to be exhaustive. The text is intended as a practical delineation of how pacemakers work and what telemetric, radiological and electrocardiographic findings are associated with normal and abnormal functions. It is these analyses that help clarify the complexity of modern cardiac pacing. We attempt not only to delineate the anomalous and normal functions but also to integrate the diagnostic capabilities of modern pacemaker systems in daily practice. We have also emphasized the utility of modern dual-chamber pacemakers that both sense and pace the atrium, a capability that has not been sufficiently emphasized in earlier volumes. In all, we have emphasized modern, practical, single- and dual-chamber pacing and the associated complications, the individual indications for each, and the operational differences between hardware.

Much has transpired in the three years since the completion of the first edition. Rate modulated pacing, in single- and dual-chamber versions occupies a very large and growing portion of implanted pacing. This is reflected in an extensive analysis and exhaustive chapter. Implanted cardioversion and defibrillation similarly is growing in importance and is described in a new chapter. Overall, much has been added and most chapters have been revised to some extent.

We hope that the reader will find that we have succeeded in the attempt to provide the sense of a practice of cardiac pacing and will consider the volume as providing an experienced "consultant" when one is needed.

The authors want to thank Joanne Lama, whose assistance in preparing this book has been integral through its completion and above and beyond the call of duty.

CONTENTS

PART I.

BASIC CONSIDERATIONS

Chapter 1

INDICATIONS FOR PERMANENT PACING

David L. Hayes

The precise criteria for the implantation of a permanent pacemaker vary from institution to institution. Some conduction disturbances generally are accepted to be definite indications for permanent pacing, and for some others, there is general agreement that permanent pacing is not necessary. In a number of conduction disturbances, the need for permanent pacing is debatable but pacing probably is necessary. Because of changes in diagnosis and therapy and research advances, the absolute indications for permanent pacing are constantly changing. Difficulties arise when an attempt is made to list rigid indications for implanted pacemaker insertion.

Before concluding that permanent pacing is in the best interest of the patient, the physician must carefully and thoughtfully analyze the patient. This analysis should include the general medical status, as well as the specifics of the cardiac rhythm disturbance. Although at one time permanent pacemakers were used solely for the treatment of atrioventricular (AV) block, pacing is appropriate for the control of any symptomatic bradyarrhythmia. Recent advances in pacemaker technology also have increased the indications for dual-chamber pacemakers. Pacemakers with antitachycardia capabilities have extended pacer treatment to include complex bradyarrhythmias and tachyarrhythmias. Controversy still exists over the implantation of pacemakers for bifascicular and trifascicular block, for new-onset bundle branch block in acute myocardial infarction, and for treatment of patients with bradycardia-related low cardiac output syndromes including, chronic congestive heart failure and others.

MEDICARE REGULATION

Guidelines for implantation of cardiac pacemakers have been set by Medicare regulation. In addition, four pacing diagnosis-related groups (DRGs) will influence pacing therapy. Under the Medicare program, cardiac pacemakers are covered as prosthetic devices, subject to several conditions and limitations. Although cardiac pacemaker implantation has been covered by Medicare for many years, specific guidelines, other than the general Medicare requirements that covered services be reasonable and necessary for the treatment of the patient's condition have been instituted. Medicare claims for pacemaker implantation are now subject to several conditions. The guidelines set by the government are based on certain assumptions about the clinical goals of pacemaker implantation. Although some uses of the pacemaker are relatively certain or unambiguous, others require considerable expertise and judgment. Medicare outlines three specific groups.

Group 1

Group 1 includes conditions under which implantation of a cardiac pacemaker is considered acceptable and necessary, provided that the conditions are chronic and recurrent and not due to transient causes, such as acute myocardial infarction, drug toxicity, and electrolyte imbalance. If the rhythm disturbance is chronic or recurrent, a single episode of a symptom such as syncope or seizure is adequate to establish medical necessity.

1. Acquired symptomatic complete AV block (syncope, seizure, congestive heart failure, dizziness, confusion, and limited exercise tolerance) (Figures 1 and 2).
2. Congenital complete heart block with severe bradycardia, significant physiological deficit, or significant symptoms due to the bradycardia.
3. Symptomatic Mobitz II AV block (Figures 3 and 4).
4. Symptomatic Mobitz I second-degree AV block with symptoms related to hemodynamic instability (Figure 5).
5. Symptomatic sinus bradycardia (syncope, seizures, congestive heart failure) or significant sinus bradycardia (heart rate of fewer than 50 bpm) associated with dizziness or confusion (Figure 6). The guidelines state that the correlation between symptoms and bradycardia must be documented or the symptoms must be clearly attributed to the bradycardia rather than to some other cause.
6. A less distinct group of patients with sinus bradycardia of lesser severity (rate, 50–59 bpm) and dizziness or confusion. Again, correlation between symptoms and bradycardia must be documented.
7. When accompanied by significant symptoms, sinus bradycardia that is the consequence of long-term required drug treatment for which there is no acceptable alternative.
8. Sinus node dysfunction with or without tachyarrhythmias or AV block. This category includes tachycardia-bradycardia syndrome, sinoatrial block, and sinus arrest.

9. Sinus node dysfunction with or without symptoms when there are potentially life-threatening ventricular arrhythmias or tachycardia secondary to bradycardia.
10. Bradycardia associated with significant symptoms and with supraventricular tachycardia and high-degree AV block unresponsive to appropriate pharmacological management. Included here are patients with carotid sinus hypersensitivity and syncope due to bradycardia who do not have a response to prophylactic medical measures.

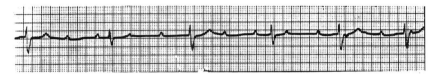

Figure 1. *Complete heart block is characterized by dissociation between atrial and ventricular activity. The atrial rate approximates 95 bpm while the ventricular rate is about 35 bpm. While antegrade conduction seems entirely lost, the fifth ventricular complex is followed by a retrograde P wave, indicating retained retrograde conduction, a circumstance which occurs in about 10% of fixed antegrade complete AV block.*

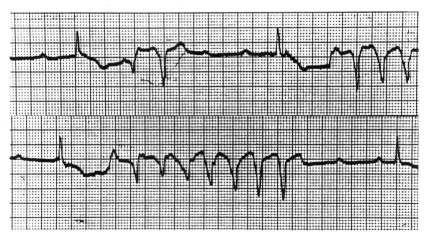

Figure 2. *Complete heart block is characterized by dissociation between atrial and ventricular activity. Several ventricular foci may exist. Symptoms of circulatory arrest follow ventricular asystole, or as in this case, ventricular tachycardia, monomorphic or polymorphic.*

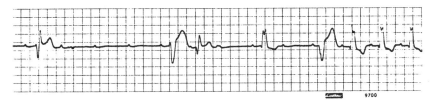

Figure 3. *Mobitz II, or high-grade, AV block in which sporadic failure to conduct from atrium through AV node results in ventricular depolarization. This is not occurring in the pattern that would be expected with Mobitz I, or Wenckebach block.*

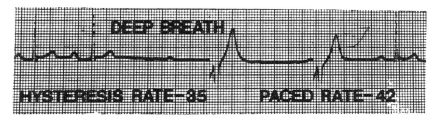

Figure 4. *A patient develops AV block during a deep breath. The pacing rate was set to be at an interval of 1440 ms (42 BPM) while the onset was set at an interval of 1680 ms (35.7 BPM). A hysteresis setting allows a longer interval from the last sensed event to the first paced event than between successive paced events.*

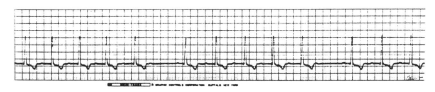

Figure 5. *Wenckebach AV block (Mobitz I) conduction defect allows progressive prolongation of the PR interval until a P wave is blocked. The cycle then recurs and is similar to the upper rate limit mechanism in some dual chamber pacemakers, hence the description (in the pacemaker) as pseudoWenckebach function.*

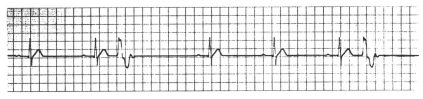

Figure 6. *Sinus bradycardia occurs at a rate of 39 BPM. The patient was symptomatic at this rate. Two coupled VPCs with coupled P waves are shown.*

Group 2

Group 2 includes conditions under which use of a cardiac pacemaker may be found acceptable or necessary, provided the medical history and prognosis of the patient can be documented and there is evidence that pacemaker implantation will assist in overall management.

1. Asymptomatic, acquired third-degree AV block.
2. Congenital complete heart block with less severe bradycardia.
3. Bifascicular or trifascicular block accompanied by syncope that is attributed to transient complete heart block after other plausible causes of syncope have been reasonably excluded.
4. Prophylactic pacemaker use after recovery from acute myocardial infarction during which there is transient, complete, or Mobitz II second-degree AV block.
5. Asymptomatic Mobitz II second-degree AV block.
6. Symptomatic sinus bradycardia (heart rate of fewer than 45 bpm) that is a consequence of long-term necessary drug treatment for which there is no acceptable alternative.
7. Overdrive pacing in patients with recurrent ventricular tachycardia to prevent the ventricular arrhythmia.

Group 3

Group 3 includes conditions that are considered unsupported by adequate evidence to benefit from permanent pacing and, therefore, generally should not be considered appropriate uses for pacemakers in the absence of indications noted in group 1 and group 2.

1. Syncope of undetermined cause. This requires vigorous investigation, including ambulatory monitoring, neurological evaluation, and electrophysiological testing, in selected patients.
2. Sinus bradycardia without significant symptoms.
3. Sinoatrial block or sinus arrest without significant symptoms.
4. Prolonged RR intervals with atrial fibrillation or other causes of transient ventricular pause.
5. Bradycardia during sleep.
6. Right bundle branch block with left axis deviation without syncope or other symptoms of intermittent AV block.
7. Asymptomatic second-degree Mobitz I (Wenckebach) AV block.

Pacing DRGs

The four pacing DRGs do not give specific indications for pacing but simply provide the diagnosis-related group for both initial and replacement procedures. The pacing DRGs are defined as follows:

115. Permanent pacemaker implant *with* primary diagnosis of acute my-ocardial infarction or congestive heart failure.
116. Permanent pacemaker implant *without* primary diagnosis of acute myocardial infarction or congestive heart failure.
117. Pacemaker replacement and revision in all cases except those in which the pulse generator is the only component being replaced.
118. Pacemaker pulse generator replacement only.

Combinations of procedures also are considered. A pacing procedure that is coupled with another cardiovascular surgical procedure is placed in the DRG with the heavier weight, for example, a patient simultaneously requiring a prosthetic heart valve and an initial implant of a pacemaker would be in the DRG of the prosthetic heart valve. The hospital would receive the reimbursement rate associated with the rate of the DRG category of the prosthetic heart valve only.

CRITERIA FOR CARDIAC PACING

The following criteria outline definite indications for permanent pacemakers, probable indications for permanent pacemakers, and conduction disturbances for which it is thought that permanent pacing is not required. Categories of conduction disturbances considered include: acquired AV block, AV block occurring with myocardial infarction, bifascicular and trifascicular block (chronic), sinus node dysfunction and sinus bradycardia, and carotid hypersensitivity. Antitachycardia pacing is discussed in chapter 13.

AV Block

AV block is defined as impairment of conduction of a cardiac impulse from the atrium to the ventricles. It can occur at different levels, depending on whether it is proximal to the AV node, at the level of the AV node, or at the level of the His-Purkinje conduction system. Electrocardiographically, AV block has been divided into first-, second-, and third-degree (complete) heart block (Table I).

First-degree heart block is a prolonged PR interval without failure of ventricular conduction. The normal PR interval is defined electrocardiographically as a range of 120–200 msec. First-degree AV block is usually secondary to a delay of impulse conduction through the AV node or the atrium. It is a nonspecific finding and not an indication for pacing (Figure 7).

Second-degree heart block (Figures 3 and 4) occurs when an atrial impulse that should be conducted to the ventricle is not. The non-

Table I
Atrioventricular Block

Degree	Pacemaker Necessary	Pacemaker Probably Necessary	Pacemaker Not Necessary
Third	Symptomatic congenital complete heart block	Acquired asymptomatic complete heart block	
	Acquired symptomatic complete heart block	Asymptomatic post-operative persistent complete heart block	
	Symptomatic persistent complete heart block postoperatively		
	Atrial fibrillation with complete heart block		
Second	Symptomatic type I	Asymptomatic type II	Asymptomatic type I
	Symptomatic type II		
First			Asymptomatic or symptomatic

conducted P waves may be intermittent or frequent, at regular or irregular intervals, and preceded by fixed or lengthening PR intervals. A distinguishing feature is that conducted P waves relate to the QRS complex in a recurrent pattern and are not random. Second-degree AV block has been classified into type I and type II Mobitz block. Typical type I second-degree AV block (Wenckebach block, Mobitz I) is characterized by progressive PR prolongation culminating in a non-conducted P wave (Figure 5). In type II second-degree AV block (Mobitz II), the PR interval remains constant before the blocked P wave

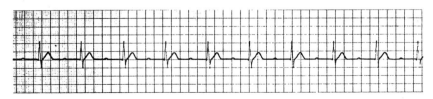

Figure 7. *First-degree AV block in which there is, by definition, prolongation of the PR interval greater than 200 ms. This conduction disturbance is benign and does not require treatment.*

(Figure 3). The AV block is intermittent and generally repetitive and may result in several nonconducted P waves in a row. Mobitz I and II are applied to the two types of block, whereas "Wenckebach block" refers to Mobitz I block only.

Separating second-degree AV block into type I and type II is important and, in most cases, can be done by ECG. Type II second-degree AV block often precedes the development of higher grades of AV block, whereas type I second-degree AV block is usually a less severe conduction disturbance and does not progress to more advanced forms of AV block. Type I AV block with a normal QRS complex usually takes place at the level of the AV node, proximal to the His bundle.

AV block that is 2:1 may be type I or type II second-degree AV block. If the QRS complex is narrow, the block is more likely to be type I, that is, located in the AV node, and one should search for transition of the 2:1 block to 3:2 block, during which the PR interval lengthens in the second cardiac cycle (Figure 8). If the QRS complex is wide, the level of block is more likely to be distal to the His bundle. The escape force in this situation is usually less reliable. If preexisting bundle branch block is present, the block may be located either in the AV node or in the His-Purkinje system.

AV block may occur simultaneously at two or more levels of the conduction system. This occurrence makes the distinction between type I and type II second-degree block difficult.

Third-degree (complete) AV block implies that there is no conduction of the atrial impulses to the ventricle. It is important to separate this from AV dissociation. In AV dissociation, a subsidiary pacemaker, usually junctional, is more rapid than the underlying sinus rate. This contrasts with third-degree AV block in which the atrial rate is faster and there is no AV nodal conduction.

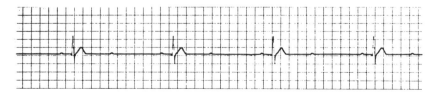

Figure 8. *AV block, 2:1, in which the QRS complex appears narrow. When the conduction ratio remains in a 2:1 pattern, it is impossible to tell from the ECG exactly where in the AV node the conduction disturbance occurs. A narrow QRS complex suggests that the conduction defect is "intra-His" as opposed to "infra-His," which would result more commonly in a wide QRS complex.*

Third-degree (complete) AV block may be congenital or acquired. In the congenital form of complete heart block, there is anatomical discontinuity in the conduction pathway. Although for many years patients with this disorder were left untreated (if no associated congenital anomaly existed) and seemingly did well with their ventricular escape rates, controversy now exists about whether these patients should receive permanent pacing especially in view of the availability of dual-chamber pacemakers. Symptomatic patients with congenital heart block should be paced.

Acquired complete heart block most commonly occurs due to aging with or without calcification of the conduction system or secondary to ischemic disease, i. e., previous myocardial infarction with damage extending to involve the conduction system. Complete heart block can also be related to a number of systemic illnesses, many of which have been described as single case reports. Table II lists categories of causes of acquired atrioventricular block.

Acquired complete heart block can be either intermittent or fixed. Patients with abnormalities of AV conduction may be symptomatic or experience severe symptoms related to profound bradycardia or ventricular arrhythmias. Decisions on the need for a pacemaker in the patient with impaired AV conduction, whether complete heart block or second-degree AV block, are influenced by a number of factors, most important of which is the presence or absence of symptoms that

---

Table II
Causes of Acquired Atrioventricular Block

Idiopathic (Senescent) AV Block
Coronary Artery Disease
Calcific Valvular Disease
Postoperative/Traumatic

Infectious	Infiltrative
Syphilis	Sarcoidosis
Diphtheria	Amyloidosis
Chagas' Disease (Trypanosoma Cruzi)	Hemochromatosis
Tuberculosis	Malignancy (Lymphomatous
Toxoplasmosis	or solid tumor)
Lyme Disease (Borrelia burgdorferi)	
Collagen-Vascular	Drug Effect
Rheumatoid arthritis	Digoxin
Scleroderma	Beta-blockers
Dermatomyositis	Calcium-blocking agents
Ankylosing Spondylitis	Amiodarone
	Procainamide

may be directly attributed to the arrhythmia. It has been well documented that patients with complete heart block and syncope have improved survival with permanent pacing.

Atrial fibrillation with a slow ventricular response is usually considered as AV block. These patients should be paced if symptoms occur (Figure 9).

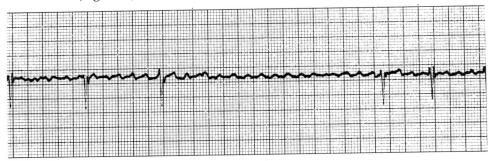

Figure 9.   *Atrial fibrillation with a slow ventricular response and a single period of asystole of approximately 3 seconds duration.*

Permanent Pacing After Acute Myocardial Infarction

Patients with myocardial infarction may experience a variety of conduction disturbances largely related to the site of the infarction and the coronary artery involved. Rigid classification is difficult because of the variations in coronary circulation (Table III).

Inferior Myocardial Infarction

Patients with an inferior myocardial infarction may have a variety of conduction disturbances. Supraventricular arrhythmias associated with an inferior myocardial infarction include (1) sinus bradycardia, (2) sinus arrest, (3) atrial fibrillation, and (4) atrial flutter.

AV nodal conduction disturbances may also occur, including (1) first-degree AV block and (2) Mobitz I (Wenckebach) AV block.

In a minority of patients, higher grades of AV block (Mobitz II and complete heart block) will develop, and these patients will require temporary pacing if they are hemodynamically unstable. Few have persistent high-grade AV block or sinus node dysfunction that requires permanent pacing.

Table III
Permanent Pacing After Acute Myocardial Infarction

Pacemaker Necessary	Pacemaker Probably Nescessary	Pacemaker Not Necessary
Persistent Complete heart block	New bundle branch block with transient complete heart block	First-degree AV block
Persistent type II second-degree AV block	Newly acquired bifascicular bundle branch block	Asymptomatic type I second-degree AV block
Persistent symptomatic bradyarrhythmias		Preexisting right bundle branch block or left bundle branch block
		New unifascicular block
		Asymptomatic sinus bradycardia

Anterior Myocardial Infarction

Anterior myocardial infarctions are more likely to be accompanied by intraventricular conduction defects or AV block (or both). Temporary pacing will be required for (1) new-onset bifascicular block, (2) bilateral bundle branch block, (3) intermittent complete heart block, and (4) persistent complete heart block.

Permanent pacing in patients with intraventricular conduction defects is predicated on the potential for development of complete heart block. In patients with newly acquired bifascicular block, transient or persistent trifascicular block requires permanent pacing.

The long-term prognosis in survivors of acute myocardial infarction who have had AV block is related primarily to the extent of myocardial injury rather than to the AV block per se. Patients with acute myocardial infarction and intraventricular conduction defect (with the exception of isolated left anterior hemiblock) have unfavorable short- and long-term prognoses and an increased incidence of sudden death.

It should be stressed that the requirement for temporary pacing in the setting of acute myocardial infarction does not constitute an indication for permanent pacing. Indications for temporary pacing are presented in chapter 7.

Chronic Bifascicular and Trifascicular Block

Permanent pacing in patients with conduction disturbances of two or more fascicles of the ventricular conduction system depends on assessment of the risk of development of complete AV block, either transient or permanent. A high mortality and a significant incidence of sudden death are known to be associated with bifascicular or trifascicular block and syncope, which, without pacing, commonly lead to complete heart block. Thus, defining the cause of syncope in patients with bifascicular and trifascicular block is important for documenting whether intermittent complete heart block is present. If this is documented, permanent pacemaker implantation should be performed. However, the incidence of progression of bifascicular block to complete heart block is low. Furthermore, no clinical or laboratory variables have proved valuable or definitive in identifying patients at a high risk of death from future bradyarrhythmia due to progression of the conduction disease. Specific controversy has arisen about patients with right bundle branch and left anterior hemiblock. Although these patients have increased cardiovascular mortality, conduction abnormalities and bradycardia are not the cause of death in a sufficiently high proportion to warrant routine prophylactic pacing.

It had been hoped that with electrophysiological testing, measurement of the H-V interval (a measure of conduction of the His-Purkinje system), would identify patients at a higher risk. In patients with H-V interval that are markedly prolonged (>100 msec), prophylactic pacing may be indicated because of an increased incidence of developing symptomatic bradycardia. For other patients with normal or a less prolonged H-V interval, this test does not reliably distinguish high-risk from low-risk groups. Thus, the clinical usefulness of routine electrophysiological studies is not proved in patients with bifascicular block. Therefore, such studies in asymptomatic patients with bifascicular block usually are not necessary (Table IV).

Sinus Node Dysfunction

Sinus node dysfunction, sick sinus syndrome, and tachycardia-bradycardia syndrome include a variety of cardiac arrhythmias that have been classified in several ways. Sinoatrial disturbances included are: (1) sinus bradycardia (Figure 6); (2) sinus arrest (Figure 10); (3)

Table IV
Chronic Bifascicular and Trifascicular Block

Pacemaker Necessary	Pacemaker Probably Necessary	Pacemaker Not Necessary
Symptomatic patients with fascicular block and significantly prolonged H-V interval by electrophysiological study	Symptomatic patients with bundle branch block despite normal H-V interval	Asymptomatic fascicular block
Symptomatic patients with block distal to His at atrial paced rates of <100–120 beats per minute	Patient undergoing electrophysiological study with block distal to His at atrial paced rates of <130 beats per minute	Asymptomatic fascicular block and first-degree AV block
Symptomatic patients with bifascicular block and intermittent type II second-degree AV block or third-degree AV block	Asymptomatic patients with fascicular block and intermittent type II second-degree AV block	

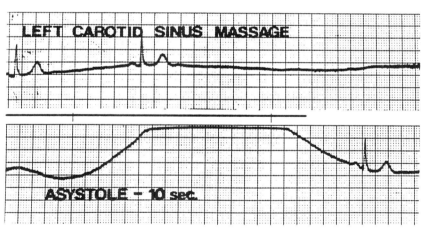

Figure 10. *Carotid sinus massage is often effective in demonstrating the basis of syncope or dizziness. Gentle massage of the carotid sinus, at the bifurcation of the common carotid artery, may produce AV block or, in this instance, prolonged sinus arrest without junctional escape. This level of sensitivity is associated with symptoms which pacing relieves. Even were a ventricular complex lost during the displaced baseline, six and one half seconds of sinus arrest with asystole will have occurred.*

sinoatrial block; and (4) paroxysmal supraventricular tachycardias alternating with periods of bradycardia or asystole (Figure 11).

The definition of bradycardia varies, but it is generally agreed to

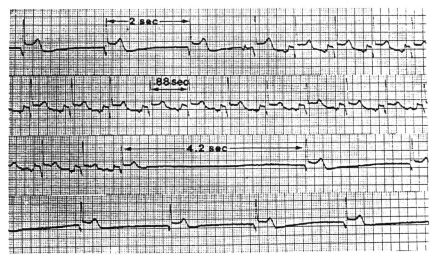

Figure 11. A continuous strip from a patient with tachycardia-bradycardia syndrome shows sinus rhythm with sudden prolonged junctional escapes of up to 4.2 sec.

Table V
Sinus Node Dysfunction

Pacemaker Necessary	Pacemaker Probably Necessary	Pacemaker Not Necessary
Symptomatic bradycardia in the tachycardia-brady-cardia syndrome	Symptomatic patient with sinus node dysfunction who has documented rates of <40–50 bpm without a clear-cut association between significant symptoms consistent with bradycardia	Asymptomatic sinus node dysfunction
Symptomatic sinus bradycardia due to long-term drug therapy of a type and dose for which there is no accepted alternative		

denote rates of less than 40–50 bpm during waking hours. There is disagreement about the absolute cycle length of an asystolic period that should require pacing. Sinus pauses of 3 sec or sustained symptomatic sinus rates below 40 bpm in the awake patient are indications for permanent pacing. Sinus bradycardia during sleep in an otherwise asymptomatic patient should not be considered an indication for pacing. Because of the uncertainty of the definition of bradycardia and the duration of sinus pauses that requires treatment, it is important to take the patient's clinical condition into consideration, including age, associated disease, medications, and symptoms.

In sinus node dysfunction, correlation of symptoms with the specific arrhythmia is essential. Patients who have episodes of both tachycardia and bradycardia and are asymptomatic require no therapy. Others become symptomatic when treated for tachycardia because the treatment produces symptomatic bradycardia. Treatment for tachycardia may, therefore, require implanted pacing for bradycardia (Table V).

Carotid Sinus Hypersensitivity

The carotid sinus reflex is the physiological response to pressure exerted on the carotid sinus. Stimulation results in activation of baroreceptors within the wall of the sinus itself. Vagal efferents then result in cardiac slowing. Although this reflex is physiological, some persons have an exaggerated or even pathological response. This reflex has two components, a cardioinhibitory response and a vasodepressor response. The former is more prominent in patients with symptoms, but mixed responses are not infrequent. The definitions of normal and abnormal responses are quite arbitrary. Ventricular asystole of 3 sec or a decrease in blood pressure of 30 to 50 mm Hg (or both) is abnormal (Table VI).

An abnormal response to carotid sinus massage occurs in 25% to 30% of patients over 50 years of age (Figure 10). Men are affected approximately twice as frequently as women, and the right carotid sinus usually is more sensitive than the left. Although most of these patients are asymptomatic during carotid sinus massage and have no clinical history of syncope, others may have had recurrent syncope. Patients with syncope may have a typical history related to a tight collar or neck extension.

Table VI
Carotid Sinus Hypersensitivty

Pacemaker Necessary	Pacemaker Probably Necessary	Pacemaker Not Necessary
Patients with recurrent syncope associated with clear spontaneous events provoked by carotid sinus stimulation in whom carotid sinus massage induces asystole of ≥3 sec	Patients with recurrent syncope without clear, provocative events who have a positive response to carotid sinus massage	Asymptomatic patients with a positive response to carotid sinus massage but without overt syncope who have only vague symptoms of dizziness or lightheadedness

Syncope secondary to isolated vasodepressor carotid sinus hypersensitivity is uncommon. In patients with carotid sinus hypersensitivity, syncope is usually secondary either to a cardioinhibitory response or to a mixed vasodepressor and cardioinhibitory response. Identifying the mixed response is very important. A permanent pacemaker eliminates syncope in patients with cardioinhibitory carotid sinus hypersensitivity but does not affect vasodepressor carotid sinus hypersensitivity. Syncope secondary to vasodepressor carotid sinus hypersensitivity is similar to that with cardioinhibitory carotid sinus hypersensitivity except that the symptoms tend to follow a more protracted course and the blood pressure may not recover for minutes.

Uncommonly, a series of vagal mediated bradyarrhythmias occur. These are usually prolonged sinus arrest without nodal or ventricular escape and may be associated with dramatic symptoms, including syncope, often undiagnosed for very prolonged periods. Syncope has been reported during swallowing, coitus, cough, micturition and respiration. Pacemaker implantation is the most effective means of controlling the event (Figures 12 and 13).

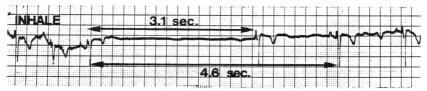

Figure 12. *Respiration can cause sinus arrest as it does in this 21 year-old woman. A modest depth of respiration causes 3.1 seconds of sinus arrest with asystole and 4.6 seconds of sinus bradycardia, before resuming a normal atrial rate.*

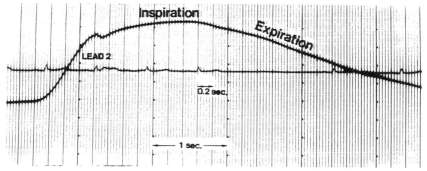

Figure 13. *Respiration may cause sinus arrest with asystole. A pneumotachograph recorded simultaneously with an ECG demonstrates that the expiratory phase produces the cardiac effect. Asystole of almost 3 seconds occurs as expiration begins and ends as expiration ends. (See Fig. 12)*

LYME DISEASE

Lyme disease is a tick borne spirochetal infection which causes an acute systemic infection, a skin eruption, erythema chronicum migrans (ECM), myalgias, arthritis, fever and in 4%–10% of those infected, carditis. The intermediate vector of the causative organism, borrelia burgdorferi is the deer tick, Ixodes dammini which is found widely in the United States, especially in the northeast and the upper midwest. Other species of ticks on the west coast also are infested with the borrelia. The tick and spirochete are carried locally by the common deer and small mammals and more remotely by birds. Infection usually occurs in summer months during outdoor activities. Lyme disease is endemic in some suburban areas such as Westchester, the heavily populated urban-surburban county immediately north of New York City.

Without antibiotic treatment over half the patients develop further complications, the most common of which is arthritis, and neurologic manifestations such as meningoencephalitis. The carditis, when it occurs, manifests as a transient myocarditis with varying degrees of atrioventricular block, non-specific ECG changes, arrhythmias and left ventricular dysfunction. Rarely, complete heart block with frightening asystole (Figure 14) may occur. In that case temporary cardiac pacing is appropriate but implanted pacing is unnecessary. All patients with reported Lyme disease, myocarditis with high degree AV block have returned to normal sinus rhythm, possibly independent of antibiotic treatment.

The diagnosis of Lyme disease with carditis has been made in patients between 2 and 88 years of age, the median age is 28 years, though in Europe the mean age (the literature is unclear) may be higher. There seems to be no discernible difference in the clinical course of those who develop arthritis or carditis or both conditions. The diagnosis of Lyme disease is clinical including the presence of

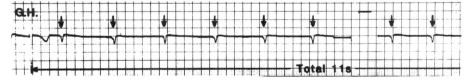

Figure 14.   *A recording of ventricular asystole with normal atrial activity during complete heart block caused by Lyme disease. The P waves are marked by arrows and while the full duration of the asystole was lost, it was at least 11 seconds.*

ECM which is pathognomonic, but may have gone unnoticed, unrecognized as to significance, or misdiagnosed. Serologic confirmation, provided by many public health services in endemic areas is helpful but is often delayed, may be insensitive and is affected by antibiotic treatment if that has been given before a specific diagnosis has been reached. Further, a positive serologic diagnosis can occur after the onset of carditis and AV block.

AV block of varying severity is the most common manifestation of carditis and occurs in 88% (43 of 49 reported cases). There is a suggestion that sinoatrial block can also occur, it has been reported once and may have been seen once at Montefiore (Figure 15). In the presence of high grade AV block a wide QRS morphology is present in about one-third of patients. Fluctuating right and left bundle branch block may exist as well as a ventricular rate below 40 beats per minute. In the few patients who have had electrophysiologic study, the block has been above the His bundle in almost all. AV block has an excellent prognosis for return to normal sinus rhythm despite the inconsistency of therapy. The block resolves within several days to two weeks, rarely remaining for six weeks at lesser levels of block. Other evidences of carditis with reduced ejection fraction, ST segment depression and T wave flattening also resolve.

Should carditis occur with AV block, hospitalization with continuous ECG monitoring is appropriate, temporary cardiac pacing may be necessary if the cardiac rate is slow or is complicated by prolonged asystole. Implantation of a cardiac pacemaker is not indicated. Three patients have been reported who have had a pacemaker implanted, in each the procedure was, almost certainly, unnecessary. It is especially important to be alert to the possibility of Lyme disease usually in a young male in whom the possibility of complete heart block is otherwise remote, who is in or from an endemic area and who has the sudden onset of complete heart block, possibly with profound asystole but who seems not to have any reason for the AV block. If

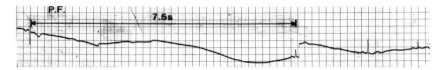

Figure 15.   *This example of prolonged (7.5 seconds) sinus arrest without ventricular escape was documented during an episode of syncope. Lyme titers were positive. No episode of asystole was recorded again. No pacemaker was implanted. No other cause of sinus arrest was found.*

the block vanishes within several days of its onset, the level of suspicion of Lyme disease should be very high.

BIBLIOGRAPHY

Bedell SE, Pastor BM, Cohen SI: Symptomatic high grade heart block in Lyme disease. *Chest* 1981; 79:236–237.

Bhandari AK, Rahimtoola SH: Indications for cardiac pacing in patients with bradyarrhythmias. *JAMA* 1984; 252:1327–28 (editorial).

Bharati S, Lev M: The anatomy and histology of the conduction system. In E. K. Chung, (Ed): *Artificial Cardiac Pacing: Practical Approach.* Williams & Wilkins Co., Baltimore 1978; pp. 8–22.

Col JJ, Weinberg SL: The incidence and mortality of intraventricular conduction defects in acute myocardial infarction. *Am J Cardiol* 1972; 29:344–50.

Davies AB, Stephens MR, Davies AG: Carotid sinus hypersensitivity in patients presenting with syncope. *Br Heart J* 1979; 42:583–86.

Del Negro AA, Fletcher RD: *Indications for and Use of Artificial Cardiac Pacemakers: Part I.* Year Book Medical Publishers, Chicago 1978, pp. 1–44.

Denes P, Dhingra RC, Wu D, et al: H-V interval in patients with bifascicular block (right bundle branch block and left anterior hemiblock): Clinical, electrocardiographic and electrophysiologic correlations. *Am J Cardiol* 1975; 35:23–9.

Denes P, Dhingra RC, Wu D, et al: Sudden death in patients with chronic bifascicular block. *Arch Intern Med* 1977; 137:1005–10.

Dhingra RC, Amat-y-Leon F, Pouget JM, et al: Infranodal block: Diagnosis, clinical significance, and management. *Med Clin North Am* 1976; 60: 175–92.

Dhingra RC, Denes P, Wu D, et al: Syncope in patients with chronic bifascicular block. Significance, causative mechanisms, and clinical implications. *Ann Intern Med* 1974; 81:302–306.

Dhingra RC, Denes P, Wu D, et al: The significance of second degree atrioventricular block and bundle branch block: Observations regarding site and type of block. *Circulation* 1974; 49:638–46.

Dhingra RC, Palileo E, Strasberg B, et al: Significance of the H-V interval in 517 patients with chronic bifascicular block. *Circulation* 1981; 64:1265–71.

Forfang K, Refsum AM, Simonsen S: Indications for permanent pacemaker treatment in 391 patients. *Scand J Thorac Cardiovasc Surg* 1978; Suppl 22:27–29.

Furman S: Cardiac pacing and pacemakers. I. Indications for pacing bradyarrhythmias. *Am Heart J* 1977; 93:523–30.

Gould L, Reddy CVR, Brevetti GC, et al: His bundle electrograms in 51 patients requiring permanent transvenous pacemakers. *J Thorac Cardiovasc Surg* 1977; 74:28–36.

Grendahl H. Sivertssen E: Endocardial pacing in acute mycardial infarction. *Acta Med Scand* 1969; 186:21–26.

Harthorne JW: Indications for pacemaker insertion: Types and modes of pacing. *Prog Cardiovasc Dis* 1981; 23:393–400.

Hindman MC, Wagner GS, JoRo M, et al: The clinical significance of bundle branch block complicating acute myocardial infarctions. 2. Indications for temporary and permanent pacemaker insertion. *Circulation* 1978; 58: 689–99.

Joint American College of Cardiology/American Heart Association Task Force on Assessment of Cardiovascular Procedures (Subcommittee on Pacemaker Implantation): Guidelines for permanent cardiac pacemaker implantation, May 1984. *J Am Coll Cardiol* 1984; 4:434–42.

Kaul TK, Kumar EB, Thomson RM, et al: Sinoatrial disorders, the "sick sinus" syndrome. Experience with implanted cardiac pacemakers. *J Cardiovasc Surg* 1978; 19:261–66.

Kay R, Estiok M, Wiener I: Primary sick sinus syndrome as an indication for chronic pacemaker therapy in young adults: Incidence, clinical features, and long-term evaluation. *Am Heart J* 1982; 103:338–42.

Kubis M, Svejda J: Indication of permanent pacing after acute myocardial infarction complicated by combined intraventricular block. *Cor Vasa* 1982; 24:295–301.

Luceri RM, Myerburg RJ: Indications for and management of cardiac pacemakers. *DM* 1985; 31:1–52.

Lüderitz B: Electrophysiology and indications for pacing in the '80's. *PACE* 1982; 5:548–60.

McAlister HF, Klementowicz PT, Andrews C, Fisher JD, Feld M, Furman S: Lyme carditis: An important cause of reversible heart block. *Ann Intern Med* 1989; 110:339–345.

Mond HG: The bradyarrhythmias: Current indications for permanent pacing (Part II). *PACE* 1981;4:538–47.

Mond HG: The bradyarrhythmias: Current indications for permanent pacing (Part I). *PACE* 1981; 4:432–42.

Moss AJ, Davis RJ: Brady-tachy syndrome: *Prog Cardiovasc Dis* 1974; 16: 439–454.

Olson LJ, Okafor EC, Clements IP: Cardiac involvement in Lyme disease: manifestations and management. *Mayo Clin Proc* 1986; 61:745–749.

Parsonnet V, Escher DJ, Furman S, et al: Indications for dual-chamber pacing. *PACE* 1984; 7:318–19.

Pinsky WW,. Gillette PC, Garson A Jr, McNamara DG: Diagnosis, management, and long-term results of patients with congential complete atrioventricular block. *Pediatrics* 1982; 69:728–33.

Reznick JW, Braunstein DB, Walsh RL, et al: Lyme carditis: electrophysiologic and histopathologic study. *Am J Med* 1986; 81:923–927.

Steere AC, Batsford WP, Weinberg M, et al: Lyme carditis: cardiac abnormalities of Lyme disease. *Ann Int Med* 1980; 93:8–16.

Steere AC, Green, J, Schoen RT, et al: Successful parenteral penicillin therapy of established Lyme arthritis. *N Engl J Med* 1985; 312:869–874.

Steere AC, Malawista SE, Newman JH, Spieler PN, Bartenhagen NH: Antibiotic therapy in Lyme disease. *Ann Intern Med* 1980; 93:1–7.

Vlay SC: Complete heart block due to Lyme disedase. *N Engl J Med* 1986; 315:1418 (letter).

Walter PF, Crawley IS, Dorney ER: Carotid sinus hypersensitivity and syncope. *Am J Cardiol* 1978; 42:396–403.

Chapter 2

BASIC CONCEPTS

Seymour Furman

THRESHOLD OF CARDIAC STIMULATION

Comprehension of the threshold of cardiac stimulation is basic to pulse generator and electrode design. The programming of and the setting of the minimum output, that will: (1) accommodate threshold; (2) set an adequate safety factor; and (3) allow maximum pulse generator longevity, is based on the comprehension of the factors concerning the long-term stability of threshold and specifically the strength-duration curve of stimulation. A variety of electrode factors are involved and each must be considered.

I. Myocardial Factors
  A. Fibrosis or local infarction increases threshold;
  B. Endocardial thickening increases threshold;
  C. Drugs, the effect is variable;
  D. Electrolyte balance, the effect is variable.
II. Lead and electrode
  A. Electrode maturity—i.e., duration of the electrode in position;
  B. Distance of the electrode from sensitive tissue (the effect of which is the same as IA and IB);
  C. Unipolar or bipolar, i.e., anodal size;
  D. Electrode surface area and shape;
  E. Electrode material;
  F. Lead insulation;
  G. Solid and porous electrodes;
  H. Steroid electrodes;
  I. Lead fixation;
  J. Anodal or cathodal stimulation;
  K. Pulse duration.

I. Myocardial Factors

A. Fibrosis or Local Infarction

Neither fibrous nor infarcted tissue is sensitive to stimulation. The nearest viable tissue will be stimulated if threshold is reached.

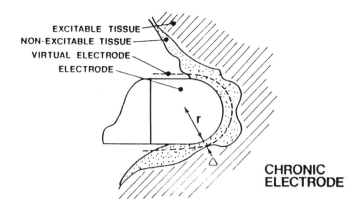

Figure 1.   *Each electrode is surrounded by an insensitive layer of fibrous tissue. Since the interface of the fibrous layer with adjacent stimulatable tissue is where stimulation actually occurs, the surface area of the "virtual" electrode is that which determines the chronic stable stimulation factors. The size of the fibrous layer may be decreased by porous electrode and local steroids.*

Extensive fibrosis or infarction about an electrode increases the size of the "virtual" electrode, which is the surface area of the encasement of such tissue about an electrode. As threshold is directly related to "virtual" electrode size, the larger the fibrotic area, the higher the threshold (Figure 1).

B. Endocardial Thickening

This separates the electrode from the stimulatable tissue as does fibrosis. The greater the distance between the stimulating electrode surface and the responsive tissue, the higher the threshold and the poorer the sensed electrogram.

C/D. Drugs, Electrolyte Balance

Changes in electrolyte concentration affect stimulation threshold. Administration of potassium (chloride) in Ringer's solution reduces threshold by as much as 20–40% consistently but briefly, while potassium in combination with insulin increases threshold by 17–30%, also briefly. Hypertonic (3%) sodium chloride increases the blood sodium concentration and threshold by 50–60% while calcium gluconate has a slight lowering effect. An increase in pO_2 has little effect, a slight decrease of pO_2 increases threshold and marked hypoxia reduces threshold. An increase in pCO_2 increases threshold and a decrease has little effect.

The glucocorticoids (methylprednisone, dexamethasone, prednisone), and epinephrine and ephedrine decrease threshold. Isoproterenol, aldactone, propanolol, verapamil, quinidine and ajmaline all increase threshold. Digitalis, morphine, lidocaine and procainamide, administered in the usual therapeutic dose range, have little effect. Still, all drug administration has little significant or sustained effect on threshold and need not be considered as a cause for threshold increase during cardiac pacing or as an effective means of long-term threshold reduction. Even where a pronounced immediate effect occurs, continued drug administration is accompanied by gradual return to the pretreatment baseline over several hours. The major problem that can occur is the acute loss of pacing during severe electrolyte imbalance. The best method of management is prompt restoration of electrolyte balance.

II. Lead and Electrode

A. Electrode Maturity

The duration of the electrode in situ affects the threshold in two ways. Early after implant the threshold of stimulation increases, i.e., more energy is required, probably because of a nonstimulatable reactive layer about the electrode. This evolution may be affected by the use of local steroids incorporated in an electrode for slow local dissemination. Early threshold increase is reduced and may be useful in avoiding the need for electrode revision. The chronic threshold of a steroid eluting lead is about the same as a similar nonsteroid electrode. As the reactive layer becomes smaller, because of decreasing edema, the threshold decreases. The threshold peak is usually reached within the first month after implant though occasional patients will evolve over a longer period, uncommonly as long as 6 months and rarely even longer (Figure 2).

B. Distance of Electrode From Sensitive Tissue

Once an electrode is in position, threshold evolves over a matter of days; but longer term evolution may occur. The peak evolution (in a nonsteroid electrode) may commonly represent a charge threshold increase of 3–5 times over that at implant and is largely determined

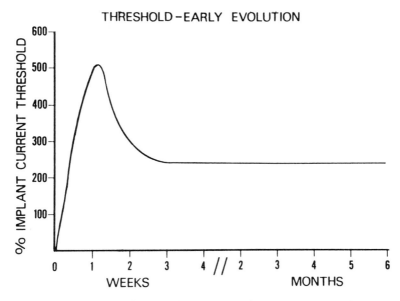

Figure 2.   *Once an electrode is placed against or within sensitive tissue, local reaction causes enlargement of its surface area as the virtual electrode is formed. As chronicity is reached, the virtual electrode is smaller than early after implant and threshold decreases. The height and duration of the threshold increase are highly variable.*

by separation of the electrode from sensitive tissue by fibrous tissue and/or local reaction. Such an increase is sufficiently small so that it will not be noted if pacer output is at conventional levels. Threshold may, in as much as 5–10% of cases, rise to 10 times that at implant. In over 90% of such instances threshold will return, within weeks or more slowly, possibly over 6 months to the usual 2–3 times threshold at implant. Even where threshold has evolved to 10 times that at implant, continued increase is very unusual but will rarely occur. The typical pattern is for return toward a lower threshold even if that level is higher than is customary (Figure 3).

Once stability has been reached it is, for all practical purposes, permanent. About 20% of chronically implanted leads will develop a slow progressive threshold increase that will not exceed the output capability of a conventional pulse generator in less than a decade. An equal number will have a drifting, but progressive decline. About 60% will remain broadly stable, increasing or decreasing about a mean with variation caused by medication, food intake, electrolyte balance, activity or sleep (Figure 4).

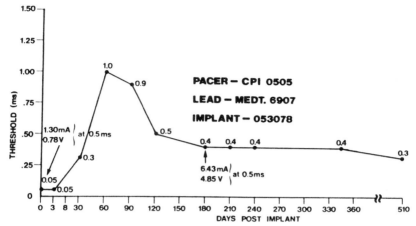

Figure 3. *Infrequently, a very high and prolonged threshold evolution will occur. Such an evolution may return to a normal threshold chronically or the threshold may be high and stable. If evolution ends with a chronic threshold within the output capability of a conventional pacemaker, the utilization of a high output pulse generator will have been very valuable*

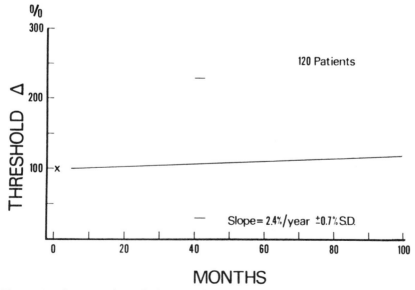

Figure 4. *Once an electrode is properly in place, prolonged and even indefinite stability of threshold can be anticipated. Progressive increase in threshold may occur, but at so slow a rate as to be practically meaningless. In this instance, 120 patients were analyzed and compared to the first threshold after implant. The rate of increase was 2.4% per year.*

C. Unipolar or Bipolar

Whether an electrode system is unipolar or bipolar makes no difference in the current threshold of stimulation, which is a function of the surface area of the cathodal electrode. The voltage threshold is somewhat higher for the bipolar compared to the unipolar lead because of the lead wire required for the second, i.e., intracardiac (anode) electrode and the relatively smaller (therefore higher impedance) anode on the lead compared to the very large anode on the pulse generator. During unipolar pacing, the cathode contacts cardiac tissues; in bipolar, both cathode and anode are in contact. In practice, the unipolar anode is usually on the pacemaker case and is adjacent to the pectoral musculature. Other possibilities exist in which the anode is not against stimulatable tissue but along a lead, lying, perhaps, in the superior vena cava. This is simply another example of unipolar pacing though in this instance, both anode and cathode are intravascular. In a recent study of stimulation threshold and electrogram amplitude, the mean atrial electrogram was found to be 4.38 mV in its unipolar version referenced to the subcutaneous tissue of the chest wall and 4.56 mV in the bipolar version. The ventricular electrogram was 11.13 mV in the unipolar and 11.09 mV in the bipolar; both were insignificant differences. The amplitude of the atrial and ventricular electrograms are, therefore, similar in unipolar and bipolar format (Table I). The amplitude of the far-field ventricular electrogram on the atrial channel is much larger in the unipolar than in a bipolar atrial electrogram. The remote atrial signal is small in both unipolar and bipolar ventricular electrograms. The unipolar and bipolar atrial and ventricular strength-duration curves are also similar, though the voltage stimulation threshold curve is higher in the bipolar than in the unipolar, reflecting the increased impedance of the

Table I
Electrogram (EGM) Amplitude
(mVolts)

Atrial			Ventricular		
Unipolar	Bipolar	P	Unipolar	Bipolar	P
4.38	4.56	NS	11.13	11.09	NS
n = 25					

bipolar lead (Figure 5). The difference between the voltage threshold of unipolar and bipolar and the difference in lead impedance between unipolar and bipolar reaches statistical significance for the voltage threshold. The difference is statistically insignificant for current stimulation thresholds. The impedances, as expected, reflect the voltage threshold difference. The unipolar impedance at each pulse duration is significantly lower than the bipolar, reflecting the higher bipolar voltage threshold. Consequently, presently available unipolar and bipolar electrodes are, for all practical purposes, interchangeable in stimulation threshold and sensing electrogram. The bipolar far-field electrograms, both for interference signals and for the ventricular electrogram on the atrial lead, are significantly attenuated. Therefore, aside from the slightly higher voltage threshold and impedance of the bipolar atrial lead, no difference exists in stimulation capability. From this perspective alone, unipolar and bipolar atrial and ventricular leads can be used interchangeably (Tables II, III).

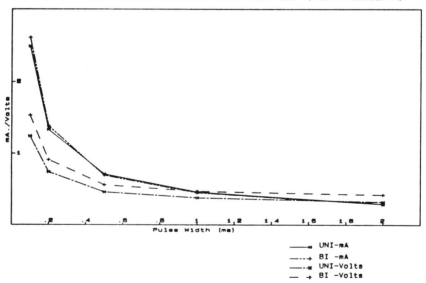

Figure 5. *Strength-duration curves for unipolar and bipolar ventricular stimulation show that current stimulation thresholds are equivalent unipolar and bipolar. The bipolar voltage threshold is slightly higher by a statistically significant margin.*

Table II
Stimulation Threshold
ATRIUM

Pulse Duration (ms)	Volts			mA		
	Unipolar	Bipolar	P	Unipolar	Bipolar	P
0.1	1.47	1.90	<.0001	3.7	3.8	NS
0.5	0.54	0.72	<.0001	1.01	1.03	NS
1.0	0.43	0.57	<.0005	0.62	0.62	NS
n = 25						

	PD	Unipolar	Bipolar
	0.1	397	500
Impedance	0.5	534	699
	1.0	693	919

Table III
Stimulation Threshold
VENTRICLE

Pulse Duration (ms)	Volts			mA		
	Unipolar	Bipolar	P	Unipolar	Bipolar	P
0.1	1.14	1.38	<.00001	2.33	2.30	NS
0.5	0.42	0.51	<.00001	0.66	0.65	NS
1.0	0.34	0.42	<.00001	0.42	0.42	NS
n = 25						

	PD	Unipolar	Bipolar
	0.1	489	600
Impedance	0.5	636	748
	1.0	809	1000

D. Electrode Surface Area and Shape

The surface area of a stimulating electrode is directly and linearly related to the current threshold of stimulation. Though the shape of the stimulating surface plays a role, its clinical significance is not clear. Smaller surface area electrodes have lower *current* and *charge* thresholds than do larger electrodes, and the current density threshold (mA/mm^2) remains relatively constant over a wide range of sur-

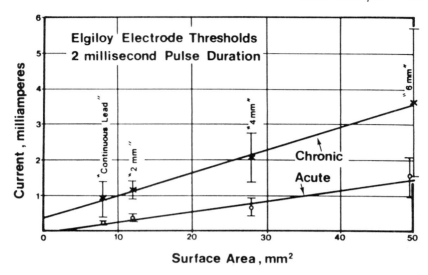

Figure 6. *There is a direct and linear relationship between current threshold and electrode size. The greater the electrode surface area the higher the current threshold.*

face areas. Voltage threshold also decreases with surface area, though not as greatly as do current and charge thresholds. These phenomena exist both at implant (acutely) and chronically (Figure 6).

The chronic-to-acute threshold ratio depends on the size, shape and material of the electrode and the thickness of the nonexcitable fibrous tissue that separates the electrode from excitable myocardium. In general, spherical solid tip electrodes have the highest chronic threshold evolution, cylindrical electrodes have lesser increases, and porous surface metal and carbon electrodes have even lower chronic threshold levels.

E. Electrode Material

CHARACTERISTICS REQUIRED FOR A PACEMAKER ELECTRODE

1. Electrochemical inertness;
2. Low overvoltage during stimulation;
3. Resistance to electrolytic destruction;
4. Low electrical resistance;
5. Low biological reactivity.

The electrode should not go into solution during passage of an electric current, at least at conventional output levels for cardiac pacing. The metal itself should be nontoxic and salt formation should not occur. If a metal meets these criteria as a cathode, but not as an anode, then it may be used only for unipolar pacing. Materials usable for implanted pacing are:

1. platinum with 10% iridium;
2. Elgiloy, an alloy of cobalt, iron, chromium, molybdenum, nickel and manganese;
3. a silver and stainless steel combination;
4. activated vitreous carbon.

Threshold is a function of the reactivity of the material and the overvoltage developed during passage of a current for cardiac stimulation. The more noble a metal, i.e., the less reactive, the lower this overvoltage and the lower the voltage and current pacing threshold. Platinum-iridium has consistently lower thresholds than the more reactive metal, Elgiloy; carbon lower than either. Nevertheless, both metals have been quite successful for long-term pacing and the difference in threshold is unimportant as a practical matter. The prolonged durability of metal electrodes is proven. Carbon, used for briefer periods, seems to behave equally well.

Some new electrodes contain a very small amount of dexamethasone (about 1 mg). The steroid is slowly eluted into adjacent tissue, reduces the local tissue reaction and maintains a low threshold acutely and chronically, and moderates the early threshold rise compared to similar, nonsteroidal electrodes.

F. Lead Insulation

Insulation material for implantable leads has long been of concern. The material must be a good insulator, must be minimally or nonreactive and noncarcinogenic. It must be durable and resist wear and the flailing of the tricuspid value. It must not undergo time-dependent spontaneous deterioration and must not be metabolized. It must not cause thrombosis.

The earliest lead material used was polyethylene. It served well and for prolonged periods, but increasing reports are that after a decade or more, insulation wear can be seen adjacent to the tricuspid valve from continual lead and valve contact. The second material introduced was silicone rubber. It is well tolerated in the soft tissue, i.e., as a myocardial lead and in the venous system. Wear seems to be a very small problem and numerous leads have been in place for 15–20 years without significant deterioration. A small and unknown number of chronically placed silicone rubber leads provoke local venous calcification that may invade the lead itself. A significant problem is that silicone rubber leads were, and are, relatively large for the venous system and may be introduced into the cephalic vein with some difficulty. This is specially true for bipolar leads and more so if two leads are to be introduced for dual-chamber pacing. Smaller diameter silicone rubber leads have been introduced in the past few years and seem to be behaving well. If lubricated at manufacture, introduction of two silicone leads may be almost as friction-free as two polyurethane leads.

Since 1979 a series of polyurethane insulated leads have been introduced and now represent the largest group of leads implanted. The leads are smaller in diameter than older rubber leads, two unipolar leads can easily be inserted into a moderate size cephalic or external jugular vein or via a plastic introducer. Of great importance is that polyurethane slides well against polyurethane while silicone rubber adheres to silicone rubber, though newer silicone leads are improved in this regard. These leads lend themselves especially well to dual-chamber implant. Since they are small, they are readily insinuated beneath a trabeculum, and threshold has been low and stable.

Polyurethane is a category of synthetic polymer, and different polyurethanes have different characteristics. At least one has been associated with a high early and late failure rate with insulation disruption, short circuit, and lead fracture (Figure 7). As this effect has

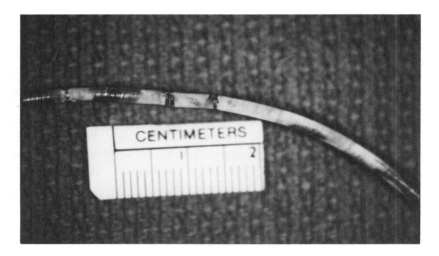

Figure 7. *A polyurethane lead that has undergone deterioration by surface cracking, whitish opacity and discoloration. Three areas of complete loss of insulation appear, two partially caused by a ligature holding the lead to the tissue. The third (left) was apparently spontaneous.*

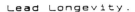

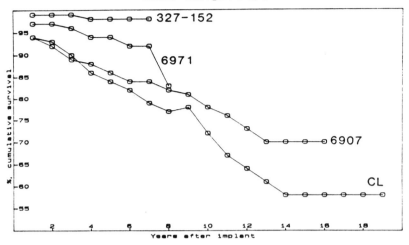

Figure 8. *Survival of individual leads is calculated on a time base of years similar to or greater than that of the longer lasting lithium anode-powered pacemakers. Patterns of wear are readily apparent. Two older silicone rubber leads (CL and 6907) have had cumulative survivals at 14 years of over 60% and 80% respectively. While some urethane leads have had very high failure rates, most have not. All urethane leads have had a far shorter exposure, but models 6971 and 327-152 have had almost 100% survival 4 years after implant, at which time the older leads had already shown a substantial failure incidence.*

been limited to several leads from one manufacturer—ventricular models 6972 and 4002, and atrial models 6990U and 6991U—either the material or the manufacturing process may have been at fault. Despite the polyurethane problems, the need for small diameter slippable leads will continue their popularity. Other polyurethane leads from a variety of manufacturers, and simultaneous and successor leads from the same manufacturer have demonstrated longevity similar to the silicone rubber leads into the short run (Figure 8). The original defective leads have caused severe clinical problems, but correction of the manufacturing problems has resulted in leads having acceptable stability.

G. Solid and Porous Electrodes

Earlier electrodes were always solid metal, whether in a tight coil, a corkscrew-like spiral or at the end of a transvenous lead of platinum-iridium, Elgiloy or silver alloy. In the past few years, new configurations have become available. These are platinum-iridium or Elgiloy porous electrodes and those of sintered carbon. The porous electrode may be a coil of fine platinum-iridium wire with interstices into which tissue grows, or a porous surface bonded into a solid base. The porous surface electrode has Elgiloy spherical powder particles bonded to each other and to a solid Elgiloy substrate. The surface is 30% porous and about 100 micrometers thick. The totally porous electrode consists of a sintered platinum-iridium fiber of 20 micrometers arranged randomly at a density of 10% and hemispherical in shape.

BENEFITS OF POROUS ELECTRODES

a. Ingrowth of fibrous tissue into the electrode interstices increases electrode anchoring;

b. A thinner fibrous capsule forms about the electrode to yield a smaller surface area "virtual electrode";

c. Increase of the effective surface area for sensing while maintaining a small area for pacing.

The activated vitreous carbon electrode produces a biocompatible porous surface electrode with pores about 10 angstroms in size and a depth of 10 microns. The fibrous capsule is thinner than that surrounding a metal electrode. The overvoltage is about 10% of that of solid tip platinum electrodes. The sensing impedance of a porous activated vitreous carbon electrode is about 10% of that of a solid tip platinum electrode. The porous Elgiloy, platinum-iridium and carbon electrodes provide:

1. lower polarization caused by overvoltage;
2. fibrous ingrowth with enhanced attachment of electrode to tissue;
3. smaller fibrous capsule;
4. lower impedance for sensing;
5. lower current and voltage for stimulation, acutely and chronically.

H. Steroid Leads

Maintenance of stable and low acute and chronic stimulation thresholds is highly desirable. Because of the effect of a fibrous tissue layer producing a "virtual" electrode, which increases stimulation threshold and reduces electrogram amplitude, a glucocorticoid steroid has been incorporated into a porous electrode tip to reduce the fibrous reaction and its consequences. Parental glucocorticoid administration has been shown to reduce threshold acutely (though not chronically) in patients with high threshold. To avoid the systemic side effects of such administration, and accomplish the maximum concentration of glucocorticoid at the electrode/tissue interface, electrode model #4003 has a porous surface surrounding a silicone rubber plug that contains approximately 1 mg of dexamethasone sodium phosphate. In contact with tissue fluids, steroid slowly elutes from the electrode in an attempt to affect those cardiac cells adjacent to the lead tip. Elution occurs over several years and 20% of the steroid remains in the electrode four years after implant.

In those in whom the lead has been implanted, the rise in threshold usually seen during the first month post-implant is ameliorated and its decline occurs somewhat earlier than with similar nonsteroid leads. At approximately 16 weeks after implantation the threshold levels between the steroid lead and nonsteroid leads remain modestly, statistically significant, and at approximately one year the thresholds for conventional and steroid leads, which are otherwise similar in electrode material and configuration, is the same (Figure 9).

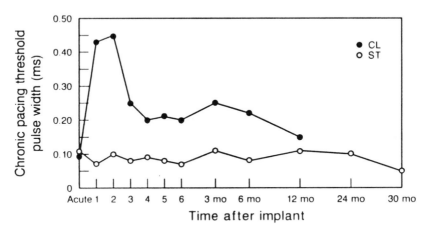

Figure 9. *Two similar leads, one with a steroid eluting electrode (open circle [ST]) and the second a similar, non-steroidal electrode (closed circle [CL]) are compared in threshold evolution following implant. The threshold at implant is similar for both, but thresholds for the non-steroid electrode rise to 4–5 times the threshold pulse duration early after implant. The steroid eluting electrode is characterized by the absence of threshold evolution and long-term stability. After early threshold rise, the non-steroid threshold declines progressively over a year to approach that of the steroid electrode. Both are stable thereafter.*

The benefit of the steroid lead seems to lie largely in the occasional problem that occurs with high threshold in the early post-implant period. Those patients who have previously demonstrated acute high threshold may have a more favorable threshold evolution when implanted with a steroid eluting lead and may, therefore, avoid early electrode revision. Whether the use of a steroid eluting lead is to be preferred to a pulse generator with a high output capability to be reduced after threshold stability occurs, is an unresolved issue. There seems to be no difficulty with the steroid eluting lead; there is no late unfavorable threshold evolution nor is there an early or late increase in displacement, which might have been associated with poor fibrous tissue formation.

I. Lead Fixation

Myocardial. Epicardial and myocardial leads have, from first usage, been actively attached to tissue. Epicardial leads have been backed by a polyester mesh sutured to the epicardium. Leads introduced into the myocardium (Medtronic 5815, 6913) have been backed by a silicone rubber plate that allows suture to the epicardium. Myocardial sutureless electrodes (Medtronic 6917 & 6917A) are screwed into the myocardium and have a polyester mesh "skirt" that provokes fibrous ingrowth to fix the electrode. This electrode has been associated with high threshold evolution and has fallen into disuse. Another sutureless design has two horizontal metal projections holding the electrode, which itself has no active attachment to the myocardium. The most recently introduced, Medtronic 4951, is harpoon-like and rests in the myocardium. It too has a suture plate designed to fix the electrode to the epicardium. In this regard, all of these electrodes can be considered as "active" fixation.

Endocardial. Over 95% of all implantations and therefore leads, are endocardial, both for atrial and ventricular use. Attachment to the endocardium is by remote control because, unlike the "epimyocardial" lead, in which the operator approaches the myocardium with the lead-electrode system, the operator never approaches the endocardial surface. The problem of displacement of the endocardial lead has existed since its earliest usage despite its ease of application and relatively stress free implantation.

The earliest (1958–1960) endocardial stimulating leads were relatively stiff and were held in place by that rigidity. Such a lead could be placed in the right ventricular apex or in the outflow tract and did not require intracardiac support. The problem of so rigid a catheter was that of ventricular perforation, loss of pacing and hemopericardium. A lead must be sufficiently rigid, aside from the stylet used to guide it, if it is to be inserted in the right ventricular apex. Leads that are excessively limp have a higher displacement rate than those that are somewhat more rigid. If excessively rigid, perforation may result. The usual solution is to have a stiff guide wire within a more flexible lead. The guide wire is withdrawn after maneuver of the softer lead into position. Early leads were cylindrical and isodiametric. As the surface was smooth, fibrous ingrowth into the lead material never occurred and the tightly fitting fibrous layer could not grip the lead itself. Two early leads, the Medtronic 5816 and the Elema-Schonander 588S had a larger diameter stimulating tip than the body of the lead. Fibrous tissue growth "glove fit" about the lead and provided a barrier to late displacement of the large tip through the fibrous neck. This provided the first, possibly inadvertant, passive fixation leads. A variety of flanges, fine tines, conical protrusions and fins (some perforated for greater attachment) about the tip of the lead have provided more modern passive fixation devices. In each instance the basis for passive fixation was the delay in actual fixation until fibrous growth from the endocardium occurs.

The bulbous tip leads suffered from two defects, high threshold after implant and a high early displacement rate though they were generally stable chronically. Parallel developments occurred that produced thinner leads, smaller electrodes and greater capacity for early fixation. The first "passive" techniques were conical "shoulders" proximal to the stimulating electrode. Once in position, a fibrous layer was laid down around the lead, trapping it in position because the fibrous "neck" is smaller than the "shoulder." Later developments were:

1. tines, or short 2–3 mm long protuberances proximal to the electrode;
2. fins, in which a conical shoulder (which is a complete conical segment), is replaced by 3 or 4 rubber or plastic slivers arranged radially around the electrode;
3. ribbing of the lead insulation proximal to the electrode;
4. a small layer of polyester velour into which fibrous tissue will grow (not a commercial product).

In all of these designs, the early fixation effect was less but the late effect more significant. The effect on early and late displacement was substantial. Probably the major residual problem is the difficulty or impossibility of late removal of the passively attached lead, once the fibrous attachment has matured. Because of the infrequent but potentially lethal occurrence of endocarditis involving tissue and a retained lead, the problem of late irremovability may be the most serious clinical pacing problem.

Active fixation leads attempt to provide immediate fixation during implant.

ACTIVE FIXATION LEADS

1. a grasping jaw mechanism;
2. a complex helical coil that can wind itself about a trabeculum;
3. an exposed metal screw which is the electrode at the end of the lead;
4. a retractable metal screw which is the electrode and is manually expelled into the endocardium
5. a retractable screw which holds the lead but which is not the electrode. The electrode is conventional at the lead tip, the screw is a fixation device only;
6. nylon whiskers which protrude from a perforated solid electrode to penetrate and grasp the endocardium. This design provided high local re-

activity and unacceptably high threshold. This lead is obsolete;

7. a balloon proximal to the electrode. The electrode is slid (hopefully) beneath a trabeculum and inflated. Once inflated with saline or contrast material the balloon holds the lead in place much as a catheter in the urinary bladder. This lead has a high late dislocation rate and high threshold. When the balloon deflates, as it must when it ruptures because of ingress of body fluid via the balloon membrane, the lead remains in a cavity from which it can be displaced. This lead is obsolete.

Active fixation leads are useful in the atrium where, in general, the early displacement rate is higher than in the ventricle and, of course, in the ventricle. At best they provide immediate stable fixation with (a) low displacement rate; and (b) potentially easy removal of a chronically implanted lead by reversal of the fixation mechanism, i.e., unscrewing it. The leads, especially with the retractable screw mechanism, seem to be relatively atraumatic, easy to use, and live up to their promise. Active fixation leads are likely to be progressively more widely used.

J. Anodal or Cathodal Stimulation

The terms unipolar and bipolar refer to the presence of the anode and cathode in the heart (bipolar) or the cathode only in the cardiac position (unipolar) and the anode at a remote site. The cathode (negative terminal) must be stimulating in all instances and threshold is a function of cathodal characteristics.

Stimulation threshold is ascertained during diastole when ventricular sensitivity has returned to a stable level before a new depolarization. During late diastole the myocardium is more sensitive to a cathodal than anodal stimulus and equally sensitive to cathodal and bipolar stimuli. Myocardial sensitivity to stimulation changes significantly immediately after the QRS complex during the relative refractory period. The phenomenon of pacemaker-induced ventricular fibrillation in which the stimulus falls into the vulnerable period of the cardiac cycle has been observed during bipolar stimulation in all published instances but two and is related to the anode of a bipolar electrode (Figure 10).

The possibility of ventricular fibrillation increases during myocardial ischemia, infarction, metabolic imbalance, and drug intoxication. Completely satisfactory pacemaker sensing of all cardiac foci, including conducted, idioventricular and aberrant, especially during

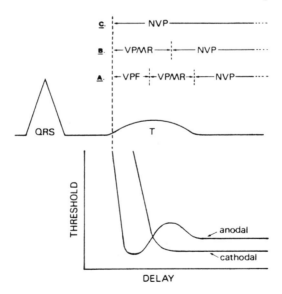

Figure 10.   *Three types of myocardial response to suprathreshold stimuli after the refractory period are observed: **A.** The vulnerable period for fibrillation (VPF) followed by one for multiple responses (VPMR), followed by the nonvulnerable period (NVP). **B.** Stimulation early in the excitable period produces multiple responses followed by a nonvulnerable period. **C.** Some animals are nonvulnerable to arrythmias, and a single stimulus produces a single response. The cathodal and anodal excitation thresholds at different delays during the cardiac cycle (strength-interval curves) are also shown.*

myocardial deterioration and infarction, does not exist. The problem of pacemaker competition with spontaneous cardiac activity has not been eliminated. Competition between premature ventricular contractions and a bipolar stimulus is especially problematic during bipolar temporary pacing following acute myocardial infarction. Most temporary pacing is bipolar. Most of implanted pacing is unipolar cathodal though bipolar pacing is becoming more common. In experimental canine cardiac stimulation during ischemia, at outputs which approximate those of conventional cardiac pacers, three distinct patterns follow the ventricular absolute refractory period:

A. some animals are *nonvulnerable* to arrhythmia (NVP), and a single stimulus (anodal or cathodal) produces a single response (NVP = *nonvulnerable period*);

B. in others, the initial sensitivity produces *multiple ventricular responses* (VPMR) to a single stimulus, followed by a nonvulnerable period (VPMR = *vulnerable period for multiple responses*);

C. in still others, the earliest response will be *ventricular fibrillation* followed by the vulnerable period for multiple responses and then the nonvulnerable period (VF = *ventricular fibrillation*).

Sensitivity to anodal stimulation occurs earlier than cathodal after the absolute refractory period, and because of the phenomenon of the "anodal dip," sensitivity is greater for a *brief* time during the vulnerable periods for multiple responses or ventricular fibrillation than it *ever* is to cathodal stimulation. In order to stimulate early with the cathode, a much higher stimulus level is required, effective only well after the beginning of anodal sensitivity (Figure 11).

The anodal refractory period, therefore, is of shorter duration than the cathodal. If the electrode stimulating surface areas are equal, and both anode and cathode lie on equally sensitive tissue, the bipolar refractory period and consequent ventricular vulnerability will equal the anodal so that a bipolar or anodal stimulus can initiate an arrhythmia over a greater portion of the cardiac cycle and at a lower threshold than can cathodal. The bipolar threshold equals the lower of the anodal or cathodal threshold so that early excitation is possible. Some temporary pacing leads are available in which the anodal surface is much larger than the cathodal, and at least one in which the anodal (ring) surface is moved to a distance of 25 cm from the cathode (tip) so that it is removed from the heart to lie in the superior vena cava.

The importance of this data lies in the relative avoidance of bipolar pacing if significant irritability is present. The possibility exists of reducing irritability, and therefore myocardial vulnerability, by changing from bipolar to unipolar where possible. When pacing is

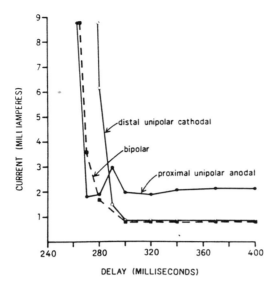

Figure 11. *Unipolar cathodal (at distal tip), unipolar anodal (at proximal ring), and bipolar stength-interval curves determined in a patient with a Cordis temporary 4F electrode. Note that the anodal and bipolar absolute refractory periods are equal and shorter than the cathodal refractory period.*

required during acute myocardial infarction, it is desirable to maintain either a large anode or one remote from the heart. Ventricular fibrillation is not a common occurrence during cardiac pacing. It does occur, but its incidence can be reduced.

FACTORS THAT REDUCE VENTRICULAR FIBRILLATION

1. Careful avoidance of excessive cardiac medication;
2. Electrolyte balance;
3. Administration of some antiarrhythmic drugs;
4. Good oxygenation and ventilation;
5. Unipolar cathodal or remote or large anodal stimulation;
6. Noncompetitive stimulation.

All newly introduced bipolar leads for implant have an anode at least ten times larger than the cathode to reduce the possibility of anodal stimulation and therefore the possibility of ventricular fibrillation.

K. Pulse Duration, i.e., The Strength-Duration Curve

Threshold varies as a function of impulse duration and the direction of this variation is dependent on the parameter measured. The

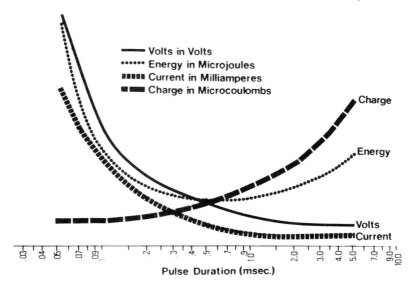

Figure 12. *Strength-duration curves of cardiac stimulation. While current and voltage requirements increase to produce cardiac response as pulse duration shortens, charge is the most significant factor in stimulation efficiency, decreasing with pulse duration. Energy at threshold is lowest at 0.5–1.0 ms pulse duration, increasing at shorter and longer durations.*

strength-duration curve is the major basis for understanding cardiac stimulation threshold. *Current, voltage, charge* (the product of current and time), and *energy* (the product of current, voltage and time [E = IVT]) all vary as a function of pulse duration. A common method of variation of output of a programmable pulse generator is by change of pulse duration. Only through comprehension of the strength-duration curve, and awareness that it is not a linear function, can the basic factors of increase of output in the presence of high threshold, and decrease of output to conserve energy be appreciated (Figure 12).

The lowest point on a stimulation curve at an infinitely long pulse duration is called *rheobase*, and the pulse duration at which threshold is twice the rheobase value is the *chronaxie* time. The knowledge of rheobase is useful in pacemaker design since a pulse duration near or beyond rheobase is a relatively or totally useless expenditure of electrical capacity.

Current.   The current flow at threshold from a constant current generator is parallel (rheobase) to the abscissa from about 1.0 ms and onward. Threshold values rise as pulse duration shortens.

Volts. Rheobase is reached between 1 to 2 ms; at shorter durations threshold rises.

Two derived functions—*charge* and *energy*—show a different pattern. *Charge* is perhaps the most useful single function since it describes threshold in the same terms in which chemical battery capacity is measured (milliampere hours or ampere hours), and its consumption is inversely related to battery longevity. *Charge* expended at threshold decreases with shortened pulse duration since the decline in time is far more rapid than increase in current flow per unit of time.

Quantification of Threshold. **The threshold of cardiac stimulation is the least cathodal electrical stimulus which, when delivered in diastole after the absolute, relative refractory and the hypersensitive periods, is able to maintain consistent capture of the heart.**

At a given pulse duration the mean current per pulse in milliamperes (mA) is the electrical impulse parameter that has been used, and should continue to be used, to quantify the threshold stimulus. The mean current is independent of the lead-heart circuit impedance. It is equally appropriate to quantify threshold by using the quantity of electricity or charge per pulse in microcoulombs (μC). Charge is found by multiplying the mean current by the pulse duration (mean current [I] $\times$ time [T]).

Voltage is an indirect measurement of threshold. The actual voltage drop across responsive myocardium and other interelectrode tissue cannot be separated from the voltage drop across lead resistance and the nonlinear polarization drop across the electrode-tissue interface. For practical purposes, voltage threshold may be the only kind obtainable because most manufacturers produce pulse generators with capacitor-coupled constant voltage output. If pulse duration is kept constant, then the variation of output voltage can be an effective means of finding threshold.

The energy threshold in microjoules (μJ) has been the most common measure of threshold and is approximated by multiplying mean current by mean voltage by pulse duration (mean current [I] $\times$ mean voltage [V] $\times$ time [T]). This is an unfortunate measure of stimulation threshold because the voltage that actually contributes to the excitation process is unknown.

Strength-Duration Curves. The strength-duration curve of stimulation is the quantity of charge, current, voltage or energy required to stimulate the heart at a series of pulse durations. These values vary signficantly as a function of pulse duration and, of these, only charge is approximately linear (Figure 13). In order to set a voltage or pulse duration for parameter output programming, the position that a specific voltage or pulse duration occupies on the curve must be known. At a 2.7 volt output approximately 0.5 ms pulse duration may be required to capture. The threshold of stimulation at a fixed voltage (2.7 or 5.0 V) is the point of intersection of the threshold and output curves. Similarly, if output voltage is varied at a constant pulse duration the voltage threshold can be determined (Figure 14). In the instance cited, the rheobase is 2.2 V. If the pacemaker had an output below 2.2 V, then no stimulus, of any duration would capture despite increasing output charge and/or energy.

A similar situation exists for current threshold. The analysis of output-to-threshold variation can be made as described above (Figure 15). During constant voltage pacing the current output decreases as the pulse duration increases. The decrease occurs because of increasing polarization and, therefore, impedance at longer pulse durations is greater than at shorter durations (Figure 16).

The relationship between threshold charge and output charge per pulse as a function of pulse duration may be easier to visualize than either the voltage or the current output-to-threshold relationships because the charge curves are nearly linear over the range of relevant pulse durations.

Safety Factor.   Safety factor refers to the amount by which the pulse generator's output exceeds the threshold at a given pulse duration.

Safety Factor:

$$= \frac{\text{Pulse Generator Output} - \text{Threshold Value}}{\text{Threshold Value}}$$

$$= \frac{\text{Pulse Generator Output}}{\text{Threshold Value}} - 1$$

As the aim of pacing is to capture the heart each time a stimulus is produced, the safety factor is used to set the output at a sufficiently high level to accommodate the variation in threshold that may occur during daily activities such as sleeping, eating and exercise, and that which may also be due to medications.

The question remains of how great the safety factor should be under various circumstances, including the period early after implantation when threshold evolution occurs. Since the threshold peak

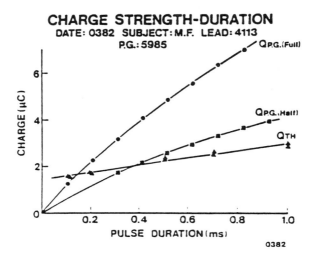

Figure 13. Output charge per pulse of a pacemaker programmed to 5 and 2.7 V, superimposed on the charge strength-duration curve. The points of intersection of the threshold with output curves determines minimum pulse duration at which capture occurs for the programmed output voltage.

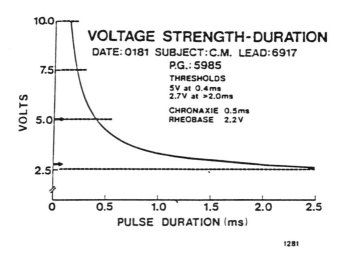

Figure 14. Mean output voltage per pulse of a pacemaker programmed to 5 V (full) and 2.7 V (half) superimposed on the voltage strength-duration curve. Capture was consistent for programmed pulse durations equal to or greater than 0.4 ms at 5 V or 2.0 ms at 2.7 V. Rheobase is at 2.2 V which means that below that output voltage, no pulse of any duration would produce capture, even though output charge and energy may be very large at long pulse durations.

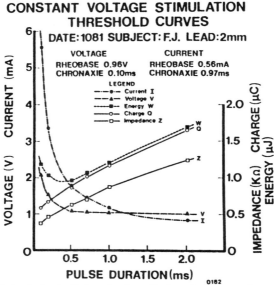

Figure 15.   *A typical set of chronic strength-duration curves for constant voltage stimulation. As pulse duration increases, charge increases, mean current and voltage threshold fall, and energy threshold is at a minimum at approximately 0.5–0.8 ms. The shortest pulse duration requires the least charge at threshold.*

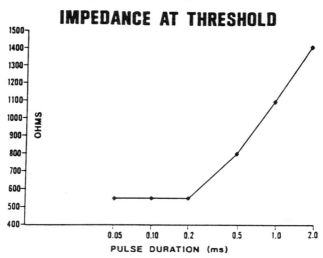

Figure 16.   *The impedance to flow of current increases with pulse duration increase. Shorter pulse durations produce much lower impedances and are therefore more efficient for stimulation. The impedance can double over the pulse duration programmable range of conventional pulse generators.*

may be five times the charge at implant, the initial output setting should be at least five times the threshold charge. The second period for which a safety factor must be considered is that of the chronic, stable threshold. As the normal physiological variation in charge threshold is no more than 30–50%, doubling the charge threshold should be adequate. The third circumstance is that of the high and, even unstable threshold. In this situation the actual threshold may be unknown (except during programming) and unpredictable. Pacemaker output should be set at a very high level to provide for maximum safety and the patient should be seen sufficiently frequently to ascertain if and when stability occurs.

The use of a safety margin of 100% of threshold charge will provide adequate patient saftey if the long-term threshold is stable. As the long-term threshold is almost always stable when chronic (6 months or more after implant, and can be expected to vary within a narrow range), 100% charge margin will be satisfactory. Even if threshold is high but stable, a safe margin can be found depending on the output capability of the pulse generator used. If threshold is actually unstable, then only very great outputs will suffice, many beyond the capability of any implantable pulse generator. In that case it is clearly desirable to revise electrode status so that a new, hopefully low and stable threshold will result.

The reasons for setting an output at some reasonable level above threshold are the reduction of output and the consequent prolongation of pulse generator longevity, and the reduction of the likelihood of local muscle stimulation if a unipolar pacer is to be used. Output programmable single-chamber pacemakers can increase or decrease the anticipated longevity by as much as 5–8 times depending on programmability capability and output setting. For dual-chamber pacemakers, the longevity range is far greater.

All output programming is based on understanding of the strength-duration curve and the various portions of the curve, the portion for voltage and current at short pulse durations, i.e., less than 0.3 ms in which relatively small changes in pulse duration make large differences in threshold, the knee in which relatively proportional changes are made between pulse duration and voltage or current threshold, and the flat portion of the curve at longer pulse durations in which large changes in pulse duration make very small changes in thresold. The charge threshold, i.e., the product of time (pulse duration) and current is low at short pulse durations and high at long pulse durations. Since it is charge that produces a cardiac event, and since it is the charge drain that should be kept to the minimum to reduce battery drain, the charge threshold should be determined and charge output kept at a minimum. All battery capacity is calculated in charge, i.e., 1 ampere hour, etc.

Atrial and ventricular thresholds are similar in principal and no difference exists in determining threshold or setting output between atrium and ventricle. For implant of dual-chamber pacemakers, similar procedures should be undertaken for atrium and ventricle if output is independently programmable. If output is not independently programmable it is likely that threshold will be lower in one chamber than the other. The output for both must be set to meet the needs of the chamber with the higher threshold, thus using battery capacity that might otherwise be conserved. It is desirable, if different output settings can be established, to set each chamber individually (Figure 17).

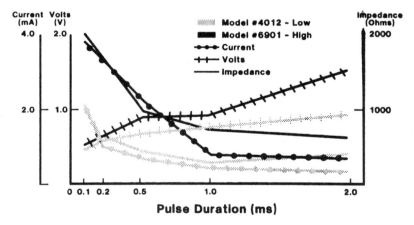

Figure 17. *The trend in electrode design has been toward lower impedance, requiring lower output voltage in the pulse generator. This graph measures the acute (i.e., at implant) behavior of a bipolar lead from 1974 (#6901) and one from 1984 (#4012). Each is graphed for three functions measured against the pulse duration. The impedance, voltage, and current at threshold of model 4012 are consistently lower throughout the range of useful pulse durations compared to that of model #6901.*

DETERMINATION OF THRESHOLD AND
SETTING OF OUTPUT

There are six different means of controlling output in an output programmable pacemaker. Pulse generators may be of constant current or constant voltage output. Most are constant voltage and four different combinations are possible. Two different combinations are possible for constant current generators.

1. Single voltage—Multiple pulse durations

This had been the most commonly available mode for single-chamber pacemakers until about five years ago. Many remain implanted. Output voltage is 5 V and pulse duration commonly from 0.05–2.0 ms. With pulse duration as the only variable, threshold is determined by progressive decrease in pulse duration until the shortest pulse duration is found that will consistently capture the heart. If 0.3 ms or less, tripling the pulse duration will provide a 100% threshold margin. (Remember that as the pulse duration is increased, threshold increases as does output.) If the threshold is 0.4 ms (the approximate voltage chronaxie) or greater, then the pulse duration should be set at 4 times threshold. So great an increase may not be available and even when it is, a full 100% safety margin may not be possible.

2. Dual voltage—Multiple pulse durations

Many pulse generators provide this capability. The two voltages are the traditional 5.0 V and 2.5 V, which is also the battery voltage before it is doubled to produce 5.0 V. Two alternative approaches are possible. Formerly, the 5 V setting alone was used, as in the single voltage unit above, and the 2.5 V setting was disregarded except when special low output or great longevity is required. Because of the recent introduction of low threshold leads, some models are delivered at 2.5 V output, and the 5 V setting is used only as a "high output" setting.

A useful approach is to set the output at 2.5 V and determine the minimum threshold pulse duration. Programming the output voltage to 5 V at that pulse duration will provide an adequate safety margin. If 2.5 V never capture no matter what the pulse duration, i.e., rheobase is above 2.5 V, threshold must be determined at 5 V, but it will certainly be high and a full 100% safety margin may not be attainable. If threshold is at 0.5–0.2 ms pulse duration at 2.5 V, then, tripling the pulse duration at 2.5 V will be safe and effective.

3. Triple voltage—Multiple pulse durations

The pulse durations usually available are similar to those of single voltage, multiple pulse duration generators. For some generators, only four pulse durations are available corresponding to the parts of the standard deviation curve in which change in pulse duration has a significant effect on threshold, i.e., 0.25 to 1.0 ms. The actual voltages available are 2.5, 5.0, 7.5–8.2, or 10 V. These represent battery voltage, the conventional doubling of battery voltage and its tripling or quadrupling. The 7.5 to 10 V output should be used as short-term expedients only. Battery capacity is consumed so rapidly at these outputs that pulse generator longevity will necessarily be very short.

The voltage setting should be at 2.5 V. Pulse duration threshold is found and the final voltage may be left at 2.5 or 5 V, as above. If capture is not 2.5 V, threshold is determined at 5 V, and the final setting is at prolonged pulse duration and 5 V or at the threshold pulse duration at 10 V. If capture is possible at a relatively short pulse duration at 5 V, it may be better to use a longer pulse duration at 5 V, knowing that a 100% margin is not possible but also recognizing the high battery drain of 7.5–10 V.

Several pulse generators have a special autothreshold procedure named "Vario." In this test process, a pulse duration and voltage are set. Application of a magnet to the generator begins a progressive reduction of output voltage by $\frac{1}{16}$ output steps. Removal of the magnet immediately restores the output to its full voltage setting. Threshold voltage is readily determined at a specific pulse duration. If this technique is available, select the shortest pulse duration and the 5 V setting. If the voltage threshold determined during the Vario process is less than half that voltage setting, leave output at 5 V. If not, increase the pulse duration until the voltage threshold is half or less than the 5 V setting. If such a setting cannot be found, a judgment will have to be made, but if possible, maintain output voltage at 5 V (Figure 18).

4. Multiple voltage—Multiple pulse durations

The present generation of CMOS (complementary metal oxide semiconductor) circuits allow very small steps in output voltage, i.e.,

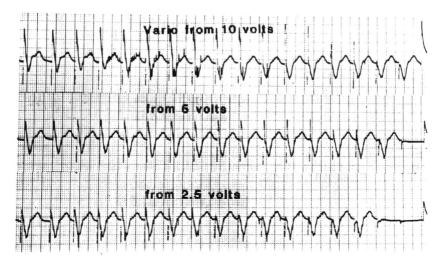

Figure 18. *Threshold can often be very accurately determined noninvasively if multiple pulse durations and output voltage settings are available. Use of the "Vario" system at three output voltages 10 V, 5 V, and 2.5 V at a pulse duration of 0.5 ms allows accurate determination of the voltage threshold.* **Top.** *Each step is 0.64 volts and capture is consistent through the fifteenth step, threshold is below 0.64 volts.* **Middle.** *Each step is 0.32 volts. One stimulus does not capture so that threshold must lie between 0.64 and 0.32 volts.* **Bottom.** *Each step is 0.15 volts. As two steps are missed, threshold is at 0.45 volts. A strength-duration curve can be constructed easily if desired.*

0.1 V, and smaller steps in pulse duration, 0.01 ms. These steps are too fine to have any practical benefit in setting output. Determining threshold, using all of this capability, can become excessively burdensome. It is probably wisest to treat such an excess of pulse duration and voltage steps as if they represented three voltage steps, i.e., 2.5, 5, and 7.5–10, and no more than 20 pulse duration steps.

Output voltage of less than 2.5 V will not represent significant benefit in reduction of battery drain and should be used for special purposes only, such as the elimination of stimulation of extracardiac tissue or local pectoral muscles. There will probably be few situations in which such low voltages will be useful.

PACEMAKER OUTPUT

A pacemaker output circuit can be readily understood by a hydraulic comparison. In those terms, the significance of high output or low output, high impedance or low impedance leads, or the effect of single- or dual-chamber pacing can all be comprehended.

The hydraulic comparison is traditional in understanding electrical circuits. Flow of water is readily compared to flow of current and the various impedances to flow can be equally compared. Many persons have difficulty comprehending electrical terms but have an intuitive understanding of hydraulic events (Figure 19).

The five major factors are energy, voltage, current, charge and impedance. They can be redefined as:

Voltage–The force moving the current. This is analogous to the height of the reservoir above the point of delivery of the current flow.
Current–The actual continuing volume of flow of electricity or of water.

PACEMAKER CIRCUIT

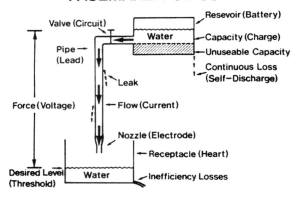

ENERGY = FORCE x FLOW x TIME
CHARGE = CURRENT x TIME (of Flow)
CURRENT = QUANTITY OF FLOW
VOLT = FORCE OF FLOW

Figure 19. *In this diagram, the battery is the reservoir of fluid above the point of delivery. The height above the point of delivery (the nozzle) is the force with which the fluid is delivered. The size of the nozzle presents a resistance to flow and the valve in the circuit represents all of the other increases or decreases in resistance to current flow. In the reservoir (i.e., the battery), water above the egress pipe is wholly useable, some below the pipe is not usable, and because the reservoir is incompletely sealed, there is some continuing loss, even if no water flows. The flow, therefore, depends on the resistance to flow, the height of the reservoir above the nozzle, the duration and rate of flow, and the usable capacity of the reservoir.*

Charge–The quantity of electricity or of water that has flowed. Because of the measurement of volume and the duration of flow, the charge is given in volume multiplied by time, i.e., Watt hours or more commonly in Coulombs, which are amperes (the quantity) multiplied by time.

Energy–This is the result of multiplying the electromotive force (voltage) by the charge (the current multiplied by the time of flow).

Impedance–This is the numerical sum of all of the resistances to the flow (either of water or of electricity). The calculation may be very complex, especially in a biological system, but in the simplest form, once a number has been selected as being reasonably accurate, calculation of the derived functions can be accomplished.

Battery capacity is given in voltage (electromotive force) and in a capacity of current delivery. The voltage is a result of the chemistry of the battery and cannot be modified once a specific chemistry is selected. The capacity of the cell to deliver current is given by the amount it will deliver for the time it will deliver. Consequently, batteries will be identified by voltage and by ampere hours, i.e., current × time. A small lithium iodine battery may have an output of 2.8 V and a capacity of 0.8 ampere (A) hours while a larger battery will have a voltage of 2.8 V and 3.0 A hours. The actual longevity of a pulse generator with either battery implanted will depend on how rapidly the battery is drained and the capacity of the battery. Because voltage is a function of battery chemistry, it declines slowly until the current is almost completely drained. In effect, it is the charge and not the voltage that is the consummable component.

The longevity of the pacemaker can be calculated from the knowledge of the battery capacity and the rate of drain caused by the sensing circuit efficiency, pacing circuit efficiency, and the factors under the control of the operator of a programmable pacemaker, which are (1) the pacemaker rate; (2) the programmed output voltage; (3) the programmed pulse duration; (4) the percent of time pacing. The current output of a pacemaker can be calculated by the output, voltage and by the impulse duration. Consequently, output can be given as energy—

Formula 1

Energy = volts × current × time;

or

volts × current × pulse duration

or

Formula 2

As current only;

or

Formula 3
As charge, i.e., current × time.

The current that will flow is a function of the resistance of the circuit to current flow and the voltage that is applied. Generally Ohm's law will be applicable, i.e.:

Formula 4
Voltage = current × resistance.

This formula may be solved for any of the three functions, i.e.,

Formula 4a
Current = voltage/resistance;
Formula 4b
Resistance = voltage/current.

It is best to calculate and give pacemaker output in charge as this (see above) is the consummable component. Giving output in energy is less meaningful because of the shape of the strength-duration curve. The pulse duration at which output occurs must always be known to appreciate its effectiveness.

ENERGY SOURCES

Many different energy sources have been used to power cardiac pacemakers. The energy to stimulate the heart under optimal and even usual circumstances is small, approximately 3 μJ though several times that amount is required for consistent, long-term stimulation.

Nuclear pacemakers powered by plutonium and promethium have been implanted. All promethium pacemakers have already been removed, none are now being implanted. The longevity of promethium pacemakers was no more than that of middle longevity lithium pulse generators because the half-life of promethium is 2.7 years. Although a few plutonium pacemakers continue to be implanted, none have been manufactured recently, and all are the technology of the 1970s. The longevity expectation of these units was 20–40 years,

---

EVALUATED ENERGY SOURCES

1. Biogalvanic
2. Piezo-electric energy
3. Photoelectric cells with trans-cutaneous light
4. Energy of glucose oxidation
5. Skeletal muscle contraction
6. Fuel cells
7. Rechargeable nickel-cadmium cells
8. Mercury-zinc cells
9. Carbon-zinc cells
10. Nuclear converters
11. Cells with a lithium anode and a variety of different cathodes.

---

and longevity experience is 88% cumulative survival 12 years after implantation. None of the developments of the past decade in cardiac pacing are available in nuclear units. Associated malignancy has not been reported. About 3000 units have been implanted worldwide and most remain functioning.

Lithium cells power all new, nonnuclear pacemakers now implanted. Five different lithium chemistries have reached commercial availability and four already are obsolete, though many pacemakers with obsolete cells (in practice only the LiCuS) will remain in service for many years. A variety of battery sizes and capacities, and therefore potential longevities, exist for the remaining lithium power source (LiI) chemistry. The user should carefully evaluate patient needs and the selection of the appropriate power source and battery capacity (Table IV).

PULSE GENERATOR LONGEVITY

Pacemaker longevity after implantation depends on many factors. Certainly it depends on the battery drain required to operate the electronic circuit, the drain required for the programmed output, and the continuous drain from the battery, the component which establishes the entity known as "shelf-life." All three factors have been improved. "Shelf-life" improvement and efficient circuit operation have been progressively accomplished and have been discussed earlier. Pulse generator output needed to achieve cardiac capture has

Table IV

Chemistry	Nominal Capacity Ah	Voltage	Estimated Longevity (Years)	Problems
LiI	0.8–3.5	2.8	4–15	1. Variable capacity
LiAgCr (Obsolete)	0.6	3.4	3–4	1. Small capacity 2. Short longevity at high drain
LiCuS (Obsolete)	0.9–1.8	2.1	4–12	1. Nonhermetic
LiPb (Obsolete)	0.9	1.9 (5.7 as manufactured)	2–3	1. Small capacity
LiSOCl (Obsolete)	0.75–1.5	3.6	3–6	1. Rapid depletion @ EOL
NiCd (Obsolete)	0.19	1.3	10(?)–20(?) Recharge monthly	1. Small capacity 2. Monthly recharge 3. Voltage & rate instability 4. Rapid self-discharge
HgZnO (Obsolete)	1.0	1.35	3–5	1. Large volume/weight 2. High self-discharge 3. Wide scatter of failures – Early/Late

also been reduced over the three decades since implanted stimulation was first used (Figure 20).

The electrodes used in 1960 required a pulse generator output of 675 μJ and longevity was about six months. The required output in 1985 for consistent stimulation was 6–10 joules and the longevity of the implantable pulse generators has increased correspondingly. Even during the mercury battery era it was known that a small surface area and a high impedance electrode would reduce the current required for stimulation and increase the effective longevity of a pulse generator. At least one manufacturer of pulse generators and leads achieved the de facto programmable reduction in output during pulse generator replacement following battery depletion by inserting a resistor in series between the lead and a constant voltage pulse generator. The higher resistance reduced pulse generator current output

LITHIUM AND NUCLEAR

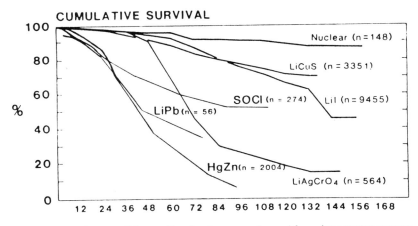

Figure 20. *The overall longevity of pulse generators with various power sources used for implantable cardiac pacemakers is given for mercury batteries, nuclear converters, and for the five different lithium batteries that have been used in devices implanted in humans. Each power source has a characteristic longevity even if used in different pulse generator designs. The longest duration source was the nuclear with a cumulative survival of 88%, 148 months after implantation. The briefest was mercury-zinc, no longer in use, with a 0% cumulative survival, 100 months after implant and 50% survival after 36 months.*

(Ohm's law). As current output determines battery drain, increased longevity occurred.

As stimulation threshold is directly related to electrode size, the progressive reduction in cathodal size and in stimulation efficiency through the introduction of porous and steroid leads have been as important in increasing pulse generator longevity as improvements in battery and electronic technology. In the case of steroid and porous leads, the reduction in current threshold has been achieved simultaneously with a reduction of electrode impedance (see above) and consequently, the same current can stimulate tissue but at a lower voltage. This has allowed lower voltage pacemakers to operate at the battery voltage rather than at a higher voltage, requiring a transformer. As voltage transformation is less than 100%, some decrease in pulse generator longevity occurred (Figure 21).

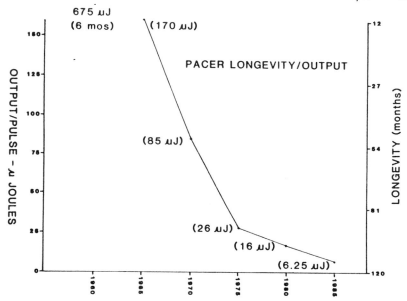

Figure 21. *The longevity of implantable pacemakers is inversely proportional to the continuous battery drain. In this diagram, the continuous battery drain is listed on the left vertical axis, the longevity is on the right vertical axis. The actual battery drain from a "typical" pulse generator of year (horizontal axis) is a function of decrease in output. A modern, programmable output pulse generator, drained at a 1960 level, would last as long.*

CALCULATION OF PULSE GENERATOR LONGEVITY

The functional longevity of an implantable pulse generator depends on a number of factors:

1. The capacity of the battery in the implanted generator

Until almost the end of the mercury-zinc era, only one battery capacity was available, i.e., each mercury cell had a capacity of 1 ampere hour. As the cells (six, five and later four) were in series, the output voltage was additive but the overall charge capacity was not.

A 3 ampere hour cell was used in one generator, had a very prolonged longevity, but the manufacturer nevertheless stopped its manufacture. During the lithium era, batteries of different chemistry have different capacities, and batteries of the same chemistry are constructed in different sizes. For example, lithium iodine batteries used in commercial pulse generators are of 0.8–3.0 A hour capacity.

The useful battery longevity is always less than the nominal capacity. As its capacity is consumed the battery voltage falls and at some point, the output voltage and current delivering capacity are insufficient to deliver the rated pacemaker output or to operate the pacemaker circuit. The useful battery capacity as opposed to its total capacity then becomes the capacity available to operate the pacemaker at settings that are consistent with normal function.

2. Battery self-discharge

The mercury cell had a very high self-discharge, approximating 10% of useful capacity per year, so that efficient operation of the pacemaker circuit and reduction of output could produce only limited benefits in prolongation of pulse generator longevity. Lithium batteries have a self-discharge of about 1% per year so that efficiency of pulse generator design and operation can be translated into increased longevity.

3. Output impedance

For a constant voltage pulse generator the impedance of the lead-electrode system influences pacemaker output. Within the limits of conventional lead impedance, lower impedance increases output and battery drain while a higher impedance lead decreases drain. As written elsewhere, the change may be sufficient to affect overall pulse generator longevity significantly. In limiting instances, a lead fracture with cessation of output preserves pulse generator longevity; lead insulation defect or conductor short circuit of a bipolar lead accelerates battery depletion. An impedance of 510 Ohms is used as the standard during calculation of output impedance and battery drain.

4. Circuit efficiency

Discrete component circuits were inefficient in operation and a great deal of battery drain was consumed in operation of the sensing and pulse forming circuits. CMOS (complementary metal oxide semiconductor) circuits are far more efficient and even far more complex than those previously available and operate at far lower battery drain. Single channel sensing pacemakers drain far less than dual-channel and triple-channel, which will soon be available.

5. Percent operation

The drain to operate the pulse generator sensing circuit is small as such circuits are efficient. The output circuit consumes much larger energies in stimulating the heart, especially at higher outputs. A pacing system that senses almost continuously will have a far greater longevity than one that paces continuously. In general, calculations of projected longevity consider stimulation 50% of the time. Wide variations in longevity can be anticipated based on the actual proportion of pacing.

6. Output programming

The most important longevity consideration during normal pulse generator operation is the output programmed for the pulse generator. Many modern single-chamber pulse generators may be programmed from 5–200 μJ. The longevity of the generator will be directly related to the change in output. Dual-chamber pulse generators, and those in which the stimulation rate changes with atrial rate or with sensor input can have the same output variation, plus an increase in the rate at which the output is delivered. At or near maximum output, a longevity of 1½ years for a modern generator may be anticipated.

7. Continuous battery drain

Considering all of the enumerated factors, a continuous battery drain is calculated and used in a formula to calculate pulse generator longevity. It is obviously subject to significant variation from the calculation. The formula for the longevity of a pulse generator is therefore:

$$\text{Longevity}_{PG} \quad = \frac{\text{Useful Battery Capacity}}{\text{Continuous battery drain}}$$

Continuous battery drain = Self discharge + continuous drain for sensing + continuous drain for circuit operation + drain for stimulation (converted to a continuous output number) + miscellaneous additional drain

$$\begin{array}{ll}\text{Longevity}_{PG} & = \dfrac{\text{Useful Battery Capacity (Ah)}}{(\text{Continuous drain})(24^*)(365^{**})} \\ \text{(Years)} & \end{array}$$

*hours per day
**days per year   PG = pulse generator

While accurate calculation of the longevity of a specific pacemaker unit depends on the factors listed and possibly others, most implanted units are set at nominal rates, outputs, and with nominal impedance leads so that, from a practical point of view, longevities fall within a relatively narrow range and the projections given will be broadly accurate.

ATRIOVENTRICULAR AND VENTRICULOATRIAL CONDUCTION

Pacemakers are implanted because of failures of atrioventricular conduction or of impulse formation with satisfactory or unsatisfactory junctional escape. The interval from the sensed or paced atrial event to the ventricular event is an important consideration in dual-chamber pacing. The appearance of the intrinsic deflections of the atrium and ventricle is different for each different atrial or ventricular focus, and the timing of the various events depends on the site at which they are sensed in the atrium and ventricle, and the site of origin of the atrial or ventricular depolarization. For example, the setting of an AV interval of 150 ms from pacing the right atrial appendage to pacing or sensing the right ventricular apex will produce timing consequences quite different from pacing the left atrial appendage and sensing or pacing the right ventricular apex. The description of AV conduction and VA conduction timing cycles are all based on the conventional implant sites of right atrial appendage and right ventricular apex. Were the implant sites different, the timing measurements would be different. None of the timing cycles will mimic closely the normal PR interval, which is not measured from intracardiac events but from the surface. The PR interval is, of course, the time from the earliest appearance of the P wave to the earliest appearance of the QRS complex in any ECG lead.

The PR Interval

The AV interval is the time that allows ventricular filling following atrial contraction. In the dual-chamber pacemaker the AV interval starts with a stimulus to the atrium from the pacemaker atrial channel or from sensing of the atrial intrinsic deflection. The intrinsic deflection begins at the SA node so that its earliest appearance is there. Atrial sensing usually occurs via a lead in the right atrial appendage, which means that by the time the atrial depolarization is sensed the atrial contraction will have begun. If sensing is from the left atrium, the atrial contraction (at least of the right atrium) will be even further advanced when the intrinsic deflection is sensed.

There are four possible AV intervals depending on different circumstances of atrial and ventricular sensing and pacing.(Figure 22).

AV INTERVALS

1. The sensed atrium to the sensed ventricle—in this instance the best AVI calculation will be from the intrinsic deflection of the atrium to the intrinsic deflection of the ventricle
2. The sensed atrium to the paced ventricle; i.e., from the intrinsic deflection of the spontaneous P wave to the ventricular channel stimulus
3. The paced atrium to the sensed ventricle—in this instance timing starts with the atrial stimulus and the P wave occurs entirely within the AV interval. To obtain a conducted QRS, a prolonged AV interval may be required
4. The paced atrium to the paced ventricle—the timing cycle starts with the atrial stimulus and ends with the ventricular stimulus. The atrial contraction is wholly within the AV interval and the effective filing time will be short (Figure 22).

Should AV conduction exist, programming the implanted dual-chamber pacemaker would allow selection of any one of these possibilities. Each change will have a different physiology to some degree.

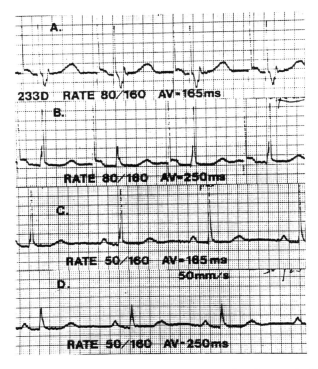

Figure 22. *Whether the atrium is paced or sensed will affect the ventricular response.* ***A.*** *The atrium is continually paced and, at an AV interval of 165 ms the ventricle is paced as well. Not enough time has elapsed for the ventricle to depolarize via AV conduction.* ***B.*** *The atrium is continually paced, but at an AV interval of 250 ms the QRS complexes are conducted. Still, the intrinsic deflection of the QRS complex is sufficiently late so that fusion beats occur.* ***C.*** *By slowing the pacing rate, the intrinsic deflection of the atrial depolarization is sensed and, at 165 ms AV interval spontaneous AV conduction occurs and pseudofusion ventricular beats occur.* ***D.*** *At 250 ms AV interval, begun by atrial sensing, both atrial and ventricular stimuli are inhibited as the ventricular intrinsic deflection falls within the AV interval.*

The physiological effect of changing the PR interval is not yet entirely understood though it is being investigated intensively. Nevertheless, the physician, who controls the duration of the PR interval by programming the AV interval, should comprehend the changes that can be made and the possible physiological consequences of AV interval programming (see Chapter 3).

Antegrade Conduction

Those implanted for sinus node dysfunction often have normal or moderately impaired AV conduction. About half of the patients implanted for sinus node dysfunction have prolonged AV conduction, defined as an interval of greater than 450 ms from the ID_A to the ID_V or the presence of Wenckebach conduction or AV block with atrial pacing below 120 bpm. The prolonged interval, i.e., 450 ms was selected because of the normally greater duration of $ID_A \rightarrow ID_V$ from the right atrial appendage to the right ventricular apex than the PR interval. It is, of course, only the $ID_A \rightarrow ID_V$ that is sensed by the pacemaker. The interval from the two spontaneous depolarizations is 40–60 ms shorter than the interval from a stimulus to the right atrial appendage to the conducted ventricular ID at similar rates. The depolarization latency is added to the AV interval during any conduction process following atrial stimulation. Because of this variation of AV interval caused by sensing or pacing the atrium, some pulse generators allow different AV intervals when pacing or sensing the atrium—longer when pacing, shorter when sensing (Figure 23).

AV DELAY AND PR INTERVAL

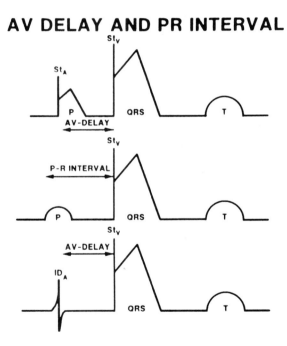

Figure 23. *The AV interval starts at the atrial stimulus or sensing of the atrial intrinsic deflection.* **Top.** *The AV interval contains the entire P wave and a briefer interval from the end of the P wave to the ventricular stimulus.* **Bottom.** *The P wave has begun spontaneously and the sensed intrinsic deflection begins the AV interval providing a longer time from the beginning of atrial contraction to the ventricular stimulus.* **Middle.** *Represents a spontaneous P wave.*

Because of the time difference between the paced atrium and the sensed atrium, the AV interval will be of different duration depending on whether the atrium has been paced or sensed. As the AV interval begins with the atrial stimulus or sensing the atrial intrinsic deflection, the difference in duration of the AV interval can be as much as 40–60 ms. Consequently, the programmed AV interval will be shorter or longer depending on whether the timing cycles are started by atrial pacing or sensing. Thus, a physiological hysteresis of the PR interval will exist unless the pacemaker responds with a longer interval when the cycle is started by a stimulus, and a shorter interval when it is started by a sensed event. Thus, there will be either hysteresis of the electronic AV interval or there will be a hysteresis of the physiological PR interval.

Retrograde (VA) Conduction

While the existence of retrograde conduction has been recognized since 1913, its effect on the implanted dual-chamber pacemaker was unexpected at the time the first pacemakers able to sense in the atrium and the ventricle were introduced. Measurement of antegrade and retrograde conduction during pacemaker implant has demonstrated that 45% of patients who require pacemaker implantation for any indication—ventricular or supraventricular tachycardia, sinus node dysfunction or AV block—have retrograde conduction at some paced rate if paced from the ventricle. If paced in the AV sequential mode by testing with extrastimuli, the incidence would be even higher. Sixty-seven percent of patients paced for sinus node dysfunction have retrograde conduction and 14% of those with fixed complete antegrade heart block have retrograde conduction. Even patients who have had AV block for many years may retain retrograde conduction. The mean retrograde conduction time from the ventricular stimulus to the atrial intrinsic deflection (ID_A) is 235 ± 50 ms and the range is 110 ms–450 ms (Table V).

The presence of retrograde (VA) conduction and the status of antegrade (AV) conduction is determined during pacemaker implantation. With the definitive pacemaker leads in place, the interval of the passive $ID_A \rightarrow ID_V$ is measured. If AV conduction exists, a clearly defined number will be found; if AV block exists, it will be apparent. The atrium is paced and the interval from the atrial pacemaker stimulus (St_A) to the ventricular (ID_V) response is evaluated at a number of paced rates, i.e., 60, 80, 100, 120, 140 and 160 bpm. The rate for the onset of AV block is ascertained (Figures 24, 25).

Table V

Primary Diagnosis	1:1 VA Conduction			VA Conduction Time at Lowest Rate
	No.	Pts	%	
Sick sinus syndrome	6	4	67	222
Sinus brady/arrest	16	11	69	214
Incomplete AV block	14	5	36	293
Complete AV block	16	4	25	210
Ventricular tachycardia	1	1	100	NA
TOTAL	53	25	47%	235 ms

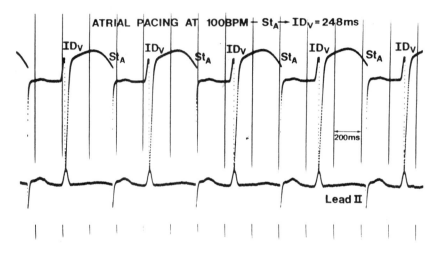

Figure 24. *Electrophysiologic testing during dual-chamber pacemaker implant involves atrial pacing to determine the stability of AV conduction. The atrial lead is used for stimulation while the ventricular response is recorded. The interval from atrial stimulus to ventricular response can be measured readily at each paced rate. Here, at a coupling interval of 600 ms (100 bpm), the conduction interval is 248 ms.*

The ventricle is then paced (St_V) at the same rates (above), the retrograde P wave recorded from the atrial channel, and retrograde conduction intervals determined (Figures 26, 27). Measurement of antegrade and retrograde conduction intervals allows evaluation of the state of AV and VA conduction as supporting evidence for pacemaker implantation and to allow the setting of the atrial refractory interval after the ventricular event to avoid retrograde conduction and the onset of the endless loop tachycardia.

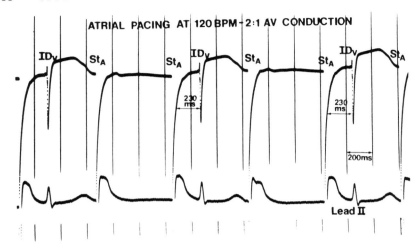

Figure 25.   *Atrial pacing at a coupling interval of 500 ms (120 bpm), results in 2:1 AV block. The consistent atrial capture and 2:1 response are clearly apparent.*

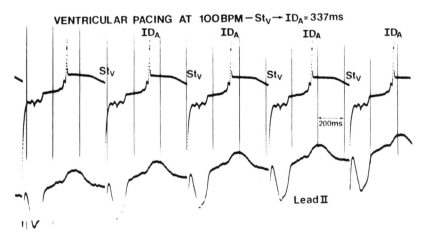

Figure 26.   *Ventricular stimulation at a coupling interval of 600 ms (120 bpm), is associated with consistent retrograde conduction at an interval of 337 ms. The measurement is from the ventricular stimulus to the intrinsic deflection of the retrograde P wave.*

Endless Loop Tachycardia

The existence of retrograde conduction via the natural pathway, and antegrade conduction via the implanted dual-chamber pace-

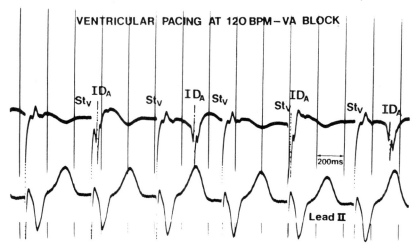

Figure 27. *Ventricular pacing at a coupling interval of 500 ms (120 bpm), results in complete retrograde block. Here, the atrial intrinsic deflections are completely dissociated from the paced QRS complexes.*

maker provides a reentry circuit that mimics the natural situation in which an accessory pathway allows a circuit movement tachycardia. This reentry tachycardia has been variously called "pacemaker reentry tachycardia," "pacemaker circus movement tachycardia," "pacemaker mediated-tachycardia," and "endless loop tachycardia." The basis of the tachycardia is the ability of the atrial channel to sense a P wave displaced from its natural position before the QRS complex. The P wave can be displaced by a ventricular premature contraction with retrograde conduction, an atrial premature contraction, a ventricular pacemaker channel escape following an ineffective atrial stimulus, a ventricular escape in an atrial synchronous pacemaker, or atrial channel triggering by electromagnetic or electromyographic interference.

Once displacement of the P wave has occurred (in order that it be sensed), the atrial refractory interval after the ventricular event must be sufficiently short so that the retrograde P wave occurs after it ends. Therefore, endless loop tachycardia cannot exist in a DVI pacemaker as the atrial channel is always insensitive. Endless loop tachycardia was described on a theoretical basis for the original atrial synchronous (VAT) pacemaker and cases apparently occurred, but may not have been recorded in the medical literature. As most of the VAT pacemakers were limited in upper rate to 100, 105 or 120 bpm with an AV interval of 165 ms, the atrial refractory interval after the ventricular event was 435, 406 or 335 ms, ample in the vast majority of patients with the only rhythm then paced, complete heart block, to avoid the reentry mechanism. With the need to increase the allowed upper rate, the atrial refractory interval was correspondingly abbreviated and the possibility increased that a retrograde P wave would occur beyond the refractory interval.

Should the P wave be displaced but fall within the atrial refractory interval, it will be unsensed and no further event will occur. If the P wave falls into the sensitive portion of the pacemaker cycle it will be sensed and begin an AV interval. As AV conduction will be via the pacemaker, the ventricular stimulus may occur when natural VA conduction does not exist. There will then be no retrograde P wave to continue the cycle and endless loop tachycardia will die out. If retrograde conduction exists, another P wave will occur and the reentry loop will be sustained. The existence of a short AV interval tends to continue VA refractoriness; a long interval tends to allow VA conduction recovery. Thus, if a psuedo-Wenckebach mechanism is programmed with a low upper rate limit, the consequent prolongation of the AV interval allows recovery of VA conduction and maintenance of the endless loop tachycardia.

The circus movement or loop occurs by ventricular escape with retrograde conduction that produces a P wave sensed by the pacemaker atrial channel which, in turn, causes a ventricular channel stimulus followed by a retrograde P wave, and so forth (Figure 28).

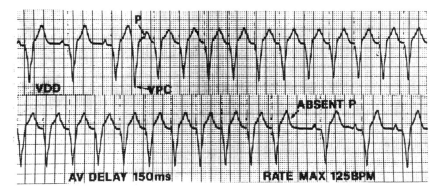

Figure 28. Endless loop tachycardia is started by a VPC that displaces a P wave and is then sustained by sensing the retrograde P at a prolonged AV interval. After progressive prolongation of the VA interval, indicative of fatigue of the retrograde conduction pathway, a P wave is not conducted and the tachycardia is terminated.

The cycle continues until:

1. retrograde conduction is lost;
2. the atrial refractory interval (ARI) is extended beyond the retrograde conduction time;
3. the atrial channel becomes refractory for a single atrial event;
4. the atrial channel becomes refractory for more than a single atrial event.

MECHANISMS FOR TERMINATION OF AN ENDLESS LOOP TACHYCARDIA

1. Programming the ARI beyond the measured retrograde conduction time;
2. Automatic extension of the ARI after a VPC (the most common cause of a displaced P wave). This does not deal with any of the other onset mechanisms of ELT;
3. Atrial insensitivity for a single event if the pacemaker operates at its upper rate limit for a specific number of paced ventricular events, 16 in one algorithm (Figure 29);
4. Atrial insensitivity for more than one atrial event such as the DVI mode followed by a full atrial refractory interval before the restoration of normal atrial sensing. This brief operation in the DVI mode may allow competition with an unsensed P wave, followed by a ventricular stimulus, a retrograde P wave and the resumption of the tachycardia;
5. Atrial insensitivity for many events, that is the resumption of the ventricular inhibited (VVI) mode which then returns to a preselected rate (fallback) with resumption then of atrial sensing (Figure 30).
6. It has been gradually recognized that antegrade and retrograde P waves have different electrical characteristics in morphology, amplitude and slew rate. Given sufficiently sophisticated analysis of all three parameters, about 95% of antegrade and retrograde P waves can be distinguished. Considering amplitude distinction only, almost 90% of antegrade P waves can be distinguished from the retrograde mate. Several pacemaker models have many atrial sensitivity levels, one has more than 20 settings, another has ten levels at each of two different frequency settings. Almost all antegrade P waves are larger than the retrograde mate. It is, therefore, possible to select a sensitivity level in which an antegrade P wave will drive the ventricle while the retrograde P wave will be too small to be sensed and cause endless loop tachycardia. Selective atrial sensing is possible and, when accomplished, very useful.

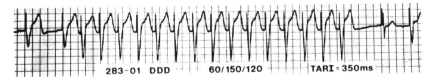

Figure 29. *This algorithm for termination of an endless loop tachycardia causes a loss of atrial sensing for a single event after sixteen ventricular channel stimuli at the upper rate limit.*

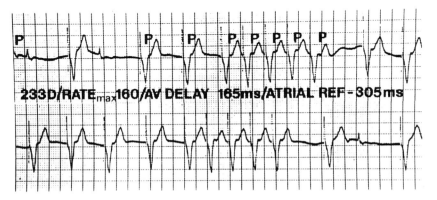

Figure 30. *The fallback response to endless loop tachycardia involves return to VVI pacing at a lower rate when the upper rate limit is reached. In this ECG, the lower rate is 80 bpm, sufficiently rapid to entrain the atrium so that when atrial sensing is automatically restored the endless loop tachycardia is immediately resumed.*

ALL MECHANISMS OF MANAGING ENDLESS LOOP TACHY-CARDIA ARE BASED ON ONE OF THESE MECHANISMS, ALL OF WHICH INVOLVE LOSS OF ATRIAL SENSITIVITY IN ONE OF A VARIETY OF FORMATS (Figure 31).

AV DESYNCHRONIZATION ARRHYTHMIA

Another dual-chamber arrhythmia recently described has been called the AV desynchronization arrhythmia (AVDA), by Barold. It is, in some ways, an analog of the endless loop tachycardia as it depends also on the presence of retrograde ventriculoatrial conduction for its mechanism. The arrhythmia occurs when a ventricular stimulus produces a ventricular contraction and a consequent retrograde P wave. If this P wave falls into an interval of atrial refractoriness it will be, of

AV UNIVERSAL
(DDD)
REF$_A$ AFTER VPC

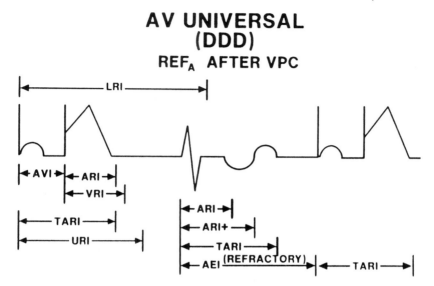

Figure 31. *The various pacemaker responses to terminate endless loop tachycardia all involve atrial insensitivity following a VPC. Several are diagrammed. ARI involves the setting of atrial refractoriness adequate to have a retrograde P wave fall within. ARI + is the production of a prolonged ARI for a single beat started by a VPC (defined as a sensed ventricular event not preceded by a sensed or paced atrial event). TARI is the establishment of a more prolonged atrial refractory interval, now including the duration of the programmed AV interval after a VPC. AEI is the start of an atrial escape interval followed by an atrial insensitive stimulus and a total atrial refractory interval. All means of preventing or terminating an endless loop tachycardia involve atrial refractoriness at the time of a retrograde or dissociated P wave.*

course, unsensed. Should the dual-chamber pacemaker be atrially refractory because of magnet placement or because of the DVI mode, the event will be continuous. In either mode the absence of atrial sensing will cause the emission of an atrial stimulus preceding the effective ventricular stimulus. If the VA conduction time is prolonged, the atrial stimulus will fall early and ineffectively after the retrograde atrial depolarization, during refractoriness of the atrial myocardium. Should this combination of events occur, the P wave cannot be re-placed into its physiological position. When atrial refractoriness ends, e.g., when the magnet is removed, the retrograde P wave persists and an endless loop tachycardia may start, usually at a more rapid rate. Such an endless loop will not end with magnet application as the AVDA will recur with magnet application, as will the endless loop when the magnet is removed. Termination of the endless loop will be by programming of mode to single-chamber operation. The AVDA is encouraged by the presence of prolonged retrograde conduction—a relatively short lower rate limit interval (rapid lower rate) and prolonged AV interval so that the atrial escape (i.e., ventricular stimulus to atrial stimulus) interval is also brief. The AVDA can be induced by any technique that loses atrial capture in the presence of sustained retrograde conduction, including a stimulus below capture threshold.

BIBLIOGRAPHY

Albert H, Glass B, Pittman B, Robichaux P: Cardiac stimulation threshold: Chronic study. *Ann NY Acad Sci* 1964; 3:889–892.

Ausubel K, Klementowicz P, Furman S: Interatrial conduction during cardiac pacing. *PACE* 1986; 9:1026–1031.

Barold SS, Ong LS, Heinle RA: Stimulation and sensing thresholds for cardiac pacing: Electrophysiologic and technical aspects. *Progr Cardiovasc Dis* 1981; 24:1–24.

Barold SS, Roehrich DR, Falkoff MD, Ong LS, Heinle RA: Sources of error in the determination of output voltage of pulse generators by pacemaker system analyzers. *PACE* 1980; 3:585–596.

Barold SS, Winner JA: Techniques and significance of threshold measurement for cardiac pacing. Relationship to output circuit of cardiac pacemakers. *Chest* 1976; 70:760–766.

Basu D, Chatterjee K: Unusually high pacemaker threshold in severe myxedema, decrease with thyroid hormone therapy. *Chest* 1976; 70:677–679.

Bink-Boelkens M, Ross B, Gillette P, Shannon C, Zinner A: The incidence of retrograde conduction in children. *PACE* 1984; 7:618–621.

Bisping HJ, Kreuser J, Birkenheier H: Three year clinical experience with a new endocardial screw-in lead with introduction protection for use in the atrium and ventricle. *PACE* 1980; 3:424–435.

Breivik K, Ohm OJ, Engedal H: Acute and chronic pulse-width thresholds in solid versus porous tip electrodes. *PACE* 1982; 5:650–657.

Breivik K, Ohm OJ, Engedal H: Long term comparison of unipolar and bipolar pacing and sensing, using a new multiprogrammable pacemaker system. *PACE* 1983; 6:592–600.

Burgess MJ, Grossman M, Abildskov JA: Fibrillation threshold of a patient with myocardial infarction treated with a fixed-rate pacemaker: Case report. *Am Heart J* 1970; 80:112–115.

Castellanos A, Lemberg L: Pacemaker arrhythmias and electrocardiographic recognition of pacemakers. *Circulation* 1973; 42:1381–1391.

Davies JG, Sowton E: Electrical threshold of the human heart. *Br Heart J* 1966; 28:231.

Dekker E, Buller J, Van Erven FA: Unipolar and bipolar stimulation thresholds of the human myocardium with chronically implanted pacemaker electrodes. *Am Heart J* 1966; 71:671–677.

Dekker E: Direct current make and break thresholds for pacemaker electrodes on the canine ventricle. *Circ Res* 1970; 27:811.

Ector H, Witters E, Tanghe L, Aubert A, DeGeest H: Measurement of pacing threshold. *PACE* 1985; 8:66–72.

Erlanger J: The physiology of heart block in mammals with especial reference to the causation of Stokes-Adams disease. *J Exper Med* 1905; 7:676.

Erlanger J, Hirschfelder AD: Further studies on the physiology of heart block in mammals. *Am J Physiol* 1905; 15:153–206.

Furman S, Cooper JA: Atrial fibrillation during AV sequential pacing. *PACE* 1982; 5:133–135.

Furman S, Fisher JD: Endless loop tachycardia in an AV universal (DDD) pacemaker. *PACE* 1982; 5:486–489.

Furman S, Garvey J, Hurzeler P: Pulse duration variation and electrode size as factors in pacemaker longevity. *J Thorac Cardiovasc Surg* 1975; 69:382–389.

Furman S, Hurzeler P, Mehra R: Cardiac pacing and pacemakers IV. Threshold of cardiac stimulation. *Am Heart J* 1977; 94:115–124.

Furman S, Hurzeler P, Parker B: Clinical thresholds of endocardial cardiac stimulation: A long term study. *J Surg Res* 1975; 19:149–155.

Furman S, Mehra R: Anodal influence on ventricular fibrillation. *Am J Cardiol* 1974; 33:137 (abstract).

Furman S, Parker B, Escher DJW: Decreasing electrode size and increasing efficiency of cardiac stimulation. *J Surg Res* 1971; 11:105–110.

Furman S, Parker B, Escher DJW, Solomon N: Endocardial threshold of cardiac response as a function of electrode surface area. *J Surg Res* 1968; 8:161–166.

Gettes LS, Shabetai R, Downs TA, Surawicz B: Effect of changes in potassium and calcium concentrations on diastolic threshold and strength-interval relationships of the human heart. *Ann NY Acad Sci* 1969; 167:693–705.

Haffajee C, Murphy J, Love JC, Vandersalm TJ, Okike N: Is routine testing for retrograde ventriculo-atrial conduction helpful prior to DDD pacemaker implantation. *PACE* 1983; 6:311 (abstract).

Hellestrand K, Nathan A, Bexton R, Milne J, Burnett P, Camm J: The effect of the antiarrhythmic agent flecainide on acute and chronic pacing thresholds. *PACE* 1983; 6:318 (abstract).

Henglein D, Gillette PC, Shannon C, Burns G: Long-term follow-up of pulse width threshold of transvenous and myo-epicardial leads. *PACE* 1984; 7:203–214.

Horowitz LN, Spear JF, Josephson ME, Kastor JA, Moore EN: The effects of coronary artery disease on the ventricular fibrillation threshold in man. *Circulation* 1979; 60:792–797.

Hughes HC Jr, Tyers GFO, Torman HA: Effects of acid-base imbalance on myocardial pacing thresholds. *J Thorac Cardiovasc Surg* 1975; 69:743–746.

Hynes JK, Holmes DR Jr, Meredith J, Trusty JM: An evaluation of long-term stimulation thresholds by measurement of chronic strength duration curves. *PACE* 1981; 4:376–379.

Irnich W: *Elektrotherapie des Herzens—physiologische und biotechnische Aspekte.* Berlin, Fachverlag Schiele & Schon, 1976.

Irnich W: The chronaxie time and its practical importance. *PACE* 1980; 3:292–301.

Jacobs LJ, Kerzner JS, Diamond MA, Berlin HF, Sprung CL: Pacemaker inhibition by myopotentials detected by Holter monitoring. *PACE* 1982; 5:30–33.

Jones M, Geddes LA: Strength-duration curves for cardiac pacemaking and ventricular fibrillation. *Cardiovasc Res Cent Bull* 1977; 15:101–112.

Kastor JA, Sanders CA, Leinbach RC, Harthorne JW: Factors influencing retrograde conduction: Study of 30 patients during cardiac catheterization. *Br Heart J* 1969; 31:580.

Kelen GJ, Bloomfield DA, Hardage M: Holter monitoring the patient with an artificial pacemaker—A new approach. *Amb Electrocardiol* 1978; 1:1–4.

Kelen GJ, Bloomfield DA, Hardage M, Gomes JA, Khan R, Gopalaswamy C, El-Sherif N: A clinical evaluation of an improved Holter monitoring technique for artificial pacemaker function. *PACE* 1980; 3:192–197.

Kistin AD, Landowne M: Retrograde conduction from premature ventricular contractions: A common occurence in the human heart. *Circulation* 1951; 3:738.

Klementowicz P, Ausubel K, Furman S: The dynamic nature of ventriculoatrial conduction. *PACE* 1986; 9:1050–1054.

Kruse IM, Terpstra B: Acute and long-term atrial and ventricular stimulation thresholds with a steroid-eluting electrode. *PACE* 1985; 8:45–49.

Lagergren H, Edhag O, Wahlberg I: A low-threshold, non-dislocating endocardial electrode. *J Thorac Cardiovasc Surg* 1976; 72:259–264.

Lapicque L: *La chronaxie et ses applications physiologiques.* Paris, Hermann & Cie, 1938.

Levy S, Corbelli JL, Labruni P, Mossaz R, Faugere G, Valeix B, Sans P, Gerard R: Retrograde (ventriculoatrial) conduction. *PACE* 1983; 6:364–371.

Lindemans FW, Zimmerman ANE: Acute voltage, charge and energy thresholds as functions of electrode size for electrical stimulation of the canine heart. *Cardiovasc Res* 1979; 13:383–391.

Luceri RM, Furman S, Hurzeler P, Escher DJW: Threshold behavior of electrodes in long-term ventricular pacing. *Am J Cardiol* 1977; 40:184–188.

Mahmud R, Denker S, Lehmann MH, Akhtar M: Effect of atrioventricular sequential pacing in patients with no ventriculoatrial conduction. *JACC* 1984; 4:273–277.

Mahmud R, Lehmann M, Estrada A, Shenasa M, Denker S, Sarwar M, Akhtar M: Facilitation of retrograde conduction with atrioventricular sequential pacing. *JACC* 1983; 1:674 (abstract).

Mehra R, Furman S: Comparison of cathodal, anodal, and bipolar strength-interval curves with temporary and permanent electrodes. *Br Heart J* 1979; 41:468–476.

Mehra R, Furman S, Crump JF: Vulnerability of the mildly ischemic ventricle to cathodal, anodal, and bipolar stimulation. *Circ Res* 1977; 41:159–166.

Mehra R, McMullen M, Furman S: Time dependence of unipolar cathodal and anodal strength-interval curves. *PACE* 1980; 3:526–530.

Michelson EL, Spear JF, Moore EN: Effects of procainamide on strength-interval relations in normal and chronically infarcted canine myocardium. *Am J Cardiol* 1981; 47:1223–1232.

Michelson EL, Spear JF, Moore EN: Strength-interval relations in a chronic canine model of myocardial infarction. *Circulation* 1981; 63:1158–1165.

Mines GR: On dynamic equilibrium in the heart. *J Physiol* 1913; 46:349–383.

Mitamura H, Ohm OJ Michelson EL, Sauermelch C, Dreifus LS: Importance of the pacing mode in the initiation of ventricular tachyarrhythmia in a canine model of chronic myocardial infarction. *JACC* 1985; 6:99–103.

Nernst W: Zur Theorie des elektrischen Reizes. *Pflugers Arch* 1908; 122:275–314.

Overdijk AD, Dekker E: Comparison of thresholds in epicardial and endocardial stimulation of the human heart by chronically implanted pacemaker electrodes. *Am Heart J* 1969; 77:172.

Preston TA: Anodal stimulation as a cause of pacemaker-induced ventricular fibrillation. *Am Heart J* 1973; 86:366–372.

Preston TA, Barold SS: Problems in measuring threshold for cardiac pacing. *Am J Cardiol* 1977; 40:658–660.

Preston TA, Fletcher RD, Lucchesi BR, Judge RD: Changes in myocardial threshold. Physiological and pharmacologic factors in patients with implanted pacemakers. *Am Heart J* 1967; 74:235–242.

Preston TA, Judge RD: Alteration of pacemaker threshold by drug and physiological factors. *Ann NY Acad Sci* 1969; 167:686–692.

Preston TA, Judge RD, Bowers DL, Morris JD: Measurement of pacemaker performance. *Am Heart J* 1966; 71:92–99.

Preston TA, Judge RD, Lucchesi BR, Bowers DL: Myocardial threshold in patients with artificial pacemakers. *Am J Cardiol* 1966; 18:83–89.

Schamroth L, Friedberg HD: Significance of retrograde conduction in AV dissociation. *Br Heart J* 1965; 27:896.

Scherf D: Retrograde conduction in the complete heart block. *Dis Chest* 1959; 35:320.

Smyth NPD, Tarjan PP, Chernoff E, Baker N: The significance of electrode surface area and stimulating thresholds in permanent cardiac pacing. *J Thorac Cardiovasc Surg* 1976; 71:559–565.

Somerndik JM, Ostermiller WE: Sleeping threshold change causing failure of artificial cardiac pacing. *JAMA* 1971; 215:980.

Sowton E, Barr I: Physiological changes in threshold. *Ann NY Acad Sci* 1969; 167:679–685.

Spear JF, Moore EN, Horowitz LN: Effects of current pulses delivered during the ventricular vulnerable period upon the ventricular fibrillation threshold. *Am J Cardiol* 1973; 32:814–822.

Starke ID: Long-term follow-up of cardiac pacing threshold using a noninvasive method of measurement. *Br Heart J* 1978; 40:530–533.

Starr DS, Lawrie GM, Morris GC Jr: Acute and chronic stimulation thresholds of intramyocardial screw-in pacemaker electrodes. *Ann Thorac Surg* 1981; 31:334–338.

Surawicz B, Chlebus H, Reeves JT, Gettes LS: Increase of ventricular excitability threshold by hyperpotassemia. *JAMA* 1965; 191:1049.

Svenson RH, Clark M, Hall D, et al: Analysis of manifest and latent retrograde conduction in patients with AV sequential pacemakers. Implications for pacer induced tachycardias. *JACC* 1983; 1:674 (abstract).

Takeshita A, Tanaka S, Nakamura M: Study of retrograde conduction in complete heart block using His bundle recordings. *Br Heart J* 1974; 36:462–467.

Thiele G, Lachmann W, Eschemann B, Wilde J: Modification of stimulus threshold increase following heart pacemaker implantation. *Zeitschrift Fur Die Gesamte Innere Medizin* 1980; 35(24):863–866.

Timmis GC, Gordon S, Westveer D, Stewart J, Stokes K, Helland J: A new steroid eluting low threshold lead. *PACE* 1983; 6:316 (abstract).

Timmis GC, Helland J, Westveer D, Stewart J, Gordon S: The evolution of low threshold leads. *CPPE* 1983; 1:313–334.

Timmis GC, Westveer DC, Helland J, Gordon S: Pacemaker stimulation thresholds and the Wedensky effect. *PACE* 1983; 6:320 (abstract).

Wahlberg I, Edhag O, Lagergren HR: Low threshold endocardial electrodes for permanent cardiac pacing. Comparison between one large and two small surface electrodes. *Acta Med Scand* 1977; 201:337–343.

Wainwright R, Davies W, Tooley M: Ideal atrial lead positioning to detect retrograde atrial depolarization by digitization and slope analysis of the atrial electrogram. *PACE* 1984; 7:1152–1158.

Walker WJ, Elkins JT, Wood LW: Effect of potassium in restoring myocardial response to a sub-threshold cardiac pacemaker. *N Engl J Med* 1964; 271:597.

Walls JT, Maloney JD, Pluth JR: Clinical evaluation of a sutureless cardiac pacing lead: Chronic threshold charges and lead durability. *Ann Thoracic Surg* 1983; 36:328–331.

Weiss G: Sur la possibilite de rendre comparable entre eux les appareils cervant a l'excitation electrique. *Arch Ital Biol* 1901; 35:413.

Wiggers CJ, Wegria R, Pinera B: The effects of myocardial ischemia on the fibrillation threshold: The mechanism of spontaneous ventricular fibrillation following coronary occlusion. *Am J Physiol* 1940; 131:309.

Winkle RA, Stinson EB, Bach SM Jr, et al: Measurement of cardioversion/defibrillation thresholds in man by a truncated exponential waveform and an apical patch-superior vena caval spring electrode configuration. *Circulation* 1984; 69:766.

Yee R, Jones DL, Jarvis E, Donner AP, Klein GJ: Changes in pacing threshold and R wave amplitude after transvenous catheter countershock. *JACC* 1984; 4:543–549.

Chapter 3

SENSING AND TIMING THE CARDIAC ELECTROGRAM

Seymour Furman

INTRODUCTION

Aside from the basic pacemaker function of cardiac stimulation, all pacemaker complexity and flexibility is based on the cardiac chambers sensed and the variety of pacemaker response. The utility and flexibility of pacemakers has increased over the years in direct proportion to the number of cardiac structures sensed and the possibility of a variety of response to sensed events. The earliest pacemakers, asynchronous ventricular, stimulated the heart but did not respond to cardiac activity. The simple timing cycles those pacemakers produced were single unmodified intervals between stimuli. If the pacemaker rate were set to be 60 bpm, a stimulus was emitted once each second. No variation existed. While stimulation is basic to pacemaker function, the ability to sense cardiac function, and the mode of response to a sensed event defines the mode of operation of the pacemaker.

All decisions concerning pacemaker design are based on the comprehension of the various intervals and timing cycles desired, and on the sensing of one or both chambers. All analysis of the ECG of pacemaker and cardiac interaction is based on the understanding of stimulation intervals (i.e, rates), refractory and blanking intervals and timing cycles of both the heart and the pacemaker. The basic principles of all pacemaker operation are identical, as are the principles of ECG interpretation. These will be emphasized. Examples concerning specific devices or ECG patterns will be used for illustrative purposes only, not to emphasize the quality of one device compared to another. The actual operation of each of the devices can be obtained from the manufacturer's literature and readily compared to the principles enunciated and analyses proposed. Without adequate sensing, all of the benefits will be unavailable.

Single-chamber pacemaker timing cycles and intervals are relatively simple, no matter how complex the device may seem, even compared to earlier pacemakers. Dual-chamber devices add far greater complexity because intervals are set for both chambers individually; both chambers must be sensed and an interval is set between the function of the two chambers and then additional intervals, such as upper and lower rate limits are set, as are intervals when the generator is insensitive (refractory) to one chamber or the other or both. Some dual-chamber pacemakers have a single timing cycle derived from sensing one chamber only (though both chambers are involved), and are therefore simpler than the designation "dual-chamber" would imply. In some units a few intervals are programmable, but others are fixed during manufacture. The operation of some pacemakers can be extensively modified following implantation, while in others, such modification is limited. If programming of atrial or refractory intervals or other timing cycles is required, it may be wiser to avoid the use of pacemakers with limited programmability. Sensing atrial and ventricular electrograms successfully is mandatory because each timing cycle begins and ends with a sensed intrinsic deflection or emission of a stimulus, and programming for consistent and reliable sensing is mandatory for appropriate pacemaker cycling. An electrogram that is unsensed will not inhibit or trigger pacemaker output, and a competitive stimulus will result.

ARTIFICIAL TEST SIGNALS

Test signals for pulse generator design have been developed by the Association for the Advancement of Medical Instrumentation (AAMI), to assist when an actual electrogram cannot be used. Such an approach provides a consistent and electronically reproducible signal to emulate the electrogram. Sensing circuits can then be designed to a standard. The standard, however, does not resemble the physiological event closely, and it may be that some undersensing occurs because of design to an artificial rather than a natural signal (Figure 1).

SENSING THE CARDIAC ELECTROGRAM

The endocardial or epicardial electrogram (EGM) is the electrical signal emitted by the heart and detected from within or upon its surface. This signal should be measured during each pacemaker implantation and pulse generator replacement. Such measurement is best done by direct recording on a physiological recorder having a band width of 0.1–2000 Hz. At the very least, a Pacing Systems Analyzer (PSA) should be used to determine the amplitude of the electrogram. Some analyzers are now sufficiently sophisticated to ap-

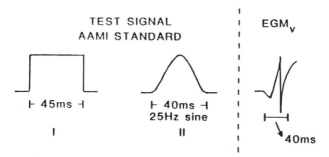

Figure 1. *AAMI recommended two standard test signals that reflect diversity in the engineering community. Standard (I) is rectangular, standard (II) is a half sine wave of approximately the same duration. The ventricular electrogram, drawn to the same scale, shows the difference between the various test signals and the electrogram.*

proach the value of a physiologic recorder. As there is no uniformly accepted standardization of the sensitivity of pacemaker circuits, it is best to measure the electrogram with an analyzer made by the manufacturer of the pacemaker to be implanted, and having the same electrode configuration (unipolar or bipolar) as the pacemaker lead that is to be used. If the electrogram is recorded on a physiologic recorder, it should be analyzed for:

1. Configuration (morphology) of the depolarization waves (QRS or P).
2. Amplitude, duration and timing   relative to the peripheral QRS or P waves   of that component of the electrogram that is called the "intrinsic deflection" (ID).
3. Slew rate (dV/dt, or rate of development) of the intrinsic deflection.
4. The presence of injury current and repolarization (S-T segments and T) waves.

If possible, the electrogram should be referenced to an ECG lead in order to relate intracardiac to surface events (Figure 2).

The "intrinsic deflection" (ID) is the rapid biphasic portion of the electrogram that occurs as the cardiac muscle adjacent to the electrode becomes electronegative with the passing depolarization wave. The intrinsic deflection exibits the highest slew rate (dV/dt) seen in the electrogram and is the only component of the electrogram with a sufficiently rapid voltage change to trigger a pacemaker. It bears only a variable relationship to the peripheral ECG since it indicates the electrical activity of only a very small area of the heart. A majority (58%) of acute unipolar ventricular electrograms have a biphasic intrinsic deflection with roughly equal R and S waves, while 30% are predominantly monophasic positive, and 12% are monophasic nega-

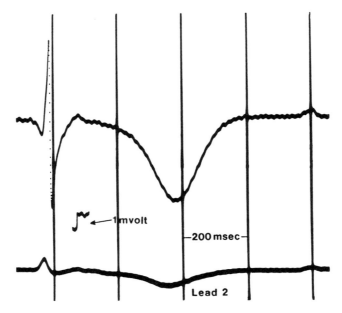

Figure 2.   *A chronic ventricular electrogram is characterized by the intrinsic deflection, i.e., the rapidly moving portion of the depolarization wave as it passes the electrode in contact with tissue. An isolectric ST segment and a deeply inverted T wave are recorded. The intrinsic deflection may appear early or late compared to the simultaneously recorded ECG.*

tive. In 88% of chronic implants the intrinsic deflection is biphasic, and in the remainder of electrograms it is monophasic negative.

"Far-field" potentials arise from electrical activity distant from the electrode and include contralateral ventricular activation, skeletal muscle potentials, and external electromagnetic interference (EMI). In the atrial electrogram, the intrinsic deflection indicates atrial activation while the ventricuclar potentials constitute far-field signals, and vice versa (Figure 3).

The "current of injury" appears as an elevation in electrical potential that follows the ID immediately in acute electrograms and represents a small area of damaged endocardium caused by electrode irritation. The current of injury appears as an elevated S-T segment during the acute period of implantation and later disappears, leaving an isoelectric chronic S-T segment (Figure 4).

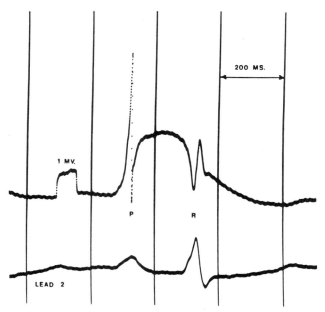

Figure 3. *An atrial electrogram is quite similar to a ventricular electrogram but its overall amplitude is smaller. In this instance, the coronary sinus electrogram is recorded approximately half way into the lead 2 P wave. The QRS complex is seen approximately 250 ms after the discrete atrial electrogram as a far-field signal.*

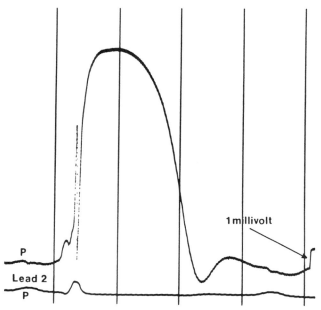

Figure 4. *An acute ventricular electrogram is characterized by the intrinsic deflection recorded simultaneously with the surface QRS complex and a current of injury, which is the domed-shaped elevation of the ST segment. The T wave is lost in the ST segment elevation. In transition from acute to chronic, the ST segment elevation will disappear.*

A statistically significant decrease in the slew rate, of about 40%, occurs as an electrode enters the chronic phase; the decrease in amplitude is not significant. The maturing electrode may, therefore, have a subthreshold signal, i.e., lacking an adequate amplitude or slew rate, or both, to trigger a pulse generator properly (Figure 5). The atrial intrinsic deflection is morphologically similar to the ventricular intrinsic deflection, differing only in overall amplitude. Its timing relative to the peripheral P wave depends on the electrode's proximity to the S-A node. Far-field ventricular potentials may be comparable in amplitude but not in slew rate to the atrial intrinsic deflection. Injury currents appear in 14% of acute atrial electrograms (Figure 6).

If lead and electrode placement is satisfactory, the best electrogram and stimulation threshold will usually coincide at one anatomic position. The amplitude of the ventricular sensing signal should be at 4 millivolts, at a slew rate of at least 1.5 millivolts per millisecond (mV/ms) to accommodate the expected 40% acute-to-chronic decrease in the slew rate. A dome-shaped S-T segment (injury potential) of at

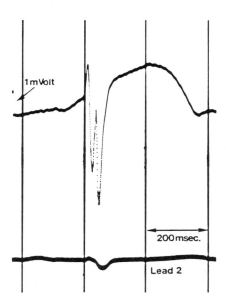

Figure 5. *A poor ventricular electrogram in distinction to a satisfactory one (see Figure 2) with a QRS complex in which the intrinsic deflection is of low amplitude, is split and reverses itself, resetting the timing mechanism of the pulse generator.*

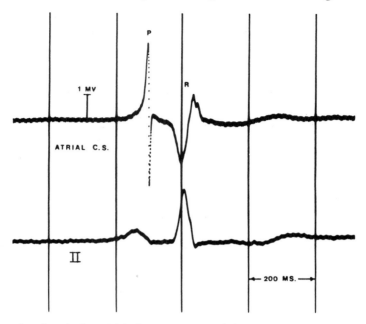

Figure 6. *A unipolar atrial electrogram recorded from the coronary sinus also records a large far-field ventricular electrogram. In this instance, the ventricular electrogram is sufficiently large so that it may be sensed from the coronary sinus lead. Note also, that the atrial electrogram appears virtually at the end of the surface P wave. This would be an example of late sensing of the atrial electrogram, far later than the beginning of the P wave in lead 2.*

least 2 mV, measured at the time of electrode placement, is a further favorable indication of adequate placement. In the absence of a suitable recorder, a pacing systems analyzer or an external pacemaker with adjustable sensitivity may be used to estimate the sensing signal.

ANTEGRADE AND RETROGRADE ATRIAL ELECTROGRAMS

Antegrade and retrograde atrial electrograms are quite different and recognizably so. Visually, it is possible to discriminate a recording of the two electrograms. In instances of amplitude difference, the pacemaker atrial sensing channel will be able to discriminate between the two and reduce the likelihood of endless loop tachycardia (see Chapter

4, Timing Cycles). In a recent evaluation of 34 patients undergoing dual-chamber pacemaker implantation, 31 had unipolar systems, 3 had bipolar. All antegrade and retrograde pairs were measurably different. All 34 had measurable antegrade/retrograde amplitude differences, thirty of the unipolar pairs (96.8%) and all bipolar cases displayed antegrade/retrograde amplitude differences of at least 0.25 mV. Thirty of the unipolar cases (96.8%) and 2 of the bipolar cases had measurable slew rate differences. Overall configuration differed in 14/ 31 (45.2%) of unipolar and all 3 bipolar cases. Using criteria of both 0.25 mV sensitivity discrimination and 0.5 V/s slew rate discrimination, all 34 antegrade atrial electrograms could be discriminated from their retrograde mates. Therefore, electronic means alone would allow the differentiation of antegrade from retrograde atrial electrograms. This approach is potentially very important as discrimination of tachycardias becomes progressively more important and antegrade and retrograde, and ectopic atrial and conducted and ectopic ventricular activity must be accurately discriminated (Figure 7).

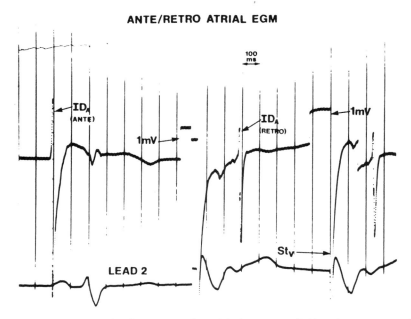

Figure 7. *An example of an antegrade atrial electrogram (left) and two retrograde atrial electrograms (right) from the same patient. The antegrade EGM (ID_a) is approximately twice the amplitude of the retrograde. The slew rate, directly related to the distance between the dots forming the intrinsic deflection, is also about twice as great. These two electrograms can be readily discriminated by presently available pulse generators.*

LATE SENSING

The electrocardiographical phenomenon of "late sensing" of a QRS complex is readily explained as sensing of the intrinsic deflection (ID) only. The intrinsic deflection is usually not coincident with the leading edge of a QRS complex or P wave in any peripheral lead. Indeed, it is likely that the position of the intrinsic deflection will be different in each lead, so that "late sensing" may appear in one lead and not in another, simultaneously recorded. In each different focus, conducted and idioventricular, the intrinsic deflection will appear at a different point in the QRS or P complex and will give the impression of different pacemaker escape intervals if it assumed that the generator senses the leading edge of the peripheral signal. Once comprehended, "late sensing" becomes a non-event and does not represent malfunction (Figure 8).

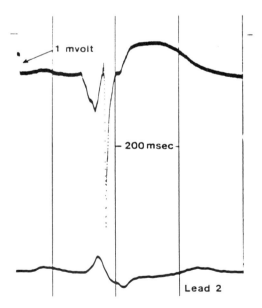

Figure 8. *The ventricular electrogram is recorded close to the end of the surface ECG. If one assumes that sensing of the surface ECG will occur at its beginning, then this electrogram will produce late sensing. Late sensing does not exist, it is simply a misinterpretation that what the pacemaker senses is the beginning of the surface QRS complex.*

THE BIPOLAR ELECTROGRAM

The bipolar electrogram is the result of the potential difference between the two intracardiac poles (electrodes), each exhibiting a unipolar pattern. If the bipolar axis is at a right angle to the depolarization pathway, simultaneous identical signals at each pole can cancel each other, yielding a small or zero bipolar result. If the bipolar axis is oriented parallel to the depolarization pathway, there will be a signal delay at one pole relative to the other, and this can result in an augmented bipolar signal greater than either unipolar component. When the proximal pole of a catheter electrode is separated from the endocardial wall, the intrinsic deflection is small, so that the tip intrinsic deflection alone dominates the bipolar waveform. Simultaneous comparison of the group of ventricular bipolar and tip unipolar signals from a single lead shows that bipolar sensing offers:

1. Either enchanced or attenuated intrinsic deflection without a difference between mean unipolar and bipolar values;
2. Intrinsic deflection durations shortened by 28%;
3. Injury currents attenuated by 37%;
4. T waves attenuated by 34%.

The only disadvantage of the bipolar sensing configuration is the possibility of intrinsic deflection attenuation or cancellation if the two electrodes become oriented 90 degrees to the direction in which the depolarization waves are propagated. In one clinical series, the bipolar intrinsic deflection was smaller than the simultaneous tip unipolar signal in 51% of cases, with 2% of the bipolar signals being too small to be sensed, while the simultaneous unipolar signal was of adequate amplitude. In 43% of cases in this series, the bipolar intrinsic deflection was larger than the tip unipolar signal, and in 6% the unipolar and bipolar signals were equal. Bipolar injury current (S-T elevation) and far-field potentials were smaller than the unipolar signal in 96% of cases. Atrial endocardial bipolar electrodes attenuate adjacent ventricular potentials by 80%, relative to simultaneous corresponding unipolar signals. When an atrial electrode is implanted for the automatic termination of supraventricular tachycardia, only a bipolar electrode should be used. Dual-chamber pacing systems now available use unipolar leads for both atrial and ventricle, some use bipolar leads, and others allow programming between unipolar and bipolar (Figures 9,10).

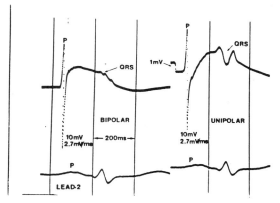

Figure 9. The major difference between atrial unipolar and bipolar electrograms is the presence of a large QRS complex in the unipolar recording and a smaller (invisible) complex in the bipolar recording. In this recording from the right atrial appendage, the unipolar electrogram has a much larger QRS complex as a far-field signal than the bipolar electrogram. The amplitude and frequency content of the two electrograms (other than far-field signals) are approximately equal.

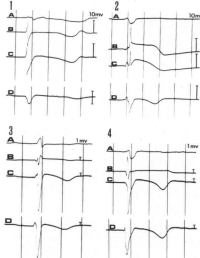

Figure 10. Four bipolar ventricular electrograms. Tracing (A) shows a simultaneously recorded lead 2 of the surface ECG; Tracing (B) the bipolar electrogram; (C) the electrogram from the tip electrode; (D) the electrogram from the ring or proximal electrode. In the first electrogram, the ring signal (D) is small and the bipolar (B) and tip (C) signals are almost identical. In the second, the bipolar signal (B) is larger than either the tip (C) or the ring (D) signal. Summation has occurred. In the third, the bipolar signal (B) is the subtraction of the tip (C) and the ring (D) signals and is somewhat smaller than either. The bipolar signal (B) in the fourth tracing is midway between the tip (C) and ring (D) signals. This is the usual situation.

BIPOLAR SENSING

To demonstrate the superior rejection of electromyographic interference, twenty pacemakers that could be programmed into unipolar and bipolar were evaluated in both unipolar and bipolar modes of operation. All implants were conventional and were free of technical or physiological complications. Four upper extremity provocative maneuvers were performed on the side of the implant. They were:

1. pushing the implant side fist into the opposite hand;
2. pulling hands (placed at mid-chest) apart with the patient's maximum effort;
3. adduction of the arm on the pacemaker side, against resistance;
4. vigorous scratching of the implant side arm across the abdomen.

There were three categories of positive response:

a. inhibition – pacemaker output inhibited (Figure 11);
b. triggering – ventricular stimulation resulted from myopotentials sensed in the atrial channel (Figure 12);
c. reversion asynchronous (noise mode) – operation in either atrial or ventricular channel or both, caused by sensed myopotentials (Figure 13).

The results of this evaluation were that no evidence of myopotential interference existed at any sensitivity setting in the bipolar configuration of either tested pacemaker in atrium or ventricle. In the unipolar configuration, all patients (20/20) had myopotential interference at the highest atrial or ventricular sensitivity setting. T wave sensing occurred at the maximum sensitivity in four patients, two only in the bipolar configuration, one in unipolar only, and one in both unipolar and bipolar (Figure 14). Twenty-five percent of patients had myopotential interference at the unipolar atrial sensing threshold, which did not allow a setting that would reject myopotential inteference while providing satisfactory atrial sensing. Twenty percent (2/10) of one model had ventricular inhibition at the least sensitivity setting (2.5 mV) of the ventricular channel, so that myopotential interference could not be avoided in the unipolar mode no matter how large the electrogram. It can be concluded from these evaluations and from the known behavior of the cardiac bipolar electrogram compared to its unipolar mate that discrete sensing and the absence of myopotential inhibition and electromagnetic interference is a characteristic of bipolar pacing, and such interference occurs substantially, even at moderate sensitivity levels during unipolar pacing.

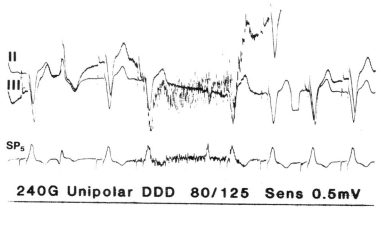

240G Unipolar DDD 80/125 Sens 0.5mV

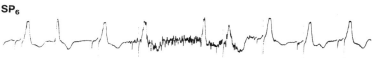

Figure 11. *Inhibition of ventricular output occurs at atrial channel sensitivity of 2.5 mV and ventricular channel sensitivity of 0.5 mV, both in the unipolar lead configuration. Onset of myopotential interference inhibits atrial and ventricular output. Following 1300 ms of asystole, the first ventricular capture is an escape beat followed by a pacemaker escape (25 mm/s). All leads 2, 3, SP5 and SP6 are simultaneous.*

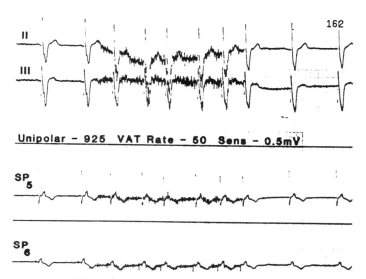

Figure 12. *In the VAT mode ventricular sensing is not present. At 0.5 mV atrial channel sensitivity, myopotential interference triggers the ventricular response above the automatic ventricular rate (25 mm/s).*

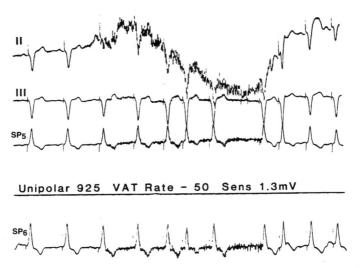

Figure 13. *In the VAT mode ventricular sensing is not present. Atrial channel sensitivity was set at 1.3 mV in the unipolar lead configuration. With the onset of myopotential interference the ventricular response is increased in rate by triggering from the sensed atrial events. In the interference mode, a single ventricular stimulus is emitted at the noise escape interval and atrial triggering then resumes for a single beat (25 mm/s).*

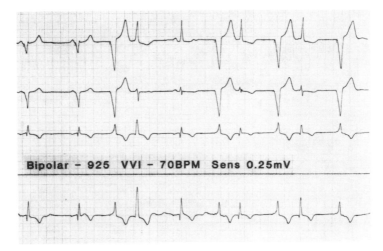

Figure 14. *Oversensing of the T wave can occur in either the unipolar or bipolar lead configuration. In the VVI mode and bipolar configuration at the maximum sensitivity (0.25 mV), the interval between beats four and five and is prolonged because of recycle from the T wave (25 mm/s). All leads 2, 3, SP5 and SP6 are simultaneous.*

ELECTROMYOGRAPHIC INTERFERENCE AND BIPOLAR SENSING

The reason that the bipolar electrode rejects electromagnetic interference is that the resultant electrogram is too small to reach the level of programmed sensitivity. Nevertheless, it is possible for a bipolar far-field electrogram to be sufficiently large (though nevertheless small) to be sensed at a high pacemaker sensitivity setting. One such event has been recorded (Figure 15) during programming of a

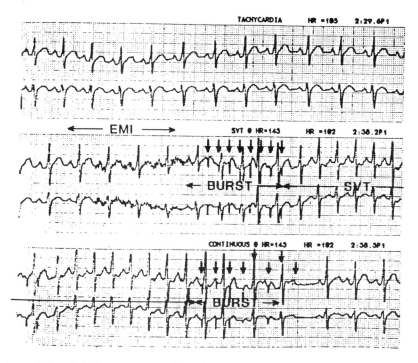

Figure 15. *Bedside monitor recording of a patient with an implanted 262-12, bipolar atrial antitachycardia pacemaker. Because of a small electrogram associated with the supraventricular tachycardia, a sensitivity of 0.4 mV was programmed. During pectoral muscle movement and normal sinus rhythm (marked EMI) a stimulus burst (arrows) was emitted that caused a recurrence of the supraventricular tachycardia. The device detected the episode and emitted a second burst (arrows) that terminated the supraventricular tachycardia. No pacemaker or lead defect was found.*

bipolar atrial antitachycardia pacemaker to its highest sensitivity when used to manage recurrent supraventricular tachycardia. The lead was in the atrial appendage, quite close to the chest wall. Pectoral movement was detected and interpreted as atrial activity. The antitachycardia mode was activated and caused supraventricular tachycardia. When that supraventricular tachycardia was later detected, it was terminated by the same stimulus burst that initiated it.

Other recorded EMI in the presence of a bipolar lead have been caused by some variety of malfunction, i.e., perforation of the electrode through the right ventricular wall to detect diaphragmatic movement or insulation defect.

THE ORTHOGONAL LEAD

The orthogonal lead is a special case of a bipolar lead system and may prove to be especially useful. In conventional bipolar leads, the tip and ring are circumferential, detect the electrogram in all directions and are separated one from the other by length along the lead system. This separation has traditionally been one centimeter or one inch but, may, of course, be any distance. The orthogonal lead uses two or three point electrodes circumferentially about a lead. One version of the orthogonal lead has the electrodes entirely circumferential, another separates the electrodes by several millimeters along the lead. In the latter, it is possible to sense two independent electrograms. In that instance, the first that reaches the sensitivity level of the pacemaker device will be sensed and will determine timing (Figure 16). These electrodes are highly directional and reject far-field signals very effectively. Consequently, because interference is so much less likely to occur, pulse generator sensitivity can be set at a much higher level. Nevertheless, lead movement within a chamber, e.g., the atrium, may result in extreme variation in the amplitude of the electrogram finally detected. Small far-field electrograms allow high sensitivity settings to detect the smallest of the signals (Figure 17).

It is important to remember that the electrogram (EGM) and the electrocardiogram (ECG) indicate intracardiac events and body surface events respectively. They have different characteristics and one cannot infer the qualities of one from the other. In the absence of pacemaker telemetry, the only occasion at which the electrogram will be available is at the time of implant or pulse generator replacement. The electrograms and surface leads should be recorded simultaneously to

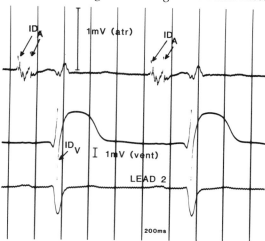

Figure 16. *An orthogonal lead electrogram (above) recorded simultaneously with a unipolar ventricular electrogram (middle) and lead 2 (below). The lead had the atrial sensing electrodes separated along its length. Two atrial electrograms were recorded, separated by about 75 ms. Because of the small size of the far-field ventricular electrogram, high sensitivity can be set to sense the diminutive atrial electrogram while rejecting the ventricular depolarization.*

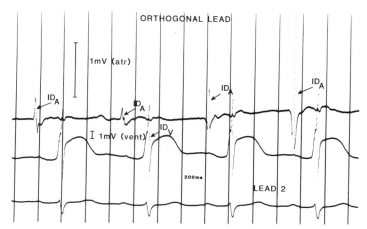

Figure 17. *This is a three channel recording of an orthogonal lead with the unipolar tip referenced to the subcutaneous tissue of the chest wall and the right ventricular apex. The atrial sensor is an orthogonal, i.e., partially bipolar electrode, in the mid-right atrium. The lead position is quite stable as indicated by the constancy of the unipolar ventricular electrogram. Because of movement of the orthogonal atrial sensor relative to the atrial wall, the amplitude of the atrial electrogram is highly variable. Atrial electrograms recorded vary between approximately 0.25 mV and 3 mV. On the atrial channel the ventricular depolarization is small relative to the ventricular electrogram so that atrial sensitivity can be made extremely high to produce satisfactory sensing of the atrial electrogram.*

determine the relationship between the two. The progressively increasing availability of electrogram telemetry will allow the post-implant determination of the quality and timing characteristics of the electrogram, and improve acumen for different diagnostic problems. Electrocardiogram interpretation channels now available in several pacemaker models trigger on the intrinsic deflection and can give an accurate indication of the exact instant of sensing. As electrocardiogram interpretation channels and a stimulus are accurate to 1 ms, pacemaker timing cycles can then be accurately determined (Figure 18). Some generators provide markers that indicate the end of a particular (atrial or ventricular) refractory interval as well as the EGM, and provide further assistance in ECG interpretation (Figure 19). Some dual-chamber generators allow the triggered mode in the atrium or the ventricle or both, allowing the marking of either P wave or QRS complex with an indication of the exact instant of sensing.

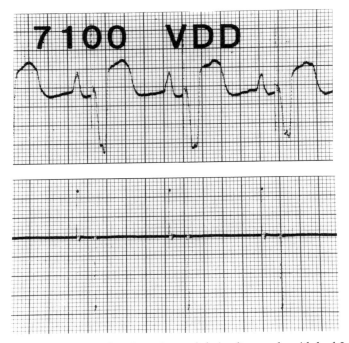

Figure 18.   *ECG interpretation channel recorded simultaneously with lead 2 for an atrial synchronous (VDD) pacemaker. In the ECG interpretation channel the sensed P wave produces an upward going stimulus at the instant of atrial sensing. The ventricular stimulus also produces a downward mark. The interval between atrial sensing and ventricular stimulus emission can be accurately determined as can the instant of atrial sensing.*

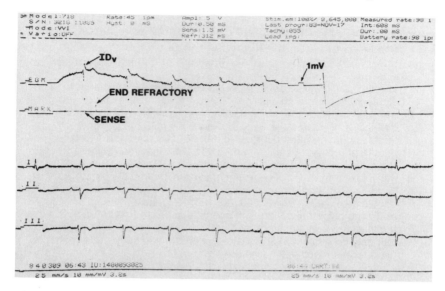

Figure 19. *A multichannel recording of pacer testing. The electrogram is of a single-chamber ventricular pacemaker recorded simultaneously with a mark for ventricular sensing and a mark for the end of the refractory period after ventricular sensing. This information is recorded simultaneously with telemetry from the pacemaker memory (above) and 3 ECG surface leads.*

When considering any timing cycles or analyzing any ECG for pacemaker function, it is necessary to analyze function as a series of intervals between sensed or paced events rather than as a continuous rate. Rate is a relatively simple designation during continuous pacing or continuous inhibition but is worthless and confusing if pacing and sensing alternate. Each event must be analyzed discretely. It must be recognized that rate is a continuum of a series of discontinuous events.

Both atrial and ventricular electrograms are readily determined via the implanted lead system. Each different site in the heart, either in atrium or ventricle, will have a different electrogram. The electrocardiogram is the sum of multiple electrograms, recorded, of course, from the body surface. The electrocardiogram and electrogram have different characteristics and those of one cannot be inferred from the other. The electrogram of importance during cardiac pacing is that sensed by the lead system in atrium and/or ventricle. Exact measurements of AV and VA conduction times can only be determined by recording and comparing the atrial and ventricular electrograms from one intrinsic deflection to the other. It is therefore necessary to record the atrial and ventricular electrograms during paced and unpaced cardiac activity. Each of the intervals determined is important to the proper setting of an implantable dual-chamber pacemaker.

With leads in place, the following measurements can be made on a multi-channel recorder with oscilloscope and hard copy recording:

1. interval from intrinsic deflection of the atrial depolarization ID_A to intrinsic deflection of ventricular depolarization ID_V ($ID_A{\rightarrow}ID_V$) (Figure 20);
2. the interval from the atrial pacemaker stimulus St_A to the intrinsic deflection of ventricular depolarization ID_V ($St_A{\rightarrow}ID_V$); optimally patients should be paced at rates of 60, 80, 100, 120 and 140 beats per minute and atrioventricular conduction time assessed (Figure 21) and the rate for onset of AV block ascertained (Figure 22);
3. the interval from the ventricular pacing stimulus St_V to the intrinsic deflection of atrial depolarization ID_A ($St_V{\rightarrow}ID_A$); optimally, patients should be paced at rates of 60, 80, 100, 120, and 140 beats per minute and ventriculoatrial conduction intervals assessed and (Figure 23) the rate for onset of VA block ascertained. Retrograde (VA) conduction can only be evaluated adequately when the ventricular rate (paced or unpaced) is more rapid than the atrial rate (Fig. 24).
4. routine measurement of atrial and/or ventricular stimulation thresholds;
5. recording and measurement of the atrial and ventricular electrograms independently.

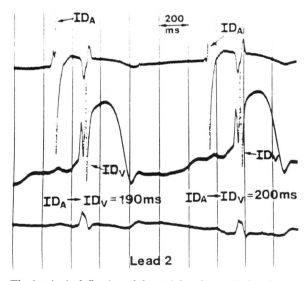

Figure 20.   *The intrinsic deflection of the atrial and ventricular electrograms are the elements sensed to recycle a pacemaker. In the dual lead system the atrial and ventricular electrograms are recorded simultaneously with the ECG (lead 2). As each focus, atrial and ventricular produce a unique electrogram, the timing of the interval from the atrial to the ventricular intrinsic deflection varies with different cardiac foci. In this three channel recording the two intervals of ID_A to ID_V are different as each electrogram originates at a different focus.*

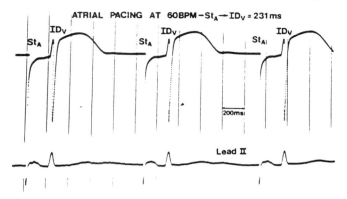

Figure 21. *The interval from the stimulus to the atrium to produce a P wave and a QRS complex that is produced in response is the interval for antegrade conduction. Here, the ventricular electrogram and ECG lead 2 are recorded simultaneously. Antegrade conduction is between the stimulus (St_A) to the ventricular response (ID_V). This varies as a function of the atrial stimulated rate. In this instance, at a cycle length of 1,000 ms (60 bpm), the interval $St_A \rightarrow ID_V$ is 231 ms.*

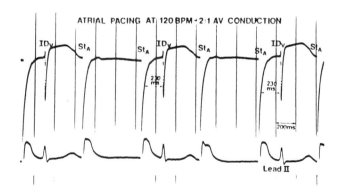

Figure 22. *Atrial pacing can be continued until AV block occurs. In this illustration, surface lead 2 is recorded simultaneously with the ventricular electrogram. The coupling interval of atrial stimulation is 500 ms (120 bpm); the atrial response to stimulation is clearly recorded, but conduction from the P wave to the QRS is at 2:1 AV block.*

In examining the recordings when the ventricle was paced, the absence of orderly atrial depolarizations, i.e., atrial depolarization that occurred independently of any ventricular activity, documented the absence of retrograde conduction (Figure 25).

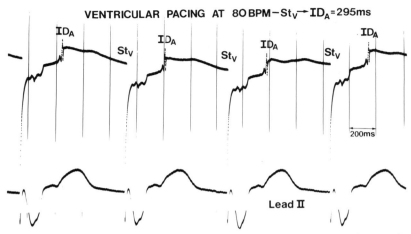

Figure 23. *The measurement of retrograde conduction is accomplished by recording surface lead 2 and the atrial electrogram. The ventricle is paced at a coupling interval of 750 ms (80 bpm) and the interval between the ventricular stimulus and the retrograde recorded P wave can be measured readily. In this instance $St_V{\rightarrow}ID_A$ is 295 ms.*

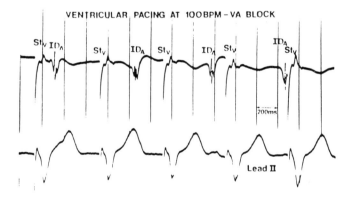

Figure 24. *In the presence of retrograde VA block the recording of the atrial electrogram will demonstrate P waves moving independently of the QRS complex. Just as with antegrade conduction this will demonstrate the absence of a relationship between ventricular depolarization and atrial depolarization.*

The mean antegrade conduction interval at rest ($ID_A{\rightarrow}ID_V$) is 212 ± 33 ms prolonged to a mean interval ($St_A{\rightarrow}ID_V$) of 312 ± 62 ms at the highest atrial pacing rate before AV block occurred. Twenty-five percent of patients with AV conduction at rest developed AV block at the lowest rate of atrial capture, 70 and 80 bpm; 25% developed AV

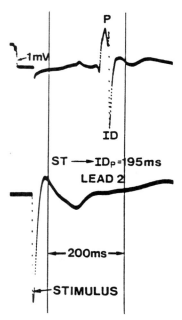

Figure 25. *Accurate measurement for the retrograde conduction time can be accomplished by measurement between the ventricular stimulus and the intrinsic deflection of the retrograde atrial depolarization. In this illustration, taken from a sequence of similarly timed retrograde atrial depolarizations, the conduction time is 195 ms.*

block at 100 bpm; 20% of patients at 120 bpm; 20% of patients at 140 bpm; 4% at 160 bpm; 4% never do develop AV block. About 50 ms of the increase in the interval during pacing can be attributed to the $St_A \rightarrow ID_A$ latency during pacing from the right atrial appendage.

A variety of retrograde conduction responses exist. In 47% of patients, 1:1 retrograde conduction is present at some ventricular paced rate; 6% of patients had retrograde Wenckebach block, and 47% of the patients had retrograde block (Figure 26). Of those patients with complete antegrade block during atrial pacing, 14% had 1:1 VA conduction at a mean VA conduction time of 235±50 ms (range 110–380 ms). Of additional patients who demonstrated 2:1 AV conduction with atrial pacing, i.e., no 1:1 antegrade conduction, 25% had intact 1:1 retrograde conduction. Therefore, 17% of patients had 1:1 retrograde VA conduction when no 1:1 antegrade conduction could be demonstrated (Figure 27).

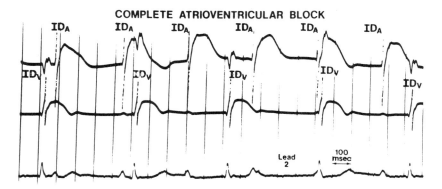

Figure 26. *An electrogram of complete AV block recorded simultaneously from atrium and ventricle. Lead 2 is below and indicates the absence of association between P waves and ventricular response. Above, the intrinsic deflection of the ventricle occurs at an approximate coupling interval of 1,000 ms and the intrinsic deflection of the atrium at coupling intervals of 800 ms. While the two rates are relatively close, the dissociation between atrial and ventricular activity is clearly indicated.*

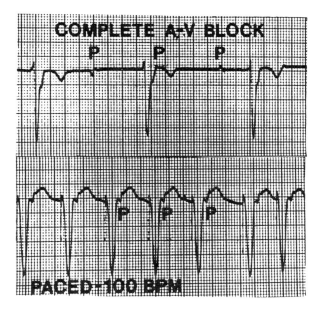

Figure 27. *Complete antegrade AV block may coexist with retrograde 1:1 conduction. In this example, the upper strip is unpaced showing complete AV block; the lower is the same patient paced at 100 bpm with consistent 1:1 retrograde conduction.*

Considering all indications for pacing, 47% of patients had some level of intact 1:1 retrograde conduction. The proportion of patients with intact VA conduction varied considerably when patients were analyzed by rhythm disturbance. In those patients with sinus node dysfunction (defined as demonstrating both tachycardia and bradycardia), 67% had intact VA conduction and 69% of patients with sinus bradycardia or sinus arrest had intact VA conduction. Thirty-six percent of patients with incomplete atrioventricular block and 17% of patients with complete atrioventricular block (spontaneously and during atrial pacing) had intact VA conduction.

. The interaction between the two chambers during implantation of a dual chamber pacemaker is all important. This interaction is based on the appropriate pacing and sensing of the two chambers and of the setting of the intervals between the atrial and ventricular channels. A variety of refractory and sensitive intervals determines the means of dealing with atrial and ventricular premature contractions and minimum and maximum atrial tracking rates. The complexity is substantial. Three intervals are of critical importance to successful management of an implanted pulse generator that senses in two chambers.

Once the pacing and sensing characteristics of the two chambers individually have been established, attention should be directed to the intervals that determine the interaction of the two chambers. The four measurements made allow determination of the spontaneous AV conduction time (if it exists), and allow the optimal setting for automatic pacemaker rate and AV delay that will permit sensing spontaneous atrial activity and permit AV conduction to drive the ventricle as frequently as is feasible. If spontaneous AV conduction varies from a desirable AV interval (probably between 160–200 ms), for the interval between the atrial and ventricular intrinsic deflection ($ID_A \rightarrow ID_V$) the pulse generator can be set at that interval deemed to be appropriate. Measurement of the atrially paced interval to the intrinsic deflection of the ventricle $St_A \rightarrow ID_V$ is determined by two distinct timing events. These are the atrial pacemaker stimulus (St_A) and the ventricular intrinsic deflection (ID_V). Two intervals are also defined. These are the latent interval between the atrial pacer stimulus (St_A) and the intrinsic deflection of the atrium (ID_A) and the interval between that stimulus (St_A) and the ventricular intrinsic deflection (ID_V), which is significantly rate dependent. The atrial latent interval does not seem to vary with the pacing rate.

The significance of recognition of the difference between $ID_A \rightarrow ID_V$ and $St_A \rightarrow ID_V$ is in maintenance of a constant PR interval. As there is a latent period of atrial stimulation and as all pacemaker timing cycles begin with a sensed event (always an intrinsic deflec-

AV DELAY AND PR INTERVAL

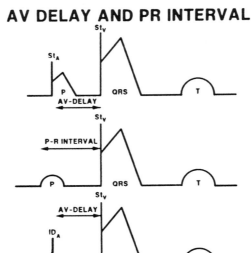

Figure 28. *Each timing cycle for an implanted pacemaker starts and ends with a sensed intrinsic deflection or the emission of a stimulus. Because the atrial electrogram recorded from the right atrial appendage is sensed well into the P wave, the AV interval between an atrial stimulus and a ventricular stimulus or a sensed atrial intrinsic deflection and a ventricular stimulus will be of different durations.*

tion) or a stimulus, always followed by a latent period, it is obvious that the interval from intrinsic deflection of the atrium (ID$_A$) to the intrinsic deflection of the ventricle (ID$_V$) is shorter than from atrial pacing stimulus (St$_A$) to the ventricular intrinsic deflection (ID$_V$) (Figure 28). In order to maintain a constant PR interval, the dual-chamber pacemaker timing cycles must be different when sensing the P wave than when pacing the atrium. If only one AV interval is available, starting with a sense or pace event, paced and sensed PR intervals will be of different duration (Figure 29).

The last measurement should be of the interval for retrograde (VA) conduction following a ventricular stimulus, once the two leads are in place. Intact retrograde conduction allows a pacemaker-mediated endless loop tachycardia and determination of its possibility, presence, and duration is required (Figure 30). Only a few conclusions can be drawn from the unpaced surface ECG concerning the existence and nature of retrograde conduction. Although the sequence of retrograde atrial activation may result in an inverted P wave in leads II, III, and AVF, the presence and morphology of a P wave is

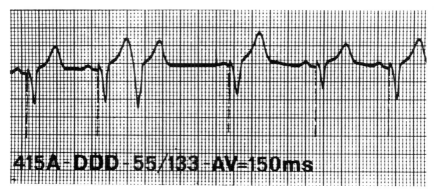

Figure 29. *In this dual-chamber pacemaker, a ventricular premature contraction after the second ventricular paced beat resets the timing cycle and the next stimulus produces a P wave and then a succeeding QRS complex. As the timing of the AV interval starts with the atrial stimulus, the P wave occurs much closer to the ventricular stimulus than it does when it is spontaneous, as it is for all other P waves seen in this ECG. Then, the P wave precedes the ventricular stimulus by a longer interval because the P wave is sensed near its peak on the ECG.*

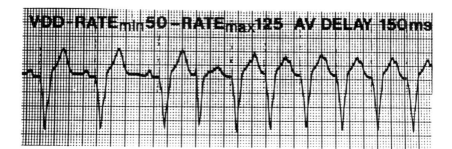

Figure 30. *Endless loop tachycardia exists because of retrograde conduction of the P wave following ventricular stimulation. Almost invariably, the endless loop tachycardia occurs at the upper rate limit and the AV interval is prolonged. The first prolongation of the AV interval occurs immediately following the VPC, the fourth ventricular complex from the left. The retrograde P wave, seen approximately 160 ms after the beginning of the VPC, causes the next ventricular stimulus that is delayed until the entire upper rate interval of the pacemaker (480 ms) has passed. Because of this requirement of delay of the ventricular stimulus, the AV interval is prolonged well above the programmed setting.*

almost impossible to discern when inscription of the QRS occurs simultaneously, and even in the ST and T segments, the presence and polarity of a P wave may be difficult to determine. Retrograde AV nodal conduction cannot be predicted from knowledge of the state of antegrade conduction. Nevertheless, during temporary or single-chamber pacing, an assessment of the state of VA conduction can sometimes be made and may be useful (Figure 31).

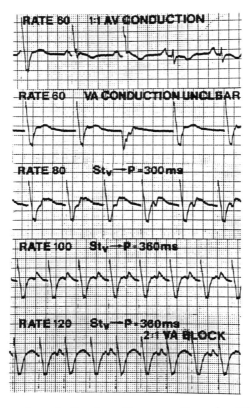

Figure 31. *Retrograde conduction is readily seen on the surface ECG when a single-chamber ventricular pacemaker is in place. Ventricular pacing must be at least 10 bpm faster than the spontaneous atrial rate. In this recording, retrograde conduction and even 2:1 retrograde block is visible. At a ventricular paced rate similar to that of the spontaneous cardiac rate, ventricular capture is seen once and 1:1 AV conduction predominates. Even with ventricular pacing (ECG #2), the ventricular paced rate is too slow to indicate whether VA conduction is present or not. As the ventricular paced rate increases to 80 bpm, the retrograde P waves are clearly seen with the peak of the P at approximately 300 ms after the ventricular stimulus. At a ventricular paced rate of 100 bpm, the retrograde conduction time increases to approximately 300 ms, and at a ventricular paced rate of 120 bpm, 2:1 VA block occurs. The state of retrograde conduction can be evaluated preoperatively in some instances.*

The characteristic arrhythmia of the pacemaker that senses the atrium and ventricle is the artificial reentry tachycardia, a pacemaker-mediated tachycardia of the "endless loop" variety. One of the most important intervals of the VDD or DDD pacemaker is the time during which the atrial channel will be refractory after a paced or sensed ventricular event. As 47% of all patients who require pacemaker implantation and 21% of those whose indication is high-degree AV block have retrograde conduction, the problem is not small. The duration of the VA conduction time demonstrates that a short atrial refractory interval after a ventricular event allows sensing of the retrograde P wave (see below).

INTERATRIAL CONDUCTION DURING CARDIAC PACING

DDD pacemakers sense and pace right-sided chambers of the heart. The activity and timing of the left atrium and left ventricle are only inferred from the sensing of right-sided events. The relationship of left-sided atrial and ventricular systole is most important for systemic hemodynamics, and effective atrioventricular synchrony is partially determined by the interatrial conduction time (IACT). At the time of DDD pacemaker implantation, interatrial conduction can be measured with an intra-esophogeal pill electrode to determine left atrial depolarization and to detect right atrial depolarization from the right atrial appendage. During stimulation of the right atrial appendage, the interatrial conduction time can thus be measured from the right atrial stimulus to the left atrial response. Mean interatrial conduction time for all patients is 95 ± 18 ms during sinus rhythm and 122 ± 30 ms during right atrial pacing ($p < 0.001$). This confirms the finding described above of the difference in AV interval between paced and sensed AV interval. In patients with P wave duration less than 110 ms, interatrial conduction prolonged from 85 ± 10 ms during sinus rhythm to 111 ± 9 ms during right atrial pacing ($p < 0.01$) compared to 114 ± 20 ms prolonging to 141 ± 17 ms ($p < 0.01$) in those patients with a P wave duration greater than 110 ms. In each patient, atrioventricular conduction prolonged with incremental right atrial pacing, but interatrial conduction times did not vary.

Interatrial conduction prolongs from the sinus rhythm baseline during atrial pacing, probably because of a latent interval between the stimulus and the local atrial depolarization, and remains constant at

all paced rates from 60–160 bpm (Table I). In addition to longer interatrial conduction times during sinus rhythm, patients with electrocardiographic P wave prolongation have longer interatrial
conduction times during right atrial pacing than do normals (p<0.001).
Based on interatrial conduction times alone, the AV interval during
DDD cardiac pacing with right atrial stimulation should be approximately 25 ms longer than when the atrium is tracked (Figures 32, 33,
34).

Several factors should be considered in determination of the optimum programmable AV interval during DDD pacing. Among them
is the interatrial conduction time (IACT). The IACT influences the
relationship between left atrial filling and contraction on the one
hand, and left ventricular systole on the other (Figure 35). Interatrial
conduction time prolongs during atrial pacing from values obtained
during sinus rhythm and remains constant in the face of increasing
atrial pacing rates. This prolongation presumably represents (right-
sided) intra-atrial propagation of the pacing stimulus that prolongs
only minimally at increasing pacing rates. This data correlates well
with earlier studies in which patients with normal P waves have had
interatrial conduction times measured at 77 ± 8 ms via coronary sinus
catheters compared to the present value of 95 ± 18 ms. Patients with
prolonged P waves on the surface electrocardiogram had prolonged
interatrial conduction times also comparable to previously reported
values (112 ± 14 ms vs 122 ± 30 ms). Of most importance is the recognition that interatrial conduction times have been constant in all studies and that a differential of approximately 25 ms between the allowed
interatrial conduction time when the patient's atrial depolarization is
sensed and the when atrial depolarization is stimulated will produce
approximately equal hemodynamic intervals.

Table I
Relative Constancy of Interatrial Conduction Time (IACT)
with Increasing Rate of Atrial Stimulation

	Sinus Rhythm		Atrial Pacing			
Rate (bpm)	65	80	100	120	140	160
IACT (ms)	95	115	118	120	122	122

Values in this table were obtained from results of 20 patients who were studied at all of
the listed pacing rates.

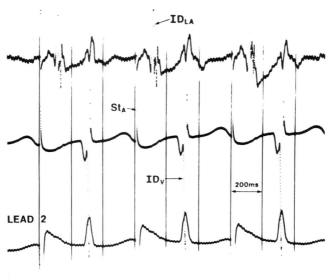

Figure 32. Intracardiac and surface recordings during pacing from the right atrial appendage. The upper tracing was recorded from the esophageal pill electrode; middle tracing from right ventricular electrode; and lower tracing from surface ECG lead 2. Interatrial conduction time was measured during atrial pacing from the atrial pacing from the atrial pacing stimulus (St_A) to the ID_{LA}.

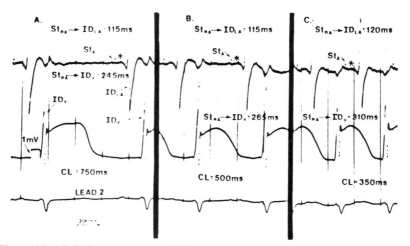

Figure 33. Relative constancy of IACT with increasing atrial pacing rates. In all three panels, upper tracing was recorded from intra-esophageal pill electrode, middle tracing from right ventricular electrode, and bottom tracing from surface ECG lead 2. Interatrial conduction time measured from $St_{RA} \rightarrow ID_{LA}$ and noted with an asterisk (*) in the tracings was approximately the same (115–120 ms) despite increasing the atrial pacing rate from 80 bpm (panel A; cycle length [CL] = 750 ms) to 120 bpm (panel B; CL = 500 ms) to 170 bpm (panel C; CL = 350 ms). Atrioventricular conduction (measured from $St_{RA} \rightarrow ID_V$) prolonged with decreasing cycle lengths.

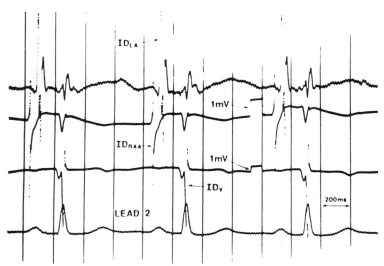

Figure 34. *Simultaneous intracardiac and surface recordings during sinus rhythm: The upper tracing was recorded from an intra-esophageal pill electrode demonstrating the intrinsic deflection (ID) of the left atrial (LA) signal. The second tracing is from an electrode in the right atrial appendage (RAA) and records right atrial activity. The third tracing, recorded from an electrode in the right ventricular apex, shows the ventricular intrinsic deflection (ID_V) coinciding with the QRS complex recording on the surface ECG lead 2 on the bottom tracing. The ID_{LA} comes at a fixed interval after the ID_{RAA} during sinus rhythm, and both are coincident with the P wave on the surface ECG. Interatrial conduction time was measured during sinus rhythm from onset of the P wave in surface ECG lead 2 to ID_{LA}.*

RIGHT / LEFT TIMING

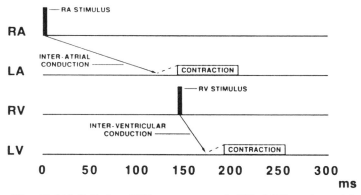

Figure 35. *Right/left timing. With a programmed AVI of 150 ms from right atrial (RA) to right ventricular (RV) pacing stimulus, the relationship of left atrial (LA) to left ventricular (LV) contraction is dependent on interatrial conduction and to a lesser degree on interventricular conduction (represented as arrows). The electromechanical delay is depicted by the dotted lines.*

PACEMAKER VARIATION OF AV INTERVAL

The AV interval during dual-chambered pacing can vary in four separate ways

1. a paced atrial event to a sensed ventricular event;
2. an atrial stimulus followed by an AV interval and a ventricular stimulus;
3. a sensed atrial event to a paced ventricular event;
4. a sensed atrial event to a sensed ventricular event (Figures 36, 37, 38).

The hemodynamic consequences of these four circumstances are distinctly different. As indicated in the text (concerning interatrial conduction time), the conduction between the right atrium and left atrium is prolonged if a timing cycle starts at an atrial stimulus rather than starting at a sensed atrial event. Several available DDD pacemakers have pairs of programmable AV intervals, one for timing cycles that start with an atrial stimulus, the other with a sensed atrial event. Because of latency following atrial stimulation and latency following ventricular stimulation, a difference of approximately 50 ms will produce the most appropriate timing cycle. Dual AV intervals of this variety are appropriate, especially at more rapid atrial rates where

AV PACING SEQUENCES

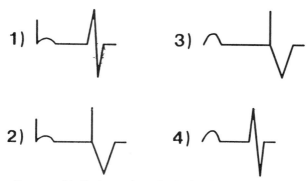

Figure 36.   *Four possible timing cycles exist during dual-chamber pacing. These are: (1) atrial stimulation with AV conduction; (2) atrial and ventricular stimulation; (3) atrial sensing and ventricular stimulation; and (4) atrial sensing and ventricular sensing. The hemodynamic AV interval of the four circumstances differs. In order to have equivalent AV intervals for hemodynamics, the intervals for each of the paced to sensed events must vary.*

AV/PR INTERVALS

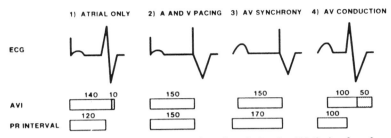

Figure 37. *The diagrammatic representation of variation in AV timing based on an unvarying programmed AV interval of 150 ms shows significant variation in the PR or physiological interval. (1) In the presence of AV conduction at a shorter interval than allowed (i.e., 150 ms), the PR interval will be briefer than programmed; (2) during pacing of both atrium and ventricle, the interval between both stimuli will be as programmed; (3) if the timing cycle begins with a sensed atrial event and ends with a paced ventricular event, the effective PR interval will be prolonged; while (4) in the presence of both atrial and ventricular sensing, the effective PR interval may be shortest of all.*

AV INTERVAL

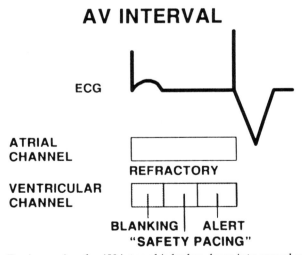

Figure 38. *During pacing the AV interval is broken down into several subintervals. Commonly, these are a brief blanking interval in which the atrial stimulus cannot inhibit ventricular output, followed in some pacemakers by a "safety pacing" interval in which a sensed event, whether an atrial stimulus, a VPC or noise produces a "committed" stimulus at some time thereafter, allowing some sensing but avoiding ventricular stimulation, and then a fully alert interval in which a sensed event normally recycles the pacemaker.*

stimulation does not occur and sensing is continuous. Determination of hemodynamics as a function of AV interval should always be performed with the knowledge of whether the AV interval has been started by a paced or a sensed event and ends with a paced or sensed event.

BIBLIOGRAPHY

Ausubel K, Klementowicz P, Furman S: The AV interval in DDD cardiac pacing. *CPEP* 1986; 4:60–66.

Bagwell P, Pannizzo F, Furman S: Unipolar and bipolar right atrial appendage electrodes: Comparison of sensing characteristics. *Med Instrum* 1985; 19:132–135.

Barold SS, Gaidula JJ: Failure of demand pacemaker from low-voltage bipolar ventricular electrograms. *JAMA* 1971; 215:923.

Breivik K, Engedal H, Ohm OJ: Electrophysiological properties of a new permanent endocardial lead for uni- and bipolar pacing. *PACE* 1982; 5:268–274.

Breivik K, Ohm OJ: Myopotential inhibition of unipolar QRS-inhibited (VV) pacemakers assessed by ambulatory Holter monitoring of the electrocardiogram. *PACE* 1980; 3:470–478.

Castillo C, Castellanos A: Retrograde activation of the His bundle in the human heart. *Am J Cardiol* 1971; 27:264–271.

Castillo C, Samet P: Retrograde conduction in complete heart block. *Br Heart J* 1967; 29:553–558.

DeCaprio V, Hurzeler P, Furman S: Comparison of unipolar and bipolar electrograms for cardiac pacemaker sensing. *Circulation* 1977; 56:750–755.

Furman S, Hurzeler P, DeCaprio V: Cardiac pacing and pacemakers. III. Sensing the cardiac electrogram. *Am Heart J* 1977; 93:794–801.

Furman S, Hurzeler P, DeCaprio V: The ventricular endocardial electrogram and pacemaker sensing. *J Thorac Cardiovasc Surg* 1977; 73:258–266.

Gabry MD, Behrens M, Andrews C, Wanliss M, Klementowicz PT, Furman S: Comparison of myopotential interference in unipolar-bipolar programmable DDD pacemakers. *PACE* 1987; 10:1322–1330.

Griffin JC: Sensing characteristics of the right atrial appendage electrode. *PACE* 1983; 6:22–25.

Griffin JC, Finke WL Jr: Analysis of the endocardial electrogram morphology of isolated ventricular beats. *PACE* 1983; 6:315 (abstract).

Kleinfeld M, Barold SS, Rozanski JJ: Pacemaker alternans: A review. *PACE* 1987; 10:924–933.

Klementowicz PT, Furman S: Selective atrial sensing in dual chamber pacemakers eliminates endless loop tachycardia. *JACC* 1986; 7:590–594.

Klementowicz PT, Furman S: Stability of atrial sensing and pacing after dual-chamber pulse generator implantation. *JACC* 1985; 6:1338–1341.

McAlister HF, Klementowicz PT, Calderon EM, Benedek ZM, Furman S: Atrial electrogram analysis: Antegrade versus retrograde. *PACE* 1988; 11:1703–1707.

Mymin D, Cuddy TE, Sinha SN, Winter DA: Inhibition of demand pacemakers by skeletal muscle potentials. *JAMA* 1973; 223:527.

Nielsen AP, Cashion R, Spencer WH, et al: Long-term assessment of unipolar and bipolar stimulation and sensing thresholds using a lead configuration programmable pacemaker. *JACC* 1985; 5:1198–1204.

Ohm OJ, Bruland H, Pedersen OM, Waerness E: Interference effect of myopotentials on function of unipolar demand pacemakers. *Br Heart J* 1974; 36:77–84.

Pannizzo F, Amikam S, Bagwell P, Furman S: Discrimination of antegrade and retrograde atrial depolarization by electrogram analysis. *Am Heart J* 1986; 112:780–786.

Pannizzo F, Furman S: Automatic discrimination of retrograde p waves for dual chamber pacemakers. *JACC* 1985; 5:393.

Pannizzo F, Mercando AD, Fisher JD, Furman S: Automatic methods for detection of tachyarrhythmias by antitachycardia devices. *JACC* 1988; 11:308–316.

Secemsky SI, Hauser RG, Denes P, Edwards LM: Unipolar sensing abnormalities: Incidence and clinical significance of skeletal muscle interference and undersensing in 228 patients. *PACE* 1982; 5:10–19.

Tomaselli GF, Nielsen AP, Finke WL, Singupta L, Clark JC, Griffin JC: Morphologic differences of the endocardial electrogram in beats of sinus and ventricular origin. *PACE* 1988; 11:254–262.

Wirtzfeld A, Lampadius M, Schmuck L: Unterdruckung von Demand-Schrittmachern durch Muskelpotentiale. *Dtsch Med Wschr* 1972; 97:61.

Wish M, Fletcher RD, Gottdiener JS, Cohen AI: Importance of left atrial timing in the programming of dual-chamber pacemakers. *Am J Cardiol* 1987; 60:566–571.

Wish M, Gottdiener JS, Cohen AI, Fletcher RD: M-mode echocardiograms for determination of optimal left atrial timing in patients with dual chamber pacemakers. *JACC* 1988; 11:317–322.

Chapter 4

COMPREHENSION OF PACEMAKER TIMING CYCLES

Seymour Furman

All comprehension of pacemaker electrocardiography depends on the interpretation of pacemaker timing cycles. What should a pacemaker channel sense and when should an event be sensed? When is either the atrial or ventricular channel refractory to an incoming electrogram? When is it sensitive? If an event is sensed, what are the primary cycles, i.e., the lower and upper rate limits? What are the atrial and ventricular refractory intervals? When will an event remain unsensed and what will be the consequences? Timing cycles must be individually interpreted. Only collectively do they make up a pacing rate. When considering any timing cycles or analyzing any ECG for pacemaker function it is necessary to analyze function as a series of intervals between sensed or paced events rather than as a continuous rate. Rate is a relatively simple designation during continuous pacing or continuous inhibition but is worthless and confusing if pacing and sensing alternate. Each event must be analyzed discretely. It must be recognized that rate is a continuum of a series of discontinuous events.

Both atrial and ventricular electrograms are readily sensed via the implanted lead system. Each different site in the heart, either atrium or ventricle will have a different electrogram. The ECG is the sum of multiple electrograms, recorded from the body surface. The ECG and EGM have different characteristics and those of one cannot be inferred from the other. The EGM of importance during cardiac pacing is that sensed by the lead system in atrium and/or ventricle. Exact measurements of atrioventricular (AV) and ventriculoatrial (VA) conduction times can only be determined by recording and comparing the atrial and ventricular EGMs from one intrinsic deflection to the other. This can best be done during the procedure of pacemaker implantation.

TIMING CYCLES

All pacemaker timing cycles begin and/or end with a sensed intrinsic deflection or a pacemaker stimulus. If a chamber is not sensed, its electrical output (ID$_A$ or ID$_V$) will not start a timing cycle and all timing in relation to the unsensed chamber will be initiated by the chamber sensed. In a DVI pacemaker, atrial activity (ID$_A$) is never sensed and never initiates a timing cycle. All timing thus originates from the sensing of the ventricle, i.e., ID$_V$. If the interval between a pacer stimulus or sensed intrinsic deflection and the next ventricular ID is less than the escape interval of the ventricular pacemaker channel, then the ventricular channel will be inhibited and a new timing cycle begun. In the single-chamber pacemaker, all timing cycles start and end by sensing the same chamber (Figure 1). In a ventricular sensing single-chamber pacemaker (VVI or VVT), that chamber determines all timing events. The generator is set at an escape interval between one event and another. The escape interval between any two events, sensed or paced, may be equal or two separate intervals may be set; one if the timing cycle is begun by a sensed event, the other if the timing cycle is begun by a pacer stimulus. Such variation is called hysteresis (Figure 2). The interval after the paced or sensed event which has begun a timing cycle is further divided into a refractory period, an insensitive portion of the interval, designed to avoid sensing the QRS complex produced by stimulus. It is usually 250–300 ms in duration for ventricular pacing, longer for atrial pacing and sensing. This is usually followed by an additional interval in which a sensed event is defined as noise and causes the emission of the pacemaker stimulus at the end of the escape interval, by extending the insensitive portion of the cycle through the normally sensitive period. Some de-

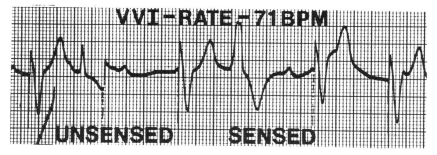

Figure 1.   *The recycle of a ventricular inhibited pacemaker is always from the intrinsic deflection of the ventricular event. In this ECG the amplitude and/or the frequency content of the second QRS complex (the conducted beat) is inadequate to recycle the pacemaker and a ventricular stimulus falls harmlessly onto the T wave. The fourth QRS complex is a ventricular premature contraction which is sensed with pacemaker recycle at the escape interval: approximately 850 ms later. Pacemaker function is normal, the electrical quality of the conducted beat is inferior to that of the VPC and below the level of sensing.*

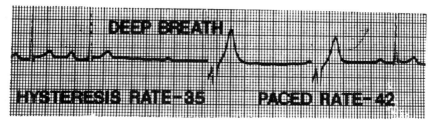

Figure 2. *A patient with AV block during a deep breath. The pacing rate was said to be at an interval of 1440 ms (42 bpm) while the onset was set at an interval of 1,680 ms (35.7 bpm). Hysteresis available in implanted pacemakers allows a longer interval from the last sensed event to the first paced event than between successive paced events.*

signs make each of the three lesser intervals (refractory, noise sampling and alert) a fixed proportion of the programmed interval between two events (i.e., the programmed pacemaker rate), in others only the sensitive interval is increased or decreased in duration by programming the rate; the refractory and noise sampling intervals are of fixed duration (Figure 3).

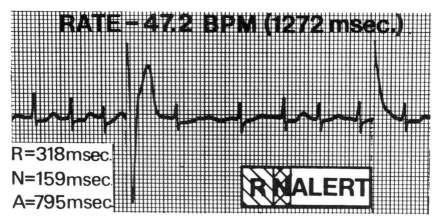

Figure 3. *The noise sampling interval is at the end of the absolute refractory interval in a single-chamber pacemaker, whether atrial or ventricular. Should a sensed event occur during the noise sampling interval, the emission of a stimulus at the escape interval will occur rather than being inhibited by succeeding sensed events during the pacemaker alert interval. In this ECG, both ventricular stimuli have been committed by previous QRS complexes, one of which fell during the noise sampling interval. Following the ventricular stimulus (left), the next QRS approximately 600 ms later inhibited and recycled the pacemaker. The second QRS once again inhibited and recycled the pacemaker. The third QRS fell during the noise sampling interval and forced pacemaker insensitivity during the alert interval. At its conclusion, the second ventricular stimulus was emitted competitively with a QRS. As the refractory interval and the noise sampling intervals are functions of the stimulus to stimulus interval, in some pulse generators the response seen above may be modified by changing the pacemaker interval (i.e. programming rate).*

If rate hysteresis is present and allows a longer interval after a sensed than a paced beat, the overall cardiac rate which inhibits such a generator will be lower (i.e., longer intervals between spontaneous cardiac events) than the pacing rate. Another version of pacemaker "hysteresis" provides a shorter interval after a sensed event thus attempting to preempt a tachycardia. In each instance, the difference between timing cycles may be a fixed amount or variable but is comprehensible only in terms of the interval between events.

DUAL-CHAMBER PACING

The single-chamber pacemaker has relatively simple timing cycles as described above. The dual-chamber pacemaker can be far more complex because, at maximum, the atrium and ventricle will both be sensed and will start timing cycles which will be both independent of each other but substantially interrelated. Each of the timing cycles begun by each chamber will have its own blanking, refractory, noise sampling and alert periods. Both sets of timing cycles, atrial and ventricular, interact with the lower rate limit which is similar to the interval which causes onset of pacing in a single-chamber unit. The lower rate limit is the longest duration without a sensed ventricular event that will be tolerated before a stimulus is emitted. In a VDD pacer, the escape will be by a ventricular stimulus, in a DVI or DDD pacemaker, escape will be by an atrial stimulus. As other intracardiac positions become timed during automatic management of tachyarrhythmias, timing cycles and their interrelationships will become ever more complex.

Both single- and dual-chamber rate modulated pacemakers have far more complex timing cycles than their single- and dual-chamber mates. Single-chamber (atrial or ventricular) rate modulated pacemakers have two sensing channels, one for the chamber and the second for the sensor. The system complexity is therefore greater than for a single rate single-chamber pacemaker. The rate modulated dual-chamber pacemakers have three sensing channels, atrium, ventricle and sensor. The timing cycle complexity for these units is far greater than in any earlier pacemakers. Such pacemaker function is described in Chapter 11, Rate Modulated Pacing.

The complexity of dual-chamber pacemaker timing is further enhanced by the programmability of the various portions of each timing cycle and of the mode of operation. Definitions of the various timing elements are necessary:

a) Lower rate limit – The longest interval between sensed events without a pacemaker stimulus.

b) Upper rate limit – The shortest interval between ventricular paced events or a sensed event followed by a paced event.

c) AV interval – The interval between an atrial pace or sense event and the succeeding ventricular pace or sense event. It is the electronic analog of the PR interval. Some pacemakers have different AV intervals depending on whether the interval is begun by a sensed or paced atrial event, i.e., AV interval hysteresis.

d) Atrial refractory interval – The interval after an atrial sense or pace event during which the atrial channel is insensitive to any incoming signal. The atrial refractory interval always consists of two consecutive portions, *the AV interval,* and a time following a ventricular pace or sense event. The atrial refractory interval after a ventricular event may be fixed or programmable and may be equal whether preceded by an atrial event or not, i.e., it may be of longer duration when initiated by a ventricular premature contraction (Figure 4).

e) Ventricular refractory interval – The interval, after a ventricular pace or sense event during which the ventricular amplifier is insensitive to in-

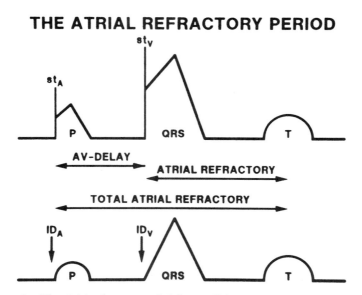

THE ATRIAL REFRACTORY PERIOD

Figure 4. *The atrial refractory period (interval) begins with sensing the atrial event (here indicated at the beginning of the P wave) or the emission of the atrial stimulus. This instant also begins the AV interval, always refractory in the atrial channel. The ventricular event, paced or sensed, begins the atrial refractory interval after the ventricular event. Both of these independently programmable, but continuous, events always comprise the total atrial refractory period (interval).*

coming signals (Figure 5). The ventricular refractory interval also sets the noise sampling period. During a rapid tachycardia, sensed QRS complexes may fall into the ventricular refractory interval, be unsensed and allow the pacemaker to function in the asynchronous and competitive or underdrive mode. While such an event normally occurs at very rapid tachycardia rates, approaching 200 beats per minute (if the ventricular refractory period is 300 ms), it is possible to lengthen the ventricular refractory interval so that slower rates will cause asynchronous stimulation especially if the duration of the refractory interval is linked to the pacing interval and changes with programmed rate. Producing competitive or "underdrive" pacing at the pacemaker "noise rate" during a tachycardia has been given the designation "dual demand" because pacing occurs if the spontaneous atrial or ventricular intervals are longer than the allowed lower rate limit, and *also,* if the intervals are sufficiently short to fall into the prolonged refractory period. Several generators can have the programmed single-chamber (atrial or ventricular) refractory set to 437 ms after the ventricular event, effectively producing a "dual demand" upper rate or onset setting of 138 beats per minute.

The duration of the atrial refractory interval determines whether a specific atrial intrinsic deflection (P wave) will be sensed or not. It is

THE VENTRICULAR REFRACTORY PERIOD

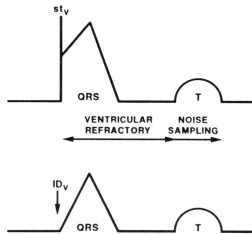

Figure 5. *The ventricular refractory interval starts with the ventricular event. In some designs, the duration of the refractory interval may be shorter if the ventricular event is sensed than if a ventricular stimulus emitted. At the conclusion of the ventricular absolute refractory interval, a noise sampling interval occurs during which a sensed event causes the emission of the next scheduled stimulus.*

obviously undesirable for a second atrial event to be sensed once the AV delay has begun. It is undesirable for an atrial event to be sensed early after the ventricular event for two reasons. The first is that some limitation must exist on the brevity of the interval allowed between two sensed atrial events. If no lower limit of the interval existed, then the ventricle could be stimulated at an infinite rate. Thus, one use for the atrial refractory interval after a ventricular event is to limit the upper rate of pacemaker response (Figure 6). The second use is that it is possible to have a retrograde conducted P wave occur following ventricular stimulation, even in the presence of fixed antegrade block. The atrial refractory interval after a ventricular event should be sufficiently long to eliminate sensing of such an atrial event. The elimination of sensing retrograde or aberrant atrial events and the setting of the level of the upper rate limit are the two critical funtions of the atrial refractory period.

f) Blanking intervals – The need for accurate timing requires a clean signal from the chamber being sensed. It is particularly upsetting to satisfactory normal timing and recycle to sense an atrial stimulus via the ventricular channel or vice versa. The consequences can be disastrous if an atrial stimulus is sensed as a ventricular event via the ventricular channel. In that event, the ventricular channel may be inhibited producing ventricular asystole. A blanking interval is in place to avoid sensing pacemaker stimuli directed at one chamber, in the opposite chamber. Blanking intervals can be considered as insensitive portions of the pacemaker cycle designed to avoid sensing hardware activity. Refractory intervals are insensitive to avoid sensing physiologic activity.

THE ATRIAL REFRACTORY PERIOD

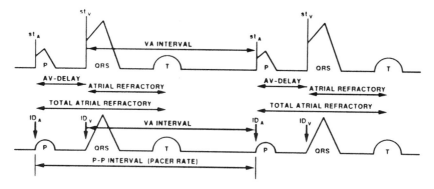

Figure 6. *This diagramatic representation is of two P-QRS sequences linked together, including the AV delay, atrial refractory interval and total atrial refractory interval. If the sensed P wave were to increase in rate, and therefore move progressively closer to the total atrial refractory interval, the upper rate of pacemaker response would be limited by the interval of total atrial refractoriness. Once the P wave entered a time of total atrial refractoriness it would be unsensed and would not begin a new cardiac cycle. The atrial refractory interval after the ventricular event is part of the total atrial refractory interval and establishes the upper rate limit.*

UPPER RATE BEHAVIOR

During bradyarrhythmia management, a pacemaker rate is set below which the ventricular rate cannot fall. This lower rate limit (LRL), i.e., the longest interval a pacemaker will allow, is basic and obvious to pacemaker operation. Equally, a pacemaker which senses and tracks the atrium requires an upper rate limit (URL), i.e., the shortest interval (between ventricular stimuli or from a spontaneous QRS to the next ventricular stimulus) at which the pacemaker will stimulate the heart. This limit is mandatory to avoid sensing or responding to excessively rapid atrial events, such as atrial fibrillation or flutter or electromagnetic or myographic interference (EMI), and produces an excessively rapid ventricular response (Figure 7). Upper

EGM$_A$– ATRIAL FLUTTER

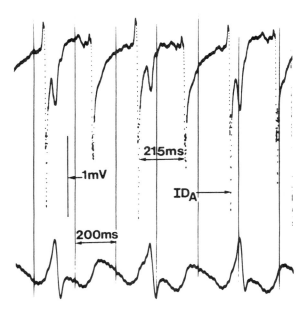

Figure 7. *A recording of an atrial electrogram during atrial flutter. The intrinsic deflections are a cycle length of 215 ms (279 bpm) with each ID of adequate amplitude to be sensed by the atrial channel. The ventricular response is limited by the atrial refractory interval and the upper rate limit established independently of the atrial refractory interval in some pacemaker pulse generators.*

rate management incorporates efforts to limit the maximum rate while maintaining the benefits of atrial synchrony throughout a range that will provide physiologic benefits for a wide range of patients. A young athlete who needs a pacemaker can tolerate and even require a ventricular rate of 175–200 bpm, i.e., ventricular coupling intervals of 300–343 ms, while the usual patient is better managed at a maximum ventricular rate of 100–150 bpm, a coupling interval of 400–600 ms. In both, the benefits of rate increase and of AV sequence are required.

A further complexity is that the implanted dual-chamber pacemaker functions as an AV conduction system, but that it may not be the only functioning AV conduction system. The natural AV conduction system may function as an antegrade system or a retrograde system or both, continually or intermittently, while implantation of a dual-chamber pacemaker, which senses the atrium, is the equivalent of the implantation of an antegrade only atrioventricular (AV) bypass tract. In managing the lower rate behavior (longest allowable interval), it is implicit that (at least) antegrade conduction by the natural AV system is interrupted or inactive. Retrograde conduction ability may be, paradoxically, intact. Pacemaker design criteria, therefore, include management under all of these circumstances. It has been recognized, with the advent of dual-chamber pacemakers, that the AV interval, the electronic analog of the PR interval, should be kept at physiologic durations. The upper rate design of each of these pacemakers must therefore accommodate all of the enumerated circumstances, i.e.,

1. Maximum rate, i.e., minimum interval appropriate for the patient;
2. Maintenance of AV synchrony;
3. Maintenance of the rate response of atrial tracking;
4. Avoidance of sensing retrograde P waves;
5. Gentle termination of a tachycardia produced by atrial arrhythmia, normal sinus activity or by sensing retrograde P waves.

The upper rate limit design is basic to all of these requirements. It must accommodate a single P wave or QRS, which may be sensed and a continuous atrial or ventricular rate which may be stable, accelerating or decelerating. Avoidance of sensing of retrograde atrial P waves is, at present, only accomplished by making the atrial channel insensitive when the anticipated P wave is to occur. Selective sensing of the atrial EGM may be attempted. A variety of mechanisms have been developed, all based on this approach. Each of these mechanisms involves loss of AV synchrony either for a single or several P waves. Review of all timing cycles for all pacemaker systems is useful.

ATRIAL SENSING

Stability of Atrial Sensing

Atrial leads are somewhat less reliable than ventricular leads. Displacement from the atrial appendage occurs more commonly than from the right ventricular apex and atrial EGMs are far smaller than ventricular, so that slight decrease in atrial EGM amplitudes or slew rate may cross the line dividing adequate from insufficient sensing.

In evaluating the long-term stability of atrial sensing and stimulation, patients were evaluated over the long-term and it was found that stimulation threshold increased by about 40% from 3 days to 1 week after implant and remained elevated for 1 to 3 months, declining thereafter and remaining stable over a year of observation. Atrial sensitivity also remained stable though considerable patient variation existed. For 54% of patients atrial sensing either improved, i.e., a lesser sensitivity was necessary, or remained stable as measured during atrial sensitivity programming. Twenty-six percent of patients required higher sensitivity programming, while for 20% the sensitivity threshold fluctuated both up and down within the programmable sensitivity range. Thus atrial charge threshold tends to follow a predictable pattern while sensing is more erratic.

Selective Atrial Pacing

Whenever antegrade and retrograde atrial activation exist the amplitude of the antegrade atrial EGM is consistently larger than the retrograde event. While the reason for this difference is unclear, pacemaker sensitivity can be set to respond to antegrade atrial EGMs while rejecting retrograde EGMs. This circumstance allows the selective rejection of retrograde P waves and provides an additional means of avoiding a pacemaker mediated tachycardia based on sensing of retrograde P waves and without the undue extension of atrial refractoriness.

TIMING INTERVALS OF DIFFERENT MODES OF PACEMAKER OPERATION

Asynchronous (VOO/AOO)

Only one timing interval exists, that between successive stimuli. While the duration of this interval may be varied, once set it is not

VENTRICULAR ASYNCHRONOUS (VOO)

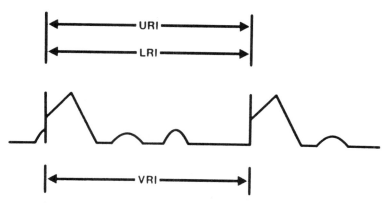

Figure 8. *In ventricular asynchronous (VOO) pacing there is no sensitivity to any cardiac activity. The upper and lower rates and ventricular refractory intervals are identical. Only the ventricle is stimulated (URI = Upper Rate Interval; LRI = Lower Rate Interval); VRI = Ventricular refractory interval).*

modified by any sensed event. As no sensing occurs, the upper and lower rate intervals are the same as the pacemaker escape interval (Figure 8).

AV Sequential Asynchronous (DOO)

Atrial and ventricular pacing is performed at fixed intervals between the atrial and ventricular stimuli and between the ventricular stimulus and the succeeding atrial stimulus. No sensing exists and no reset of timing occurs. Upper and lower rate and escape intervals are all equal (Figure 9).

Inhibited (VVI, AAI)

Stimulus emission is at the set escape rate in the absence of spontaneous activity. If spontaneous activity is sensed after the end of the pacemaker refractory interval, pacer output is inhibited and a

AV ASYNCHRONOUS (DOO)

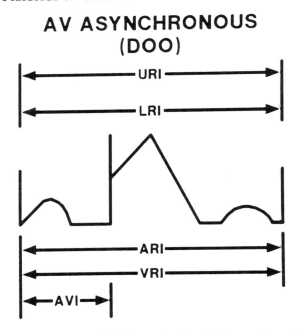

Figure 9. *AV asynchronous (DOO) pacing is of atrium and ventricle without sensing either chamber. The atrial and ventricular refractory intervals extend throughout the cardiac cycle. The upper rate interval and lower rate intervals are equal, and both equal the atrial and ventricular refractory intervals. The atrial ventricular interval (AVI), between atrial refractory interval (TARI) and the upper rate interval (URI).*

new timing cycle begun. The new timing cycle may be of different duration depending on whether it was begun by a paced or sensed event. This differential timing is referred to as hysteresis. The lower and upper rate intervals may be equal unless hysteresis exists (Figures 10, 11).

Triggered (VVT, AAT)

The same operation exists as in a single-chamber inhibited pacemaker. The difference is that a spontaneous cardiac event produces a pacemaker stimulus onto the P or QRS, simultaneously with the intrinsic deflection. The unit is not inhibited. There is a lower rate

VENTRICULAR INHIBITED
(VVI)

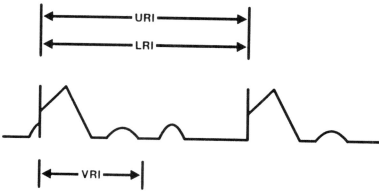

Figure 10. *In ventricular inhibited (VVI) pacing the ventricular refractory interval (VRI) extends for part of a cycle beginning with the ventricular event. During the ventricular alert interval, ventricular activity is sensed and can recycle the pulse generator. Upper rate and lower rate intervals are identical unless hysteresis is designed into the system.*

ATRIAL INHIBITED
(AAI)

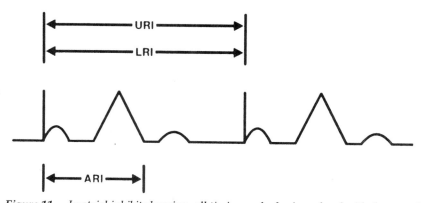

Figure 11. *In atrial inhibited pacing, all timing cycles begin and end with the sensed atrial event. The upper and lower rate intervals are equal as pacemaker output is inhibited by the sensed atrial event. The atrial refractory interval starts with an atrial sensed or stimulated event and ends before the lower rate interval ends. This allows for an alert interval between the end of the atrial refractory interval and the end of the lower rate interval, when the next atrial stimulus must be emitted.*

interval (i.e., the pacemaker escape interval) and an upper rate interval beyond which the pacemaker will not respond to a sensed event.

AV Sequential, Ventricular Inhibited (DVI)

The atrium is paced and then the ventricle is paced after a set AV interval (AVI). The atrium is never sensed and all cycles are begun by a ventricular pace or sense event. There are two different versions of this mode of operation; one allows ventricular sensing after the atrial stimulus (during the AVI), the other must stimulate the ventricle if the atrium is stimulated and is therefore referred to as "committed".

In the "non-committed" version the timing cycle begins with the establishment of the AV interval upon emission of an atrial stimulus. As the atrium is never sensed, no timing cycle ever begins with atrial sensing. Sensing continues in the ventricular channel throughout the AV interval. A sensed ventricular event during the AV interval inhibits ventricular output and begins the fixed duration ventriculo-atrial (VA) interval. The VA interval consists of the ventricular refractory interval during which no ventricular (and of course no atrial) activity will be sensed, and the ventricular alert interval during which ventricular activity will inhibit and recycle both atrial and ventricular channels. Once the ventricular event is sensed, the VA interval is begun. Competition between atrial stimuli and atrial contraction is possible if a P wave falls during the ventricular refractory or alert intervals of the ventricular interval. Thus, there are two major intervals, the AV interval and the VA interval (Figures 12, 13).

In the "committed" version of the AV sequential (DVI) pacemaker, a single timing cycle begins with the atrial stimulus. The ventricular channel is refractory during the AV interval and for the ventricular refractory interval thereafter. As the atrium is never sensed and the AV interval is refractory for both atrium and ventricle, this pacemaker has only one timing cycle that is begun by the ventricular pace or sense event. The single timing cycle may be of different duration depending on whether it starts from a pace or sense event. Both "committed" and "non-committed" units can be competitive with atrial activity as the atrium is never sensed, but as an atrial stimulus forces a ventricular stimulus after the AV interval, a committed device is readily competitive with spontaneous ventricular activity (Figure 14).

All pacemakers that do not sense the atrium or if they do, do not stimulate the ventricle have an upper rate limit interval which equals

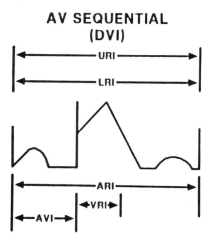

Figure 12. *The AV sequential (DVI) pacemaker has no atrial sensing, i.e., the atrial refractory interval (ARI) extends throughout the pacemaker timing cycle. As the ARI sets the upper rate interval (URI), the ARI and URI are equivalent and the pacemaker does not increase its rate in response to atrial activity. Only one rate exists for pacing, i.e., URI = LRI. The ventricular refractory interval (VRI) occurs after the ventricular event. Thereafter, the ventricular channel is alert, i.e., during the AVI, the interval between the atrial paced event and the ventricular paced or sensed event.*

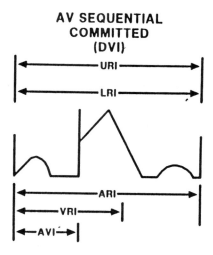

Figure 13. *The committed AV sequential (DVI) pacemaker has no atrial sensing, i.e., the atrial refractory interval (ARI) extends throughout the pacemaker timing cycle. It differs from the noncommitted DVI unit by extension of the ventricular refractory interval (VRI) throughout the AV interval (AVI). Consequently, once the atrial stimulus has been emitted, neither atrial nor ventricular sensing occurs during the AV interval. Absence of sensing of ventricular activity during the AV interval is the timing cycle difference between committed and noncommitted DVI modes.*

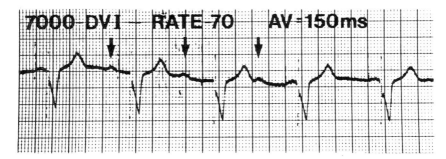

Figure 14. *Because of the lack of atrial sensing in the DVI mode, competition with spontaneous atrial activity can readily occur. If a ventricular stimulus is emitted, unless an event is sensed during the alert portion of the ventricular cycle, the next atrial stimulus must be emitted. In this instance, competition between spontaneous atrial activity and pacemaker stimuli in the atrial channel exists.*

the stimulation interval. Except in the instance of pacemaker lower rate hysteresis (in which a longer interval without a sensed event is allowed than between two paced events) the lower rate interval equals the upper rate interval, which in turn equals the pacing interval and the pacemaker escape interval.

AV Sequential, Atrial and Ventricular Inhibited (DDI)

An additional mode of pacer operation is analogous to the DVI mode in which the atrium is unsensed and all sensing and recycling derives from the ventricular channel. The major benefit of the DVI mode is that the ventricular rate cannot increase above the programmed pacemaker rate because the atrium is unsensed and ventricular activity inhibits both ventricular and atrial output. The major defect is that the atrium is not sensed and that therefore, pacemaker atrial channel activity can be competitive with spontaneous atrial activity. This is so because the emission of a ventricular stimulus in either the committed or non-committed DVI modes forces the next atrial stimulus unless there is an intervening ventricular event that inhibits and recycles the generator.

In dual-chamber pacemakers that sense the atrium, a dual function has traditionally been present, atrial sensing with inhibition of atrial channel output and the start of the AV interval. This allows increase in the ventricular stimulation rate in response to a sensed atrial event. In the DDI mode, sensing of the atrium only inhibits atrial channel output, it does not start an AV interval. Thus a spontaneous P wave falling during the alert interval of the atrial cycle inhibits atrial output but does not start an AV interval and does not increase the ventricular rate in response to the atrial rate (Figure 15).

During DVI pacing, continuous stimulation in the ventricular channel will produce continuous stimulation in the atrial channel and, if the spontaneous atrial rate is more rapid than the pacemaker rate, competition with atrial activity will result. In the DDI mode, atrial activity will inhibit atrial channel output. In both DVI and DDI there is no ventricular rate response. If the atrial rate is slower than the pacemaker rate AV synchrony is restored, and if the atrial rate is more rapid than the ventricular rate competition occurs in DVI and does not occur in DDI pacing. The more rapid the atrial rate the less AV Synchrony exists with either mode (Figure 16).

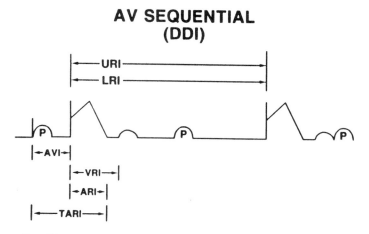

**AV SEQUENTIAL
(DDI)**

Figure 15.   *The AV sequential (DDI) mode differs from the DVI mode in that the atrium is sensed. It differs from the DDD mode in that sensing a spontaneous atrial event does not begin a timing cycle, which must end with a sensed or paced ventricular event. Atrial competition is thus avoided, but the rate response of the DDD pacemaker is also avoided. An atrial event after the atrial refractory interval causes inhibition of atrial output but does not trigger a ventricular response.*

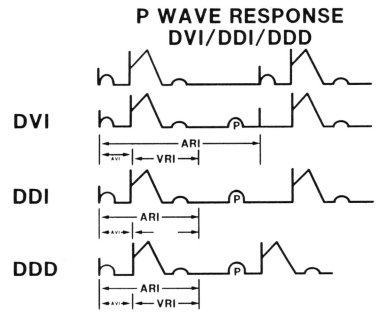

Figure 16.   *The diagramatic response of DVI, DDI and DDD pacemakers to a spontaneous P wave shows that in DVI, a spontaneous P wave is unsensed and an atrial stimulus may occur at the atrial escape interval. In the DDI mode, the P wave is sensed and the atrial channel is inhibited and recycled, and an AV interval is not begun. In the DDD mode, the atrial channel output is inhibited and an AV interval is begun, the ventricular rate is increased.*

Atrial Synchronized (VAT)

This dual-chamber pacemaker senses the atrium and stimulates the ventricle. The ventricle is never sensed. There are two timing cycles. One cycle begins with the sensed atrial event. After the set AV interval the ventricular stimulus is emitted. If no P wave is sensed, stimulation returns to a second interval established between ventricular stimuli, the lower rate or ventricular escape interval. The atrial refractory interval (ARI) (the upper rate limit interval) begins at atrial sensing and continues beyond the ventricular event. The upper rate limit may be set by the atrial refractory interval only or it may be set independently of the ARI, with the upper rate limit as one interval and the atrial refractory period as another yielding a pseudo-Wenckebach response at the upper rate limit. This was the first unit to sense only a single-chamber in which both a lower rate limit interval be-

AV SYNCHRONOUS
(VAT)

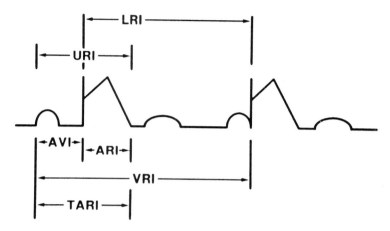

Figure 17. Atrial synchronous pacing without ventricular sensing establishes an upper rate interval, which is equivalent to the duration of the total atrial refractory interval and a lower rate interval between ventricular events. The ventricular refractory interval (VRI) extends throughout the entire timing cycle so that ventricular sensing does not occur at any time.

tween ventricular stimuli and an upper rate limit interval between ventricular events was required (Figure 17).

Management of the upper rate response is a problem in any pacemaker that senses the atrium. The problem existed in the atrial synchronous (VAT) pacemaker, which did not sense the ventricle, but as the unit is now obsolete, it need not be considered further. In modern devices, upper rate management is a problem for the atrial synchronous (VDD) and AV universal (DDD) pacemakers. These will be discussed and analyzed further.

Atrial Synchronized, Ventricular Inhibited (VDD)

This dual-chamber pacemaker senses the atrium and paces and senses the ventricle. It is inhibited and recycled by a ventricular contraction. There are four major timing cycles:

1. The AV interval (AVI) starting at an atrial sense event;
2. The VA interval (VAI) starting at a ventricular pace or sense event;

3. The lower rate interval (LRI) between ventricular events;
4. The upper rate interval (URI) between ventricular events.

   The AV, lower and upper rate intervals begin with the sensed atrial event. During the AV interval the atrial channel is refractory, as it is for a time after the ventricular event. The ventricular pace or sense event begins the VA interval, of which the ventricular refractory interval and the atrial refractory interval are part. The atrial and ventricular refractory intervals are coinicident in part, but one may be longer than the other. In the absence of atrial activity, the AV interval is not begun and ventricular stimuli are emitted at the ventricular lower rate interval—if no ventricular activity is sensed during the ventricular alert interval. The upper rate, at which atrial activity will be tracked, is limited by the sum of the atrial refractory interval before the ventricular event (the AV interval) and that after the ventricular event, which together add up to the total atrial refractory interval (Figure 18).

AV SYNCHRONOUS (VDD)

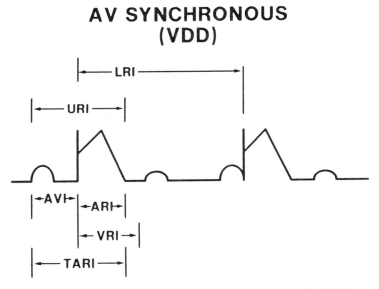

Figure 18. *The AV synchronous (VDD) pacemaker is similar to the VAT pacemaker with similar upper and lower rate intervals but with, in addition, ventricular sensing. Cardiac sensing thus exists in the atrial and ventricular channels. The total atrial refractory interval (TARI) consists of the AV interval (AVI) and the atrial refractory interval (ARI). The upper rate interval (URI) is here coincident with TARI and the lower rate interval (LRI) is via a ventricular stimulus escape, i.e., from one ventricular stimulus to the next. The major timing difference between VAT and VDD is that the ventricular channel is refractory throughout the entire pacemaker timing cycle in the VAT mode.*

FORMULA 1

Atrial Refractory + AV Interval = Total Atrial Refractory
Interval   Interval

ARI   +   AVI   =   (TARI)

If, for example, the AV interval is fixed at 150 ms and the atrial refractory interval after a ventricular event is 250 ms, the total atrial refractory interval will be 400 ms and the maximum tracking rate 150 impulses per minute. Calculation of the upper rate interval, if the TARI is known, is by formula 2.

FORMULA 2

60,000/TARI = Upper Rate Limit (BPM)

Two different approaches exist for the upper rate limit. One is that of setting the upper rate limit independently of the TARI, the other is to set the TARI and allow the upper rate limit to result from the TARI. A consequence of the independent upper rate limit is the pseudo-Wenckebach mode in which the AV delay cannot be fixed but consumes the time differential between the TARI and the upper rate limit interval. While the AV interval cannot be abbreviated below its programmed setting (unless a nonconducted, aberrant or early conducted contraction occurs), it can lengthen. In the AV block approach no prolongation of the AV delay occurs and a P wave that falls into any part of the TARI is unsensed, and sudden AV block results without previous lengthening of the AV interval (Figure 19). The pseudo-Wenckebach approach produces a plateau at the upper rate limit before AV block occurs. In both, a P wave that falls into the TARI will be unsensed and will be blocked. In the pseudo-Wenckebach approach, one more interval exists, the Wenckebach interval between the TARI and the independently programmed URI of greater duration than TARI. The maximum ARI after a ventricular event is kept short to allow high upper rates, generally in the range of 175–180 bpm (coupling interval of 333–343 ms). The TARI will be as long as in the AV block mode because of the lengthening of the AV interval (which is part of the TARI). When the AV interval prolongs in the pseudo-Wenckebach mode of upper rate behavior, the TARI is being prolonged. When the ARI after the ventricular event and the minimum AV interval are set to limit the upper rate, AV block will result. If the total of the minimum AV interval and the ARI after a ventricular event allow a higher rate than the independently set upper rate limit,

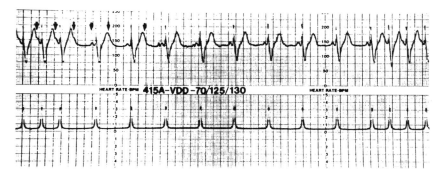

Figure 19. *A VDD pacemaker operating in the AV block mode, recorded during Holter monitoring. As the P waves move closer to the preceding ventricular stimulus, they eventually fall into the atrial refractory interval after the ventricular event. The second P wave (arrow) is unsensed as are the marked fourth and sixth P waves. The patient remains in 2:1 AV block until the atrial rate slows and atrial synchronization returns. Paradoxically, the ventricular rate increases as the atrial rate decreases. The AV interval between a sensed P wave and a ventricular stimulus it causes is constant.*

then the pseudo-Wenckebach response, i.e., prolongation of the AV interval, will result. The degree of prolongation will be the difference between the upper rate interval and the minimum TARI (Figure 20).

AV INTERVAL PROLONGATION

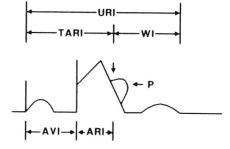

TARI	-	TOTAL ATRIAL REFRACTORY INTERVAL
URI	-	UPPER RATE INTERVAL
AVI	-	AV INTERVAL
ARI	-	ATRIAL REFRACTORY INTERVAL
WI	-	WENCKEBACH INTERVAL

Figure 20. *The Wenckebach upper rate limit response is the result of an upper rate interval that is longer (therefore setting a lower rate) than the total atrial refractory interval. The difference between the two intervals (TARI–URI) is the Wenckebach interval. It is the equivalent of the duration of the rate plateau from the onset of the upper rate interval to the onset of AV block, and it is the duration of the potential prolongation of the AV interval during upper rate operation.*

FORMULA 3

Upper Rate Limit (URI) − TARI = Prolongation of AV =
Interval   Interval

Wenckebach Interval (WI)

The upper rate limit can be set by one of two intervals. The first is the total atrial refractory interval (TARI). As no P wave falling during any part of the TARI can be sensed, total atrial refractory interval = upper rate limit interval (TARI = URI). The other possibility is that the desired upper rate limit will be lower (URI will be longer) than that imposed by the TARI. In that event, the upper rate interval (URI) will be set independently of the TARI. The difference between the two intervals can be called the Wenckebach interval (WI). A P wave that falls into the TARI will be unsensed; one that falls after the upper rate limit interval will start a timing cycle that incorporates an AV interval of programmed duration. A P wave that falls into the Wenckebach interval (the difference between TARI and URI) will be sensed and will start a timing cycle, the ventricular stimulus of which cannot be emitted until the URI has passed. Depending on duration and when the P wave is sensed in the Wenckebach interval, the AVI may actually be prolonged or nevertheless, be of normal duration (Figure 21).

If the TARI sets the upper rate (i.e., TARI = URI), sudden AV block will result. If the URI sets the upper rate below that set by the TARI, then pseudo-Wenckebach results. For example, if the independently set URI is at a cycle length interval of 343 ms (175 bpm), and that interval is of shorter duration than the TARI, e.g., 400 ms (150 bpm), a P wave will fall into the TARI before it can fall into the upper rate interval. AV block results and Wenckebach block is impossible.

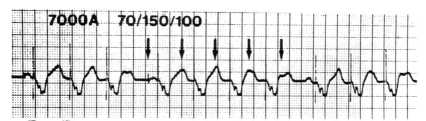

Figure 21. *Wenckebach upper rate behavior occurs when the atrial rate is more rapid than the controlled ventricular pacemaker response. The minimum response is 70 bpm, the maximum is 100 pbm and the AV interval is 150 ms. As the atrial rate is more rapid than the allowed ventricular response, the P waves (marked by a vertical arrow) move progressively closer to the preceding ventricular stimulus, prolonging the AV interval until the fifth P wave falls into the atrial refractory interval after the ventricular event and is blocked, i.e., produces no response. The next, spontaneous P wave, begins the cycle again.*

Formula 3 can be further interpreted so that if a positive number results, pseudo-Wenckebach behavior can occur; if a negative number results (negative time is impossible), AV block occurs (Figure 22).

Pseudo-Wenckebach AV behavior depends on a short ARI after a ventricular event. If the ARI is programmable, then the longer it is made, the less will be the extension of the AVI, and the more likely it will be that the AV block mode will occur. The unique mode of behavior of pseudo-Wenckebach operation is that of a rate plateau between the upper rate limit and the rate at which AV block occurs. Once again, this is a matter of the timing cycles involved. For example, if the TARI is 385 ms (156 bpm), and the upper rate interval is 480 ms (125 bpm), then the interval between 480 ms and 385 ms (a rate of 125–156 bpm) will be one of a rate plateau with prolongation of the AV interval. When the P wave falls into TARI, i.e., at an interval less than 385 ms, it will be blocked (Figure 23).

WENCKEBACH

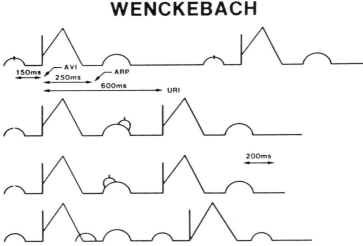

Figure 22. *Pseudo-Wenckebach operation depends on stabilization of the upper ventricular rate below the actual atrial rate, i.e., with the upper rate limit interval longer than the total atrial refractory interval. In this diagram, the P wave is sensed at the mark. ABOVE: TARI (AVI + ARP) is 400 ms giving a maximum follow rate of 150 bpm. As the upper rate limit interval is 600 ms the maximum allowed ventricular response will be 100 bpm. There is a 200 ms Wenckebach interval (URI–TARI). The P wave is sensed after TARI and URI and provokes a normal ventricular response. NEXT: The P wave falls within the URI, at a time when a response at the normal AV interval will not violate the URI. No prolongation of the AV interval occurs. NEXT: The P wave occurs earlier but beyond the TARI. A normal AV interval would cause a stimulus that would violate the URI; the stimulus is, therefore, delayed. BELOW: The P wave falls into the atrial refractory interval, it is unsensed and the next P wave produces the ventricular response.*

In the pseudo-Wenckebach approach, the atrial refractory interval after a ventricular event is fixed (though it may be programmable). The AV interval is flexible and may be extended but not shortened. In the hierarchial design of such a unit, the set upper rate limit is at a higher priority than the constancy of the AV interval. If the shortest interval between ventricular stimuli is set at 600 ms (URI), but that allowed by the TARI is 300 ms, any sensed atrial event that occurs after the end of the atrial refractory interval but which, after the set AV interval would cause a ventricular stimulus before the end of the upper rate interval, will be delayed so that a stimulus does not occur before 600 ms (from one ventricular event to the next) have elapsed. This delay is added to the programmed AV interval so that in this instance, to the AV interval (possibly programmed to 150 ms) from the

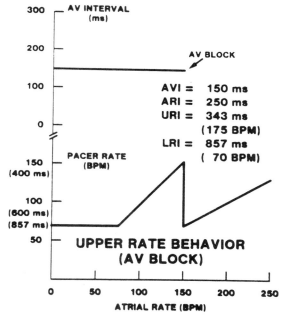

Figure 23. *A graphic illustration of the AV block upper rate limitation in which the total atrial refractory interval is the upper rate interval. Two simultaneous events, the ventricular rate and AV interval, are dependent upon the actual numerical settings. In this instance, taken from a commercially available pacemaker, the AV interval is set at 150 ms and the atrial refractory interval at 250 ms. The total atrial refractory interval is 400 ms and the maximum follow rate is 150 bpm. The URI has been independently set at 343 ms (175 bpm), a number which is, in this setting, irrelevant, as the pacemaker cannot track at an atrial coupling interval of 343 ms. At an atrial rate of less than 70 bpm (857 ms) the atrium is driven. Between 70 and 150 bpm (857–400ms) there is a 1:1 response at a constant AV interval (above). When a P wave falls into the atrial refractory interval it is unsensed and the ventricular response is to the next P wave, i.e., AV block.*

sensed atrial event would have been prolonged from the programmed 150 to 450 ms. Time is moved from after the ventricular event
to before the ventricular event (the AVI), but the TARI still determines the upper rate limit (Figure 24). Two additional events occur:
The sudden production of AV block after a stable AVI, characteristic

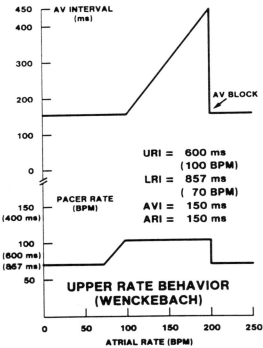

Figure 24. *A graphic illustration of the effect of Wenckebach upper rate limitation
involves two simultaneous events and is dependent upon the actual settings and numerical relationships of the various intervals. In this interval, the upper rate limit is
at an interval of 600 ms, the lower rate interval is 857 ms, the AV interval and the
atrial refractory interval each equal 150 ms and total 300 ms. If not for the independent
rate limitation at 100 bpm, this pacemaker could respond at 200 bpm. BELOW: Until
the atrial rate exceeds 70 bpm (857 ms) the atrium is paced. Between an interval of 857
ms and 600 ms (rate of 70–100 atrial bpm) there is a 1:1 ventricular response and the
AV interval remains as programmed, in this instance, 150 ms. As the ventricular rate
is stabilized at an interval of 600 ms, this will be maintained as the P-R interval decreases. Simultaneously, the AV interval prolongs (above) with the addition of each
millisecond of the Wenckebach interval, which is consumed by a P wave moving toward
the ventricular event and added to the AV interval. Because of the numbers chosen in
this example (taken from the capability of a formerly commercially available pulse generator) the maximum duration of the AV interval can be 450 ms. When a P wave falls
into the ARI, it is unsensed, the rate plateau ends, and the AV interval returns to
normal. If the atrial rate maintains its relationship to the URI, the cycle resumes.*

of the AV block upper rate limit, is replaced by a prolonged Wencke-bach period between the programmed upper rate limit and the upper rate limit imposed by the actual refractory intervals. The ventricular rate is stabilized by prolongation of the AV interval while the AVI is prolonged.

The AV interval may also be shorter than programmed if the atrial event occurs at a time when emission of a ventricular stimulus, following the programmed AV interval, would occur after the passage of the entire lower rate interval. In this circumstance, the lower rate interval (which is between ventricular events) takes hierarchial precedence over the evolution of the entire AV interval. The AV interval will appear to be short but only because the pacemaker has not allowed a full AV delay to occur, i.e., has disregarded the P wave as a time-setting event (Figure 25). In some designs, no longer available, the AV interval takes hierarchial precedence over the lower rate limit.

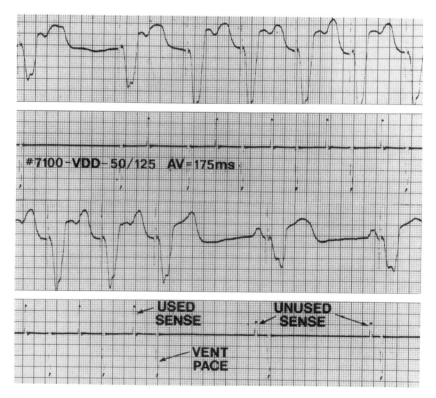

Figure 25.   *An endless loop tachycardia recorded simultaneously with an ECG interpretation channel in a VDD pacemaker. The lower rate limit is 60 bpm (1,000 ms), the paper speed is 50 mm/s. The onset of the tachycardia is by a ventricular (continued)*

A sensed P wave will start the AV interval and can extend the lower rate interval beyond its set duration. In most designs, an atrial event that occurs so late that a cycle which it starts would occur after the end of the lower rate limit, will be sensed but disregarded in the timing of the ventricular stimuli.

AV Universal (DDD)

The AV universal pacemaker senses and paces both atrium and ventricle. There are at least four different timing cycles:

1. The AV interval (AVI), starting at a sensed or paced atrial event;
2. The VA interval (VAI), starting at a sensed or paced ventricular event;
3. The lower rate interval (LRI) between atrial events;
4. The upper rate interval (URI) between ventricular events.

In addition to these basic timing cycles, each channel has refractory and blanking periods that determine the response to an atrial or ventricular event at a particular time in the cardiac or pacemaker cycle. In effect, the pacemaker is a combination of the AV sequential (DVI) and AV synchronous (VDD) pacemakers. The combination of sensing and pacing two chambers leads to far greater complexity of function than pacing and sensing in one channel, i.e., single-chamber pacing or pacing in two channels and sensing in one (AV sequential–DVI) or even sensing in two channels and pacing in one (VDD).

DDD pacing shares with DVI and VDD the restoration of AV synchrony, but the lower rate interval is started either from the atrial event (paced or sensed) or from a ventricular event rather than from the ventricular event only as it is in VDD pacing. It shares with the VDD mode an additional capability, that of the production of a tachycardia mediated by the pacemaker when the two parallel conduction systems allow antegrade conduction in the pacemaker and retrograde conduction via the natural AV conduction system.

Figure 25. (cont.) escape and a retrograde P wave (upper left). The marks below the line are ventricular channel stimulation indicators. The upward marks are atrial channel sensing indicators. The taller marks indicate an atrial event sensed by the pacemaker, in this instance the retrograde P, which is sensed 260 ms after the ventricular stimulus. The AV interval is also clearly indicated as 220 ms, prolonged beyond the programmed 175 ms. At the lower right retrograde conduction fatigues, the tachycardia ends with a ventricular escape. The P waves occur too late to start the timing cycle as an AV delay after a sensed P would have required a longer interval than 1,000 ms between ventricular stimuli. Though the P waves are sensed they are not used to start a timing cycle and the marks are, therefore, lower to indicate a sensed but unused event.

In the VDD mode, atrial pacing does not exist so that pacemaker escape is only in the ventricular channel. Should retrograde conduction exist, a retrograde conducted P wave may occur, be sensed and cause a consequent ventricular stimulus. If the P wave is closely coupled to the ventricular event but beyond the ARI it will be sensed, and if the URI is set to produce a low upper rate, (prolonged URI), the AVI will be prolonged via the pseudo-Wenckebach mode so that the mechanism for recovery of VA conduction and endless loop tachycardia exists. This mechanism is likely for the VDD mode but less likely for the DDD mode because the pacemaker escape is not via the ventricular channel, but via the atrial channel. The atrial stimulus produces a P wave before the ventricular stimulus produces a QRS complex. The result is a greater likelihood of avoiding the tachycardia because displacement of the P wave is limited. Nevertheless, if the ventricular event is idioventricular, i.e., not produced by the pacemaker or conducted from a preceding P wave, then a retrograde P wave is possible and will initiate the tachycardia. If retrograde conduction exists and the P wave is closely coupled to the ventricular event and within the ARI, consistent retrograde conduction can occur.

ENDLESS LOOP TACHYCARDIA

The endless loop tachycardia (ELT) is the pacemaker analog of a natural reentry tachycardia. As the reentry tachycardia depends on the presence of two pathways, antegrade and retrograde, a pacemaker mediated reentry arrhythmia (the endless loop tachycardia) requires the pacemaker as the antegrade pathway and the natural pathway as the retrograde conduction pathway. Fortunately, retrograde conduction via the pacemaker itself cannot occur (Figure 26).

Endless loop tachycardia is only one of a series of pacemaker-mediated tachycardias. Other such tachycardias include pacemaker electronic tachycardias, autonomic pacemaker tachycardia in which the pulse generator timing circuit senses P and QRS at a time when a pacemaker tachycardia is produced and the circuit is caught or "latched" in that mode. Echo beats, atrial premature contractions and

---

Figure 26. (Next page) In this atrial synchronous ventricular inhibited (VDD) pacemaker (model 7100), the atrial refractory period after a ventricular sensed or paced event is 120 ms, guaranteeing that any retrograde P wave will be sensed. The patient had antegrade 2:1 block. The duration of the endless loop tachycardia depends on the number of factors, including the ability to sustain retrograde conduction. In each of the three ECGs, the endless loop tachycardia is started by the application of the magnet,

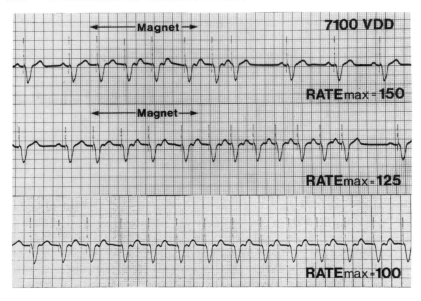

Figure 26. (cont.) *which converts the pacemaker to the asynchronous (VOO) mode of operation. Because the magnet rate of 85 bpm is faster than the spontaneous atrial rate, the P waves are forced into the retrograde position. The AV delay is set at 125 ms. The tachycardia, in each instance, is started by application of a magnet with entrainment of the P waves retrograde. The irregularity of ventricular stimuli with the magnet in place is caused by a timing cycle variation as part of magnet operation in this pulse generator. In the upper strip, in which the maximum allowed pacemaker rate is 150 per minute (400 ms), the tachycardia is sustained for only one beat because the P wave meets a refractory VA conduction pathway. The maximum pacemaker rate (minimum interval) is set by the total of the AV delay and the atrial refractory period. Because the atrial refractory period is fixed, the AV delay is prolonged by the pacemaker to meet the maximum programmed rate. As the allowed AV delay is shortest at the most rapid maximum rate, it is very likely that the conduction pathway will be refractory. The middle ECG has a maximum pacemaker rate of 125 bpm (480 ms). The AV delay is prolonged compared to that of the upper strip, because no two ventricular stimuli may be separated by less than 480 ms no matter where the retrograde P wave occurs. The AV delay is prolonged compared with that of the upper strip, and the retrograde pathway is less likely to be refractory. The endless loop tachycardia thus is briefly sustained, in this instance for six beats, before the retrograde pathway becomes refractory. The lowest ECG has a maximum pacemaker rate of 100 bpm (600 ms). The VA delay is prolonged as the retrograde conduction time remains the same as above but the delay between the sensed P and the next allowed ventricular stimulus is greater. Because recovery of the retrograde conduction system is possible, endless loop tachycardia is sustained. Initially it may be assumed that, in the presence of possible endless loop tachycardia, the minimum rate should be set to protect the patient. In this instance, as in others in which retrograde conduction exists but is unreliable, setting a higher rate may fatigue retrograde conduction fast enough to eliminate endless loop tachycardia. (Courtesy of Dr. S. Amikam)*

atrial fibrillation and flutter in the presence of heart block are other possible pacemaker-mediated tachycardias.

Endless loop tachycardia is most commonly initiated by a spontaneous ventricular premature contraction, electromagnetic interference or electromyographic interference, a programmed ventricular stimulus, an asynchronous ventricular stimulus (magnet) or a ventricular stimulus after a non-capture atrial stimulus. This latter may result in retrograde atrial activation during an alert period of the pacemaker cycle. The common denominator is that the P wave is displaced from its normal relation to the QRS complex. The endless loop tachycardia may also begin with an end diastolic, normally timed, atrial premature complex and a P wave that occurs retrograde after a normal antegrade P wave. In some instances, endless loop tachycardia may begin spontaneously, i.e., following a normally timed paced atrial beat or normally timed spontaneous P wave, in some cases followed by a paced QRS complex. Retrograde atrial activation may nevertheless be present in such instances. In other instances, in the absence of a pacemaker, a retrograde P wave may occur immediately after an antegrade P wave and a conducted QRS complex (Figure 27).

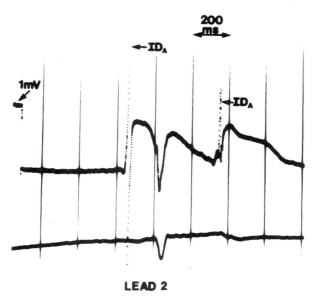

LEAD 2

Figure 27. *It is entirely possible for a retrograde P wave to occur after a normal spontaneous antegrade P wave. This electrogram is of an antegrade P wave of approximately 4 mV amplitude preceding a QRS by about 200 ms, to be followed by a retrograde P wave of approximately 1 mV amplitude about 350 ms later.*

Endless Loop Tachycardia Caused By An Atrial Premature Complex

During sinus rhythm with the right atrial appendage electrode, the atrial depolarization waveform reaches the AV node. Potential retrograde conduction finds the AV junctional tissue normally refractory. If an atrial premature complex arises from an atrial ectopic focus near the AV junction, the AV node depolarization may occur before the depolarization wave front reaches the atrial sensing electrode and the pacemaker interval will then be initiated. Should this occur, a significantly longer interval from AV node depolarization to the arrival of the returning retrograde, i.e., ventriculoatrial impulse occurs and retrograde (VA) conduction is allowed. This retrograde P wave may be sensed and endless loop tachycardia will then follow. The same mechanism is applicable to left as well as right atrial ectopic atrial activity (Figures 28, 29).

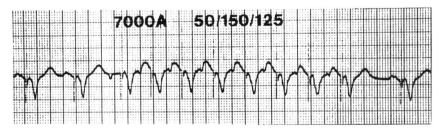

Figure 28. Lead II. The third P wave is aberrant and starts an endless loop tachycardia that ends when the retrograde pathway is fatigued and a P wave is not conducted.

Differentiation of Endless Loop Tachycardia From Primary Supraventricular Tachycardia

An endless loop tachycardia (or pacemaker-mediated endless loop tachycardia) differs from a supraventricular tachycardia, with conduction via the pacemaker, in a variety of ways:

1. The endless loop tachycardia is almost always **exactly** at the upper rate limit of the pacemaker, the coupling interval is **exactly** that of the upper rate limit interval. This exactness is caused by the highly accurate timing mechanism of the pacemaker and not by the exactness of the supraventricular tachycardia. Infrequently (see below) the endless loop tachycardia rate may be below the upper rate limit, never above.

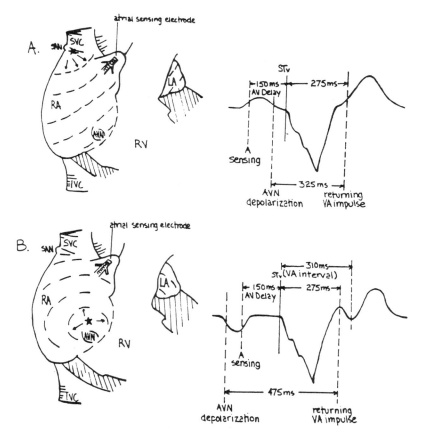

Figure 29.   *Mechanisms of induction of tachycardia. **A.** During sinus rhythm, atrial sensing precedes AV node (AVN) depolarization. A relatively short interval (325 ms) elapses between AV node depolarization and the arrival of the retrograde (VA) impulse. **B.** If an atrial premature complex arises from the area of the AV node, AV node depolarization may precede atrial sensing. A longer interval elapses (475 ms) from AV node depolarization to the arrival of the retrograde (VA) impulse. The AV node has recovered and retrograde conduction is allowed. ASE = atrial sensing electrode; IVC = inferior vena cava; LA = left atrium; RA = right atrium; RV = right ventricle; SAN = sinoatrial node; STv = ventricular pacing stimulus; SVC = superior vena cava. (Courtesy of Dr. H. Frumin)*

2. If the supraventricular tachycardia is slower than the upper rate limit, the pacemaker rate will be slower and the tachycardia can be sustained. The possibility of sustaining an endless loop tachycardia at a rate below the upper rate limit exists and the name given has been of a balanced endless loop tachycardia (BELT). Such a tachycardia is particularly important because the algorithms that exist in several pacemakers to terminate an endless loop tachycardia are based on the diagnostic criterion of stability at the upper rate limit interval.

3. If a supraventricular tachycardia is more rapid than the upper pacemaker rate, a Wenckebach or AV block mechanism of upper rate limitation, depending on the variety of pacemaker implanted and its technique of upper rate management, is invoked. If the atrial rate substantially exceeds the upper rate limit, the Wenckebach mechanism may be obvious. If it exceeds the upper rate only marginally, the Wenckebach cycle may be so prolonged as to be almost invisible. In either event, whether at a rapid evolution, i.e., 3:1; 4:1; 5:1; etc., or at a very slow evolution, 15–20:1, it is a Wenckebach mechanism of upper rate limitation (Figure 30). Programming the upper rate limit down may produce Wenckebach operation and clarify the tachycardia.

An atrial rate below the upper rate limit does not prolong the AV interval; only when the upper rate limit has been reached does AV interval prolongation begin. At exactly the upper rate limit the AV interval is as programmed. A longer AV interval in the endless loop tachycardia is required to sustain the tachycardia because the endless

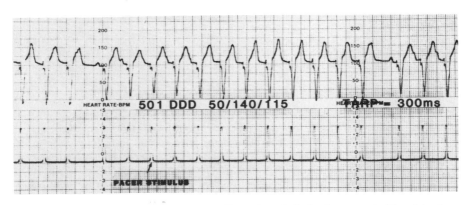

Figure 30. This Holter monitor recording of a relatively slow pseudo-Wenckebach cycle may not be recognized for what it is. The first three beats to the left are the end of the preceding cycle. Because the P wave is blocked, the fourth complex starts with a P wave and succeeding P waves are seen to move progressively closer to the pacemaker stimulus. As the atrial rate and the upper rate limit of the pacemaker are relatively close to each other, this progression is by only a few milliseconds for each beat, and the movement of the last P wave into the atrial refractory period after the ventricular event, to the right, occurs over twelve QRS complexes. The pseudo-Wenckebach cycle ends with a blocked P wave and the next cycle resumes with an escape P wave.

loop tachycardia is based on retrograde conduction with a need to allow the AV conduction pathway to recover after the retrograde P wave so that it will conduct retrograde once again. No such prolongation of AV interval is necessary for supraventricular tachycardia in which the atrial rate is sustained on a basis other than the pacemaker-mediated reentry.

All of these characteristics, tachycardia rate exactly the same as the pacemaker upper rate limit, AV interval prolongation, absence of the Wenckebach mechanism and prompt termination of a tachycardia when it is forced to be sustained at a lower rate, all strongly suggest endless loop tachycardia instead of primary supraventricular tachycardia.

Spontaneous Endless Loop Tachycardia

Spontaneous endless loop tachycardia may be initiated following a normally timed atrial event either spontaneous or paced and syn-

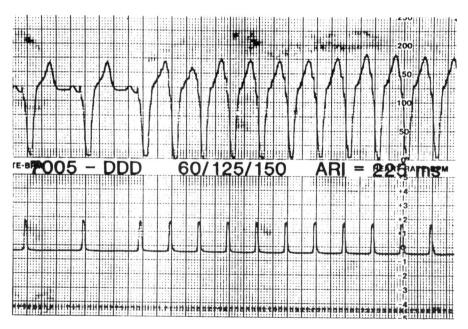

Figure 31. *Endless loop tachycardia begins after the third spontaneous P wave causes the third pacemaker-produced QRS complex. The retrograde P waves occur 200 ms after the ventricular stimulus, and as the upper rate limit interval is 400 ms, the resultant AV interval is also approximately 200 ms. (Model – Mode-lower rate/AV interval/upper limit-atrial refractory after ventricular event.*

chronized with a ventricular paced beat. Patients need not have a known or demonstrated bypass tract or other evidence of spontaneous reentry tachycardia. The spontaneous endless loop tachycardia may begin after a spontaneous P wave that produces a ventricular stimulus, and then a retrograde P wave after the end of the atrial refractory period following the ventricular event. Such a tachycardia can then be sustained until fatigue terminates retrograde conduction (Figure 31). An endless loop tachycardia may begin following retrograde conduction following an atrial stimulus with atrial capture and a ventricular stimulus with ventricular capture. This will occur if retrograde conduction occurs at an interval greater than the programmed atrial refractory period after the ventricular event (Figure 32).

Spontaneous episodes of endless loop tachycardia may begin following a spontaneous P wave that precedes the ventricular stimulus by a somewhat prolonged AV interval, i.e., 200 ms. With a low upper rate limit, i.e., 500 ms (120 bpm), an AV interval may be prolonged to 200 ms allowing easy maintenance of retrograde conduction. Should a tachycardia-terminating algorithm be in effect, the tachycardia may end only to begin a few beats later via the same mechanism (Figure 33).

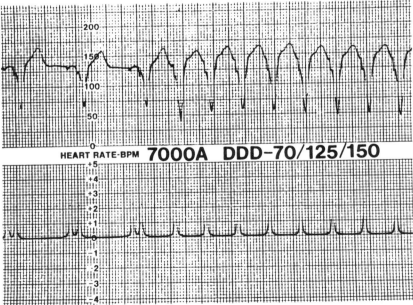

Figure 32. An endless loop tachycardia starts with retrograde conduction following an atrial stimulus with atrial capture and a ventricular stimulus with ventricular capture. Retrograde conduction occurred at an interval greater than 235 ms.

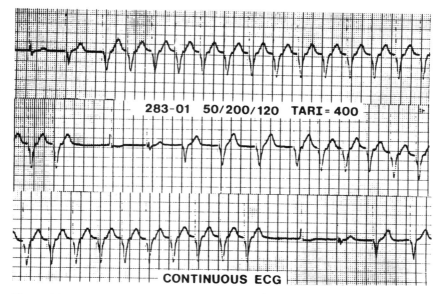

Figure 33. *Two spontaneous episodes of endless loop tachycardia are each begun following a spontaneous P wave that precedes the ventricular stimulus by 200 ms. As the upper rate coupling interval is 500 ms, the AV interval is 300 ms. Each tachycardia ends after 15 intervals at the upper rate limit. The tachycardia terminating algorithm causes atrial channel insensitivity for one event after the sixteenth ventricular stimulus.*

BALANCED ENDLESS LOOP TACHYCARDIA

As previously described, most endless loop tachycardias operate exactly at the upper rate limit. But this is not necessarily the case. The existence of endless loop tachycardia below the upper rate limit is important because it defeats those tachycardia-terminating algorithms that depend on sustained ventricular stimulation exactly at the upper rate limit, and because of the recognition of the importance of exact timing in any decision making process that uses a specific event (e.g.. upper rate) as an absolute determinant of a tachycardia. The cycle length of a balanced endless loop tachycardia is determined by the sum of the ventriculoatrial conduction time and the atrioventricular interval (Figure 34). When an endless loop tachycardia occurs below the upper rate limit, ventriculoatrial conduction can be calculated by subtracting the atrioventricular interval from the tachycardia cycle length. The ventriculoatrial conduction time cannot be determined by this method when the tachycardia is at the upper rate limit

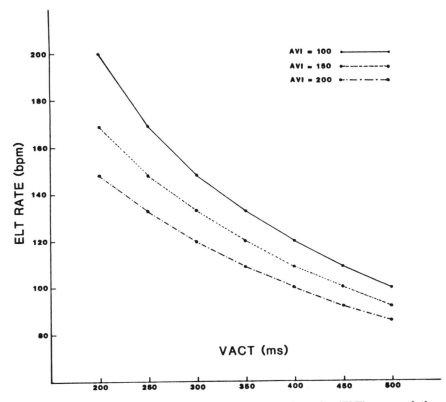

Figure 34. *Relationship between the endless loop tachycardia (ELT) rate and the programmed atrioventricular interval (AVI) and the ventriculoatrial conduction time (VACT). With longer ventriculoatrial conduction time for each atrioventricular interval, the tachycardia rate is slower. Similarly, at a given ventriculoatrial conduction time, as the atrioventricular interval increases, the tachycardia rate decreases.*

because the AV interval may be extended to maintain the selected upper ventricular rate.

The necessary condition for occurrence of this tachycardia (Figure 35) is either preserved retrograde conduction at rapid pacing rates or a very long ventriculoatrial conduction time. Retrograde conduction can occur at higher pacing rates (140–160 bpm) in approximately 20% of patients tested at implant. Prolonged retrograde conduction times occur infrequently. Routine programming of long atrial refractory periods after a ventricular event will therefore avoid most but not all of these tachycardias. But, such prolongation will force a lower upper rate limit.

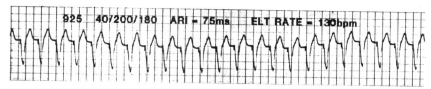

Figure 35. *Endless loop tachycardia (ELT) occurring at a rate slower than the pacemaker upper rate limit. This tachycardia was induced in a patient with pacemaker model 925, programmed to a minimum rate of 40 bpm, an upper rate limit of 180 bpm, an atrioventricular interval of 200 ms and an atrial refractory interval (ARI) of 75 ms. The tachycardia is at an approximate rate of 130 bpm, well below the upper rate limit of 180 bpm.*

Consequently, during management of an endless loop tachycardia, its origin should be determined and may result from any one of the listed mechanisms. Further, a tachycardia may be spontaneous in that it may occur without any one of the mechanisms known to induce an endless loop tachycardia. It may be sustained over a prolonged period, especially if the upper rate limit is low, prolonged VA conduction exists and prolonged AV conduction is encouraged. It may be at exactly the upper rate limit allowing the invocation of a tachycardia-terminating algorithm or it may be below the upper rate limit defeating efforts at its control and even making its diagnosis difficult if it is assumed that all such tachycardias operate exactly at the upper rate limit.

In the endless loop tachycardia, depolarization of the ventricle may penetrate the His-Purkinje system and, if the pathway is not refractory, retrograde conduction can occur and another P wave will be produced. This P wave can, in turn, be sensed by the pacemaker atrial channel and stimulate the ventricle after the programmed AV interval. The reentry loop may thus be perpetuated as long as the retrograde pathway is not fatigued and as long as some algorithm designed to make the atrial channel refractory is not activated by the pacemaker circuit. In actual practice, the tachycardia may be incessant or prolonged as it is with natural reentry tachycardias or it may be self-limited after a brief episode.

The upper rate behavior of the pacemaker has a direct bearing on the existence of ELT. As in the natural tachycardia in which one pathway is used as the antegrade limb and the other as the retrograde, the natural pathway in the presence of a pacemaker acts as the retrograde limb. The retrograde pathway has a conduction refractoriness that is a function of a variety of factors, including the prematurity of the ventricular stimulus, the state of sympathetic and parasympathetic tone, the circulating catecholamine level, whether atrium and ventricle are being paced and presumably others as well. Despite these factors, the retrograde (VA) conduction interval is well defined at any one time, though it may be no more constant than antegrade (AV) conduction. If retrograde conduction of a ventricular contraction produces a P wave after the ventricular event, it will be sensed or unsensed depending on whether the atrial channel is refractory at the time, and the sensitivity setting of the atrial channel. If the atrial channel is refractory, it will be unsensed; if the atrial channel is not refractory and is adequately sensitive, the atrial contraction will be sensed.

The two conditions that encourage ELT are: (1) short atrial refractory interval (ARI) after a ventricular event; (2) prolongation of the AV interval (Figure 36).

The first allows sensing of a retrograde P wave; the second allows recovery of the tissue of the His-Purkinje system so that a ventricular contraction meets a nonrefractory retrograde pathway. Both factors are conditions of the pseudo-Wenckebach mode of upper rate limit

ENDLESS LOOP TACHYCARDIA

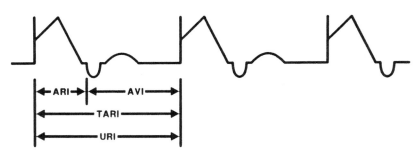

Figure 36. A diagramatic representation of the endless loop tachycardia involves a constant atrial refractory interval (ARI) and the establishment of an upper rate interval (URI) independently of the total atrial refractory interval (TARI). Because the retrograde P is sensed and produces the next ventricular stimulus, at the conclusion of the URI, the AV interval (AVI) is extended. As the AV interval is always part of the total atrial refractory interval, that interval is now prolonged to equal the upper rate interval. Once again, in this instance, the upper rate limit is set by the total atrial refractory interval, in this instance prolonged by the prolongation of the AV interval.

management. Should ELT occur, management is by one of these means:

1. An algorithm that stops atrial sensing, restoring DVI or VVI pacing at the atrial rate with restoration of the AV synchrony later;
2. Recognition that a displaced P wave, i.e., one that does not precede a QRS complex is the most common cause of ELT, so that the ARI is prolonged after a ventricular event not preceded by an atrial event;
3. Programmed prolongation of the ARI for each ventricular event so that a retrograde P wave always falls into the ARI;
4. Programming atrial sensitivity so that antegrade atrial EGMs, almost always larger, are sensed while retrograde EGMs, almost always smaller, are rejected.
5. Differentiation by pattern recognition by the pacemaker between an antegrade and retrograde P wave. This approach is hypothetical only at this time.

    If a retrograde or dissociated P wave is sensed, the AVI is begun. If the AVI is fixed, then a P wave will be followed by a ventricular stimulus after the programmed AV interval. If the AVI is at a "normal" interval then it is unlikely that a retrograde P wave can occur. If, however, the AVI is unfixed, i.e., the upper rate limit is the pseudo-Wenckebach mode, then the AVI will prolong, so that the next ventricular stimulus occurs after the entire upper rate interval. If this prolongation is sufficient, the retrograde AV pathway will not be refractory and continuation of the tachycardia will result. The only method that effectively stops ELT is by the first four means listed, effectively stopping sensing of P waves through one means or another.

All presently available choices that are designed to stop or prevent the endless loop pacemaker-mediated tachycardia involve loss of sensing of one or more retrograde atrial beats (Figure 37). The common feature of all endless loop tachycardia management techniques is the loss of atrial sensing. All of the approaches are attempts to combine a high upper rate capability with insensitivity to retrograde P waves and to ameliorate the sudden deceleration associated with reaching the upper rate limit. A technique referred to as "rate smoothing" is one such, in which, at the upper rate limit and potential AV block onset, the ventricular rate is slowly decelerated by allowing a programmable percentage of rate change only. Sudden halving of the rate with onset of AV block becomes a programmable feature and may be replaced, for example, by a 3% or 12.5% allowable decline. After all fallback and smoothing operations have been completed, endless loop tachycardia may resume unless a P wave falls into a refractory interval.

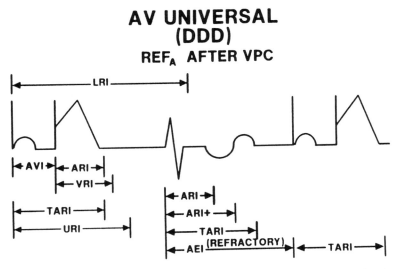

Figure 37. *Four different approaches are illustrated for the prevention of endless loop tachycardia (ELT) by making the atrial channel refractory. As most (but not all) ELT starts with a P wave displaced by a ventricular premature contraction, atrial channel refractoriness begins with a VPC. ARI is used in pacemakers with AV block upper rate limitation and provides that the atrial refractory interval is programmed to exceed the retrograde conduction interval after each ventricular event. ARI + is used in Wencke-bach upper rate limitation with the atrial refractory interval kept relatively short but prolonged by a set duration after a VPC. TARI   After each VPC a total atrial refractory interval is begun. This approach is often used in devices in which no clear programming distinction is allowed between the ARI before the ventricular event (i.e., the AVI) and that after the ventricular event. AEI + TARI   An entire atrial escape (ventriculoatrial) interval is made refractory succeeded by the establishment of a new TARI, following which normal atrial sensitivity is resumed.*

PSEUDO-WENCKEBACH AND AV BLOCK

From the previous discussion it is now clear that whether an atrial-sensing pacemaker operates in the pseudo-Wenckebach or the AV block mode is a function of the timing cycles selected during upper rate behavior. Briefly stated, the upper rate limit of any pace-maker can be set by the TARI only; if this is so then the AV block mode will be present (Figure 38). If the TARI is sufficiently short so that the upper rate interval is set independently, then the difference between URI-TARI = Wenckebach Interval. In a pulse generator in which the ARI is fixed, i.e., not programmable, the only part of the TARI that will be programmable is the AVI. As long as the TARI is of

AV UNIVERSAL (DDD)

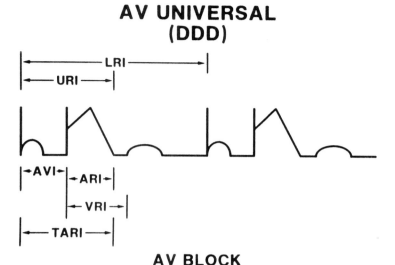

AV BLOCK

Figure 38. *The AV universal (DDD) pacemaker can consist of a variety of modes all of which have the common denominator of sensing and pacing atrium and ventricle. Diagram of the usual mode, in which a spontaneous event in either chamber inhibits its output and in the atrium triggers a ventricular response. In the AV block mode of upper rate limitation, the AV begins with the sensed or paced atrial event. It ends with a sensed or paced ventricular event. The ARI begins with a sensed or paced ventricular event and together they add up to the TARI, which establishes the upper rate limit (URI). The VRI begins with a ventricular event and is coincident with the ARI, which also begins with a ventricular event, though they need not be of similar duration. The lower rate interval (LRI) is programmed independently and is the interval between the ventricular event and the next atrial event or between two atrial events. Unlike the VDD mode, escape is from the atrial not the ventricular channel. Note that the TARI establishes the upper rate limit (LRI); it is not established independently of atrial refractoriness.*

shorter duration than the URI, a Wenckebach interval will exist. If a P wave falls during this interval, prolongation of the AVI can occur.

If, however, the ARI is programmable then the upper rate limit may be set by the TARI or by the URI depending on whether the ARI is programmed to be of shorter or longer duration. If the total of ARI and AVI, i.e., the TARI, is less than the URI then the upper rate mode will be pseudo-Wenckebach as a P wave will enter the Wenckebach interval before entering the completely refractory interval (Figure 39).

If by programming the ARI the TARI becomes longer than the URI, a P wave will enter a zone of absolute refractoriness from one of

AV UNIVERSAL
(DDD)

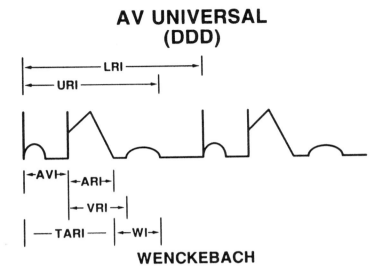

WENCKEBACH

Figure 39.   *The AV universal (DDD) pacemaker in which the upper rate limit is via the pseudo-Wenckebach mechanism operates in a similar fashion to that of the AV block mode. Both AV block and the pseudo-Wenckebach approaches are interchangeable upon selection of the appropriate timing cycles. Unlike the AV block mode in which the URI is established by the TARI, in this mode the URI is programmed independently. As an independently programmed URI must be at a lower rate (longer interval) then TARI, the difference between the two intervals is the Wenckebach interval (WI). If a P wave falls in the Wenckebach interval, the subsequent ventricular stimulus is delayed until the end of the URI. AV block and pseudo-Wenckebach upper rate management are interchangeable depending on the duration of the URI and the TARI. As the TARI occupies a greater portion of the URI, the WI correspondingly decreases in duration. When TARI equals URI, no pseudo-Wenckebach effect exists.*

complete sensitivity. AV block will result. Thus, programmability of the ARI will allow a pacemaker to operate in the AV block or pseudo-Wenckebach modes.

As an example, if the AVI is set to be 150 ms and the ARI 155 ms, the TARI will be 305 ms as will the URI, and the upper rate limit will be 197 bpm. If the upper rate limit is independently programmed to 150 bpm, i.e., 400 ms, the Wenckebach interval is 95 ms, which is also the maximum prolongation of the AVI. If now the ARI is prolonged from 155–250 ms the TARI becomes 400 ms yielding an URL of 150 bpm. No Wenckebach interval can exist and no prolongation of the AVI is possible. If the ARI is prolonged beyond 250 ms the TARI becomes longer than the URI. A P wave will enter a zone of absolute refractoriness, the TARI, before it reaches the independently programmed URI. No Wenckebach function is possible.

With the introduction of ARI programming in all atrial sensing dual-chamber pacemakers, the physician is able to select between two upper rate behaviors, pseudo-Wenckebach or AV block. This option will add flexibility to patient management. In the presence of retrograde conduction, pseudo-Wenckebach is less desirable than AV block and will, in any event be less likely because a prolonged AVI will be selected to encompass the retrograde conduction time. For those patients, usually without retrograde conduction, in whom a relatively low maximum ventricular rate is desired and in whom a moderate prolongation of AVI can be tolerated hemodynamically, the pseudo-Wenckebach mode can be programmed. As long as programmability of both AVI and ARI is possible, the physician can select one or the other.

INCREASING THE UPPER RATE LIMIT

In recent dual-chamber units the absolute upper rate limitation imposed by TARI, i.e., total atrial refractoriness, (the AV interval plus the atrial refractory interval after the ventricular event) has been partially circumvented by the mechanism of automatic reduction of TARI. As delineated earlier, retrograde conduction commonly (but not universally) disappears at more rapid ventricular paced rates. Consequently, the atrial refractory interval after the ventricular stimulus can be reduced in duration. As the PR interval is normally reduced in duration at more rapid rates, this can be mimicked by reduction of the AV interval during atrial tracking in DDD (or VDD) pacing or during rapid atrial pacing in rate modulated, i.e., DDDR pacing. The abbreviation of the AV interval is translated into an equivalent abbreviation of TARI and thus to a higher upper rate limit. For example: If the TARI is 450 ms consisting of 150 ms of AV interval and 300 ms of PVARP (postventricular atrial refractory period), the absolute upper rate limit will be 133 bpm. As that rate is approached, were the AV interval to be abbreviated to 125 ms, TARI would be 425 ms and upper rate 141 bpm. If AVI were reduced to 100 ms, TARI would be 350 ms and URL 150 bpm. Further extensions of the URL might be achieved by simultaneous reduction in the duration of PVARP to take advantage of the reduction in retrograde conduction at more rapid rates, though this might cause some difficulty were retrograde conduction time to increase with increasing paced rate rather than resulting in VA block.

LOWER RATE BEHAVIOR

In a single-or dual-chamber pacemaker the intervals begun by paced or sensed events can be equal or unequal. Formerly, most intervals were equal in duration. With the advent of electronic circuits in which it is easy to provide either an unequal or equal interval, many single-chamber pacemakers provide a programming capability for hysteresis. All that is changed is the interval between successive events depending on whether the cycle begins with a paced or sensed event. Hysteresis usually allows a longer interval between successively sensed events. An interval that ends with a paced event starts a shorter interval before emitting a stimulus and requires a still shorter interval for a spontaneous beat to begin a longer cycle. Hysteresis can be available in a DDD pacemaker as a longer escape interval in the atrial channel.

HYSTERESIS

During customary hysteresis operation, a lesser rate (i.e., longer coupling interval) inhibits the pacemaker. Should a single allowed interval be exceeded, pacing begins at a shorter coupling interval (i.e., a greater rate). During continuous pacing, a single ventricular interval shorter than the pacing interval is required to resume the lower rate. Because such a single event may be infrequent, prolonged, possibly unnecessary pacing may occur. A recently introduced hysteresis variant called "search hysteresis" extends the pacing interval to the duration of the hysteresis interval every 256 continuous pacing cycles. With such prolongation, a spontaneous event may occur and inhibit pacing. If a spontaneous event does not occur, pacing resumes at the usual interval. If an event does occur, the pacemaker is inhibited until the hysteresis interval is exceeded when pacing will resume, testing once again after each 256 consecutive paced events.

In the DDD mode, escape is by an atrial stimulus that occurs at the ventricular escape interval minus the AVI. This interval is the VA interval. For example, if the ventricular escape interval (which is the same as the lower rate interval) is 1000 ms and the AVI is 150 ms, the ventriculoatrial interval, VAI (assuming no hysteresis) will be 850 ms from the preceding ventricular event. A P wave that occurs during the ventricular escape interval, i.e., during that 850 ms interval will start a new AVI, a new LRI and a new URI.

In the DVI mode, the absence of atrial sensing means that during LRI and URI which, in the absence of deliberate or accidental hysteresis, are identical, all sensing is from the ventricular channel, but the atrial channel escape is at the VA interval, that is the ventricular escape interval minus the AVI.

SENSOR DRIVEN INTERVALS

The newly available sensor driven, (rate modulated or adaptive-rate or rate-responsive) pacemakers have an interval in addition to those that now are used to operate the device. The normal operation of a single-chamber, SSI device or a dual-chamber DDD device is as usual. In the single-chamber device, the lower rate or escape interval is as in an AAI or VVI pacemaker. In such a device there is no means of abbreviating the escape interval. In the rate modulated single-chamber device, a sensor allows abbreviation of the escape interval just as the sensed P wave causes abbreviation of the escape interval in a VDD pacemaker. Indeed, the most widely used rate modulated (activity sensing) device was a direct modification of an atrial synchronous, ventricular inhibited pulse generator. As the sensor is not sensitive to a stimulus visible on the ECG, there may be no clear indicator of why a specific response occurs. Nevertheless, the lower rate limit is the escape interval and the sensor driven interval (SDI) and the upper rate interval (URI) are identical (Figure 40).

VENTRICULAR INHIBITED
SENSOR DRIVEN
VVIR

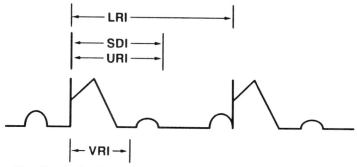

Figure 40. *Single-chamber rate modulated, sensor driven pacing differs from single-chamber inhibited pacing by the presence of an upper and a lower rate. The lower rate is the analog of the set rate of the single rate pacemaker. In the rate modulated device, the set duration of the interval between stimuli can be modified by the sensor of physiology. The timing diagram is similar to that of the VVI device with the addition of a sensor driven interval (SDI), which is the equivalent of the upper rate interval (URI).*

The dual-chamber sensor driven pacemaker is similar to the DDD pacemaker. In this instance, the lower rate limit is an atrial escape stimulus. Two stimuli set the upper rate limit. Should the sensor driven (SDI) upper rate interval be shorter than the atrial coupling interval (i.e., the atrial rate) the atrium will be paced and spontaneous atrial activity will be suppressed. If AV conduction occurs from the spontaneous or paced atrial event, the ventricular stimulus will be suppressed. If the atrial coupling interval is briefer than the SDI, it will take precedence and the sensor rate modulation and spontaneous atrial synchrony will occur (Figure 41).

Other options exist. For example, the programmed AV interval may be a function of the atrial or sensor driven rate or both. In that event, the AVI may be one value at the lower rate limit and another at the upper rate limit. This feature is likely to become more common as new devices are made available.

Another possibility is that atrial synchrony during dual-chamber pacing will be preserved at relatively lower rates and will then be sacrificed at higher rates. In such an instance, for example, the mechanism described above of dual sensors, atrium and another physiological sen-

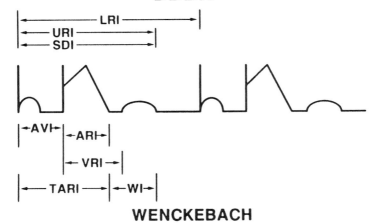

AV UNIVERSAL-SENSOR DRIVEN DDDR

WENCKEBACH

Figure 41. *The dual-chamber rate modulated device provides a sensor driven interval (SDI), the equivalent of the upper rate interval. In the dual-chamber device diagrammed, the timing cycles are those of the conventional dual-chamber pacemaker. In the DDD device, the atrium drives the ventricular stimulus to the upper rate interval (URI). In the rate modulated device, the upper rate interval is driven by the sensor and by the atrium, which is sensed or paced depending on which, sensor drive or atrium, is at the briefer interval.*

sor may be used up to a rate of perhaps 100 bpm, i.e., a coupling interval of 600 ms. Thereafter, if the sensor directs a shorter coupling interval, i.e., a higher rate, the atrial channel would be inactive and neither sensing nor stimulation would occur. The ventricular drive will then be from the sensor and no attempt at atrial synchrony would exist. Other timing events are likely as single-chamber and dual-chamber sensor driven, i.e., rate modulated pacemakers are developed.

MULTIPLE SENSING CHANNELS

With the introduction of sensor driven dual-chamber pacing, an additional channel of sensitivity has been added to pacemaker capability. It is possible to view evolution in pacing as relative to the increase in the amount of data received via the sensing channels rather than in any other way. Certainly it is readily possible to stimulate via one or many channels, sensing and correlating the responses of more than one channel becomes progressively more complex. Sensing a single channel, first the atrium and then the ventricle, was critical in pacemaker development. Until two channels could be sensed and logically handled, dual-chamber pacing and the practical restoration of atrial synchrony was not possible. The single-chamber rate modulated pacemaker was not more complex than dual-chamber pacing. Sensitivity to atrial activity was replaced by sensitivity to another event. The introduction of three channels of sensitivity, i.e., ventricle, atrium and an additional sensor marks a new level of complexity and sophistication.

BIBLIOGRAPHY

Ausubel K, Gabry MD, Klementowicz PT, Furman S: Pacemaker-mediated endless loop tachycardia at rates below the upper rate limit. *Am J Cardiol* 1988; 61:465–467.

Barold SS: Clinical significance of pacemaker refractory periods. *Am J Cardiol* 1971; 28:237–239 (editorial).

Barold SS, Carroll M: "Double reset" of demand pacemakers. *Am Heart J* 1972; 84:276–277.

Barold SS, Falkoff MD, Ong LS, Heinle RA: Interpretation of electrocardiograms produced by a new unipolar multiprogrammable "committed" AV sequential demand (DVI) pulse generator. *PACE* 1981; 4:692–708.

Barold SS, Gaidula JJ: Evaluation of normal and abnormal sensing functions of demand pacemakers. *Am J Cardiol* 1971; 28:201–210.

Barold SS, Gaidula JJ, Banner RL, Litman GI, Goldstein S: Interpretation of complex demand pacemaker arrhythmias. *Br Heart J* 1972; 34:312.

Barold SS, Gaidula JJ, Castillo R, Masood A, Keller JW: Evaluation of demand pacemakers by chest wall stimulation. *Chest* 1973; 63:589–606.

Barold SS, Gaidula JJ, Lyon JL, Carroll M: Irregular recycling of demand pacemakers from borderline electrographic signals. *Am Heart J* 1971; 82:477.

Barold SS, Levine PA: Autointerference of demand pulse generators. *PACE* 1981; 4:274–280.

Barold SS, Linhart J, Samet P: Reciprocal beating induced by ventricular pacing. *Circulation* 1968; 38:330–340.

Barold SS, Ong LS, Falkoff MD, Heinle R: Inhibition of bipolar demand pacemaker by diaphragmatic myopotentials. *Circulation* 1977; 56:679–683.

Batey RL, Calabria DA, Shewmaker S, Sweesy M: Crosstalk and blanking periods in a dual-chamber (DDD) pacemaker: A case report. *CPPE* 1985; 3:314–318.

Bathen J, Gundersen T, Forfang K: Tachycardias related to atrial synchronous ventricular pacing. *PACE* 1982; 5:471–475.

Bertuso J, Kapoor AS, Schafer J: A case of ventricular undersensing in the DDI mode: Cause and correction. *PACE* 1986; 9:685–689.

Burchell HB: Analogy of electronic pacemaker and ventricular parasystole with observations on refractory period, supernormal phase, and synchronization. *Circulation* 1963; 27:878–889.

Castellanos A, Bloom MG, Sung RJ, Roxanski JJ, Myerburg RJ: Mode of operation induced by rapid external chest wall stimulation in patients with normally functioning QRS-inhibited (WI) pacemakers. *PACE* 1979; 2:2–10.

Castellanos A, Lemberg L: Disorders of rhythm appearing after implantation of synchronized pacemakers. *Br Heart J* 1964; 26:747–754.

Castellanos A, Lemberg L: Pacemaker arrhythmias and electrocardiographic recognition of pacemakers. *Circulation* 1973; 42:1381–1391.

Castellanos A, Lemberg L, Arcebal AG, Berkovits BV, Hernandez-Pierotti O: Repetitive firing produced by pacemaker stimuli falling after the T wave. *Am J Cardiol* 1970; 25:247–251.

Castellanos A, Lemberg L, Jude JR, Berkovits BV: Repetitive firing occurring during synchronized electrical stimulation of the heart. *J Thorac Cardiovasc Surg* 1966; 51:334–340.

Castellanos A, Lemberg L, Jude JR: Depression of artificial pacemakers by extraneous impulses. *Am Heart J* 1976; 73:24–31.

Castellanos A, Lemberg L, Rodriguez-Tocker L, Berkovits BV: Atrial synchronized pacemaker arrhythmias: Revisited. *Am Heart J* 1968; 76:199–208.

Castellanos A, Maytin O, Lemberg L, Berkovits BV: Part VIII. Rhythm disturbances and pacing. Pacemaker induced cardiac rhythm disturbances. *Ann NY Acad Sci* 1969; 167:903–910.

Castellanos A, Ortiz JM, Pastis N, Castillo C: The electrocardiogram in patients with pacemakers. *Prog Cardiovasc Dis* 1970; 13:190–205.

Castellanos A, Spence M: Pacemaker arrhythmias in context. *Am J Cardiol* 1970; 25:372 (editorial).

Castellanos A, Waxman HL, Moleiro F, Berkovits BV, Sung RJ: Preliminary studies with an implantable multimodel AV pacemaker for reciprocating atrioventricular tachycardias. *PACE* 1980; 3:257–265.

Castillo A, Berkovits BV, Castellanos A, Lemberg L, Callard G, Jude JR: Bifocal demand pacing. *Chest* 1971; 59:360–364.

Castillo C, Lemberg L, Castellanos A, Berkovits BV: Bifocal (sequential atrioventricular) demand pacemaker for sinoatrial and atrioventricular conduction disturbances. *Am J Cardiol* 1970; 25:87 (abstract).

Center S, Samet P, Castillo C: Synchronous, standby, and asynchronous pervenous pacing of the heart. *Ann Thorac Surg* 1968; 5:498–507.

Den Dulk K, Lindemans FW, Bar FW, Wellens HJJ: Pacemaker related tachycardias. *PACE* 1982; 5:476–485.

Den Dulk K, Lindemans, FW, Wellens HJJ: Noninvasive evaluation of pacemaker circus movement tachycardias. *Am J Cardiol* 1984; 53:537–543.

Echeverria HG, Luceri RM, Thurer RJ, Castellanos A: Myopotential inhibition of unipolar AV sequential (DVI) pacemaker. *PACE* 1982; 5:20–22.

Edwards LM, Hauser RG: Dual mode sensing by a variable cycle ventricular synchronous pulse generator. *PACE* 1981; 4:309–312.

Falkoff M, Ong LS, Heinle RA, Barold SS: The noise sampling period: A new cause of apparent sensing malfunction of demand pacemakers. *PACE* 1978; 1:250–253.

Freedman RA, Rothman MT, Mason JW: Recurrent ventricular tachycardia induced by an atrial synchronous ventricular-inhibited pacemaker. *PACE* 1982; 5:490–494.

Frohlig G, Dyckmans J, Doenecke P, Sen S, Bette L: Noise reversion of a dual-chamber pacemaker without noise. *PACE* 1986; 9:690–696.

Frumin H, Furman S: Endless loop tachycardia started by an atrial premature complex in a patient with a dual-chamber pacemaker. *JACC* 1985; 5:707–710.

Furman S: Dual-chamber pacemakers: Upper rate behavior. *PACE* 1985; 8:197–214.

Furman S: Inhibition of a ventricular synchronous pacemaker. *Am Heart J* 1977; 93:581–584.

Furman S: Retreat from Wenckebach. *PACE* 1984; 7:1–2 (editorial).

Furman S, Fisher JD: Endless loop tachycardia in an AV universal (DDD) pacemaker. *PACE* 1982; 5:486–489.

Furman S, Fisher JD: Repetitive ventricular firing caused by AV universal pacing. (letter) *Chest* 1983; 83:586.

Furman S, Hayes DL: Implantation of atrioventricular synchronous and atrioventricular universal pacemaker. *J Thorac Cardiovasc Surg* 1983; 85:839–850.

Furman S, Huang W: Pacemaker recycle from repolarization artifact. *PACE* 1982; 5:927–928.

Furman S, Reicher-Reiss H, Escher DJW: Atrio-ventricular sequential pacing and pacemakers. *Chest* 1973; 63:783.

Harthorne JW, Eisenhauer AC, Steinhaus DM: Pacemaker-mediated tachycardias: An unresolved problem. *PACE* 1984; 7:1140–1147.

Johnson CD: AV universal (DDD) pacemaker-mediated reentrant endless loop tachycardia initiated by a reciprocal beat of atrial origin. *PACE* 1984; 7:29–33.

Kristensson BE, Kruse I, Ryden L: Clinical problems in atrial synchronous ventricular inhibited pacing: A long-term follow-up of 54 patients. *PACE* 1984; 7:693–701.

Kruse I, Ryden L, Duffin E: Clinical evaluation of atrial synchronous ventricular inhibited pacemakers. *PACE* 1980; 3:641–650.

Lamas GA, Antman EM: Pacemaker-mediated tachycardia initiated by coincident P-wave undersensing and ventricular blanking period. *PACE* 1985; 8:436–439.

Levine PA: Confirmation of atrial capture and determination of atrial capture thresholds in DDD pacing systems. *CPPE* 1984; 2:465–473.

Levine PA: Postventricular atrial refractory periods and pacemaker mediated tachycardias. *CPPE* 1983; 1:394–401.

Levine PA, Brodsky SJ, Seltzer JP: Assessment of atrial capture in committed atrioventricular sequential (DVI) pacing systems. *PACE* 1983; 6:616–623.

Levine PA, Lindenberg BS, Mace RC: Analysis of AV universal (DDD) pacemaker rhythms. *CPPE* 1984; 2:54–73.

Levine PA, Seltzer JP: AV universal (DDD) pacing and atrial fibrillation. *CPPE* 1983; 1:275–282.

Levine PA, Seltzer JP: Fusion, pseudo-fusion, pseudo-pseudofusion and confusion: Normal rhythms associated with atrioventricular sequential "DVI" pacing. *CPPE* 1983; 1:70–80.

Levine PA, Seltzer JP: Runaway or normal pacing? Two cases of normal rate responsive (VDD) pacing. *CPPE* 1983; 1:177–183.

Luceri RM, Castellanos A, Zaman L, Myerburg R: The arrhythmias of dual-chamber cardiac pacemakers and their management. *Ann Intern Med* 1983; 99:354–359.

Luceri RM, Parker M, Thurer R, Castellanos A, Myerburg R: Particularities of management and follow-up of patients with DDD pacemakers. *CPPE* 1984; 2:261–271.

Luceri RM, Ramirez AV, Castellanos A, Zaman L, et al: Ventricular tachycardia produced by a normally functioning AV sequential demand (DVI) pacemaker with "committed" ventricular stimulation. *JACC* 1983; 1:1177–1179.

Medina-Ravell V, Castellanos A, Portillo-Acosta B, Maduro-Maytin C, Rodriguez-Salas L, et al: Management of tachyarrhythmias with dual-chamber pacemakers. *PACE* 1983; 6:333–345.

Nathan D, Center S, Wu C, et al: Synchronization of the ventricle and atrium in complete heart block by self-contained implantable pacer. *Circulation* 1962; 26:767.

Oseran D, Ausubel K, Klementowicz PT, Furman S: Spontaneous endless loop tachycardia. *PACE* 1986; 9:379–386.

Rozanski JJ, Blankstein RL, Lister JW: Pacer arrhythmias: Myopotential triggering of pacemaker mediated tachycardia. *PACE* 1983; 6:795–797.

Seltzer JP, Levine PA, Watson WS: Patient-initiated autonomous pacemaker tachycardia. *PACE* 1984; 7:961–969.

Spurrell RAJ, Sowton E: An implanted atrial synchronous pacemaker with a short atrioventricular delay for the prevention of paroxysmal supraventricular tachycardias. *J Electrocardiol* 1976; 9:89–96.

Sung RJ, Castellanos A, Thurer RJ, Myerburg RJ: Partial pacemaker recycling of implanted QRS-inhibited pulse generators. *PACE* 978; 1:189–195.

Tolentino AO, Javier RP, Byrd C, Samet P: Pacer-induced tachycardia associated with an atrial synchronous ventricular inhibited (ASVIP) pulse generator. *PACE* 1982; 5:251–259.

Van Cleve RB, Sung RJ, Maytin O, Castellanos A: Notes on ventricular tachycardia occurring during magnet waving and on the function of the Omni-Ectocor pacemaker. *Eur J Cardiol* 1978; 8:543–551.

Whalen RE, Starmer CF, McIntosh HD: Electrical hazards associated with cardiac pacemaking. *Ann NY Acad Sci* 1964; 111:922–931.

Yokoyama M, Wada J, Barold SS: Transient early T wave sensing by implanted programmable demand pulse generator. *PACE* 1981; 4:68–74.

Chapter 5

HEMODYNAMICS OF CARDIAC PACING

David R. Holmes Jr.

Symptomatic bradycardia is the most common indication for placement of a permanent cardiac pacing system. Symptoms in patients with bradycardia may occur at rest from the slow rate itself; the loss of atrioventricular (AV) synchrony seen, for example, in AV block; the development of ventriculoatrial (VA) conduction with AV valve regurgitation; the onset of escape tachyarrhythmias, or the instability of the escape rhythm itself. Symptoms may also occur with exercise for these same reasons. In addition, symptoms with exercise may occur because of inability to increase the heart rate with exercise (chronotropic incompetence). This chronotropic incompetence may be the result of a fixed rate VVI pacemaker in the presence of AV block, the result of a "physiologic pacemaker" with inappropriate upper rate response such as 2:1 block, or because of sinus node dysfunction with failure of the sinus node to increase its rate with exercise. In the latter case, even DDD pacing fails to provide the means to increase the heart rate with exercise. The aim of cardiac pacing is to prevent these manifestations of symptomatic bradycardia and restore more normal hemodynamics over the wide range of physiologic demands.

Circulatory hemodynamics are complex because of the many interrelationships of variables, and the effect of disease states on these variables. Review of the increasingly large body of literature dealing with the hemodynamics of cardiac pacing yields often confounding, contradictory data. Some of the agreements and disagreements are the result of small but significant differences in protocols or methodology used for the individual studies, some are the result of different patient populations included, for example, patients with congestive heart failure or valvular heart disease versus structurally normal hearts with primary electrical problems, and, finally, some are the result of small numbers of patients. The problems are complicated by the inability to isolate various components, for example, AV interval, atrial contractions, and rate, and thereby study their individual importance.

These difficulties notwithstanding, the hemodynamics of cardiac pacing have attracted increasing interest. This interest has been stimulated in part by the recognition that some patients have limitations and problems with ventricular pacing. Although fixed rate ventricular pacing results in a stable ventricular rhythm and prevents asystole, it compromises AV synchrony, may result in VA conduction, and is unable to increase in response to physiologic demands. This interest in hemodynamics has also been stimulated by the development of new technology that allows for combined atrial and ventricular pacing, and more recently by the development of physiologic sensor driven, rate modulating pacemakers. These pacemakers currently have the ability to maintain ventricular rate responsiveness with exercise. Units being tested now will allow atrial and ventricular rate responsiveness and maintenance of AV synchrony, thus more closely simulating the normal physiology of the intact cardiovascular system.

The use of these rate modulating or responsive pacemakers has rekindled interest in assessing the relative roles and merits of maintaining AV synchrony versus ability to increase rate in a physiologic response to increased demands. Understanding the basis of the normal adaptive physiologic mechanism is important for assessing the potential and real impact of these newer pacemakers. The relative importance of each has been studied in small groups of patients and an increasing amount of information has been documented. For the individual patient, predicting the relative importance of AV synchrony versus rate responsiveness, however, is more problematic.

DETERMINANTS OF CARDIAC OUTPUT

Heart Rate

Changes in cardiac output are an important means by which the normal cardiovascular system responds to changing demands, such as exercise. The cardiac output is the product of heart rate and stroke volume. The relationship of each of these is variable for a given patient and depends upon the level of exercise and the presence or absence of underlying cardiovascular disease, and the specific characteristics of the disease, for example, the degree of compliance of the ventricular muscle relative to normal. Demands for an increase in cardiac output, such as those with exercise, are usually met primarily by an increase in heart rate and to a lesser extent by an increase in stroke volume (Figure 1). During exercise, some persons, such as

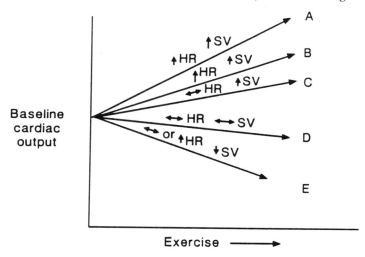

Figure 1.   *Potential responses in heart rate (HR) and stroke volume (SV) to increasing exercise. **A.** Response in trained athletes during exercise. Large increase in cardiac output is result of increase in heart rate but a larger increase in stroke volume. **B.** Response in normal persons. There is larger relative increase in heart rate but also some increase in stroke volume. **C.** Response in patient with AV block or sinus node dysfunction but normal ventricular function who is unable to increase heart rate. Increase in cardiac output is result of increase in stroke volume. **D.** Response in patient with fixed heart rate and stroke volume who is unable to increase cardiac output with exercise or in whom cardiac output falls somewhat. **E.** Response of patient with markedly impaired ventricular function that worsens with exercise.*

highly trained athletes, can increase their stroke volume more proportionately to increase cardiac output. These highly trained athletes are able to increase stroke volume during exercise; their heart rates also increase, but peak heart rate may be less than that in sedentary persons. On the other hand, in patients with left ventricular dysfunction secondary to coronary artery disease or cardiomyopathy, conditions not uncommon in patients with permanent cardiac pacemakers the ability to increase stroke volume may be limited or even be absent. In these persons, the ability to increase heart rate in response to increased demands is of paramount importance.

Stroke Volume

Factors affecting stroke volume are more complex. The stroke volume is the amount of blood ejected with each ventricular contraction, that is, end-diastolic volume minus end-systolic volume. The end-systolic volume depends upon two major factors—myocardial contractility and afterload. Myocardial contractility is difficult to assess alone because it depends upon both the afterload and the end-diastolic volume. It can be assessed by evaluation of the ejection fraction or with more sophisticated invasive techniques, such as pressure and volume changes over time. The ejection fraction is most commonly used and can be determined by echocardiography, left ventricular angiography, or nuclear medicine techniques; it gives an estimate of contractility. In patients with abnormal hearts, ventricular dysfunction, and decreased contractility, other compensatory mechanisms must be recruited to maintain cardiac output, and even these may not be sufficient.

Afterload is a measure of the systolic ventricular wall stress required to eject blood. The resistance circuit into which the ventricle ejects blood is an important determinant of afterload. Although blood pressure is sometimes used to quantitate afterload, it is the peripheral vascular resistance that is more important. The cardiac output (CO), blood pressure (BP), and systemic vascular resistance (SVR) are related in the following equation:

$$CO = \frac{BP}{SVR}$$

The concept of afterload is of particular importance in patients with hypertension or ventricular dysfunction. In the latter group, impaired contractility results in decreased cardiac output. This, in turn, results in compensatory physiologic changes in an attempt to maintain perfusion by an increase in systemic vascular resistance. These changes, however, may further impair ventricular function by increasing the wall stress required to eject blood.

The end-diastolic volume depends primarily on filling pressure, filling time, and diastolic compliance. The well-known Frank Starling curves (Figure 2) relate the degree of ventricular muscle stretch (preload) to a measure of performance, for example, cardiac output at a given level of myocardial contractility. Although the stretch of a muscle fiber (preload) can be easily measured experimentally, it cannot be quantitated clinically. Stretch can be correlated with diastolic volume. In turn, diastolic volume can be measured at angiography by nuclear medicine techniques or with echocardiography. More often, preload is assessed by measurement of the left ventricular end-diastolic pres-

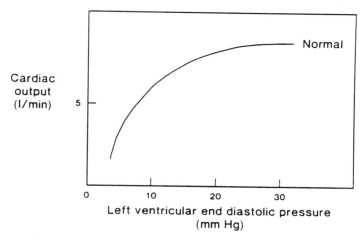

Figure 2. Frank Starling curve of cardiac output compared with left ventricular end-diastolic pressure.

sure. The relationship between volume and pressure is a measure of the compliance of the ventricle. Patients with hypertrophied, stiff, noncompliant ventricles require a higher pressure to achieve the same diastolic volume (stretch) as that required in a normal ventricle.

In addition to preload and afterload, ventricular function also affects cardiac output. Depending upon the underlying contractility, a change in the preload may significantly improve cardiac performance or change it very little (Figure 3). In a patient with significant left ventricular impairment and an increased left ventricular end-diastolic pressure, increasing the preload further may not alter cardiac output.

In addition to determinants of cardiac output, the concept of VA conduction is essential to the understanding of hemodynamics. Activation of mechanoreceptors (stretch receptors) within the walls of the atria and pulmonary veins results in peripheral vasodilatation and a decrease in systemic blood pressure (Figure 4). Either ventricular systole when the AV valves are open or atrial systole when the AV valves are closed can result in activation of these receptors.

In each patient, the relative roles of heart rate, stroke volume, and VA conduction vary. The relationship of these variables is confounded by the presence or absence of structural heart disease with impaired ventricular function, by the fluid status of the patient, and by the effect of cardioactive and vasoactive medications. In Table I, some potential combinations of stroke volume and heart rate changes are shown.

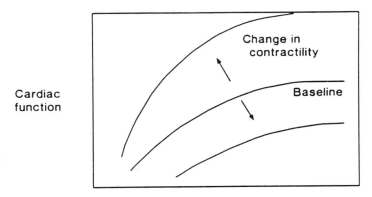

Figure 3. *Schematic of a family of ventricular function curves. Changes in contractility affect the relationship between myocardial fiber stretch (preload) and cardiac performance.*

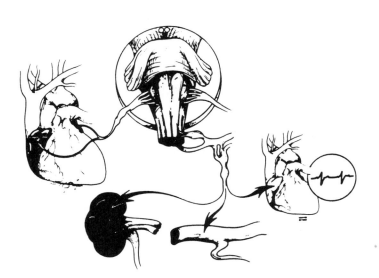

Figure 4. *Potential reflex mechanisms important in evaluation of VA conduction. VA conduction results in activation of stretch receptors in atria and pulmonary veins (upper left). Activation of stretch receptors results in reflex sinus bradycardia (lower right), peripheral vasodilatation, and a decrease in systemic blood pressure (lower middle). Activation of these stretch receptors could also result in changes in renal blood flow (lower left). By permission of Mayo Foundation.*

Table I
Relationship Among Stroke Volume (SV), Heart Rate (HR), and Cardiac Output (CO)

HR × SV = CO	
↑HR × ↑SV = ↑CO	Usual response to exercise
↑HR × ↑SV = ↑CO	Highly trained athlete
HR fixed × ↑SV = ↑ CO	Response to exercise in patient with fixed-rate ventricular pacemaker and normal ventricle
HR fixed × SV fixed or ↓ = ↔ CO or ↓CO	Response to exercise in patient with fixed-rate ventricular pacemaker and abnormal left ventricular function
↑HR × SV↑ or ↔ = ↑CO	Response to exercise in patient with rate-responsive pacemaker

VENTRICULAR PACING

The earliest indication for cardiac pacing was high- grade or complete heart block with recurrent Stokes-Adams attacks. In patients with this disorder, establishing a stable ventricular rhythm was life-saving and prevented catastrophic asystole. This fact alone overshadowed the observation that although ventricular pacing changed the rhythm from a ventricular escape focus with a rate of 35–70 beats per minute and improved cardiac output or patients' symptoms, normal function did not return in these patients. In addition, some patients with intermittent heart block actually experienced symptomatic hemodynamic deterioration with ventricular pacing (Figure 5). This was

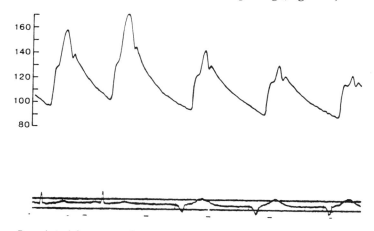

Figure 5. *Arterial pressure changes at onset of ventricular demand pacing. The first two normal sinus beats result in a systolic blood pressure of 160–170 mm Hg. With the onset of ventricular demand pacing, the systolic blood pressure falls to 125 mm Hg.*

even more of a problem in patients paced for symptomatic intermittent sinus bradycardia, who as a group have a high incidence of intact VA conduction.

From the original indication (complete heart block) the selection criteria have broadened. The change in indications for pacing has been accompanied by a change in the expectations of patients and physicians. The basic goal of preventing symptomatic bradycardia or asystole remains but now includes restoring as closely as possible the normal adaptive features of the cardiovascular system. As previously mentioned, ventricular pacing, although providing a stable, reliable ventricular rate, in some patients it is not optimal in preventing symptoms, because (1) it compromises AV synchrony, (2) it may result in VA conduction, and (3) it results in a fixed heart rate.

Compromise of AV Synchrony

The maintenance of normal AV synchrony has many potential beneficial effects. These have been documented to include reducing oxygen requirements, increasing cardiac output, and improving ventricular filling. In addition, in patients requiring permanent pacing, maintenance of AV synchrony can help to prevent many of the arrhythmias associated with single-chamber pacemakers. Ventricular-demand pacing compromises AV synchrony. The importance of AV synchrony for the specific patient depends upon the volume status, the status of ventricular function, and the level of cardiac output required (Table II, III).

Table II
Maintenance of AV Synchrony
Resting State

Normal ventricular filling and normal or noncompliant ventricle
    a) maintains optimal preload
    b) contributes up to 20% of cardiac output compared to ventricular
       pacing
    c) prevents elevation of venous pressure seen with atrial systole against
       a closed AV valve or ventricular systole with an open AV valve
    d) prevents AV valve regurgitiation seen with ventricular systole and an
       open AV valve
Left ventricular impairment and elevated filling pressure
    a) diminishing effect on cardiac output inversely proportional to the
       degree of left ventricular impairment
    b) prevents AV valve regurgitation seen with ventricular systole against
       an open AV valve

Table III
Maintenance of AV Synchrony

Moderate–Maximal Exercise

Normal ventricular filling and normal or noncompliant ventricle
    a) maintains optimal timed preload
    b) contributes only small amount of increased cardiac output (<10%)
       compared to rate matched asynchronous pacing
    c) prevents AV valve regurgitation seen with ventricular systole against
       an open AV valve
Left ventricular impairment and elevated filling pressure
    a) little effect on improving cardiac output
    b) prevents AV valve regurgitation seen with ventricular systole against
       an open AV valve

Atrial Systole

Atrial systole has been studied in detail in experimental preparations and in patients with and without structural cardiovascular disease. Atrial systole has several functions. In the low-pressure venous circulation, atrial systole maintains a reduced pressure and improves venous return. It acts as a pump to enhance ventricular filling. Atrial systole may contribute up to 20–30% of the cardiac output under certain clinical conditions (Figure 6). The specific size of this contribution depends heavily on the basic physiologic principles previously discussed. By enhancing ventricular filling, atrial systole increases preload and may improve myocardial performance. Improvement depends, however, on the level of myocardial contractility and the initial preload or fiber stretch. In a failing ventricle with an end-diastolic pressure that is markedly elevated, a further increase in preload may not improve cardiac output at all. However, in patients with a more normal left ventricular end-diastolic pressure and a hypertrophied, noncompliant ventricle, such as those with myocardial hypertrophy, increasing preload by restoration of normal atrial systole may significantly increase cardiac output.

AV Synchrony

The timing of AV valve closure is also of great importance. In the absence of AV synchrony, atrial systole may occur against a closed AV valve, or ventricular systole may occur with open AV valves. In the former, atrial systole results in elevation of venous pressure, whereas in the latter, both AV valve insufficiency and elevation of venous pressure occur.

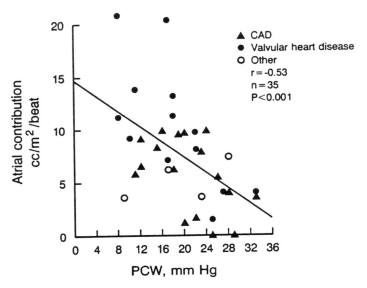

Figure 6. The importance of the atrial contribution depends on the filling pressure. There is an inverse relationship between absolute atrial contribution and the level of pulmonary capillary wedge pressure that reflects end-diastolic pressure. From Greenberg B, Chatterjee K, et al: The influence of left ventricular filling pressure on atrial contribution to cardiac output. From Am Heart J 98(6):742-751, 1979, with permission.

The interval between atrial and ventricular systole is also important. This may vary from patient to patient depending upon the pacing rate and on ventricular compliance. Ventricular filling occurs in two phases with passive filling immediately after the opening of the AV valve, and active filling during atrial systole. Maximizing ventricular filling, particularly during the active phase, results in optimal preload and thereby achieves the optimal cardiac output. In patients without congestive heart failure, cardiac output is optimal at an AV interval of 100–150 msec during pacing at rates from 80–120 beats per minute. As can be seen, with shorter AV intervals (<75 msec), the cardiac output is less (Figure 7). With such a short AV interval, the lower cardiac output may be the result of suboptimal ventricular filling during atrial systole, or from AV valve regurgitation. At longer AV intervals, there is also deterioration of cardiac output. In patients with impaired left ventricular function and high filling pressures, the role of AV synchrony is less important than the ability to increase heart rate. In patients with normal AV conduction, the PR interval shortens as the heart rate increases. In an effort to optimize hemodynamics and more closely simulate normal conduction, newer dual

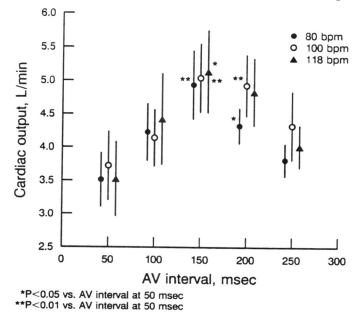

Figure 7. *Relationship between AV interval and cardiac output at different rates (80, 100, 110 bpm). In this study, the maximal cardiac output was seen at an AV interval of 150 msec. From Haskell RJ, French WJ: Optimum AV interval in dual chamber pacemakers. From PACE 9:670-675, 1986, with permission.*

chamber pacemakers allow progressive shortening of the programmed AV interval as the atrial rate increases.

The effect of the atrial and ventricular activation sequence must also be considered. Cardiac output varies with pacing from different ventricular sites. Atrioventricular sequential pacing with pacing activation of the right ventricular apex is not equivalent to atrial pacing at the same AV interval with conduction through the AV node. In patients with dual-chamber systems, it may be best to maximize the potential for normal AV node conduction by making the pacemaker AV interval as long as possible. As mentioned, however, in patients with dual-chamber pacing and complete AV block, optimal AV intervals is approximately 150±25 msec.

VA Conduction

The importance of VA conduction has become increasingly well recognized (Table IV). In patients with permanent pacemakers, intact

Table IV
Effects of Ventricular Pacing with
Retrograde Ventriculoatrial Conduction

Reciprocal (ECHO) beats
Cannon waves
Elevation of:
    Mean right atrial pressures
    Pulmonary wedge pressures
Decrease cardiac output

VA conduction may result in pacemaker-mediated arrhythmias. In patients with ventricular pacemakers, VA conduction may result in the pacemaker syndrome (Table V). VA conduction, as previously mentioned, may result in AV valve insufficiency and abnormal venous pulsations that may be bothersome to the patients. More importantly, VA conduction can result in activation of stretch mechanoreceptors in the walls of the atria and pulmonary veins. Vagal afferents transmit these impulses centrally, and the result is reflex peripheral vasodilatation, which may cause dizziness, near-syncope, or syncope. This constellation of symptoms, characterized by abnormal venous pulsations, weakness, dizziness, and hypotension occurring with the onset of ventricular pacing, has been termed the "pacemaker syndrome" (Table V; Figure 8). In addition to the VA conduction, loss of AV synchrony and the atrial contribution to ventricular filling may be important.

Table V
Pacemaker Syndrome

Symptoms
    Jugular venous distension and pulsations
    Weakness, dizziness, near-syncope
    Hypotension
    Precordial distress
Physiology
    "Cannon waves" in the jugular venous system
    "Cannon waves" in the pulmonary venous system
    Cyclic variation in cardiac output, arterial
        pressure, peripheral vascular resistance
Etiology
    Intact VA conduction with activation of arterial
        stretch receptors
    Loss of AV synchrony

ATRIAL SYNCHRONOUS

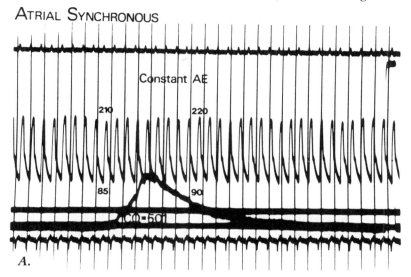

A.

V-PACED

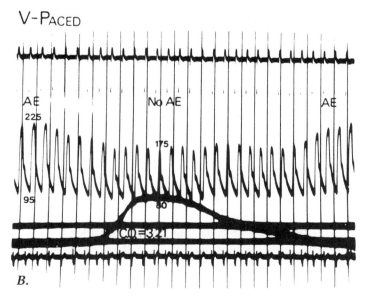

B.

Figure 8. *Composite hemodynamics.* **A.** *During atrial synchronous pacing, blood pressure is constant at 210/85, with cardiac output of 5 liters/min.* **B.** *During ventricular pacing, blood pressure decreases from 225/95 to 175/80, and cardiac output is 3.2 liters/min. AE = atrial and ventricular synchrony.*

Increasing knowledge about the hemodynamics of pacing, recognition of the limitations of ventricular demand systems, development of reliable atrial lead systems, and advances in pacemaker technology have all contributed to the increasing interest in pacing systems that more closely simulate normal sinoatrial, AV nodal, and His-Purkinje function. None of the current units function as well as normal "standard equipment," that is, a normal conduction system, but new technology approaches normal physiology by allowing restoration of AV synchrony and rate responsiveness.

HEART RATE REGULATION

The importance that an increase in heart rate plays on the ability to respond to exercise has received increasing interest. It has also been the subject of conflicting opinions based upon the degree of exercise and the presence or absence as well as severity of ventricular dysfunction. Early reports documented "at comparable heart rates, a disappointingly small but significant increase in cardiac index with atrial triggering, rather than with ventricular pacing."* This was of academic interest in studying the physiology of the circulatory response to exercise. It, however, has become of practical concern with the development of rate responsive pacemakers. Subsequent studies have focused on the relative role of rate responsiveness versus AV synchrony and have found that the ability to increase heart rate accounts for most of the increase in cardiac output seen with either exercise or an increase in paced rate. This rate responsiveness is of even more importance in patients with ventricular dysfunction. They are already operating at a high filling pressure and further augmentation by atrial systole is less important. In addition, in these patients the ventricular dysfunction often precludes the ability to increase stroke volume in response to exercise.

ATTEMPTS TO MAINTAIN PHYSIOLOGIC RESPONSE TO EXERCISE

Interest in simulating or restoring the normal response of the cardiovascular system to increasing demands such as exercise dates to the 1950s. Attempts at restoring atrial synchrony by sensing of the

---

*Escher DJW, Schwedel JB, Schwartz LS, Solomon N: Transvenous electrical stimulation of the heart. Annals New York Academy of Science 11:988, 1964.

atrium and pacing of the ventricle were the first steps. These attempts were limited by the lack of stable, reliable transvenous leads for atrial sensing and pacing. Early systems allowed atrial sensing but had no ventricular sensing circuits. The development of leads which permitted stable atrial pacing then fostered widespread attempts at restoration of AV synchrony with AV sequential units. In these units, rate responsiveness was lacking. Attempts to simulate the normal response to exercise have expanded with the use of DDD units. These units return to the concept of atrial sensing and tracking with maintenance of AV synchrony. Development continues with sensor driven, single and dual chamber, rate-responsive pacemakers. Dual chamber, sensor driven, rate-responsive pacemakers (DDDR) may be the optimal units for simulating the normal response to exercise.

Atrial Pacing (AAI)

Atrial pacing systems were among the first devices used. Their application was initially limited by technologic problems with inability to maintain a permanent atrial lead with adequate pacing and sensing thresholds. These problems have been solved. Use of these systems, however, continues to remain limited because patients with sinus bradycardia who would otherwise be excellent candidates may have associated AV nodal disease that could be progressive and result in unstable and unreliable AV conduction.

Atrial pacing preserves AV synchrony, maintains the normal AV nodal conduction sequence, optimizes cardiac output, reduces myocardial oxygen consumption at a given work load, and prevents VA conduction. In addition, it prevents atrial bradycardia and may decrease supraventricular arrhythmias by suppressing escape or ectopic focus discharge. These factors are of particular importance in patients with left ventricular dysfunction. However, patients in whom atrial pacing would be considered, for example, sinus node dysfunction, may have chronotropic incompetence and atrial demand pacing (AAI) would not restore rate responsiveness.

Atrial Synchronous Pacing (VAT, VDD)

Atrial synchronous pacemakers were introduced in 1962 and 1963. These units sense atrial activity and then pace the ventricle after a preset AV interval. Early units were limited by the instability of atrial leads, the requirement for thoracotomy, and the lack of ventricular sensing (VAT). Later units incorporated a second sensing circuit for ventricular sensing (VDD), a feature that decreased the potential for ventricular competition.

The major advantage of these systems is the ability to track increasing atrial rate and match it with an increase in ventricular rate in a 1:1 fashion at a normal AV interval. Normal AV synchrony is thereby maintained both at rest and during exercise and allows for improved hemodynamics with a more normal increase in cardiac output due to an increase in heart rate (Figures 9, 10). Atrial synchronous (VDD) units are not widely used, since atrial synchronous function is part of normal DDD function.

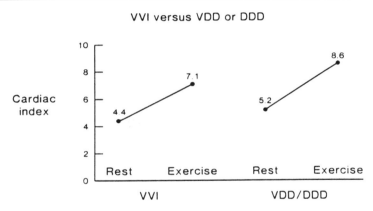

HEMODYNAMIC RESPONSE TO EXERCISE

Figure 9. Hemodynamic response to exercise in 13 patients programmed to either VVI or VDD/DDD pacing. When programmed to VVI mode, with exercise the peak cardiac index was lower at 7.1 liters/min/m², compared to 8.6 liters/min/m² when the pulse generator was programmed to VDD/DDD mode.

AV Sequential Pacing

In the past, AV sequential pacing was used more frequently than atrial inhibited and atrial synchronous, ventricular inhibited pacing. The major advantages of AV sequential pacing are that it maintains AV synchrony, prevents sinus bradycardia, and, because of the lack of atrial sensing, eliminates some of the unfavorable consequences of VA conduction. Both temporary and permanent AV sequential systems have been documented to increase cardiac output over that produced by ventricular pacing alone (Figure 11).

The major disadvantages of AV sequential pacing are the lack of

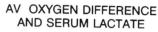

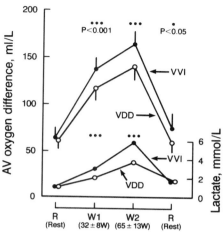

Figure 10. Comparison of AV oxygen difference and serum lactate in patients with VVI versus VDD pacing. The latter is associated with an improved hemodynamic response to the demands of exercise. From Kruse, et al: Circulation 65:846, 1982, with permission.

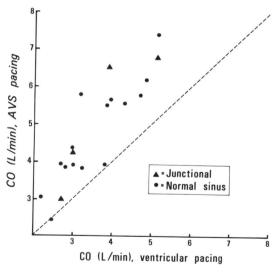

Figure 11. Hemodynamic effect of AV sequential (AVS) pacing compared with ventricular demand pacing. Cardiac output (CO) is improved with AVS pacing. By permission of Mayo Foundation; Curtis J, Maloney J, Hartzler G.

rate responsiveness, that is, the lack of P-synchronous pacing, and the potential for atrial arrhythmias due to competitive atrial pacing. The lack of response to physiologic atrial rate increases with exercise is a major problem in some patients, particularly those with a very active life style.

DDD Systems

DDD systems were developed to overcome the limitations of previous pacing methods. Specifically, they provide atrial pacing during atrial bradycardia, ventricular pacing during ventricular bradycardia, and atrial and ventricular pacing during combined atrial and ventricular bradycardia. In addition, they provide an atrial synchronous mode. These features more closely approximate the normal response to exercise by permitting a rate increase in response to exercise in patients with normal chronotropic response (Figure 12). This increase improves cardiac output in patients with normal or noncompliant ventricles and facilitates maintenance of AV synchrony (Figure 9). In active, vigorous patients, these accomplishments are both important in maintaining a more normal response to physiologic stress, such as that associated with exercise.

DDD pacing devices have clear-cut theoretical advantages and, in specific patients, definite practical advantages. These advantages have resulted in the widespread use of these devices. There are trade-offs, however. Because the timing cycles for each chamber are initiated by either a sensed or a paced beat, the cycles are independent but closely related, and multiprogrammability is available, analysis of function may be very difficult. As was true with VDD units, the potential for pacemaker-mediated tachycardia exists, although with optimal patient selection and the extensive programmability available, particularly programmability of the atrial refractory period, this possibility can be minimized. Finally, the upper rate behavior or inappropriate programming (see Chapter 17) may result in symptoms. If the pacemaker goes into 2:1 block at the upper rate when a patient is exercising, significant symptoms may result. The development of upper rate fallback or rate smoothing mechanisms and Wenckebach behavior is an important feature in minimizing such symptoms

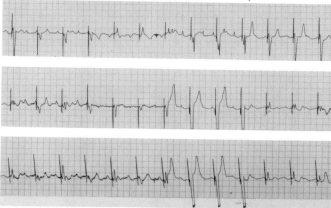

A. Peak Exercise in VVI mode Sinus rate ≃ 175 BPM

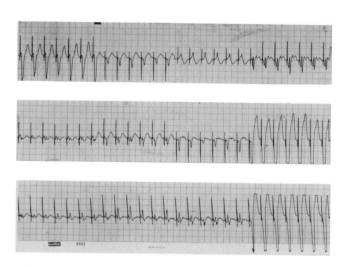

B. 1:1 pacing in DDD mode during exercise (HR = 150 BPM)

Figure 12.   *Exercise response with pacemaker programmed VVI and then programmed DDD.* **A.** *At peak of exercise with VVI pacing, atrial rate is approximately 175 beats per minute (bpm), whereas ventricular rate is fixed.* **B.** *At peak of exercise with DDD pacing, there is atrial tracking up to 150 bpm and 1:1 AV conduction.*

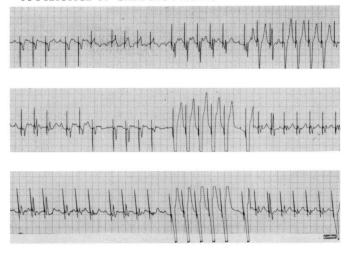

Upper rate limit exceeded producing Wenckebach effect during exercise

Figure 13. *Response of DDD pacemaker when programmable upper rate is exceeded during exercise. Wenckebach effect is produced.*

(Figure 13). The advantages of preserving as closely as possible the normal cardiovascular response to exercise must be balanced by the increased cost and complexity of the units themselves.

Although current DDD units can maintain AV synchrony and have an atrial synchronous mode, they have no rate response mode in patients with persistent sinus bradycardia. A rate responsive dual-chamber mode would be ideal in this regard.

Rate Responsive Pacemakers

A wide variety of physiologic sensors are either in use or under clinical investigation (see Chapter 11). The ideal sensor should accurately reflect cardiac output, allow for an increase in rate within 30–60 seconds after the onset of exercise, and should allow for a closed feedback loop. Single-chambered activity sensing units are now the most commonly implanted pacemakers (Figure 14). These allow for an increase in heart rate with exercise and an increase in cardiac output which closely, although not completely, equates that seen with atrial triggered pacing. In the patient with sinus node dysfunction and chronotropic incompetence, with high filling pressures and impaired left ventricular function, in whom the importance of AV synchrony is

AAI Activitrax
Without magnet

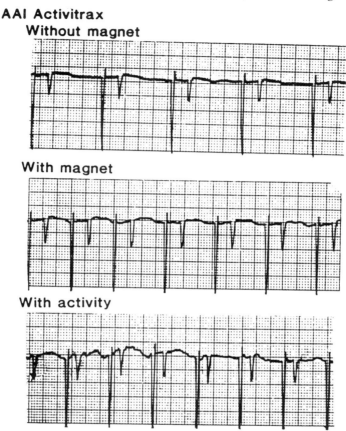

With magnet

With activity

Figure 14.   *Electrocardiographic tracings from a patient with an activity sensing rate modulated pacemaker used in the AAIR mode. Upper tracing is non-magnet tracing with atrium paced at 60 ppm. Middle panel shows atrium paced at 85 ppm with magnet application. Lower panel demonstrates response to activity. The atrium is being paced at approximately 100 ppm with each paced atrial depolarization followed by intrinsic QRS complex.*

less, these rate responsive units are more "physiologic" than current DDD pacemakers which are only rate responsive in a VDD mode. These single-chamber units, however, do not prevent the deleterious effect of VA conduction with AV valve regurgitation, elevation in venous pressure, and activation of baroreceptors due to atrial stretch. Dual-chamber multisensor pacing units should allow for rate responsiveness as well as maintenance of normal AV synchrony.

The options available for patients requiring permanent pacemakers have increased substantially. Selection of the optimal unit for a specific patient has accordingly become more complex. Given the importance of selecting the optimal unit and avoiding the unit that will not yield optimal clinical and hemodynamic results, considerable care must be taken prior to implantation. It is essential to understand the hemodynamics of cardiac pacing. This must be modified by the understanding that predicting the response of a specific patient is difficult. Selection of a physiologic pacing system for any given person must be based upon the clinical setting, the conduction disturbance requiring pacing, associated disease states, and expected hemodynamic benefit or adverse consequences of the pacing system selected. The frequency with which specific physiologic systems are used varies widely among institutions. A blanket policy dictating the use of only ventricular demand pacemakers or exclusive physiologic pacemakers is suboptimal. The best approach is to select the right pacemaker with the proper flexibility to meet the patient's clinical needs and to optimize the clinical situation.

BIBLIOGRAPHY

Akhtar M: Retrograde conduction in man. *PACE* 1981; 4:548–562.

Ausubel K, Furman S: The pacemaker syndrome. *Ann Int Med* 1985; 103:420–429.

Baller D, Hoeft A, Korb H, Wolpers HG, Zipfel J, Hellige G: Basic physiological studies on cardiac pacing with special reference to the optimal mode and rate after cardiac surgery. *Thorac Cardiovasc Surg* 1981; 29:168–173.

Benchimol A, Duenas A, Liggett MS, Dimond EG: Contribution of atrial systole to the cardiac function at a fixed and at a variable ventricular rate. *Am J Cardiol* 1965; 16:11–21.

Benchimol A, Ellis JG, Dimond EG: Hemodynamic consequences of atrial and ventricular pacing in patients with normal and abnormal hearts: Effect of exercise at a fixed atrial and ventricular rate. *Am J Med* 1965; 39:911–922.

Benditt D, Mianulli M, Fetter J: Single chamber cardiac pacing with activity-initiated chronotropic response: Evaluation by cardiopulmonary exercise testing. *Circulation* 1987; 75:184–189.

Brockman SK, Collins HA, Bloomfield DA, Sinclair-Smith BC, Gobbel WG: Physiological studies and clinical experience in patients with synchronous and asynchronous pacemakers. *J Thorac Cardiovasc Surg* 1966; 51: 864–872.

Edhag O, Fagrell B, Lagergren H: Deleterious effects of cardiac pacing in a patient with mitral insufficiency. *Acta Med Scand* 1977; 202:331–334.

Erlebacher JA, Danner RL, Stelzer PE: Hypotension with ventricular pacing: An atrial vasodepressor reflex in human beings. *JACC* 1984; 4:550–555.

Fananapazir L, Bennett DH, Monks P: Atrial synchronized ventricular pacing: Contribution of the chronotropic response to improved exercise performance. *PACE* 1983; 6:601–608.

Furman S: Therapeutic uses of atrial pacing. *Am Heart J* 1973; 86:835–840.

Gilmore JP, Sarnoff SJ, Mitchell JH, Linden RJ: Synchronicity of ventricular contraction: Observations comparing haemodynamic effects of atrial and ventricular pacing. *Br Heart J* 1963; 25:299–307.

Greenberg B, Chatterjee K, Parmley WW, Werner JA, Holly AN: The influence of left ventricular filling pressure on atrial contribution to cardiac output. *Am Heart J* 1979: 98:742–751.

Hartzler GO, Maloney JD, Curtis JJ, Barnhorst DA: Hemodynamic benefits of atrioventricular sequential pacing after cardiac surgery. *Am J Cardiol* 1977; 40:232–236.

Hayes D, Furman S: Stability of AV conduction in patients with implanted atrial pacemakers. *Am Heart J* 1984; 107:644–647.

Humen DP, Kostuk WJ, Klein GJ: Activity-sensing, rate-responsive pacing: Improvement in myocardial performance with exercise. *PACE* 1985; 8:52–59.

Johnson AD, Laiken SL, Engler RL: Hemodynamic compromise associated with ventriculoatrial conduction following transvenous pacemaker placement. *Am J Med* 1978; 65:75–79.

Karlöf I: Haemodynamic effect of atrial triggered versus fixed rate pacing at rest and during exercise in complete heart block. *Acta Med Scand* 1975; 197:195–206.

Kristensson BE, Arnman K, Smedgård P, Rydén L: Physiological versus single-rate ventricular pacing: A double-blind cross-over study. *PACE* 1985; 8:73–84.

Kroetz FW, Leonard JJ, Shaver JA, Leon DF, Lancaster JF, Beamer VL: The effect of atrial contraction on left ventricular performance in valvular aortic stenosis. *Circulation* 1967: 35:852–867.

Kruse IB, Arnman K, Conradson TB, Rydén L: A comparison of the acute and long-term hemodynamic effects of ventricular inhibited and atrial synchronous ventricular inhibited pacing. *Circulation* 1982; 65:846–855.

Kruse IB, Rydén L: Comparison of physical work capacity and systolic time intervals with ventricular inhibited and atrial synchronous ventricular inhibited pacing. *Br Heart J* 1981; 46:129–136.

Leinbach RC, Chamberlain DA, Kastor JA, Harthorne JW, Sanders CA: A comparison of the hemodynamic effects of ventricular and sequential A-V pacing in patients with heart block. *Am Heart J* 1969; 78:502–508.

Levine PA, Mace RC: Hemodynamic concepts applied to cardiac pacing. In: Levine PA, Mace RC (eds). Pacing Therapy: A Guide to Cardiac Pacing for Optimum Hemodynamic Benefit. Mount Kisco, New York: *Futura Publishing Company*, 1983: 19–40.

Linden RJ, Mitchell JH: Relation between left ventricular diastolic pressure and myocardial segment length and observations on the contribution of atrial systole. *Circ Res* 1960; 8:1092–1099.

Little RC: Effect of atrial systole on ventricular pressure and closure of the A-V valves. *Am J Physiol* 1951; 166:289–295.

Mitsui T, Hori M, Suma K, Saigusa M: Optimal heart rate in cardiac pacing in coronary sclerosis and non-sclerosis. *Ann NY Acad Sci* 1969; 167:745–755.

Morris JJ Jr, Entman M, North WC, Kong Y, McIntosh H: The changes in cardiac output with reversion of atrial fibrillation to sinus rhythm. *Circulation* 1965; 31:670–678.

Narula OS, Samet P, Javier RP: Atrioventricular conduction defects in patients with sinus bradycardia. *Circulation* 1971; 44:1096–1110.

Nishimura RA, Gersh BJ, Vlietstra RE, Osborn MJ, Ilstrup DM, Holmes DR Jr: Hemodynamic and symptomatic consequences of ventricular pacing. *PACE* 1982; 5:903–910.

Ogawa S, Dreifus LS, Shenoy PN, Brockman SK, Berkovits BV: Hemodynamic consequences of atrioventricular and ventriculoatrial pacing. *PACE* 1978; 1:8–15.

Panidis I, Dreifus LS, Michelson EL: Hemodynamic effects of cardiac pacing. *Cardiovasc Clin* 1983; 14(no. 2):1–11.

Perrins EJ, Morley CA, Chan SL, Sutton R: Randomised controlled trial of physiological and ventricular pacing. *Br Heart J* 1983; 50:112–117.

Rahimtoola SH, Ehsani A, Sinno MZ, Loeb HS, Rosen KM, Gunnar RM: Left atrial transport function in myocardial infarction: Importance of its booster pump function. *Am J Med* 1975; 59:686–694.

Raza ST, Lajos TZ, Bhayana JN, Lee AB Jr, Lewin AN, Gehring B, Schimert G: Improved cardiovascular hemodynamics with atrioventricular sequential pacing compared with ventricular demand pacing. *Ann Thorac Surg* 1984; 38:260–264.

Reiter MJ, Hindman MC: Hemodynamic effects of acute atrioventricular sequential pacing in patients with left ventricular dysfunction. *Am J Cardiol* 1982; 49:687–692.

Rickards AF, Donaldson RM, Thalen HJ: The use of QT interval to determine pacing rate: Early clinical experience. *PACE* 1983; 6:346–354.

Rosen KM, Loeb HS, Sinno MZ, Rahimtoola SH, Gunnar RM: Cardiac conduction in patients with symptomatic sinus node disease. *Circulation* 1971; 43:836–844.

Ryden L, Kruse B: Hemodynamic aspects of physiologic pacing. In: Barold SS (ed). Modern Cardiac Pacing. Mount Kisco, New York: *Futura Publishing Company*, 1985; 19–32.

Samet P: Hemodynamic sequelae of cardiac arrhythmias. *Circulation* 1973; 47:339–407.

Samet P, Bernstein WH, Levine S: Significance of the atrial contribution to ventricular filling. *Am J Cardiol* 1965; 15:195–202.

Samet P, Bernstein WH, Medow A, Nathan DA: Effect of alterations in ventricular rate on cardiac output in complete heart block. *Am J Cardiol* 1964; 14:477–482.

Samet P, Bernstein WH, Nathan DA, López A: Atrial contribution to cardiac output in complete heart block. *Am J Cardiol* 1965; 16:1–10.

Samet P, Castillo C, Bernstein WH: Hemodynamic sequelae of atrial, ventricular, and sequential atrioventricular pacing in cardiac patients. *Am Heart J* 1966; 72:725–729.

Samet P, Castillo C, Bernstein WH: Hemodynamic consequences of sequential atrioventricular pacing: Subjects with normal hearts. *Am J Cardiol* 1968; 21:207–212.

Samet P, Castillo C, Bernstein WH, Fernandez P: Hemodynamic results of right atrial pacing in cardiac subjects. *Dis Chest* 1968; 53:133–137.

Shapland JE, MacCarter D, Tockman B, Knudson M: Physiologic benefits of rate responsiveness. *PACE* 1983; 6:329–332.

Simon AB, Janz N: Symptomatic bradyarrhythmias in the adult: Natural history following ventricular pacemaker implantation. *PACE* 1982; 5:372–383.

Sutton R, Morley C, Chan SL, Perrins J: Physiological benefits of atrial synchrony in paced patients. *PACE* 1983; 6:327–328.

Vallin H, Edhag O: Associated conduction disturbances in patients with symptomatic sinus node disease. *Acta Med Scand* 1981; 210:263–270.

van Mechelen R, Hagemeijer F, de Boer H, Schelling A: Atrioventricular and ventriculo-atrial conduction in patients with symptomatic sinus node dysfunction. *PACE* 1983; 6:13–21.

Chapter 6

PACEMAKER CODES

Seymour Furman

ICHD CODE

Implantable pacemakers have a variety of different modes of operation. They may pace atrium or ventricle and be insensitive to the chambers paced. They may sense and pace one chamber, sense one chamber and pace the other, sense one and pace both, or pace and sense both. Pacemaker codes were designed to indicate pacemaker function so that, despite the model pacemaker or pacemaker name, the mode of operation will be known. The first pacemaker code was published in 1974 by the pacemaker committee of the Intersociety Commission for Heart Disease Resources and has been widely adopted and used internationally for pulse generator designation. It is well understood and has been adopted by regulation in some jurisdictions. The code is so widely used that some know what the three-position describes about a specific generator without being aware of the meaning of each letter of the three positions. The code was modified in 1981 by the members of the original committee under NASPE auspices and extended to five positions. The revised code was then reemphasized in a second ICHD report in 1983. The first three positions are basic to the code and constituted a complete designation. The latest revision, i.e., the 1987 NBG code, requires four positions for completeness (Table I).

NBG CODE

The rapid evolution in bradycardia and tachycardia pacing has necessitated a revision in the existing ICHD/NASPE five-position code. To maintain its usefulness, the code has undergone three revisions since its introduction in 1974. The initial revision was an expansion from three to five positions to represent programmability in position IV and tachycardia management in position V. The latest revision (1987) expands its utility into rate-modulated pacemakers and refines the description of techniques of tachycardia management in position V.

Table I
The Five-Position ICHD Code

Position	I	II	III	IV	V
Category	Chamber(s) paced	Chamber(s) sensed	Modes of response(s)	Programmable functions	Special antitachyarrhythmia functions
Letters used	V—ventricle	V—ventricle	T—triggered	P—programmable (rate and/or output)	B—bursts
	A—atrium	A—atrium	I—inhibited	M—multiprogrammable	N—normal rate competition
	D—double	D—double	D—double*	C—communicating	S—scanning
		O—none	O—none	O—none	E—external
			R—reverse		A—active antitachycardia fixation otherwise undefined
Manufacturer's designation only	S—single chamber	S—single chamber		Comma optional here	

*Triggered and inhibited response.

Modified and reprinted with permission of Futura Publishing Company from Bernstein et al: Report of the NASPE Mode Code Committee. *PACE* 7:396, 1984.

The basic grammar of the code has remained unchanged since its introduction. Letters have been added to each of the positions and some letters have been removed in order to increase the utility of the code as needs have changed. In the instance of tachycardia management, the letter "R" had been placed in position III to indicate a pacemaker that was inhibited at normal or slow cardiac rates but functions in a "reverse" mode in response to a tachycardia. As no such pacing mode now exists, and as all tachycardia management is now in position V, "R" was removed from position III and the letter has been used once again, now in position IV, to indicate the function of adaptive rate pacing or rate modulation.

Position V has been troublesome since its introduction, largely because of uncertainty and evolution in the field of tachycardia management. While the earlier version of the code allowed description of various modes of antitachycardia pacing, all have now been consolidated into an indication of stimulation output levels. The letter "O" indicates the absence of any antitachycardia function. The second letter "P" is for output at the microJoule or traditional pacing level and the third letter "S" is for output of one or more Joules, and is an abbreviation of "shock." The fourth letter "D" is a combination of pacing and shock, i.e., P + S, in anticipation of devices soon to be available.

It is hoped that this simplification will increase the utility of the code while avoiding attempts at specific description of techniques that may soon be obsolete. In order to provide a code for a pacemaker that has been programmed to the OFF mode, i.e., entirely inactive, the letter "O" has been allowed in each of the five positions. As each position must have a letter, just as a multidigit number requires a digit in each position, i.e., 150 differs from 1050, the placement of "O" in each of the five positions allows a meaningful sixth position when it becomes necessary.

POSITION I—designates the chamber(s) paced. Five letters are possible: "A" for atrium, "V" for ventricle, "D" if both atrium and ventricle are paced, and "O" if the unit is shut down and no pacing is to occur. The letter "S" is for manufacturer's use only and indicates that the device paces a single chamber only, but that the chamber may be either atrium or ventricle.

POSITION II—designates the chamber(s) sensed. Five possibilities exist and consequently five letters. If the atrium alone is sensed, the letter "A" is used, if the ventricle, "V." If both atrium and ventricle are sensed, the letter "D" is used, and if the pacemaker is used in either atrium or ventricle, but only in a single chamber at a time, a manufacturer may use the letter "S." "O" indicates that the pacemaker is insensitive to incoming signals. This may be used as part of the totally inactive state with an "O" in position I or a unit may be insensitive while pacing.

POSITION III—designates the response to a sensed signal. "I" indicates that pacemaker output is inhibited by a sensed event, "T" that a stimulus is triggered by a sensed event, and "D" that a stimulus may be triggered by a sensed event in one chamber and inhibited by a sensed event in the other. In practice this means ventricular inhibited and atrial triggered. The letter "O" in this position indicates that there is no mode of response to the lack of sensitivity indicated by the "O" in position II.

The three-position code is often used by manufacturers to indicate the intended use of the pulse generator. Programmable pulse generators commonly have sensitivity and refractory periods that allow use of the same generator in the atrium or the ventricle as a single-chamber device. Dual-chamber devices are, of course, used in both atrium and ventricle. To allow manufacturers to designate a pulse generator as single-chamber pacing and sensing as opposed to one that is designed for use in the atrium or the ventricle but should not be used in both chambers, the letter "S" exists in positions I and II. "S" in either position indicates that a single chamber is being paced (position I) and sensed (position II). The mode of response to sensing in position II, as the pacemaker is delivered, is designated in position III. As positions IV and V are used to indicate programmability and antitachycardia functions, the same letters available to physicians are used by manufacturers.

The increasing complexity of pacemakers has necessitated the addition and then the modification of two additional positions, IV and V.

POSITION IV—describes two different device characteristics: the degree of programmability and the presence or absence of a rate modulation mechanism. The letters are hierarchial, from the absence of function in this channel to the most complex. The assumption is that the next higher level will incorporate all of the features of all lower levels. Five letters are possible in this position. The letter "O" in this position indicates that the device is not programmable and does not provide rate modulation. The letter "P" indicates simple programmability, almost always, in practice, change in rate or output or both. "M" indicates multiprogrammability, i.e., more than two functions. The presence of sensitivity programmability will make a "P" device into an "M" device. The addition of telemetry (in practice telemetry is always added to multiprogrammable capability) allows the use of the letter "C" which is the abbreviation for "communicating." The obvious letter "T" was avoided as it had been previously used for "triggered function" in position III. The degree of programmability refers to antitachycardia features as well as (and even in the absence of) antibradycardia pacing. The last letter in this position is "R" (rate modulation) which indicates sensor-driven variation of the antibradycardia escape interval in response to a physiological or nonphysiological stimulus other than the atrium. Such stimuli include the interval from pacemaker emission to repolarization (i.e., the QT interval), respiratory rate, central venous temperature, right ventricular dP/dt, and others. Excluded are all means of upper rate limitation including AV block, Wenckebach, rate smoothing, etc.

POSITION V—indicates the presence of one or two antitachycardia functions activated manually or automatically in an implanted device when a tachycardia is anticipated or has occurred. "O" once again indicates the absence of any such capability; "P" indicates a pacing modality and includes underdrive, burst, and scanning, but at a level of electrical output of a cardiac pacemaker, i.e., in the microJoule range. "S" indicates a shock to terminate the tachyarrhythmia, i.e., at the level of Joules or several orders of magnitude above pacer output. The letter "S," used previously to indicate "single chamber," has been redefined for position V but this should offer little confusion. If the device is capable of pacing level and shock level output either simultanenously and/or successively, the letter "D" indicates both pacing and sensing (i.e., P + S).

Position V has been devised to allow its use for any electrical stimulating device that provides either bradycardia or tachycardia management or both. Unlike the earlier versions of the code, position V may be used for a bradycardia pacemaker, or for a simple, i.e., nonprogrammable defibrillator or cardioverter incapable of pacing, or for an antitachycardia device with bradycardia and tachycardia pacing functions, multiprogrammability, and the capability of emitting a shock to terminate a tachycardia (Table II).

It is important when using the code that each letter be properly positioned. The position is as important as it is in a number. The "O" designation is thus as critical as in the number system. A comma may be used (optional) after the first three positions, much as in a long

Table II
The NASPE/BPEG Generic (NBG) Pacemaker Code

Position	I	II	III	IV	V
Category	Chamber(s) paced	Chamber(s) sensed	Response to sensing	Programmability, rate modulation	Antitachyarrhythmia function(s)
	O = None	O = None	O = None	O = none	O = None
	A = Atrium	A = Atrium	T = triggered	P = Simple Programmable	P = Pacing (antitachyarrhythmia)
	V = Ventricle	V = Ventricle	I = Inhibited	M = Multiprogram-mable	S = Shock
	D = Dual (A + V)	D = Dual (A + V)	D = Dual (D + I)	C = Communicating	D = Dual (P + S)
				R = Rate modulation	
Manufacturer's designation only	S = single (A or V)	S = single (A or V)			
				Comma optional here	

Note: Positions I through III are used exclusively for antibradyarrhythmia function.

number. A complete code consists of four or five positions. Fewer than four positions is incomplete. Examples of the new code are given in Table III.

Some who write about or design pacemakers are anxious to use the code with additional letters, such as an "X" in one position or another. As the "X" is an undefined letter in this system, little clarity is added and obscurity may be caused. Because many pulse generators now being introduced have a maximum capability of pacing and sensing in both chambers, such a multiprogrammable

Table III
Examples of the NASPE/BPEG Generic (NBG) Code

Code	Meaning
VOOO or VOOOO	Asynchronous ventricular pacing. no adaptive rate control or antitachyarrhythmia functions (also VOO in clinical use but not in device labelling
DDDM or DDDMO	Multiprogrammable "physiologic" dual-chamber pacing. No adaptive rate control or antitachyarrythmia capability
VVIPP	Simple-programmable VVI pacemaker with antitachyarrythmia-pacing capability
DDDCP	DDD pacemaker with telemetry and antitachyarrythmia-pacing capability
OOOPS	Simple-programmable cardioverter, defibrillator, or cardioverter-defibrillator
OOOPD	Simple-programmable cardioverter, defibrillator, or cardioverter-defibrillator with antitachyarrythmia-pacing capability
VVIMD	Multiprogrammable VVI pacemaker with defibrillation (or cardioversion), or cardioversion and defibrillation and antitachyarrythmia-pacing capabilities
VVIR or VVIRO	VVI pacemaker with escape interval controlled adaptively by one or more unspecified variables
VVIRP	Programmable VVI pacemaker with escape interval controlled adaptively by one or more unspecified variables, also incorporating antitachyarrhythmia-pacing capability
DDDRD	Programmable DDD pacemaker with escape interval controlled adaptively by one or more unspecified variables, also incorporating antitachyarrythmia pacing capability and cardioversion (or defibrillation, or cardioversion and defibrillation) functions

unit may be designated as DDD,M but may be used in a lesser mode after implant, i.e., AAI, VVI, DVI, VDD, etc. The practice of designating the pacemaker maximum capability as well as its actual operation is useful.

THE NASPE SPECIFIC CODE

While the ICHD code and the NBG modification have been very useful and have achieved widespread acceptance, the growing complexity of cardiac pacemakers and especially the increasing availability of dual-chamber devices have necessitated another code that will, more specifically, indicate pacemaker function in management of bradyarrhythmias. The NASPE specific code can deal with this complexity. A problem with the first three positions of the ICHD code is that they may be inadequately specific for dual-chamber modes. For example, there are four possible modes in which both atrium and ventricle are sensed and paced. In one mode, a spontaneous P wave inhibits the atrial channel and triggers the ventricle. It is referred to as DDD. In another mode, a spontaneous QRS complex produces triggered responses without delay, while the P wave also triggers a stimulus in the atrium and the ventricle after a delay. No pacemaker inhibition occurs at any time. The mode is DDT. The "T" in position III indicates that no inhibition of pacemaker function ever occurs. However, there are two additional modes, one in which the atrial channel is triggered and the ventricular channel is inhibited and the other in which the atrial channel is inhibited (although sensing a P wave triggers a ventricular response) and the ventricular channel is triggered. The ICHD code cannot accommodate these two modes. They can be described clearly with the NASPE specific code.

Atrial and ventricular channel functions are described in the numerator and denominator of a ratio or fraction format. If the code is limited to one printed line, a virgule (slash) separates the atrial (numerator) from the ventricular (denominator) designation. A letter code describes pacemaker activity.

O = No antibradycardia activity in the chamber
P = Pacing
S = Sensing
I = Inhibited in response to a sensed event

T = Triggered in response to a sensed event
A = Atrial activity
V = Ventricular activity

A subscript of the chamber affected is appended to indicate the chamber in which the activity is sensed and which causes the triggered or inhibited pacemaker response. By convention, pacing is indicated first, sensing next, followed by an inhibited response (I_v or I_a), and then a triggered response (T_a or T_v). Atrial activity is listed first. The omission of a letter designation in either chamber means that it does not apply. While the order of activity is maintained, the code would be equally comprehensible if the order were not maintained. For example, P, S, I_a, I_v (correct) is no more comprehensible than I_v, P, S, I_a (incorrect).

Antitachyarrhythmia functions also are readily specified by the chamber in which they occur. The function is indicated by an uppercase letter in the chamber in which it occurs. The subscript is the chamber that prompts the specific response, much as the bradycardia is inhibited (I) or triggered (T).

U = Underdrive—pacing at a rate lower than that of the tachyarrhythmia.

B = Burst—overdrive; fixed rate pacing of limited duration at a rate greater than that of the tachyarrythmia.

R = Ramp—asynchronous pacing of limited duration and systematically varying rate, both chosen by the user

X = Extrastimulus—stimulus or stimuli synchronous with a previous event sensed by the device, with fixed or variable coupling and/or interstimulus intervals.

C = Cardioversion—delivery of a synchronized shock of preselected energy.

D = Defibrillation—delivery of an asynchronous shock of preselected energy.

The following lower-case modifiers may be applied as appropriate to any of the antitachyarrhythmia modes represented by U, B, R, X, C, and D;

a = atrial (initiated by sensing of an atrial event);
v = ventricular (initiated by sensing of a ventricular event);
e = external (activated by the user).

Each upper-case letter antitachyarrhythmia function or symbol or combination of symbols is followed by a subscript modifier. One example of combined antibradyarrhythmia and antitachyarrhythmia pacemakers can be described as follows in combined format.

A ventricular inhibited single-chamber pacemaker would be indicated as follows:

Bradyarrhythmia
atrial channel−no activity O
ventricular channel−P,S,I$_v$
The equivalent ICHD code is VVI;
the NASPE code $\dfrac{O}{P,S,I_v}$.

If this unit also has antitachycardia functions, only in the ventricle, and only prompted by external control, these would be added to the numerator. If burst (B) pacing were available under external control while defibrillator occurred automatically in response to ventricular sensed events, B$_e$D would be added to the denominator making this device. $\dfrac{0}{P,S,I_v(B_eD)}$ Antitachycardia symbols are in parentheses. Other designations are possible (Table IV).

ICHD Code	Modified Generic Code	NBG Code	NASPE Specific Code	Description
VOO	VOO	VOO	$\dfrac{O}{P}$	Ventricular pacing, asynchronous
VVI,P	VVI,P	VVI,P	$\dfrac{O}{PSI_v}$	Ventricular pacing inhibited by sensing in ventricle, simple programmable
VVI,M	VVI,M	VVI,M	$\dfrac{O}{PSI_v}$	Ventricular pacing inhibited by sensing in ventricle, multiprogrammable
VVI,C	VVI,C	VVI,C	$\dfrac{O}{PSI_v}$	Ventricular pacing inhibited by sensing in ventricle, telemetry and multiprogrammable
VVI,M	VVI,M	VVI,R	$\dfrac{O}{PSI_v}$	Ventricular inhibited multiprogrammable pacing with rate modulation
AAI,M	AAI,M	AAI,R	$\dfrac{PSI_a}{O}$	Atrial inhibited multiprogrammable pacing with rate modulation

Table IV
Examples

(Continued)

Table IV
Examples (continued)

ICHD Code	Modified Generic Code	NBG Code	NASPE Specific Code	Description
DVI,M	DVI,M	DVI,M	$\dfrac{PI_v}{PSI_v}$	Atrial pacing inhibited by sensing in ventricle; ventricular pacing inhibited by sensing in ventricle
VDD,M	VDD,M	VDD,M	$\dfrac{S}{PSI_vT_a}$	Ventricular pacing triggered by sensing in atrium, inhibited by sensing in ventricle
DDD,M	DDD,M	DDD,M	$\dfrac{PSI_aI_v}{PSI_vT_a}$	Atrial pacing inhibited by sensing in atrium or ventricle; ventricular pacing triggered by sensing in atrium, inhibited by sensing in ventricle
DDD,M	DDD,M	DDD,M	$\dfrac{PST_aI_v}{PSI_vT_a}$	Atrial pacing triggered by sensing in atrium, inhibited by sensing in ventricle; ventricular pacing triggered by sensing in atrium, inhibited by sensing in ventricle
DDD,M	DDD,M	DDD,R	$\dfrac{PSI_aI_v}{PSI_vT_a}$	Atrial pacing inhibited by sensing in atrium or ventricle; ventricular pacing triggered by sensing in atrium inhibited by sensing in ventricle with rate modulation
DDD,M	DDD,M	DDD,MS	$\dfrac{PSI_aI_v}{PSI_vT_a}$	Atrial pacing inhibited by atrial or ventricular sensing; ventricular pacing triggered by atrial sensing, inhibited by ventricular sensing; shock termination of tachyarrythmia
DDD,C	DDD,CB	DDD,CD	$\dfrac{PSI_aI_v}{PSI_vT_a(D)}$	Atrial pacing inhibited by atrial or ventricular sensing; ventricular pacing triggered by atrial sensing, inhibited by ventricular sensing; pacing termination in atrium or vetnricle of tachyarrythmia followed by a high output shock to terminate a tachyarrythmia if necessary
VVI,MB	VVI,MA	VVI,MP	$\dfrac{O}{PSI_v(B_v)}$	Ventricular pacing inhibited by sensing in ventricle; bursts in ventricle activated by tachycardia detection in ventricle

(Continued)

Table IV
Examples (continued)

ICHD Code	Modified Generic Code	NBG Code	NASPE Specific Code	Description
AAR,ON	OOO,OA	OOO,OP	$\dfrac{O(UA)}{O}$	Underdrive in atrium activated by tachycardia detection in atrium
VVI,MB VVI,MN VVI,ME	VVI,MA		$\dfrac{O}{PSI_v(B_eU_eR_eBX_eX_e)}$	Pacing in ventricle inhibited by sensing in ventricle; burst, underdrive, ramp, burst plus extrastimulus, or extrastimulus in ventricle activated externally
DDD,CB DDD,CN	DDD,CA	DDD,CP	$\dfrac{PSI_aI_v(B_aB_vU_v)}{PSI_vT_a(U_v)}$	Atrial pacing inhibited by atrial or ventricular sensing; ventricular pacing triggered by atrial sensing, inhibited by ventricular sensing; bursts in atrium or ventricle; underdrive in atrium and ventricle activated by tachycardia detection in ventricle

BIBLIOGRAPHY

Bernstein AD, Brownlee RR, Fletcher R, Gold RD, Smyth NPD, Spielman SR: Report of the NASPE mode code committee. *PACE* 1984; 7(I):395–402.

Bernstein AD, Camm AJ, Fletcher R, Gold RD, Rickards AF, Smyth NPD, Spielman SR, Sutton R: The NASPE/BPEG generic pacemaker code for antibradyarrhythmia and adaptive-rate pacing and antitachyarrhythmia devices. *PACE* 1987; 10(I):794–799.

Bernstein AD, Parsonnet V: Notation system and overlay diagrams for the analysis of paced electrocardiograms. *PACE* 1983; 6:73–80.

Bredikis JJ, Stirbys PP: A suggested code for permanent cardiac pacing leads. *PACE* 1985; 8:320–321.

Brownlee RR, Shimmel-Golden JB, DelMarco CJ, et al: A new symbolic language for diagramming pacemaker/heart interaction. *PACE* 1982; 5:700–709.

Brownlee RR, Shimmel JB, DelMarco CJ: A new code for pacemaker operating modes. *PACE* 1981; 4:396–399.

Furman S: Coding for pacemaker leads. *PACE* 1985; 8:319 (editorial).

Furman S: Pacemaker codes. *PACE* 1981; 4:357 (editorial).

Irnich W: Development of coding system for pacemakers. *PACE* 1984; 7:882–901.

Kruse I, Markowitz T, Ryden L: Timing markers showing pacemaker behavior to aid in the follow up of a physiological pacemaker. *PACE* 1983; 6:801–805.

Olson WH, McConnell MV, Sah RL, et al: Pacemaker diagnostic diagrams. *PACE* 1985; 8:691–700.

Parsonnet V, Furman S, Smyth NPD: A revised code for pacemaker identification. Five-position pacemaker code (ICHD). *PACE* 1981; 4:400–403.

Parsonnet V, Furman S, Smyth NPD: Implantable cardiac pacemakers: Status report and resource guideline. A report of the Inter-society Commission for Heart Disease Resources. *Am J Cardiol* 1974; 34:487–500.

Parsonnet V, Furman S, Smyth NPD, et al: Optimal resources for implantable cardiac pacemakers. Report of Inter-society Commission for Heart Disease Resources. *Circulation* 1983; 68:226a–244a.

PART II.

CLINICAL CONSIDERATIONS

Chapter 7

TEMPORARY CARDIAC PACING

David R. Holmes, Jr.

Familiarity with temporary cardiac pacing is essential for those involved in the preparation for permanent cardiac pacing, and the treatment of patients in coronary care units and postsurgical wards. Knowledge of the indications, techniques, and routes of implantation, postinsertion management, and risk-benefit ratio for each patient is required for safe, reliable pacing.

INDICATIONS

The indications for temporary pacing are less controversial than those for permanent pacing (Table I). Because temporary pacing is an invasive procedure with a potential, albeit minimal, for serious complications, it is essential to analyze the benefits and the risks.

Table I
Indications for Temporary Pacing

Third-degree atrioventricular block
   Symptomatic congenital complete heart block
   Symptomatic acquired complete heart block
   Asmptomatic acquired complete heart block of new onset
   Asymptomatic complete heart block postoperatively
   Symptomatic complete heart block postoperatively
Second-degree atrioventricular block
   Symptomatic Type I
   Symptomatic Type II
   Asymptomatic Type II
Acute myocardial infarction
   Newly acquired bifascicular block
   New bundle branch block with transient complete heart block
   Type II second-degree atrioventricular block
   Complete heart block
Sinus node dysfunction
   Symptomatic bradyarrhythmias
Tachycardia—Prevention or Treatment
   Bradycardia-dependent arrhythmias
   Re-entrant arrhythmias

The indications for temporary pacing include both bradycardia and tachycardia. There are three general categories.

1. Patients with symptomatic bradycardia or symptomatic conduction defects (or both)—the indication is clear.
2. Patients with asymptomatic bradycardia or conduction defects—the decision to proceed with temporary pacing depends on assessment of the risk of development of symptomatic bradycardia.
3. Patients with tachycardia—in selected patients, temporary pacing may be used to terminate or prevent tachycardia. This is a temporary therapeutic maneuver until the tachycardia can be prevented with medications, surgery, or, in some patients, permanent pacing.

Symptomatic Bradycardia or Conduction Defects

Patients with symptomatic bradycardia with recurrent Stokes-Adams attacks, and syncope or near-syncope require temporary pacing. Patients in this category include those with second- or third-degree atrioventricular (AV) block. Block may occur in chronic conduction system disease or in acute myocardial infarction, drug intoxication, or electrolyte imbalance. Patients with sinus dysfunction and symptomatic bradycardia also may require temporary pacing. For patients in these groups with fixed conduction system lesions, the temporary pacemaker may be placed before and discontinued after permanent cardiac pacing. For patients in whom symptomatic bradycardia is reversible, for example, by discontinuing administration of drugs, the temporary pacemaker is used until an acceptable rhythm returns.

Asymptomatic Bradycardia or Conduction Defects

In patients with asymptomatic bradycardia, assessment of the risk-benefit ratio is essential, because the decision to proceed with pacing depends on the risk of *symptomatic* bradycardia developing. Patients with asymptomatic acquired complete heart block that develops postoperatively should also undergo temporary cardiac pacing. In these persons, the reliability of the escape focus is often uncertain, and the risk of symptomatic bradycardia developing outweighs the risk of temporary pacing.

Temporary pacing in patients with acute myocardial infarction is

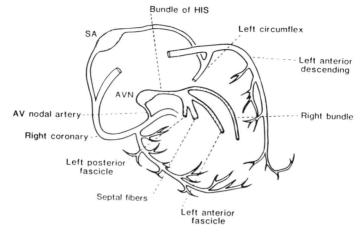

Figure 1. *Blood supply to the cardiac conduction system. The sinoatrial (SA) node is supplied by a branch of the right coronary artery in 60% of patients, and the left circumflex coronary artery in 40% of patients. During inferior infarction, if the right coronary artery is occluded proximal to the origin of SA nodal artery, sinus node dysfunction may occur. The atrioventricular (AV) node (AVN) is supplied by a branch of the right coronary artery in 90% of patients. During inferior infarction, occlusion of the right coronary artery may result in AV block, which is usually at the level of the AVN. Anterior infarctions may result in conduction defects, which usually indicate more extensive infarction with involvement of the conduction system distal to the AV node.*

somewhat more controversial. In these patients, the decision to proceed with temporary pacing is based on knowledge of the blood supply of the conduction system, the location and extent of infarction, and the presence of a preexisting conduction system disease (Figure 1). All of these factors influence the risk of symptomatic bradycardia developing. It is important to try to assess the level of the conduction abnormality.

Conduction Abnormalities Proximal to the His Bundle (Table II)

Conduction disturbances proximal to the bundle of His are most commonly associated with an inferior infarction. The escape rhythms often have a narrow QRS complex, although they may be wide, and they tend to be faster and more stable than distal escape rhythms. If AV block develops, it is usually gradual in onset and transient. A typical clinical occurrence would be Wenckebach AV block followed

Table II
Atrioventricular Conduction Abnormalities Associated With
Acute Myocardial Infarction

	Anterior infarction	Inferior infarction
Conduction abnormality proximal to His bundle	–	Yes
Conduction abnormality distal to His bundle	Yes	–
Degree of necrosis	Extensive	Less extensive
Escape rhythm	Wide QRS Rate <40 bpm Less stable	Narrow QRS Rate 40–50 bpm Stable
Progression of atrioventricular block	Rapid	Gradual

by higher grades of block in a patient with inferior myocardial infarction. In patients with inferior infarction and high-grade block, the indication for pacing is a rate persistently less than about 40 bpm, or the development of symptoms such as a low output state or recurrent bradycardia associated with angina or ventricular irritability. In other asymptomatic patients with conduction abnormalities proximal to the His bundle, temporary pacemakers need not be inserted prophylactically.

Conduction Abnormalities Distal to the His Bundle

Distal abnormalities usually occur in association with anterior infarctions. A wide spectrum of electrocardiographical patterns can be seen, including bundle branch block and high-grade AV block. The escape rhythms usually have a wider QRS complex, are slower, and are less stable than the proximal escape rhythms. In addition, unlike proximal conduction abnormalities, distal abnormalities often progress rapidly to complete AV block. If the patient has an anterior infarction and significant conduction abnormalities, the degree of myocardial damage usually is extensive and often is associated with pump failure. The progression to complete heart block, however, contributes independently to morbidity and mortality in some patients. In patients with high-grade AV block, the decision to proceed with temporary pacing is straightforward. In patients with only bundle branch block, the decision to proceed is based on the risk of AV block developing. In patients at high risk, placement of a temporary

Table III
Indications for Temporary Pacing in Acute Myocardial Infarction and Distal Conduction Disturbances

High-grade AVB (Type II second-degree AVB or CHB)
RBBB and either LAFB or RBBB and LPFB (new or indeterminate onset)
RBBB or LBBB and first-degree or second-degree AVB (Type 1 AVB)
Alternating RBBB and LBBB (irrespective of time of onset)
RBBB with alternating LAFB and LPFB (irrespective of time of onset)
"Old" or preexisting RBBB and new LAFB and first-degree AVB

AVB = atrioventricular block; CHB = complete heart block; LAFB = left anterior fascicular block; LBBB = left bundle branch block; LPFB = left posterior fascicular block; RBBB = right bundle branch block

pacemaker is recommended. Table III gives our generally accepted criteria for placement of temporary pacemakers in patients with acute anterior infarction.

Tachycardia

The placement of temporary pacemakers in patients with tachycardia is useful in several ways. The ability to simultaneously record atrial deflections and the surface ECG on a two-channel monitor facilitates analysis of the relationship between the atrial and the ventricular electrograms (Figure 2). Such recording is important particularly in patients with wide-complex tachycardia. Documenting ventriculoatrial (VA) block or VA dissociation in this situation is often helpful in the differential diagnosis of supraventricular and ventricular tachycardia. It is also helpful in patients with supraventricular tachycardia; for example, recording atrial rates of 300 bpm establishes the diagnosis of atrial flutter. In addition to diagnostic uses, in selected patients with re-entrant tachycardia (either supraventricular or ventricular), burst pacing can be used to terminate tachycardia (see Chapter 13). In these patients, temporary pacing can be used until an effective drug regimen is instituted or until the clinical factors responsible for the arrhythmia have been controlled, as in patients with drug- or electrolyte-induced arrhythmias. In occasional patients, overdrive pacing can be very useful in the prevention of arrhythmias. For overdrive pacing, the rate required varies with the underlying rhythm. It must exceed the spontaneous rate by approximately 10–25% to effect complete capture. As the arrhythmia subsides or responds to drug therapy, the overdrive rate is reduced or pacing is

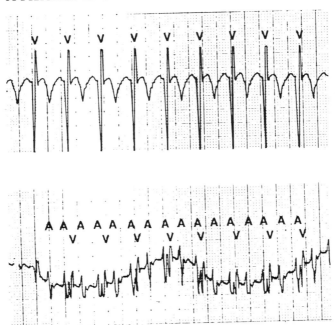

Figure 2. *A simultaneous two-channel electrocardiogram. The ECG (top) demonstrates tachycardia at a 480 ms coupling interval (125 bpm). No clear-cut atrial activity is seen. The simultaneous atrial recording (bottom) documents atrial activity at a rate of 250 bpm (240 ms), and 2:1 atrioventricular block. V = ventricular depolarization; A = atrial depolarization.*

discontinued. Such pacing is usually a temporizing maneuver. Temporary pacing is valuable in patients with temporary transvenous lead systems in coronary care units, and in patients with temporary epicardial electrodes after cardiac surgery.

TEMPORARY PACING MODE

For the treatment of symptomatic bradycardia or asystole, safe, temporary ventricular pacing is lifesaving. Although it remains the most common type of temporary pacing, alternatives are being used with increasing frequency.

Atrial Pacing

Atrial pacing is used in selected patients, including some with sinus node dysfunction without AV block. In these patients, pacing can be used for overdrive suppression of supraventricular tachycardia, overdrive burst pacing for treatment of tachycardia, or treatment of symptomatic bradycardia. In this clinical setting, permanent pacing often is eventually required, but temporary pacing may be very helpful in the interim. In addition, in patients with possible drug-induced symptomatic sinus bradycardia, temporary atrial pacing may be used until the specific need for the drug in question is determined. Finally, in some patients with prolonged Q-T syndromes (either drug-induced or spontaneous) and recurrent ventricular tachycardia, temporary atrial pacing may help to prevent the arrhythmia by shortening the Q-T interval and suppressing ventricular ectopy.

Dual-Chamber Pacing

Advances in technology have occurred along with our increased knowledge about the hemodynamics of pacing. These two factors have been responsible for the increased use of temporary dual-chamber pacing. Both temporary AV sequential and recently, temporary DDD units have become available. These are particularly useful in patients with noncompliant ventricles in whom the atrial contribution to ventricular filling is essential. In patients with AV block and acute myocardial infarction, dual-chamber pacing may maintain optimal hemodynamics. Another use of temporary dual-chamber pacing is to assess the need for a permanent dual-chamber system or upgrade of a ventricular demand system. Measurement of blood pressure and cardiac output with different temporary pacing modes may help to document the need for a specific permanent pacing mode in equivocal cases.

TEMPORARY PACEMAKER PLACEMENT

Temporary pacing usually is performed by a transvenous approach. The clinical setting determines the urgency with which pacing is required and, to a certain extent, the venous access chosen.

The basic equipment required for temporary transvenous pacing includes a surgical pack with instruments to obtain venous access, a pacing catheter, an external pulse generator, and under usual circumstances, a procedure room for placement.

Catheters

Several catheters are available (Table IV and Figure 3), each of which has advantages and disadvantages. The mode of pacing selected determines, in part, the catheter system used (Table V). Al-

Table IV
Temporary Pacing Systems

Route	Requirements for Use	Reliability
Transvenous		
Rigid catheter	Fluoroscopy	Excellent
Flexible, balloon-tipped	ECG monitoring or fluoroscopy, or both	Fair to Good
Noninvasive		
Transthoracic	External shock	Good, but patient discomfort a problem

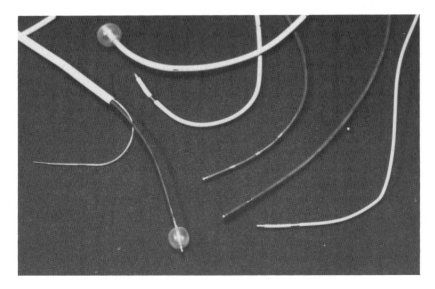

Figure 3. Representative types of temporary pacing leads. Clockwise, from left: (1) Single-pass lead with atrial "J" and balloon-tipped ventricular lead; (2) balloon-tipped flotation catheter; (3) atrial "J" lead; (4) quadripolar woven Dacron lead; (5) bipolar woven Dacron lead; (6) flexible bipolar lead.

Table V
Modes of Temporary Pacing

Mode	Equipment
Single-chamber	
Atrial	Atrial "J" lead
Ventricular	Balloon-tipped lead
	Flexible bipolar lead
	Quadripolar lead
	(see Figure 3)
Dual-chamber	Separate atrial and ventricular catheters
	Single multi-electrode catheter for both atrial and ventricular pacing
	Dual electrode system, single sheath

though both unipolar and bipolar catheters are available, the overwhelming majority of temporary pacing systems are bipolar.

There are two major types of catheter design. The first is a more rigid, firm catheter, usually made of woven Dacron. The use of this catheter requires fluoroscopic imaging during the procedure for safe and proper placement. Because this catheter remains somewhat firmer after placement, it is more reliable in maintaining temporary pacing.

The other major type of catheter is very flexible and may have a balloon tip. Balloon flotation catheters do not require fluoroscopy for insertion, and are particularly useful during emergencies. For placement of these catheters, the balloon is inflated after it enters the central circulation. If fluoroscopy is not available or not used at the time of placement, intracardiac electrograms can be used to position the leads. Intracardiac electrograms are strikingly different from surface ECGs. When the lead enters the right atrium, large P waves are seen. Passage of the lead across the tricuspid valve into the right ventricle is associated with recording of large QRS complexes, which indicate ventricular position. Contact with the endocardium is manifested by elevation of S-T segments with a current of injury (Figure 4). Because they are so flexible, these balloon flotation catheters do not maintain stable pacing positions as well as the more rigid catheters.

In addition to catheters for ventricular placement, there are now atrial "J" catheters that can be used for right atrial appendage placement. Finally, single-pass catheters are available for dual-chamber pacing (Figure 3).

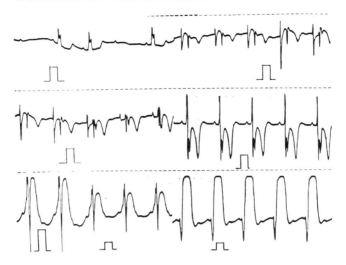

Figure 4. *Passage of a transvenous bipolar electrode with ECG control involves recognition of the electrograms of different intracardiac positions.* **Upper left:** *Intermittent AV block.* **Upper right:** *The electrode is in the right atrium with P waves larger than the QRS complexes.* **Middle left:** *The electrode is moved into the inferior vena cava where the P waves are reduced in size, now smaller than the QRS complexes.* **Middle right:** *Within the right ventricle, past the tricuspid valve, the QRS complexes are enlarged, the P waves small, and the T waves inverted.* **Lower left:** *The P waves virtually disappear, the ventricular electrogram is 6 mV in amplitude (the standardization has been reduced by half).* **Lower right:** *Increase in pressure on the endocardium increases electrogram amplitude and the elevation of the ST segment.*

External Generators

There are also several external pulse generators (Figure 5). The most commonly used are single-chamber, constant-current devices with variable output up to 20 mA, variable rate up to approximately 180 bpm, and variable sensitivity. In addition to these single-chamber units, AV sequential pacemakers and, more recently, a modified DDD pacemaker are available for selected patients. Finally, programmable stimulators are available for patients in whom the indication for pacing is termination of tachycardia. These stimulators can be used for burst pacing and for the introduction of one or more extrastimuli.

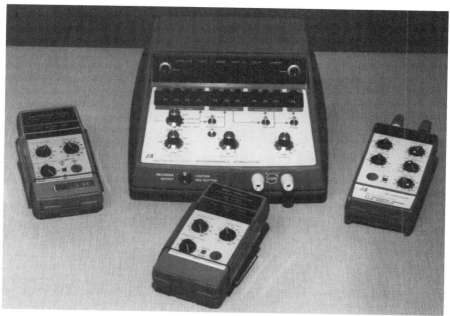

Figure 5. *External pulse generators.* **Left:** *Single-chamber.* **Center-top:** *Programmable stimulator capable of rapid burst pacing and programmed stimulation. Center-bottom: High-output single-chamber pulse generator.* **Right:** *Atrioventricular sequential pulse generator.*

Venous Access and Placement

Access to the venous system for placement of temporary pacing catheters is possible from several sites, including subclavian, external and internal jugular, brachial, and femoral veins (Figure 6). Selection of the specific approach depends on the clinical conditions and the experience of the operator. At our institutions, a central venous approach is preferred because of ease of insertion, percutaneous placement, and stability.

Insertion should be done under sterile, aseptic conditions. Electrocardiographical monitoring, plus emergency equipment including a defibrillator are essential. If a rigid transvenous catheter is to be used, the patient must be on a radiolucent table with fluoroscopy available. The insertion site should be thoroughly prepared and draped, and an instrument pack with equipment for percutaneous entry or venous cutdown should be available.

Selection of the specific vein (subclavian, jugular, brachial, or

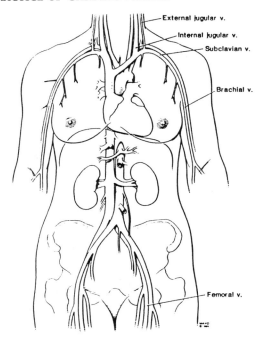

Figure 6. *Sites of venous access for temporary pacing. Selection of a specific approach depends on clinical conditions and the experience of the operator. (Reproduced by permission of Mayo Foundation.)*

femoral) depends on the patient's condition and the operator's experience. Usually, the subclavian (Chapter 8) or jugular (Figure 7) vein is used, because the catheter is more stable, and the incidence of dislodgment is lower. There are risks with each approach; they must be balanced against the benefits.

Whenever possible, a percutaneous technique is used. Local anesthesia is administered to the subcutaneous and deeper structures, and a small puncture is made with a scalpel blade. With the use of a hemostat, the subcutaneous tissues are dissected bluntly in the direction the introducer will follow. A thin-walled needle, usually 18 gauge, is used to enter the vein (Figure 7). Blood is aspirated after venous entry to document placement within the lumen. A guide wire is then advanced through the needle into the venous circulation, and the needle is removed. The dilator and venous sheath are then advanced over the wire. Several introducer kits of different sizes are available commercially; they include the needle, guide wire and syringe, and dilator-introducer. We prefer to use sheaths that have a

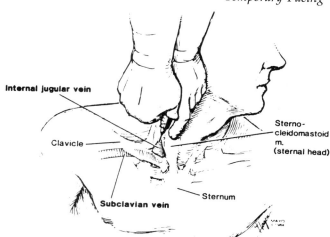

Internal jugular vein

Clavicle

Subclavian vein

Sterno-
cleidomastoid
m.
(sternal head)

Sternum

Figure 7. *Approach used for internal jugular venipuncture: use of this or the sub-clavian approach has been associated with lower dislodgment rates than with periph-eral venous access, for example, the antecubital vein. (Reproduced by permission of Mayo Foundation.)*

sidearm for fluid administration, and a diaphragm to prevent back-bleeding. The pacing catheter can be advanced into the central circulation through this sheath.

If two central lines are needed, i.e., a pulmonary artery catheter and a temporary pacing wire, two sheaths can be placed with a single central venous puncture. After placing a single sheath, two guide wires can be placed through the diaphragm of the sheath, advanced into the central vein, and the sheath removed. Two separate sheaths can then be placed over the two indwelling guide wires.

Rarely is a cutdown necessary to identify and cannulate the venous entry site. The cutdown approach was most commonly used for the brachial veins. We prefer to avoid this approach if possible, because it is very difficult to immobilize the arm and thereby, to stabilize the lead position.

Subclavian Approach

The techniques for subclavian venous entry for temporary pacing are identical to those for permanent pacing (see Chapter 8). The vein is entered at the junction of the middle and inner thirds. Placing the patient in the reverse Trendelenburg position, or positioning a towel between the scapulae often helps to facilitate venous entry. Infiltration of the subcutaneous and deeper tissues, particularly the ligament between the clavicle and the first rib, and the periosteum, is important for patient comfort. If permanent pacemaker implantation is anticipated, use of a vein other than the subclavian—for example, the internal or external jugular—is preferred. After placement of a sheath with a sidearm and diaphragm, the pacing lead can be advanced into the central venous circulation.

Internal Jugular Approach

The internal jugular venous approach also allows easy access to the central circulation (Figure 7). The patient's head is turned away from the side of venipuncture. There are several approaches to the internal jugular vein. We prefer to infiltrate the apex of the triangle formed by the medial and lateral borders of the sternocleidomastoid muscle with a local anesthetic. A small incision is made with a scalpel blade, and the subcutaneous tissue is dissected bluntly in the direction of the vein, which lies lateral to the carotid artery. A 23-gauge needle is used to identify the location of the vein. Care must be taken to avoid puncture of the apical pleura or carotid artery. After the vein has been identified with the smaller needle, a short 18-gauge needle is used for venipuncture. The guide wire and introducer and valved venous sheath are placed successively. The pacing lead then can be advanced into the right side of the heart.

External Jugular Venous Approach

Either external jugular vein can provide easy access for temporary pacing, although the right external jugular vein is the more direct approach. The vessels often can be seen, particularly in patients with elevated venous pressure, or during a Valsalva maneuver. The external jugular veins course inferiorly toward the middle third of the clavicle, just beneath the platysma muscle. Their position and course can be marked with an indelible pen, and then the area is prepared and draped for venipuncture. After infiltration with a local anesthetic, a small incision is made over the vein with a scalpel. The vein often is very superficial, and care must be taken to avoid laceration. The vein is then entered, and a venous sheath is placed.

Femoral Venous Approach

Temporary pacing through the femoral vein is less common, because more immobilization of the patient usually is required than with a jugular or subclavian approach. The incidence of infection may be increased slightly. The vein is medial to the femoral artery

(Figure 8). It is entered 1–2 cm distal to the inguinal ligament. This ligament runs along a line between the anterosuperior iliac crest and the superior pubic tubercle. The inguinal crease is a rough approximation of the ligament. After infiltration of the site with a local anesthetic, the vein is entered with a long 18-gauge needle (Figure 9). Care must be taken to avoid arterial damage, since in some patients the vein is very close to the artery. In patients who have had femoral arterial or venous punctures, femoral arterial surgery, or cannulation of the femoral artery for bypass, there may be considerable fibrous tissue impeding entry into the femoral vein. After placement of the venous sheath, the pacing lead can be introduced. In some patients, the lead enters a small parallel vein and buckles, causing local low back or pelvic pain. Withdrawing the lead, and rotation usually allow passage up the femoral vein into the inferior vena cava. In patients who require temporary pacing immediately before implantation of a permanent pacemaker, we may avoid a central venous approach and use the femoral vein. This route allows easy access to the central circulation, and optimal flexibility in selection of a site for placement of the permanent pacing lead.

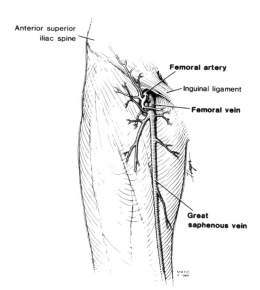

Figure 8. *Anatomy of venous access to the femoral vein. The femoral vein is entered one to two fingerbreadths inferior to the inguinal ligament. (Reproduced by permission of Mayo Foundation.)*

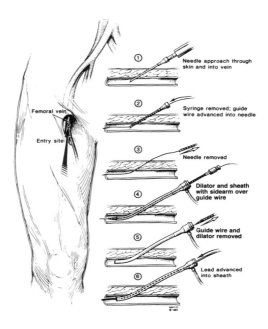

Figure 9. *Entry in the femoral vein is accomplished by puncture with a thin wall needle on a syringe. Once the needle is within the vein, as shown by free flow of venous blood, the syringe is removed and a guide wire introduced. A dilator and sheath with a sidearm are placed over the guide wire, and then the guide wire and dilator are removed. The lead is then introduced via the remaining sheath. The sheath can later be withdrawn from the femoral vein. (Reproduced by permission of the Mayo Foundation.)*

Brachial Venous Approach

A brachial venous approach usually is avoided because of the problems of immobilization and dislodgment; in some instances, however, it may be necessary. If possible, a percutaneous approach is used to enter the brachial vein. If a cutdown is required, the area should be prepared and draped as it would be for percutaneous insertion. After infiltration of the subcutaneous and deeper tissues with a short-acting local anesthetic, an incision is made over the antebrachial crease. A tourniquet may be placed proximally to distend the veins. Superficial veins are used if possible. If none are identified, blunt dissection must be carried deeper toward the brachial artery, which lies beneath the bicipital aponeurosis. Care must be taken to avoid injury to arterial or neural structures. Adequate veins are usually located in this region.

The vein is isolated with ligatures and the distal vein is tied. A venotomy is made, and the pacing lead is introduced. Upper extremity veins draining into the cephalic system should be avoided if possible, because it may be difficult to pass the catheter through the angle where the cephalic vein enters the subclavian vein.

CATHETER PLACEMENT

Ventricular Placement

Placement of a temporary ventricular pacing lead involves consideration of the type of lead selected, the venous access used, and specific patient factors, for example, right atrial enlargement and tricuspid insufficiency. For placement from the subclavian or jugular vein, the more rigid woven Dacron catheters can be passed with a gentle curve through the tricuspid valve into the right ventricular apex. In some patients, a loop is fashioned within the right atrium and then is rotated counterclockwise across the tricuspid valve. In some patients, a loop may be made within the right atrium and backed across the tricuspid valve (see Chapter 8, Permanent Pacemaker Implantation). For placement from the femoral venous approach, a gently curved lead can be passed toward the tricuspid valve, and may cross and be easily positioned in the right ventricular apex. In other patients, a loop must be fashioned in the right atrium and then rotated anteriorly across the tricuspid valve. Avoiding undue pressure on the right atrium is important because it is thin and may be perforated. For balloon flotation leads, the balloon is inflated in the superior vena cava, inferior vena cava, or right atrium, and the catheter then is flow-directed across the tricuspid valve into the right ventricle. Occasionally, rotation of a loop of catheter may be required. Once the lead is within the right ventricle, the balloon is advanced to a stable ventricular position and is deflated.

The most stable position is the right ventricular apex. This usually provides adequate pacing and sensing thresholds. Pacing thresholds should be less than 1 mA, and the position should be stable despite deep breaths and coughing.

Atrial Placement

For dual-chamber or atrial pacing, several options are available. The atrial lead is usually placed in the right atrial appendage, because this position allows for stable, reliable pacing. The currently available temporary "J" leads (Figure 3) can be easily inserted from the subclavian or jugular vein. Advancing the lead from the superior vena cava into the right atrium with medial rotation allows the "J" to form, and facilitates right atrial appendage intubation. Right atrial appendage placement from the femoral vein is accomplished by a straight passage through the right atrium, and rotation toward the spine. Slow advancement with medial rotation usually results in right atrial intubation, which is characterized by the typical medial and lateral movement during atrial systole.

Dual-chamber pacing ordinarily involves placement of two separate catheters (Figure 10). Alternatives exist, including the use of a hexapolar catheter with electrodes that can be placed against the right ventricle and lateral border of the right atrium, a single-pass catheter with expandable flexible wires for atrial pacing, and a balloon-tipped catheter for right ventricular pacing (Figure 3).

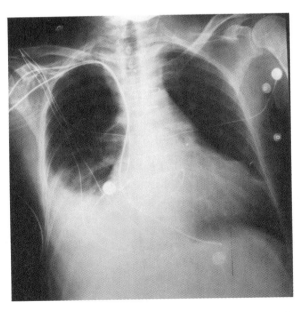

Figure 10.   *Chest radiograph of patient with temporary dual-chamber pacing system. "J" lead is in right atrial appendage, and ventricular lead is in right ventricular apex.*

CATHETER FIXATION

After placement of the catheter, and documentation of satisfactory pacing thresholds, the catheter is fixed to the skin at the entry site with secure nonabsorbable sutures. If the sidearm of the sheath is to be used for drug administration, the sheath is also sutured; if not, the sheath is withdrawn to the lead bifurcation. The site is covered with antiseptic or antibiotic ointment.

The pacing lead is connected to the external pulse generator, and the pacing rate and mode are selected. The maintenance stimulation current is set at two or three times the threshold, or usually 3–5 mA. The rate selected depends on the clinical setting. For uncomplicated heart block, a rate of 70 bpm is usual. The patient's bed and other equipment must be properly grounded, because the pacing lead provides a low-resistance circuit through which current can flow to the heart and produce significant arrhythmias. An insulating cover should be maintained over any exposed ends of the pacing wires.

After placement of the catheter, a chest radiograph should be obtained to document catheter position. The chest radiograph must also be evaluated for complications such as pneumothorax, related to the procedure. An ECG should also be made to document the paced QRS complex, and adequate pacing and sensing. The baseline chest radiograph and ECG are essential for follow-up after placement so that any changes in pacing can be assessed.

CARE AFTER PACEMAKER PLACEMENT

For continued safe and reliable temporary pacing, meticulous attention must be paid to the insertion site and the pacing system itself. It must be kept in mind that the more prolonged the period of temporary pacing, the greater the risk of complication. Temporary pacing from a single site can usually be maintained for seven to ten days if meticulous attention is paid to detail.

Monitoring

All patients with transvenous temporary pacemakers have continuous electrocardiographical monitoring to ensure continued reliable pacing, and to detect any other significant arrhythmias.

Before permanent pacemaker implantation or termination of

temporary pacing, and intermittently during the course of temporary pacing, the underlying cardiac rhythm and the ECGs are evaluated while the pacemaker is turned off. Discontinuance may present a problem in patients who have become dependent on the temporary pacemaker. In these patients, an AV rhythm usually can be induced if the paced rate is reduced gradually. A spontaneous rhythm may be slow to appear and may begin at a very slow rate, but if sustained, it usually will rise to 30–40 bpm.

Pacing and sensing thresholds must be checked daily. Changing thresholds may be the first manifestation of lead dislodgment. Chest radiographs and ECGs should be obtained periodically, and physical examination should be performed daily to identify any complications or change in pacing function. If the patient's intrinsic rate is overriding the pacemaker's, the pacemaker rate is increased to approximately 10 beats above the intrinsic rate so that the paced activity can be evaluated. The stimulation current is then slowly decreased until capture is lost. The point at which capture is lost is noted on the chart. The output is then increased to at least three times the threshold value, usually at least 3–5 mA.

Nursing Care

Meticulous nursing care is essential for patients with transvenous pacemakers. As previously noted, the patient is constantly monitored, and notation is made of the rate, clinical condition, and on/off status of the temporary pacemaker. After the patient moves significantly, the nurses evaluate the electrocardiographical monitoring strips to confirm normal pacemaker function. The external pulse generator is pinned to the patient's gown or to the bed so that it cannot be inadvertently moved away from the patient. Even though the temporary pacing wire is secured to the skin, any undue pressure placed on the pacing wire, for example, application of pressure to the external pulse generator connected to the temporary pacemaker, could result in dislodgment. All connections are checked daily to be certain that they are secure.

The entry site should be redressed daily. The old dressings are removed, the exposed catheter is cleansed with alcohol, and an ointment such as povidone-iodine is applied. The exposed wires are coiled, and a protective dressing is applied. Careful attention to site care signficantly reduces the potential for infection. The pacing catheter should be immobilized as much as possible at the skin entry site. With femoral or brachial vein approach, immobilization of the extremity is usually required. With jugular or subclavian vein placement, the patient is less restricted. The junction between the temporary lead and the pulse generator should be protected with insulation, and the noninsulated connecting tip of the lead must be shielded.

Post-insertion Practices

If possible, the patient should not receive anticoagulants at the time the temporary pacing lead is placed. If a temporary pacing procedure is performed as an emergency in a patient known to be receiving anticoagulants, a femoral or antecubital site may be safer because any bleeding may be easier to control.

After the temporary pacemaker is in place, anticoagulation, if indicated, can be carried out cautiously. The insertion site should be watched closely for evidence of bleeding. Activity is as tolerated for those with subclavian or external jugular leads.

Antibiotics are not used prophylactically when a temporary pacemaker is placed. Antibiotic solutions and ointments may be used locally in site care, but they probably are not necessary if sterile techniques are used to cleanse the site thoroughly every day.

EPICARDIAL SYSTEMS

Epicardial temporary pacing systems are used exclusively in patients undergoing cardiac surgery. In some institutions, these systems are placed prophylactically in all patients undergoing cardiac surgery. In other institutions, epicardial electrodes are placed only in patients in whom AV block develops during the procedure. Temporary epicardial pacing systems can be used for the treatment of symptomatic bradycardia. With atrial or ventricular wires, or both, any combination of pacing, including VVI, AAI, DVI, or DDD, can be used as described for temporary transvenous systems. The selection of the specific mode depends on the clinical setting. In addition to pacing for bradycardia, temporary epicardial systems are of particular use in the evaluation and even treatment, of tachycardia. Electrograms can be recorded to document the relationship between atrial and ventricular depolarizations. Recording rapid atrial rates with 2:1 or greater AV block allows ready documentation of atrial flutter (Figure 2).

The electrodes used for temporary epicardial pacing are stainless steel teflon-coated wires that are sutured loosely onto the epicardium and brought out through the chest wall. Usually, pairs are put on the atrium and the ventricles, and one or more skin ground wires may be placed. The atrial and ventricular wires should be carefully distinguished, either by marking or distinctive placement; for example, atrial leads may be brought out to the right side of the chest, and ventricular leads to the left side. The leads should be fixed to the skin to prevent inadvertent traction or displacement. As is true with transvenous pacing, maintaining an insulating cover over the exposed ends of the pacing wires is essential.

Postpacemaker Placement Care

Patients who have temporary epicardial wires in the postoperative period are monitored for the duration the pacing leads are connected to an external pulse generator. If the pulse generator is disconnected before the temporary pacing wires are removed, the patient does not need continued monitoring.

The exit sites for the epicardial wires should be redressed daily with an antiseptic or antibiotic ointment to avoid infection. Stimulation thresholds with epicardial wires tend to increase rapidly, and the result may be failure to pace. Thresholds, both pacing and sensing, should be checked daily, particularly in patients who are pacemaker-dependent. In pacemaker-dependent patients, early conversion to temporary or implanted transvenous pacing systems should be considered. During atrial pacing, a ventricular wire should never be used as the anodal ground.

The only significant difference in care between patients with temporary epicardial wires and those with temporary transvenous pacing systems is that the former are allowed to ambulate normally without restrictions on movement, while with femoral or brachial leads, immobilization is required.

EMERGENCY PACING TECHNIQUES

In patients whose need for temporary pacing is an emergency because of severe bradycardia with hemodynamic instability or asystole, cardiopulmonary resuscitation should be carried out until some type of emergency temporary pacing can be established. In the past, balloon flotation pacing catheters or transmyocardial pacing have been used in the emergency situation until a standard pacing catheter could be placed with fluoroscopic guidance. Transmyocardial pacing—

placement of an intracardiac cannula through the chest wall into the ventricle should no longer be used. The technique was rarely successful, and carried with it significant potential risks, i.e., laceration of a coronary artery. This technique has been supplanted by external/ transcutaneous pacing. Ballon flotation pacing catheters are still used by some, but external/transcutaneous pacing should now be considered the technique of choice in the emergency situation.

External Transcutaneous Pacing

External cardiac pacing devices have become accepted as necessary emergency equipment in recent years after having been introduced by Zoll, more than 25 years ago. For patients in whom cardiac arrest is precipitated by a bradyarrhythmia, external cardiac pacing can be lifesaving.

External cardiac pacing devices are designed for easy and rapid application and are especially helpful in the following ways: (1) to support symptomatic bradyarrhythmias until a transvenous pacemaker can be placed; (2) on a standby basis for patients at an increased risk for developing ventricular asystole (that is, patients with a myocardial infarction and a new conduction abnormality); and (3) for potential backup pacing during cardioversion of atrial tachyarrhythmias.

External pacing can be quite uncomfortable for the patient. However, it can usually be tolerated until a temporary transvenous device can be placed.

COMPLICATIONS

Complications of temporary cardiac pacing are frequent, occurring in 15–20% of patients. Fortunately, complications are usually minor and not associated with either major morbidity or mortality. The complication rate depends on the skill of the physician, the duration of temporary pacing, and the attention given to the care of the system.

Intracardiac Lead Dislodgment

The most common complication with temporary pacing is movement of the lead. Temporary pacing leads are not as reliable as permanent leads. They cannot always be placed as accurately as permanent leads, and do not have active or passive fixation devices. Movement of the electrode tip may cause failure to pace. In other instances, pacing may continue but stimulation thresholds may rise, or there may be changes in the configuration of the QRS complex. In some cases, maintenance of pacing, despite significant intraventricular motion, can be achieved with a greater output of current. This increase can be continued without danger in most patients; however, if there is evidence of significant movement of the electrode, repositioning usually is required (Figure 11).

If the electrode tip moves towards the tricuspid or pulmonary valve area, or to the free cavity of a large right ventricle, extremely high currents may be required to maintain pacing. Displacement to the pulmonary artery or right atrium results in loss of ventricular capture. In this case, pacing artifacts are still present on the ECG, but no ventricular capture is evident.

If one suspects that the temporary pacing lead has moved, an ECG and a chest radiograph should be obtained if the situation permits. This radiograph then can be compared with the one obtained immediately after temporary pacemaker placement. If dislodgment has occurred, the lead must be repositioned.

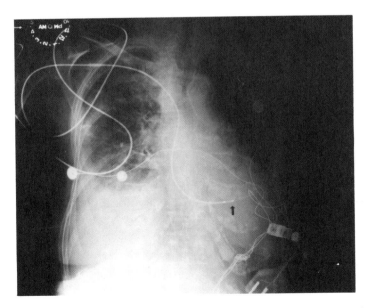

Figure 11.   A. Portable AP chest X-ray showing a temporary pacing wire positioned in the vicinity of the right ventricular apex.

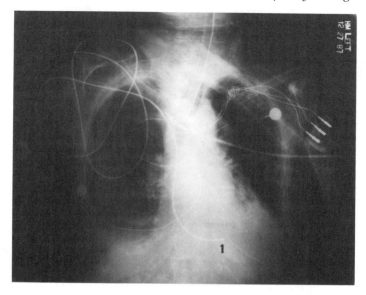

Figure 11B. *A subsequent chest X-ray shows slight but definite movement of the temporary wire.*

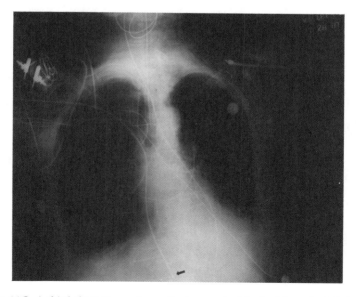

Figure 11C. *A third chest X-ray shows displacement of the lead into the inferior vena cava.*

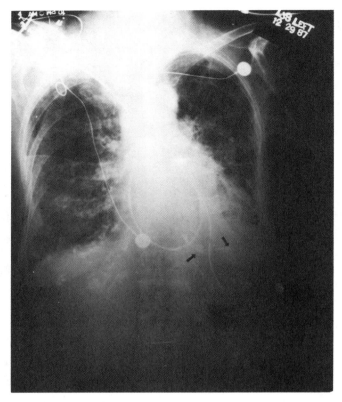

Figure 11D. *A final chest X-ray is obtained after placing a pulmonary artery catheter, which has a port for a ventricular pacing wire to be passed into the ventricle.*

Perforation

Perforation of the right ventricle is a well-recognized complication of temporary pacing. If perforation is suspected during placement of the lead, the lead usually can immediately be withdrawn into the right ventricular cavity without significant consequences. Late perforation results from continuous or intermittent pressure of the catheter on a thin right ventricular apex or the right ventricular free wall. Although the overall incidence of perforation is low, the incidence is higher with the standard semirigid, temporary lead than with a floating temporary lead that is more flexible. If the brachial or femoral route is used, excessive motion of the extremity also may increase the incidence of perforation.

Perforation may become evident clinically because of a postin-sertion friction rub, loss of pacing, diaphragmatic stimulation, a change in the QRS complex (specifically, ventricular pacing contin-ued, but development of a right bundle branch block pattern), and, rarely, by pericardial tamponade. When perforation is suspected, the lead should be repositioned.

Pneumothorax

Pneumothorax occurs only when the subclavian or internal jug-ular venous puncture is used. This complication is directly related to the experience of the operator. If pneumothorax occurs, one should proceed as outlined in chapter 14, "Pacemaker Complications."

Arterial Entry

Inadvertent entry into an adjacent artery may occur with a sub-clavian, internal jugular, or femoral venous approach. If it occurs, the needle should be withdrawn promptly, and pressure placed over the puncture site to control bleeding. This complication also depends on the experience of the operator. After local hemostasis, the same venous site can be used.

Arrhythmias

As with placement of any catheter in an intracardiac position, a temporary pacing lead may induce certain arrhythmias, the most common of which is ventricular ectopy. Any patient may be affected, but ventricular ectopy is of most concern in those with recent myo-cardial infarctions, in whom there may be significant underlying my-ocardial irritability. If significant ventricular ectopy occurs during placement of a temporary pacing lead in a patient with an acute infarction, it should be treated with an intravenously effective anti-arrhythmic agent.

In patients with left bundle branch block in whom a temporary pacing catheter is being placed, mechanical trauma to the right bun-dle branch may result in complete heart block. The incidence is very low. If block does occur, rapid passage of the intracardiac electrode into the right ventricle should establish effective ventricular pacing.

In patients with temporary atrial pacing, as in patients with per-

manent atrial pacing, if stimulation occurs during the vulnerable period after intrinsic atrial depolarization, atrial fibrillation may result.

Local Skin or Suture Area Infection

Skin or suture area infection of clinical significance rarely occurs
in patients with temporary pacing if attention is paid to skin care,
which includes daily cleaning of the placement site and dressing
change. A small amount of purulence at the site of skin suture rarely
is significant and usually heals as soon as the sutures are removed.
Systemic antibiotics rarely are required or used as long as the infection remains local.

Bacteremia

If sterile conditions are not maintained during placement of a
temporary pacing lead, or if the temporary pacing lead is left in place
for prolonged periods without adequate care of the system, bacere-
mia may result. We prefer not to leave a transvenous temporary pacing lead in for longer than one week.

If bacteremia does occur, it is treated by identification of the
responsible organism and treatment with appropriate antibiotics. The
pacing leads should be removed as soon as possible, and a culture
should be done at the time of removal. If temporary pacing is still
required, a new temporary pacing lead may be inserted by another
venous route during antibiotic therapy.

BIBLIOGRAPHY

Austin JL, Preis, LK, Cramptom RS, et al: Analysis of pacemaker malfunction
    and complications of temporary pacing in the coronary care unit. *Am J
    Cardiol* 1982; 49:301–306.
Del Negro AA, Fletcher RD: Indications for and use of artificial cardiac pace-
    makers. Part II. *Curr Probl Cardiol* 1978 Nov; 3:1–43.
Falk RH, Zoll PM, Zoll RH: Safety and efficacy of noninvasive cardiac pacing:
    A preliminary report. *N Engl J Med* 1983; 309:1166–1168.
Furman S, Escher DJW: *Principles and Techniques of Cardiac Pacing.* Harper &
    Row, Publishers, New York, 1970; 62–112.
Furman S, Robinson G: The use of an intracardiac pacemaker in the correc-
    tion of total heart block. *Surg Forum* 1958; 9:245–248.
Hartzler GO, Maloney JD, Curtis JJ, et al: Hemodynamic benefits of atrio-

ventricular sequential pacing after cardiac surgery. *Am J Cardiol* 1977; 40:232–236.

Hill PE: Complications of permanent transvenous cardiac pacing: a 14-year review of all transvenous pacemakers inserted at one community hospital. *PACE* 1987 10(3 Part 1):564–70.

Hindman MC, Wagner GS, JaRo M, et al: The clinical significance of bundle branch block during infarction for temporary and permanent pacemaker insertion. *Circulation* 1978; 58:689–699.

Horowitz LN: Temporary cardiac pacing: Indications, techniques and management. In: A-H Hakki (Ed): *Ideal Cardiac Pacing*. WB Saunders Company, Philadelphia, 1984; pp 86–105.

Hynes JK, Holmes DR Jr, Harrison CE: Five-year experience with temporary pacemaker therapy in the coronary care unit. *Mayo Clin Proc* 1983; 58:122–126.

Jacob AS, Schweiger MJ: A method for inserting two catheters, pulmonary arterial and temporary pacing, through a single puncture into a subclavian vein. *Cathet Cardiovasc Diagn* 1983; 9:611–615.

Kersschot IE, Goethals MA, Vanagt EJ, et al: Temporary AVI pacing by chest wall stimulation. *PACE* 1985; 8:4–5.

Kersschot IE, Vanagt EJ, Vrints CJ, et al: Temporary A-V sequential pacing using chest wall stimulation. *PACE* 1984; 7:668–670.

Klein RC, Vera Z, Mason DT: Intraventricular conduction defects in acute myocardial infarction: Incidence, prognosis, and therapy. *Am Heart J* 1984; 108:1007–1013.

Lang R, David D, Klein HO, et al: The use of the balloon-tipped floating catheter in temporary transvenous cardiac pacing. *PACE* 1981; 4:491–496.

Linos DA, Mucha P Jr, van Heerden JA: Subclavian vein: A golden route. *Mayo Clin Proc* 1980; 55:315–321.

Littleford PO: Physiologic temporary pacing: Techniques and indications. *Clin Prog Pacing Electrophysiol* 1984; 2:236–254.

Littleford PO: Physiologic temporary pacing: Techniques and indications. In SS Barold (Ed): *Modern Cardiac Pacing*. Futura Publishing Company, Mount Kisco, New York, 1985, 231–255.

Littleford PO, Curry RC Jr, Schwartz KM, et al: Clinical evaluation of a new temporary atrial pacing catheter: Results in 100 patients. *Am Heart J* 1984; 107:237–240.

Littleford PO, Pepine CJ: A new temporary atrial pacing catheter inserted percutaneously into the subclavian vein without fluoroscopy: A preliminary report. *PACE* 1981; 4:458–464.

Littleford PO, Schwartz KM, Pepine CJ: A temporary external DDD pacing unit. *Am J Cardiol* 1984; 53:1041–1043.

Lumia FJ, Rios JC: Temporary transvenous pacemaker therapy: An analysis of complications. *Chest* 1973; 64:604–608.

Mooss AN, Ross WB, Esterbrooks DJ, et al: Ventricular fibrillation complicating pacemaker insertion in acute myocardial infarction. *Cathet Cardiovasc Diagn* 1982; 8:253–259.

Olson CM, Jastremski MS, Smith RW, et al: External cardiac pacing for out-of-hospital bradyasystolic arrest. *Am J Emerg Med* 1985 3:129.

Paris PM, Stewart RD, Kaplan RM, et al: Transcutaneous pacing for brady-asystolic cardiac arrests in prehospital care. *Ann Emerg Med* 1985; 14:320–323.

Parsonnet V, Bhatti M: A technique for postoperative application of a newly designed temporary bipolar dual-chamber pacemaker electrode. *J Thorac Cardiovasc Surg* 1985; 89:456–458.

Roberts JR, Greenberg MI, Crisanti JW, et al: Successful use of emergency transthoracic pacing in bradyasystolic cardiac arrest. *Ann Emerg Med* 1984; 13:277–283.

Scheinman MM: Treatment of cardiac arrhythmias in patients with acute myocardial infarction. *Am J Surg* 1983; 145:707–710.

Schnitzler RN, Caracta AR, Damato AN: "Floating" catheter for temporary transvenous ventricular pacing. *Am J Cardiol* 1973; 31:351–354.

Sharkey SW, Chaffee V, and Kapsner S: Prophylactic external pacing during cardioversion of atrial tachyarrhythmias. *Am J Cardiol* 1985 55:1632.

Sugrue DD, McLaran C, Hammill SC, et al: Refractory supraventricular tachycardia in the neonate: Treatment with temporary antitachycardia pacing. *Mayo Clin Proc* 1985; 60:169–172.

Syverud SA, Dalsey WC, Hedges JR: Transcutaneous and transvenous cardiac pacing for early bradyasystolic cardiac arrest. *Ann Emerg Med* 1986 15(2):121–4.

Waldo AL, Henthorn RW, Epstein AE, et al: Diagnosis and treatment of arrhythmias during and following open heart surgery. *Med Clin North Am* 1984; 68:1153–1169.

Weinstein J, Gnoj J, Mazzara JT, et al: Temporary transvenous pacing via the percutaneous femoral vein approach: A prospective study of 100 cases. *Am Heart J* 1973; 85:695–705.

Zoll PM: Resuscitation of the heart in ventricular standstill by external electric stimulation. *N Engl J Med* 1952 247:768.

Zoll PM, Zoll RH, Falk RH, et al: External noninvasive temporary cardiac pacing: Clinical trials. *Circulation* 1985; 71:937–944.

Chapter 8

PERMANENT PACEMAKER IMPLANTATION

David R. Holmes, David L. Hayes, Seymour Furman

The transthoracic approach for the placement of epimyocardial pacing electrodes dominated pacemaker implantation until the introduction of implantable transvenous systems in 1965. Increased experience with the transvenous approach, coupled with the development of active and passive fixation leads that greatly decrease the frequency of dislodgment has resulted in the current approach to cardiac pacing in which transvenous systems account for approximately 95% of all pacemaker implants. For the most part, thoracotomy implantation is now limited to that done at the time of thoracotomy for other reasons, for example, open heart surgery.

IMPLANT FACILITY

Requirements for the rooms, personnel, and equipment in which permanent cardiac pacemakers are implanted were described in the 1983 Intersociety Commission for Heart Disease Resources report. Pacemakers should be implanted in a surgical environment, whether a specially equipped operating room or a catheterization suite. Requirements include excellent fluoroscopy, electrocardiographic monitoring, and standby defibrillator and life-support equipment. Additional desirable features are facilities for lateral and anteroposterior fluoroscopy projection, and equipment to measure intra-arterial pressure and ventriculoatrial (VA) and atrioventricular (AV) conduction intervals.

ANESTHESIA

Local anesthesia is used for all patients unless contraindicated. Pediatric or very elderly patients undergoing permanent pacing and other special circumstances may require general anesthesia. Supplemental parenteral sedatives are used as needed for patient comfort.

ANATOMIC APPROACH

Before 1979, transvenous pacing leads were almost always placed through a cephalic vein cutdown in the deltopectoral groove. If the cephalic vein was too small or friable or had previously been used for implantation or if a second lead was required, the ipsilateral external or internal jugular vein was used. Rarely, subclavian or axillary vein cutdowns were performed. Deep dissection demanded precise surgical techniques, a disadvantage for medical cardiologists who implanted pacemakers. Each approach has its own particular advantages and disadvantages. The subclavian puncture and cephalic cutdown approaches are most commonly used today. Placement through the external or internal jugular veins, in addition to more local dissection, requires the operator to tunnel the lead over or under the clavicle to the pulse generator itself. The external jugular approach has with it the potential for erosion, and the internal jugular approach requires more extensive dissection.

Subclavian Approach

In 1979, an introducer approach that used subclavian venipuncture became well known. Because this technique is fast and usually causes minimal trauma, is useful when the cephalic vein is absent, and facilitates placement of multiple leads, it has become the procedure of choice in many institutions. The basic procedure, a modification of the Seldinger technique, requires detailed knowledge about the route of the subclavian vein and the relationship of the vein to the clavicle, first rib, subclavian artery, and apex of the lung (Figure 1). The ease, efficacy, and safety of the technique are directly related to adherence to specific guidelines (Table I) and to the expertise of the physician performing the venipuncture.

After infiltration with a local anesthetic agent, a 5–8 cm incision is made approximately 2 cm below and parallel to the clavicle, beginning at the junction of its middle and inner thirds. This incision is carried down to the pectoralis fascia. By use of blunt and sharp dissection, a prepectoralis fascial pocket is fashioned for the pulse generator. This pocket should be generous in size and allow for an adequate fit of the pulse generator and the leads selected. It should be

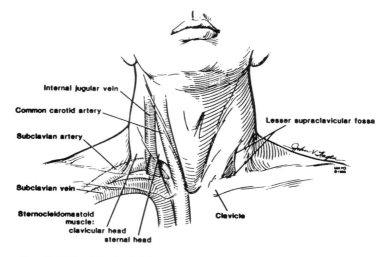

Figure 1. Relationship of calvicle, subclavain artery, and vein and of carotid artery and internal jugular vein. (Reproduced by permission of Mayo Foundation.)

Table I
Principles of Subclavian Puncture

Know the anatomy
Distend the subclavian vein
 Hydration
 Trendelenburg's position
Use as small a needle as possible (18 gauge)
Approach the vein as medially as possible: Start at
 junction of middle and lateral thirds of clavicle
Avoid repeated punctures

---

placed medially rather than laterally near the axilla to prevent migration of the pulse generator and impingement on the anterior axillary fold. Care should be taken to avoid either an excessively tight pocket, which may result in erosion, or an excessively large pocket, which may permit pacemaker migration. After dissection and development of the pocket, a sponge soaked with antibiotic solution may be kept within it during placement of the leads.

Prepackaged kits containing a needle, guide wire, dilator, and peel-away sheath are available (Figure 2). The subclavian vein is en-

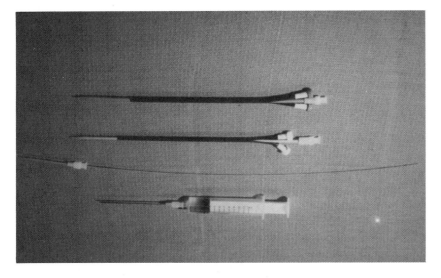

Figure 2.   *Prepackaged kit for subclavian venipuncture; contains needle, guide wire, dilator and peel-away sheath.*

tered through the infraclavicle incision with an 18-gauge needle (Figure 3A). Placing the patient in the Trendelenburg position may facilitate entry because the subclavian vein may be somewhat flattened in the recumbent patient with normal venous pressure. This is even more of a problem if the patient has been fasting for several hours prior to the procedure and is volume depleted. The vein is entered at the junction of the middle and inner thirds of the clavicle; more lateral venipuncture has greater potential for damage to the apex of the pleural space. An introducer guide wire is then advanced through the needle and into the right side of the heart under fluoroscopic control (Figure 3B). On occasion, this guide wire enters the jugular system and ascends. This error can be corrected by manipulation under fluoroscopy. After removal of the needle, the introducer, dilator, and peel-away sheath are advanced over the guide wire into the superior vena cava (Figure 3C). Selection of the appropriate size (ranging from 8F to 14F) is based on the size of the lead or leads to be used. After removal of the dilator and guide, the pacing lead or leads are advanced through the sheath into the right side of the heart. One should take care to avoid air embolism during this procedure by pinching the sheath ends closed and by having the patient hold respiration until passage of the lead into the right side of the heart. The sheath is then peeled away (Figure 3D).

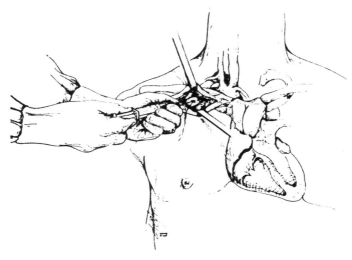

Figure 3A.   *The subclavian vein can be used for single- or dual-lead placement. Initial step involves puncturing the vein with an 18-gauge needle. Blood is aspirated to ensure proper positioning in venous structure.*

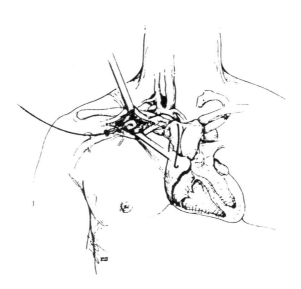

Figure 3B.   *Syringe is removed and flexible guide wire is passed through needle, passing proximal end of the wire into region of right atrium.*

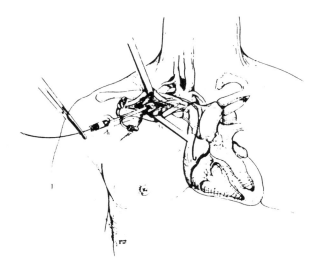

Figure 3C. *With guide wire in place, needle is pulled back and off the guide wire. Dilator and peel-away sheath are then placed over guide wire and passed into subclavian vein. Sizes of dilator and peel-away sheath depend on size of lead(s) to be used. As dilator and sheath are being passed into vein, a hemostat is placed on guide wire to prevent guide wire from being lost into venous circulation.*

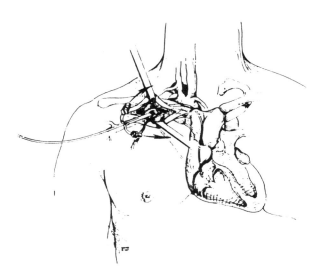

Figure 3D. *Guide wire and dilator are removed from sheath, and pacing lead is quickly passed through sheath into right heart. Arrow indicates pulling of the peel-away introducer away from the lead.*

In some patients, the space between the clavicle and the first rib is tight or the costoclavicular ligament is fibrotic and calcified. This can be recognized by problems with needle entry into the vein or problems with advancement of the dilator. Although lead placement can be achieved, it may be suboptimal. Insulation defects have been identified at this site. These defects may be due to continued pressure on the lead or traction because the lead is fixed in the right ventricle and also at the space between the clavicle and first rib. When such a tight space is identified during implantation, consideration should be given to repositioning the venous entry laterally or using a cephalic approach. Subclavian venous entry carries with it potential complications, among others, including pneumothorax, hemopneumothorax, lung laceration, inadvertent arterial puncture, and air embolism. Meticulous attention is required to minimize these risks.

Cephalic Approach

Although the subclavian venipuncture technique accounts for most implants in many centers, it cannot be used in some patients. In addition, some institutions prefer the cephalic or jugular approach, which avoids the risks of subclavian venipuncture. The cephalic vein always lies within the delto-pectoral groove. The delto-pectoral groove is a constant anatomic site and lies between the deloid and pectoralis major muscles. The cephalic vein is commonly sufficiently large for a single bipolar lead and often large enough for two unipolar and even two bipolar leads. The operative skills required for the cephalic approach are modest and can be readily taught to anyone sufficiently skilled to perform subclavian puncture or other invasive cardiovascular procedures. Cannulation of the cephalic vein is free of significant complications. If damaged, it can be ligated with prompt cessation of bleeding. In addition, the normal venous pressure and the venous valves prevent aspiration of air into the central circulation.

If the cephalic vein is too small to accommodate even a single lead, a guide wire technique may be useful. To perform the guide wire technique the cephalic vein is opened in the usual manner, but instead of attempting to pass the lead, a guide wire is placed through the opening into the superior vena cava or right atrium. The introducer is then placed over the guide wire, as in a conventional subclavian approach, and a lead or leads introduced. A modification of this technique can be used if a single lead is passed into the cephalic vein and the vein will not accommodate a second lead necessary for dual-chamber pacing. In this case, the guide wire is passed into the subclavian vein along side the initially placed lead. An introducer can then be placed over the guide wire and a second lead introduced (Figure 4).

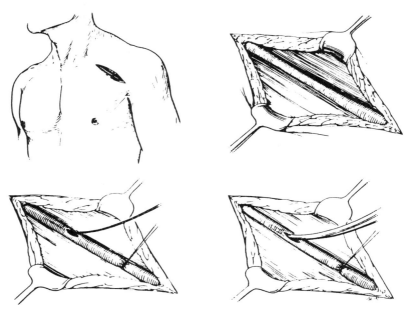

Figure 4.   *A partial cephalic cutdown, introducer technique involves exposure of the cephalic vein in the delto-pectoral groove (upper left, upper right). If the vein is too small to accept a lead, a guide wire is placed (lower left) and the introducer over it (lower right).*

Jugular Approach

If the external or internal jugular vein is selected, two incisions are required. An incision is made immediately above the clavicle, over the area between the posterior border of the sternocleidomastoid muscle and the anterior border of the trapezius muscle. External jugular access to the heart usually is easier by the right external jugular vein than by the left, because the vessel is often less tortuous. If no satisfactory external jugular vessel is found, the incision is extended to a point anterior to the sternal head of the sternocleidomastoid muscle. The carotid sheath is exposed after the superficial fascia is opened behind the posterior border of the sternocleidomastoid mus-

cle. The muscle is then elevated to visualize the carotid sheath optimally. On occasion, the clavicular head of the sternocleidomastoid
muscle must be divided to expose the carotid sheath (Figure 5). The
carotid sheath is then opened; the internal jugular vein is identified
and isolated with nonabsorbable ligatures. After venotomy, the lead
or leads can be introduced. Use of either the external or the internal
jugular vein requires that the lead be tunneled down to the pulse
generator site, either superficial or deep to the clavicle. The external
jugular approach has the potential for erosion of the pacing lead,
whereas the internal jugular procedure requires more extensive dissection with the possibility of damage to the subclavian artery and
vein and the recurrent laryngeal nerve. Should the cutdown route be
attempted before subclavian puncture, use of the cephalic and external jugular veins for introduction of lead systems remains consistent
and reliable. Of all primary dual-chamber implants by one of the
authors (S. Furman), the cephalic vein was used for two unipolar
leads in 61% of instances, the external jugular and cephalic veins in
8%, while subclavian puncture alone was required for only 16% of

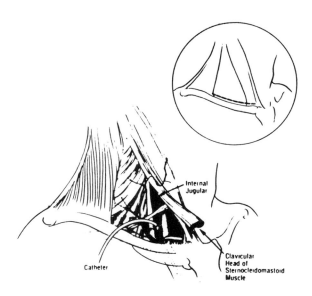

Figure 5. *Approach to internal jugular vein. Incision (insert) is made immediately
above clavicle. The carotid sheath is exposed and then opened (see text for details).
(Reproduced by permission of Annals of Thoracic Surgery.)*

implants. During dual-chamber bipolar implant, the cephalic vein alone was used 43% of the time, the external jugular 14% of the time, and subclavian puncture for 7% of implants. For unipolar lead systems, the cephalic and external jugular venous routes alone were used in 78% of implants, for bipolar leads, 72%.

VENTRICULAR LEAD PLACEMENT

Successful placement of a reliable right ventricular pacing system requires knowledge of, and experience with the specific lead used as well as knowledge of right heart anatomy and catheterization techniques. Great care must be taken during implantation to avoid damage to the lead. The lead stylet, in particular, should not be forced, as the result may be perforation of the insulation within the lead. Several placement techniques are used; all must result in stable right ventricular catheter position with adequate pacing and sensing thresholds. Usually, the right ventricular apex is selected. Other sites are used, however, because of local myocardial problems, such as those seen in patients with coronary artery disease and prior inferior-apical infarction (Figure 6).

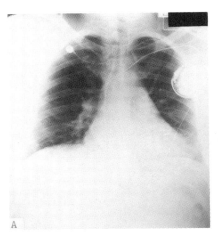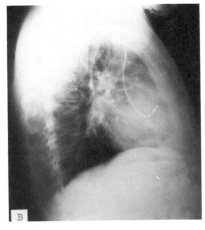

Figure 6. *Postero-anterior (A) and lateral (B) chest x-ray demonstrating a ventricular lead positioned in the right ventricular outflow tract.*

Once the ventricular lead is in the superior vena cava it should move freely. The stylet should be withdrawn about 5 cm and the lead moved inferiorly. It will often catch in the right atrium and be deflected towards the tricuspid valve (Figure 7). If it passes the tricuspid valve it will be in the inflow tract of the right ventricle. It may cause several premature ventricular contractions as it passes through the outflow tract but these usually cease as the catheter passes into the main pulmonary artery. All of this is readily visible fluoroscopically and, if seen, assures that the lead has traversed the right ventricle. The lead will occasionally enter the coronary sinus as it exits the right atrium. A lead within the coronary sinus may appear to be within the right ventricle, but the passage will not be superiorly but rather more laterally toward the left cardiac border. Should the lead begin to curl about the left cardiac border, then it is certainly in the coronary sinus. Attempts at entering the pulmonary artery will be unsuccessful, but the most important clue will be in the lateral fluoroscopic view. The outflow tract of the right ventricle is an anterior structure, and a lead in it will be seen in the retrosternal position. The coronary sinus is on the posterior wall of the heart, and a lead within it will be visualized on the posterior cardiac border.

If the lead cannot be deflected across the tricuspid valve, the stylet should be removed and a curve placed on its distal 5 cm. This is accomplished by wetting the stylet and the gloved index finger and thumb and pulling the wire through the apposed fingers while rotating the fingers to impart a curve to the wire. This curve will be helpful in introducing the lead through the tricuspid valve. Alternatively, the lead tip can be projected against the lateral atrial wall and the curved portion of the lead backed into the tricuspid valve. This technique works best with the leads that have a conical shoulder or fins or a fixation mechanism as part of the electrode, as opposed to tined leads, which tend to catch on the chordae tendinae and impede entry of the tip into the right ventricular outflow tract. Once the lead tip is in the outflow tract, the curved guide wire should be replaced by a straight stylet which, once again, should extend to about 5 cm from the tip. Slow withdrawal of the lead will then cause the lead tip to fall toward the right ventricular apex. The stylet should be advanced up to 2 cm from the lead tip, and then the patient should be asked to breathe deeply. This will cause the right ventricular apex to descend with the diaphragm and the lead can then be advanced. If an atrial lead is not to be implanted, the guide wire can be removed from the ventricular lead and the lead can once again be checked for stability with deep breathing and/or coughing (Figure 8).

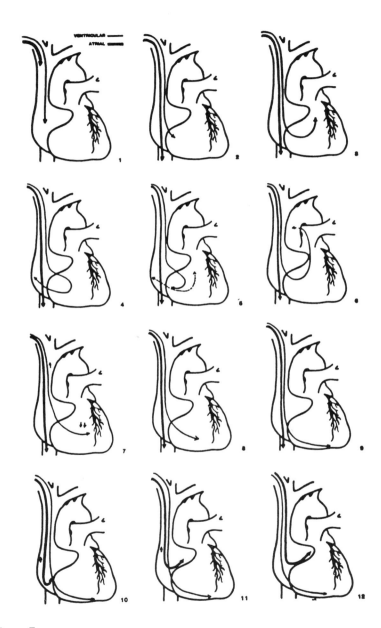

Figure 7

Figure 7. (Opposite page) Intracardiac manipulation is basic to successful pacemaker implantation. Implantation of a dual-chamber pacemaker involves placement of an atrial and ventricular lead. 1) Both leads may be introduced via the subclavian, cephalic or external jugular veins. Initially both will be in the superior vena cava or the right atrial appendage. 2) As ventricular stimulation is more important than atrial stimulation, the atrial lead guide wire, which makes it a straight catheter should be placed into the upper inferior vena cava. The ventricular lead can then be directed through the tricuspid valve. 3) Once past the valve and in the mid-right ventricle it should be advanced into the pulmonary artery so that it is clear that it has not entered the coronary sinus (Panel 6). 4) If the lead tip will not pass the tricuspid valve, entry via a curve, deflected from the lateral atrial wall may be successful. 5) Advancing the bowed lead, in the right ventricle, and then the guide wire within the bow, can flip the lead tip into the right ventricular outflow tract. Note that during this entire maneuver the atrial lead is "parked" in the inferior vena cava. 6) As above, the lead is passed into the pulmonary artery. 7) Once there, the lead is slowly withdrawn so that it falls toward the right ventricular apex. 8) Once at the diaphragmatic surface of the ventricle, it is advanced into the apex. A deep breath is a useful maneuver as it angulates the apex downward and allows easier access. 9) When the ventricular lead has been positioned properly, the guide wire is allowed to remain withdrawn about one inch from the tip to hold it in position while the atrial lead is being manipulated. 10) As the two leads will often adhere lightly, one to the other, when manipulating one lead the other should be held so that it is not inadvertently displaced. The lead should be pulled into the low right atrium and the guide wire withdrawn about 7 cm. The "J" will form. 11) The atrial lead should then be pulled upward slowly. Entry into the base of the atrial appendage will be recognized by straightening of the "J" with pull on the lead. 12) Additional pulling is stopped and the lead advanced into the tip of the atrial appendage.

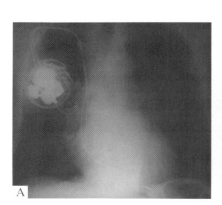 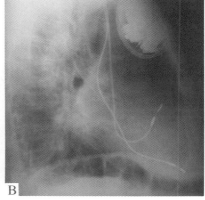

Figure 8. Posterior (A) and lateral (B) views of permanent endocardial pacing leads in the right atrial appendage and optimal right ventricular apical position.

SECURING THE LEAD

If pacing and sensing thresholds are satisfactory and there is no diaphragmatic stimulation measured with pacing at 10 V, the integral silicone rubber sleeve is positioned over the lead or leads at the point of entry into the vein (Figure 9). Nonabsorbable ligature is used to fix the sleeve to the lead and to the muscle or the vein itself. It is essential to use the sleeve and not affix the lead directly to the adjacent tissue. Ligatures applied directly to the lead may damage the insulation and act as a fulcrum, and lead fracture at the fixation site may eventually result (Figure 10).

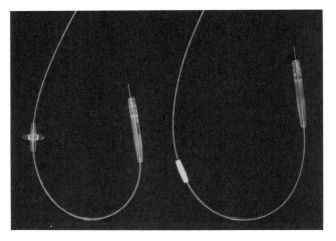

Figure 9. Several different types of sleeves are used to fix the lead to adjacent tissue. These protect the lead from damage induced by ligature.

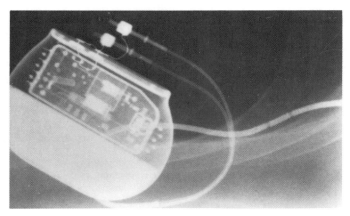

Figure 10. Close-up radiograph shows that two ligatures (arrows) have been tied around the lead without a protective sleeve. These may damage lead insulation.

DUAL-CHAMBER PACEMAKER IMPLANTATION

The subclavian introducer technique can be used for placement of two leads. With this technique, two thin leads (one for atrial and one for ventricular placement) can be advanced through the same introducer sheath into the right side of the heart (Figure 11). The atrial lead is held in a stable position in the right atrium, while the ventricular lead is positioned in the right ventricular apex. After stable ventricular placement is achieved to allow ventricular pacing during the remainder of the procedure, the right atrial catheter is positioned. Alternatively, (Figure 12) two subclavian venipunctures can be used, one for each catheter to be inserted, the ventricular lead being placed first. This technique reduces the problem of displacement of one lead while the other is being positioned (as sometimes occurs with the single cannulation technique), but does require two separate venipunctures. In a third variation, one venipuncture is performed and one lead is introduced, and the guide wire is reintroduced before peeling away the sheath (Figure 13A); a new introducer is placed over the retained guide wire to accommodate the second lead (Figure 13B).

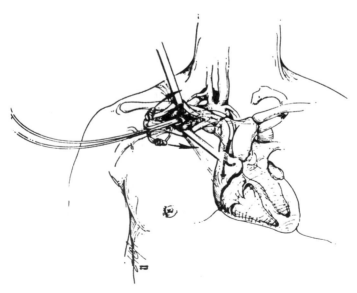

Figure 11.   *If two pacing leads are necessary, both leads can be inserted simultaneously if a peel-away introducer large enough to accommodate both leads is used. With straight stylets in place, one lead is staggered 1–2 cm behind the other lead, and they are passed simultaneously into the right heart and the introducer is then peeled away.*

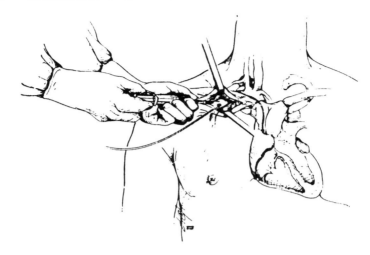

Figure 12. *If a second lead is to be used, a second subclavian puncture can be performed parallel to the already placed pacing lead. Care should be taken to avoid puncturing the indwelling lead.*

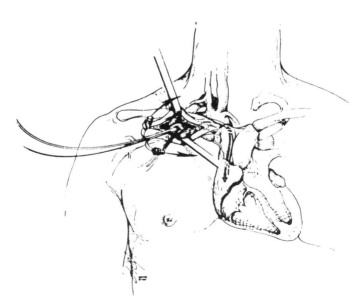

Figure 13A. *Two leads can be placed without a second subclavian puncture and without simultaneously passing the leads. As dilator and guide wire are removed and initial pacing lead is passed into right heart, guide wire is reinserted through peel-away introducer alongside the pacing lead. Introducer is then peeled away and pacing lead and guide wire are left in place.*

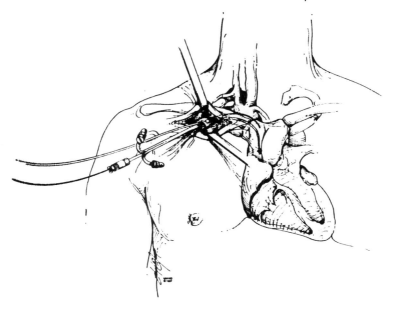

Figure 13B. *A second introducer is then passed over replaced guide wire and sub-sequently the second lead is placed. (Reproduced by permission of Mayo Foundation.)*

Atrial Lead Placement

Placement of the atrial lead is identical for either single-chamber or dual-chamber pacemakers. Satisfactory pacing can be achieved from the right atrial appendage, the atrial wall or occasionally from the coronary sinus. The right atrial appendage is used most commonly. In patients with previous cardiac surgery in whom the appendage has been cannulated or amputated, finding a stable position in the atrial appendage may be more difficult but it is usually still possible.

The usual technique for atrial lead placement is to straighten the atrial lead with a straight stylet and pass the lead into the mid right atrium. (If the atrial lead is being placed as part of a dual-chamber pacemaker implant, it is usually easiest to pass both leads into the central circulation at the onset. The atrial lead tip should be left in the inferior vena cava while the ventricular lead is positioned.) The atrial lead may have passive fixation in which case it will be "J" in shape when the guide wire is removed. The tip of the lead should be placed into the low right atrium (Figure 14A) and the straight guide wire

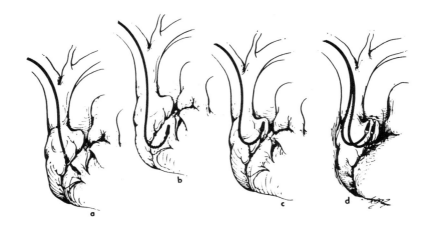

Figure 14. **A.** *Atrial "J" lead at middle of right atrium with straight stylet in place.* **B.** *Straight stylet is removed; removal allows catheter to assume the preformed "J" configuration.* **C.** *Entire lead is pulled back and tip of electrode is allowed to enter right atrial appendage.* **D.** *Characteristic to-and-fro motion of lead when positioned in right atrial appendage. (Reproduced by permission of Mayo Foundation.)*

withdrawn about 10 cm (Figure 14B). The "J" will be formed spontaneously and the entire lead can be drawn upward into the right atrial appendage (Figure 14C). Entry into the appendage is indicated by a rhythmic to and fro, medial and lateral motion of the "J" portion of the lead (Figure 14D). The PA fluoroscopic projection may show the lead medial or lateral, and a lateral projection will show the lead to be anterior at approximately the same level as a lead in the right ventricular apex. If the atrial lead is being placed as part of a dual-chamber procedure, the ventricular lead should be carefully observed so that it is not inadvertently displaced.

Active fixation atrial leads may be "straight" or in a "preformed "J" configuration. If a lead of the "preformed J" variety is used, the screw mechanism can be advanced with the straight stylet fully extended or with the stylet pulled back into the body of the lead, i.e., withdrawn from the "J" portion of the lead. If a straight active fixation lead is used, a "J" curved stylet will be needed to enter the atrial appendage. The stylet is introduced into the atrial lead in the low right atrium and the assembly pulled into the right atrial appendage. The active fixation lead is fixed in place by releasing the screw mechanism. Once fixed, the "J" guide wire is gently withdrawn so as not to displace from the point of attachment. Sensing and pacing thresholds should be checked. If adequate, the lead should be secured as previously described.

As noted above, locations other than the right atrial appendage may be used for atrial lead positioning. The right atrium can be explored, particularly when lateral fluoroscopy is available, to find optimal positioning for lead placement. With active fixation leads, the lead can be placed in the atrial septum (Figure 15A and 15B) or in the free atrial wall (Figure 16A and B). Coronary sinus placement is rarely used (Figure 17A and B). Specific problems with coronary sinus pacing include entry into the ostium itself, which may be difficult, accurate positioning within the coronary sinus, and ventricular pacing or inappropriate sensing of ventricular potentials due to proximity to the ventricle. Coronary sinus leads are not fixed but move within the coronary sinus.

Special circumstances may call for innovative placement of the atrial lead. Placement of an atrial endocardial lead through the atrial wall at the time of open heart surgery has been described with stable atrial pacing being maintained without complication (Figure 18).

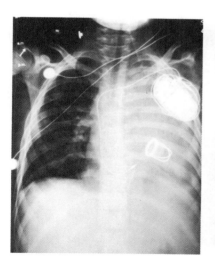 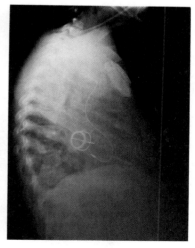

Figure 15.   *Atrial septal implantation. **A.** (left) Postero-anterior view. **B.** (right) Lateral view.*

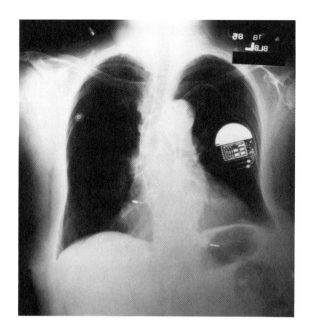

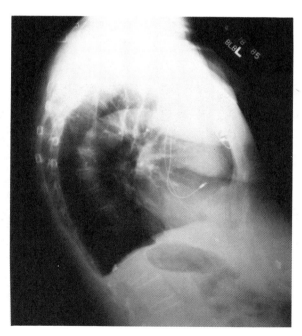

Figure 16. *Atrial lateral wall. Active fixation atrial lead positioned in lateral aspect of right atrium. Postero-anterior (**A, top**) and lateral (**B, bottom**).*

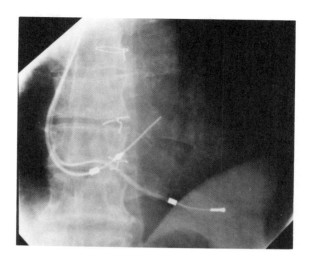

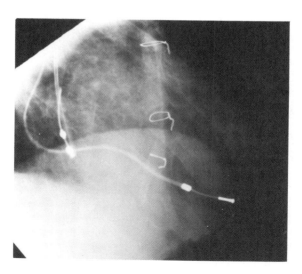

Figure 17. *Postero-anterior (A, top) and oblique (B, bottom) radiographs in a patient with previous cardiac surgery and an atrioventricular sequential pacemaker. Atrial lead is positioned in coronary sinus.*

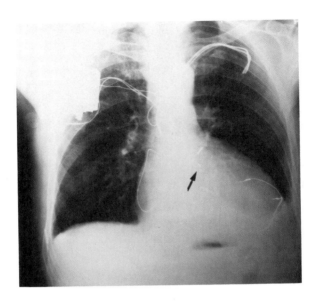

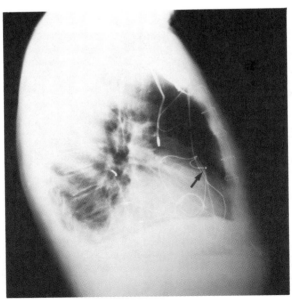

Figure 18.   Postero-anterior (**A, top**) and lateral (**B, bottom**) chest x-ray demonstrating ventricular epicardial leads (2) and an atrial endocardial lead that has been passed through the atrial wall.

MEASUREMENT OF PACING AND SENSING THRESHOLDS

Knowledge and measurement of pacing and sensing thresholds are integral parts in the placement of permanent pacemakers. The equipment used and measurements made vary from laboratory to laboratory. In some institutions, pacing systems analyzers (PSA) are used. These are available from the pacemaker manufacturers (Figure 19). It is best to match the PSA with the pulse generator itself. In some laboratories, physiological recorders with band widths of 0.1–2,000 Hz are used to assess intracardiac electrograms.

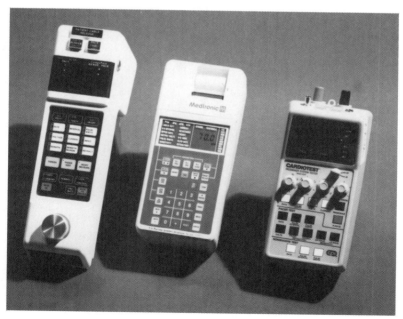

Figure 19. *Representative pacing systems analyzers from three manufacturers. It is recommended that analyzer be matched with pulse generator to be implanted.*

Determination of Pacing Threshold

The pacing threshold is the minimal electrical stimulus required to produce consistent cardiac depolarization. It should be measured with the same electrode configuration (unipolar or bipolar) as the lead and pulse generator that are to be used. During pacing, the output of the PSA is gradually decreased from 5 V down to the point at which loss of capture is documented. The pacing rate selected during this measurement is important. The rate should be just fast enough (approximately 10 bpm faster) to override the intrinsic rhythm. In some patients, pacing during measurement of thresholds suppresses intrinsic rhythm and results in the lack of a stable ventricular escape focus, or even asystole, when pacing is discontinued. The implanting physician may decide to position a temporary pacemaker in these patients. The lower the stimulation threshold, the better. Acceptable acute thresholds are less than 1 V for both ventricular and atrial leads at 0.5 ms pulse duration. Typical acute thresholds for ventricular leads at 0.5 ms pulse duration would be approximately 0.5 V and 1.4 mA, and typical thresholds for atrial leads would be 0.9 V and 1.8 mA.

The duration of pacemaker stimulus is an important determinant of pacing threshold. "Strength-duration" curves (see Chapter 2) are plotted at the time of implantation (Figure 20). Two approaches exist.

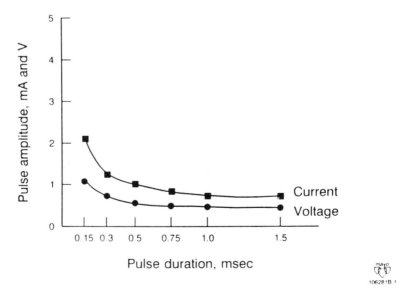

Figure 20. *Sample strength-duration curve plotted at time of implantation. This allows selection of optimal stimulation parameters (pulse duration, output voltage) that result in safe pacing but conserve battery life.*

The output voltage is fixed and the pulse duration is varied; the pulse duration is fixed and the output is varied. The two techniques are equivalent and allow derivation of the current and voltage thresholds at a specific pulse duration.

The impedance of the pacing electrode is also measured, usually by Ohm's law, in which volts equal current times resistance. Measurement of volts and current allows calculation of the lead resistance, which is usually 300–700 ohms. Impedances should always be measured under standardized conditions of output and pulse duration. All PSAs measure impedance as a standard pulse duration and output and not at pacing threshold. The finding of unsuspected low impedance raises the possibility of an insulation failure in the lead.

Determination of Sensing Threshold

Measurement of sensing thresholds is equally important. If a PSA is used, it is best to measure the electrogram with the analyzer made by the manufacturer of the pulse generator to be used, since there is not standardization of the sensitivity of pacemaker circuits. Adequate sensing thresholds are essential to avoid the problem of undersensing or oversensing after implantation. The pacemaker senses intracardiac events, not the events seen on the surface electrocardiogram (Figure 21). The intrinsic deflection is that component of the intracardiac electrogram that is sensed. It is the amplitude of this

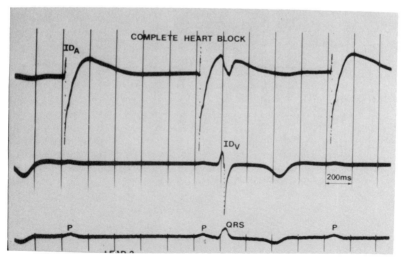

Figure 21.   *Intracardiac electrograms obtained at time of pacemaker implantation in patient with complete heart block. Pacemakers sense intracardiac electrograms, specifically intrinsic deflection of either ventricle (IDᵥ) or atrium (IDₐ). Slew rate is measure of dV/dt (see text for details).*

intracardiac signal in the chamber to be paced that is measured. The result is expressed as a voltage. The ventricular electrogram sensed for adequate long-term sensing should be more than 4 mV. More commonly, the ventricular signal is 6–10 mV, a range that provides excellent sensing. In the past, atrial sensing has been more of a problem. A signal of at least 2 mV is needed for stable, acceptable atrial sensing, and usually 2–3 mV is the range with an adequate atrial position.

In addition to peak amplitude, other aspects of sensing should be considered. The change in voltage with time (dV/dt) the slew rate—of the intrinsic deflection is also important. Usually, this is most important in patients with borderline sensing voltages. If an R wave of 10 mV is measured, the result almost always will be accurate sensing. In patients with low voltages (3–6 mV), the slew rate measurement is very important. Some patients with a QRS of 3 mV but a slow slew rate may have undersensing, whereas other patients with a QRS of 3 mV but a normal slew rate will have normal sensing. Some PSAs now offer the capacity to measure electrograms and slew rates. In the past, a physiological recording system was required.

If electrograms are assessed, an added feature is evaluation of current of injury at the time of pacemaker placement. The current, appearing as an elevation in the electrical potential that immediately follows the intrinsic deflection, represents a small area of damaged endocardium (Figure 22). This finding indicates adequate contact with the endocardium.

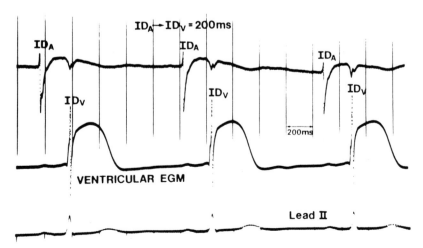

Figure 22. *Intracardiac electrograms at time of pacemaker implantation. In addition to assessment of magnitude and relationship of intrinsic deflection of atrium and ventricle (ID$_A$, ID$_V$), a current of injury is identified. This current of injury, which is manifested as an elevation in electrical potential after intrinsic deflection, indicates adequate endocardial contact. EGM = electrogram.*

Additional Measurements

At the time of dual-chamber implantation, measurements in addition to pacing and sensing thresholds and electrograms for both atrium and ventricle are required (Table II). Atrioventricular (AV) nodal conduction must be assessed. The atrium is paced at rates nearly equal to the sinus rate and then at incremental rates up to approximately 150 bpm. A typical sequence might be 80, 100, 120, 140 and 160 bpm. The rate at which Wenckebach, or higher grade AV block occurs is recorded, as is the AV interval. These values are helpful in setting the pacemaker AV interval and upper rate.

Table II
Studies During Dual-Chamber Implantation

Threshold of stimulation
  Atrium
  Ventricle
Measurement of electrogram
  Atrium
  Ventricle
Measurement of antegrade conduction
  AV conduction interval ($St_A \rightarrow ID_V$)
  Coupling interval for onset of AV block
Measurement of retrograde conduction
  VA conduction interval ($St_V \rightarrow ID_V$)
  Coupling interval for onset of VA block

ID_A = intrinsic deflection of atrial depolarization; ID_V = intrinsic deflection of ventricular depolarization; St_A = atrial pacing stumulus; St_V = ventricular pacing stimulus.

THE PACEMAKER POCKET

Design of the pacemaker pocket is an integral part of pacemaker implantation. The pocket commonly is developed in the prepectoralis fascia (Figure 23). It should be placed medially, rather than laterally, and be large enough to allow for easy placement of the pulse generator and leads. It is important to avoid a tight pocket, which can cause erosion, or a loose pocket, which can permit excessive movement and migration. One of our centers routinely uses a snugly fitting Dacron pouch to encase the pulse generator and leads within the pocket to reduce migration and prevent torsion of the pacing system (Figure 24). The pacemaker itself should be placed deep to adipose tissue in the subcutaneous space. This placement is comfortable and mini-

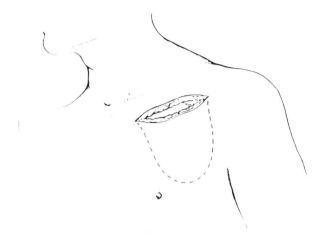

Figure 23. *Location of subcutaneous pacemaker pocket in upper left aspect of chest. Note that incision is made parallel to and several centimeters below lower clavicular margin. (Reproduced by permission of Mayo Foundation.)*

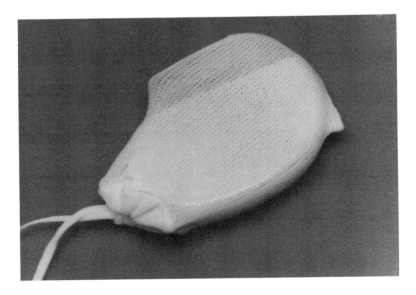

Figure 24. *Dacron pouch used to reduce migration of pulse generator.*

mizes the chance of erosion. In general, the smallest pulse generator appropriate for the patient should be selected. This is of particular importance in pediatric patients, young adults, and thin patients. If the prepectoral position is not suitable because the optimal pulse generator is too large, or because there are cosmetic or other considerations, there are several choices. The pacemaker can be placed deep to the pectoral muscle. This location may result in a higher incidence of pectoral muscle stimulation or muscle inhibition of a unipolar system; therefore, in this situation, a bipolar position is preferred.

Another option is retromammary implantation, which is a useful approach in the young woman. It may be used for cosmetic purposes or, in the thin woman, for protection of the implant site by the fatty layer of the breast. Implantation of the modern small pulse generator of a 20–30 ml volume can be accomplished with no deformity of the breast. Often there is so little difference in breast size that it is barely visible. There is no interference with lactation.

For retromammary placement, implantation should be done under light general anesthesia (Figure 25A-D). Complete relaxation is not required. Subclavian puncture or approach to the cephalic vein is

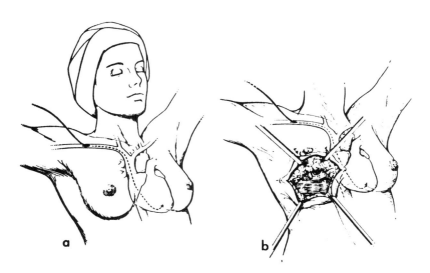

Figure 25. *Placement of pacemaker in retromammary position. **A.** Subclavian puncture and lead placement peformed through limited (2–3 mm) incision. **B.** Inframammary incision is made and dissected to pectoral fascia. Breast is then lifted from fascia.* ***C.*** *Pacing lead or leads are tunneled deep to breast and connected to pulse generator.* ***D.*** *Skin is closed routinely.*

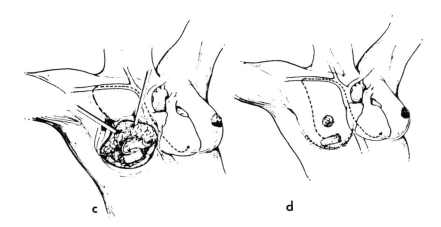

Figure 25 C-D

accomplished routinely. Puncture may be preferable because the incision adjacent to the clavicle may be limited to a length of 2 or 3 cm. Once the leads are in place, they are fastened to the pectoralis fascia with nonabsorbable ligature about the sleeve. An incision is then made in the inframammary fold, which is clearly visible when the breast is elevated. The incision is carried down to the pectoral fascia behind the breast, and the breast is lifted from the fascia. After a long instrument is introduced deep to the breast and brought through the upper small incision, the lead (or leads) are brought to the retromammary incision and are connected to the pulse generator. It is wise to use the Dacron pouch and to suture it lightly to the pectoral fascia with two or three sutures. Mammary tissue is resutured anatomically inferior to the pulse generator to provide an additional cushion, and the skin is closed routinely. Hemostasis is especially important. The pulse generator will be barely palpable and probably not visible. The inframammary incision is invisible when the patient is standing. The pulse generator can be readily replaced through reopening of the inframammary incision.

COMPLICATIONS

Complications of the transvenous approach to permanent pacing include two major groups: (1) those related to venous access and entry and (2) those related to placement of the lead. Both groups of complications are minimized by meticulous attention to detail.

Venous Access and Entry

Complications of entry, inherent in any approach to venous structures, include damage to associated arterial or neural structures, extensive bleeding, air embolism, and thrombosis. In the subclavian approach, the potential of pneumothorax also exists; it can be minimized by knowledge of the patient's anatomy and attention to details. Recent experience indicates that fewer than 0.5% of introducer implantations are associated with serious complications. In some patients, the subclavian vein may be difficult to locate. Contrast material infused through the ipsilateral arm during the search for the vein may be helpful (Figure 26).

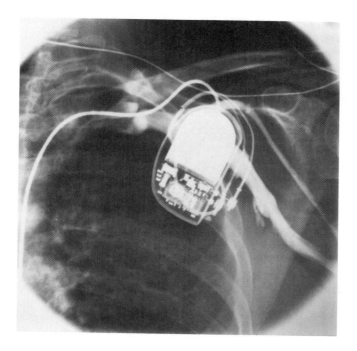

Figure 26.   *Contrast material infused into ipsilateral arm may make subclavian vein identification easier under fluoroscopic visualization.*

Lead Placement

Complications of lead placement result from catheterization of the heart and from placement of a permanent lead itself.

Dislodgment

In the past, the most common complication of transvenous pacing was lead dislodgment. Extensive use of active and passive fixation leads has significantly reduced this complication both for atrial and for ventricular pacing. Secondary intervention rates for all reasons should be well below 2% for ventricular leads and below 5% for atrial leads.

Perforation

Perforation with at least the potential for cardiac tamponade also exists. Ventricular perforation is caused by improper force on the lead. It may be a particular problem in a patient with a thin-walled right ventricle. It usually presents only as diaphragmatic, anterior chest, or abdominal wall stimulation and high thresholds, although tamponade may result rarely. Perforation of the atrium and coronary sinus also has been described. Again, meticulous attention to detail minimizes these risks.

Arrhythmias

A frequent complication is development of supraventricular or ventricular arrhythmia related to lead manipulation. These effects are usually transient, stopping promptly when the lead position is changed. On occasion, they may be sustained. Atrial manipulation may result in sustained atrial tachycardia, fibrillation, or flutter, which complicates placement of a permanent atrial system. Atrial tachycardia may revert to normal sinus rhythm with a tap by the electrode against the atrial wall or may be paced to sinus rhythm if a temporary burst device is available. Management of atrial flutter or fibrillation is more difficult and may require intravenous administration of a drug, such as procainamide hydrochloride (Pronestyl), to restore normal sinus rhythm, or if that fails, cardioversion. Brief ventricular arrhythmias are more common, particularly during lead manipulation. They are usually easily controlled. However, patients with a history of spontaneous sustained ventricular tachycardia may experience these during lead manipulation. For this reason, all patients are monitored and life-support equipment and a defibrillator are immediately available.

In addition to tachycardia, bradyarrhythmias may occur. In patients with intermittent AV block and left bundle branch block, catheter trauma to the right bundle may result in an AV block. More commonly bradycardia results from overdrive suppression of an escape ventricular focus during threshold testing. In a patient at risk for development of asystole or complete heart block during the procedure, a temporary pacemaker should be placed prior to implantation.

Pacemaker Pocket

Complications of the pacemaker pocket can be grouped into early and late. Local hematoma formation is common but usually is minor. It occurs particularly in patients receiving anticoagulants or antiplatelet agents. Aspirin is a major, and often unrecognized, offender. Careful local hemostasis is essential. In patients requiring oral anticoagulants, the prothrombin time should be normal before implantation. Administration of anticoagulants can be resumed 48–72 hours after implantation if there is no evidence of significant hematoma formation. Should a significant hematoma occur, local conservative treatment is preferred. If at all possible, needle aspiration or placement of a drain should be avoided, so that the risk of infection is minimized. If evacuation of the hematoma is required to manage local pain or stop progression, it should be undertaken as a thoroughly sterile procedure.

Late complications, including erosion and migration, are often the result of suboptimal initial surgery. These can be minimized by careful technique at the time of initial pacemaker implantation and by the formation of an adequate pocket.

EPIMYOCARDIAL SYSTEMS

Epimyocardial systems account for no more than 5% of pacemaker implantation procedures. This shift from implantation by thoracotomy to the transvenous route occurred because of the higher morbidity and mortality with epicardial lead systems, the higher incidence of wire fracture, a lack of reliable atrial leads, and the increasing reliability of transvenous pacing systems with active and passive fixation leads. Three groups of patients still undergo placement of epicardial systems.

1. *Patients undergoing cardiac surgery for another indication.* In these patients, permanent epicardial leads may be placed at the time of surgery. Alternatively, some of these patients have temporary pacing until recovery from open-heart surgery. Before dismissal from the hospital, they may undergo placement of a transvenous pacing system. This latter approach is preferable, since transvenous leads have proved to be more reliable than epimyocardial leads.
2. *Patients with recurrent dislodgment of transvenous system.* The number of these patients has declined greatly with the use of active and new passive fixation leads, and it is now rare to see patients with recurrent dislodgment of a transvenous system.
3. *Patients with a prosthetic tricuspid valve, a congenital anomaly, or atresia of the tricuspid valve.* In these patients, epimyocardial ventricular leads are usually required. Prosthetic porcine valves are, however, compatible with transvenous implant.

Several surgical procedures have been described; the two most commonly used are: (1) a subxiphoid or left costal approach and (2) left lateral thoracotomy. A sutureless electrode is most commonly used.

Subxiphoid and Subcostal Approaches

These approaches allow epimyocardial pacing without the need for a formal thoracotomy. Through an upper abdominal incision with xiphoid resection, the diaphragmatic surface of the heart can be approached. With this approach, electrodes can be placed on the diaphragmatic surface of the heart, that is, the right ventricle and some portion of the left ventricle. The amount of left ventricle exposed depends on the anatomy of the patient. Left ventricular placement is preferred for improved sensing. Because of the small and uncertain portion of the left ventricle available with the subxiphoid approach, some surgeons favor the use of a left subcostal incision, which allows better exposure of the left ventricle. Great care must be taken with these approaches to avoid laceration of the right or left ventricle, which requires emergency full thoracotomy for control of bleeding and treatment. Deaths have occurred from this complication.

Left Lateral Thoracotomy

With left lateral thoracotomy (Figure 27), left ventricular implantation is favored. The heart usually is approached through the fifth

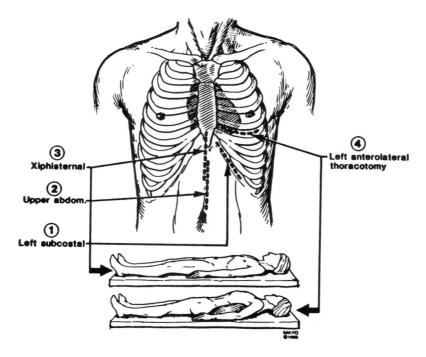

Figure 27. *Incisions and positions of patient used for placement of epimyocardial systems (see text for details). (Reproduced by permission of Mayo Foundation.)*

left intercostal space. An incision is made from the left parasternal border to the left anterior axillary line. Sutureless electrodes can be placed into the left ventricular myocardium through this incision. Care must be taken to implant these at a distance from the phrenic nerve to avoid phrenic stimulation.

Both of these epimyocardial approaches commonly require general anesthesia. Because of the potential surgical complications with these techniques as well as the higher historical incidence of system malfunction, the frequency with which epimyocardial pacing is used has declined significantly. The overwhelming majority of these implants occur in patients undergoing heart surgery at which time the leads are placed.

HARDWARE ADAPTATIONS

Connectors

The connector is the portion of the lead and the pulse generator header that provides the permanent but reversible connection between the two. The portion of the connector on the header holds that portion which is the extravascular end of lead. The connector has undergone substantial evolution since the earliest pulse generators. The first generators introduced had an integral lead system. The presumption was that the patient would not outlive the implanted pulse generator, predicted to have a longevity of 5 years. There was soon a rude awakening. Pulse generators had a longevity of only several months and it was not until the era of lithium powered pulse generators that greater longevity was achieved. It became quickly apparent that despite frequent lead fracture, the lead was a relatively more permanent element than the pulse generator. The need for the ability to disconnect the generator from the lead became clear and was soon introduced.

In Europe, the first connector type was the bare proximal end of the conductor wire. The receptacle, part of the pulse generator, was a set screw overlying a metal or plastic slot for the wire. The wire was inserted, the screw tightened and the lead held. Pulse generator replacement was accomplished by transsecting the lead adjacent to the connector and replacing the freshly cut end into the receptacle.

In the United States, the earliest connectors consisted of a pin (1.6 mm diameter) to fit into the receptacle in the pulse generator and a silicone rubber plug immediately distal to the pin, which was 4.5 mm in diameter (referred to as 5 mm). The lead system was bipolar and two such connectors (one for each lead) were required. A second variety was a unipolar system in which a plug with two pins could be placed into the header. It was designed for an atrial synchronous system in which two connections were required, one of the atrium, the other for the ventricle, and correct placement of each was necessary. With the introduction of transvenous leads, the plug connector became progressively more unwieldly and bipolar transvenous leads required a bifurcation, each leg of which fit into each of the pulse generator receptacles. The receptacle was replaced with a pin and plug combination. The plug was 5.5 mm in diameter (commonly referred to as 6 mm) and the diameter of the pin was somewhat larger (2.25 mm) than that associated with the 5 mm connector.

These two varieties have come to dominate all connectors of all other manufacturers, even those who had introduced other varieties. While other plug and twist lock connectors had been introduced, all eventually yielded to these two varieties. All manufacturers eventually provided leads with these two connectors and most with a receptacle in the header, capable of accepting both.

With the advent of lead systems for dual-chamber pacemakers and especially bipolar leads, the size of the header (now requiring 4 plugs for a dual bipolar system) became as large (or potentially larger) than the electronic battery portion of the generator. The need for smaller connectors became obvious and unipolar and bipolar coaxial (or "in-line") leads were introduced with a plug diameter of 3.2 mm. This new size was incompatible with the two earlier "standards" and the connectors introduced were incompatible with each other. Following a brief era during which lead systems had largely become compatible and interchangeable, incompatibility was again present. The industry then attempted, for the first time in a concerted effort, to produce a connector small enough for modern bipolar lead systems and interchangeable between manufacturers. The result was the series of VOLUNTARY STANDARD-1 connectors. These have been accepted by the entire industry, and new leads and pulse generators, unipolar and bipolar, as they are introduced, will be of this connector configuration.

Many older connector leads remain in service. As pulse generator replacement is required, adapters will be necessary. Some pulse generators are now made specifically to accommodate pulse generator replacement. Some of the newest model generators are available only in a VS-1 or IS-1 connector format, and use with an older lead will require adaptation and often considerable ingenuity.

An attempt should be made to match polarity and design of the pacing lead and pulse generator, i.e., a bipolar in-line lead to a bipolar in-line pulse generator; a bifuracated bipolar lead to a bipolar pulse generator, etc. It is progressively more necessary to use mismatched hardware. Special adaptors are necessary to allow use of polarity mismatched lead and pulse generator. Table III outlines possible combinations and adaptors necessary. Each adaptor is numbered and the numbers correspond to the numbers in Figure 28, which pictures the adaptors. Again, every attempt should be made to match lead and pulse generator hardware (adaptors).

Incompatibility between lead size and pacemaker connector size has long been a source of confusion for the physician implanting pacemakers. This has become more confusing with the introduction of in-line bipolar leads. In an effort to achieve compatibility and interchangeability between pacemakers and leads, a voluntary stan-

Table III

Pulse generator \ Lead	Unipolar	In-line bipolar	Bifurcated bipolar
Unipolar	ō	Low profile adaptor sleeve[1]	End cap[2]
In-line bipolar	Low profile lead to bifurcated pulse generator[5] and an indifferent electrode[4]	ō	Bifurcated lead to in-line generator adaptor[3]
Bipolar with bifurcated connector	Indifferent electrode[4]	Low profile lead to bifurcated pulse generator adaptor[5]	ō

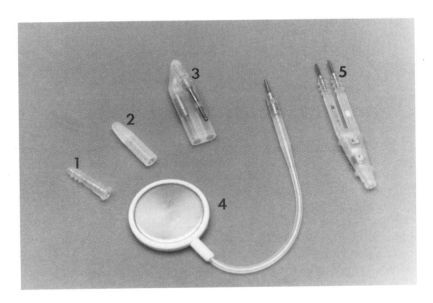

Figure 28. Various adaptors used for pacing lead/pulse generator mismatches. The numbers (1 to 5) correspond to Table III, which outlines specific adaptors needed for specific combinations. 1 = bipolar in-line sleeve adaptor; 2 = end cap; 3 = bifurcated lead to in-line connector; 4 = indifferent electrode; 5 = in-line lead to bifurcated connector.

dard (VS-1) has been developed by an Ad Hoc Committee of pace-maker manufacturers. An international standard (IS-1), which is controlled by the International Standards Organization has also been designated.

This terminology need not be confusing. Dimensions are the same for both unipolar and bipolar VS-1/IS-1 leads and pacers. There is only one configuration for VS-1 and IS-1 lead connectors. The VS-1 and IS-1 designs have provisions within the pacer connector for 3 functional opinions. These are as follows:

VS-1/IS-1	Accepts only VS-1/IS-1 leads.
VS-1A/IS-1A	Accepts VS-1/IS-1 leads and Cordis style 3.2 mm in-line leads (incorporates a longer bore pin).
VS-1B/IS-1B	Accepts VS-1/IS-1 leads. Cordis, Medtronic, CPI and Telectronics style 3.2 mm in-line leads (incorporates a longer pin bore and sealing rings) (Figure 29).

VS1/IS1 CONNECTOR

SEALING RINGS

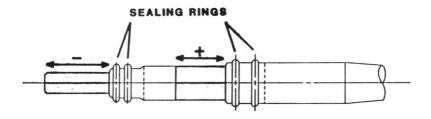

Figure 29. *The VS1/IS1 connectors are intended to restore universal interconnection of all leads and pulse generators via the newly standardized 3.2 mm connectors. The pin (shaded in gray) is connected to the negative output, the ring (also shaded in gray) is connected to the positive terminal in the pulse generator header. Unipolar leads of similar configuration exist but without a positive terminal and are of the same size and are interchangeable with a bipolar receptacle. The four ridges represent the sealing rings, which prevent the ingress of fluid into the header.*

SPECIAL CONSIDERATIONS IN
PEDIATRIC PATIENTS

Permanent pacing in the pediatric population raises specific issues including the size of the patient, expected growth of the patient, the presence of associated congenital heart disease, need for long-term pacing and often a need for dual-chambered pacing systems.

Transvenous systems are used most frequently and have been shown to be superior to epicardial systems. Previous studies have shown that survival of endocardial leads in the pediatric pacemaker population is superior to that of myoepicardial leads.

In the pediatric patient undergoing permanent pacing, it is helpful to know prior to the implant if a persistent left superior vena cava is present. This can usually be determined echocardiographically. If concern exists, angiography is diagnostic (Figure 30). Advancing the

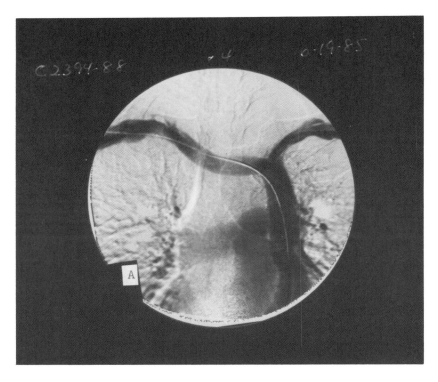

Figure 30A. *Contrast injection into the right side shows absence of the right superior vena cava and presence of a left superior vena cava.*

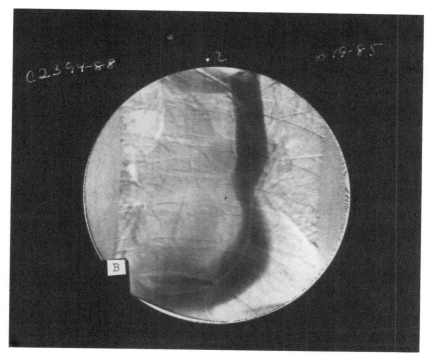

Figure 30B.   *The dye enters the coronary sinus and then the right atrium.*

pacing lead into a persistent left superior vena cava will result in coronary sinus placement. While pacing has been accomplished from this position, it is unstable and generally not reliable for permanent pacing. To avoid the problems associated with a persistent left superior vena cava, the right subclavian vein should be used routinely.

In placement of the leads it is important to allow some redundancy, which provides for stable pacing despite patient growth (Figure 31). During follow-up, the leads must be evaluated periodically. It had once been thought that perhaps the lead could be advanced to accommodate growth. Because of entrapment of the lead in the vein (subclavian or cephalic depending on the venous route used), it may not be possible to advance a lead that has been in place for a long period of time. Although a variety of clinical situations may occur when the patient truly "outgrows" the pacing system, more commonly intermittent sensing abnormalities may occur as tension develops on the lead at the electrode/tissue interface.

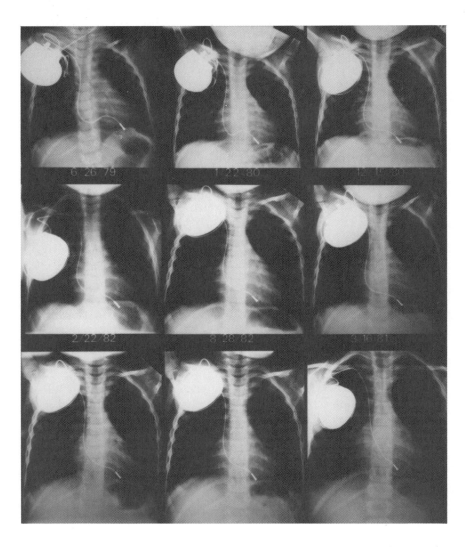

Figure 31.   *Serial radiographs of a transvenous pacemaker in a child show that initial lead redundancy becomes less with growth.*

It is of particular importance to select the smallest pulse generator that allows the desired pacing mode for the pediatric patient. Current pacemakers are now available as small as 22 grams. The small weight and dimensions of these pacemakers will allow their implantation in a prepectoral position in almost any sized patient (Figure 32). In very small infants, in whom there is a concern that there is not enough subcutaneous tissue to protect the pacemaker, consideration may be given to placing the pacemaker in a subpectoral position. In our experience this is not often necessary. Prior to the advent of very small pulse generators, the transvenous lead was occasionally tunneled subcutaneously from the pectoral entry site to an area in the abdomen or flank where the pulse generator could be placed more easily (Figure 33). This, too, is rarely necessary with the small size of currently available pulse generators.

Traditional pacing lead implantation techniques can be used in the pediatric patient. That is, the subclavian puncture technique with placement of 1 or 2 leads via the subclavian vein is usually possible. Two leads can also be placed via direct cutdown on the cephalic vein.

Although any standard pacing lead can be used in the pediatric patient, many prefer the use of active fixation leads in the pediatric population for three specific reasons. An active fixation lead may allow additional stability of the lead in the immediate post-implant period when it is difficult to control the activities of a pediatric patient as compared to the adult patient. The pediatric patient may require several pacing systems during the growth years. While a noninfected lead may be abandoned and left in place, it is reasonable to attempt removal of abandoned leads in the pediatric patient so that the patient will not accummulate an excessive amount of hardware throughout a lifetime. Some preference has therefore been given to active fixation leads because of the relative ease of removal of a chronic active fixation lead compared to a chronic passive/fixation lead.

Active fixation leads can be placed in a greater variety of positions than passive fixation leads. This is important in the patient with associated congenital heart disease in which the anatomy may be quite distorted. An active fixation lead allows placement in all portions of the atrium, not the atrial appendage alone. Active fixation leads have been used in patients following a Mustard procedure, placing the leads across the intra-atrial baffle and pacing the left atrium (Chapter 12, Figure 25).

A specific problem in pediatric pacing involves cardiac pacing after the Fontan procedure. As postoperative anatomy precludes transvenous endocardial ventricular pacing, dual-chamber pacing in these patients has been accomplished by placing a ventricular epicar-

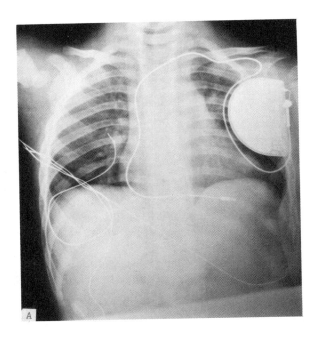

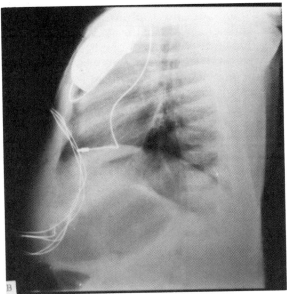

Figure 32.   *Postero-anterior (A, **top**) and lateral (B, **bottom**) chest x-ray showing the relationship of pacemaker size to chest wall size in a 10.8 kg child. The pacemaker appears very large in relationship to chest size but was easily accommodated by tissues in the prepectoral position.*

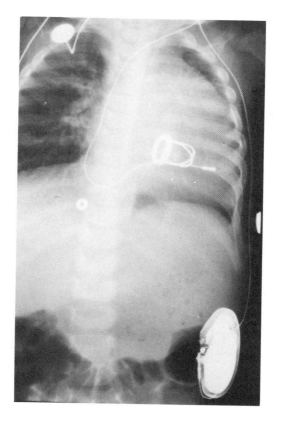

Figure 33. *An implanted transvenous lead system in which there is inadequate prepectoral tissue for pulse generator placement. The lead has been tunneled to flank for pulse generator placement.*

dial lead at the time of surgery and subsequently placing an atrial endocardial lead and tunneling the 2 leads to a common prepectoral position to be attached to a dual-chamber pacemaker (Figure 34).

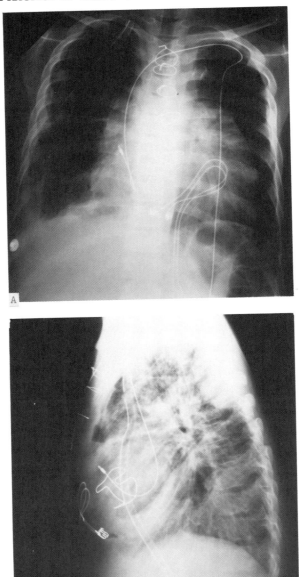

Figure 34.   *Posteroanterior (**A, top**) and lateral (**B, bottom**) views from a patient with dual-chamber a pacemaker. The ventricle is paced from the epimyocardial position and the atrium is paced from the endocardial position. The atrial lead is then tunneled subcutaneously to the abdomen where the pulse generator is implanted.*

PERMANENT PACING AFTER CARDIAC TRANSPLANTATION

As increasing numbers of cardiac transplantations are performed, information is emerging regarding special considerations in pacing this population. Sinus node dysfunction, specifically sinus bradycardia, is not uncommon in the early post-transplant period. This is most likely caused by trauma/damage to the donor atrium at the time of harvesting and transplant. In some patients sinus node dysfunction remits spontaneously several weeks following the procedure, but in some patients permanent pacing has been required.

Implantation of the pacemaker can be accomplished in the usual fashion but special consideration must be given to placement of an atrial lead. After cardiac transplantation there is a remnant of the recipient atrium as well as the donor atrium. Present experience suggests that it is preferable and perhaps easier to place the atrial lead in the donor atrium.

The mode of pacing chosen depends on the rhythm disturbance necessitating permanent pacing. The patients with sinus node dysfunction can, and have been paced in the AAI and AAIR modes if there is no associated atrioventricular nodal disease. Ventricular pacing as well as dual-chamber pacing has been described in this population.

Few specific complications can be anticipated. Cyclosporine, a mainstay of immunosuppressive therapy in the transplant patient, may cause tremors. Such tremors have been reported to cause myopotential inhibition in paced transplanted patients. This may favor pacing transplanted patients in a bipolar configuration, which is less susceptible to myopotential interference.

Rejection episodes in the transplanted patient can alter the intracardiac electrogram and could potentially cause sensing abnormalities. Telemetered electrograms have, in fact, been used to detect rejection episodes.

BIBLIOGRAPHY

Belott PH, Bucko D: Inframammary pulse generator placement for maximizing cosmetic effect. *PACE* 1983; 6:1241–1244.

Bisping HJ, Kreuzer J, Birkenheier H: Three-year clinical experience with a new endocardial screw-in lead with introduction protection for use in the atrium and ventricle. *PACE* 1980; 3:424–435.

Bognolo DA: Recent advances in permanent pacemaker implantation techniques. In SS Barold (Ed): *Modern Cardiac Pacing*. Futura Publishing Company, Mount Kisco, New York, 1985, pp 199–229.

Bognolo DA, Vijayanagar R, Eckstein PF, et al: Two leads in one introducer technique for A-V sequential implantations. *PACE* 1982; 5:217–218.

Byrd C: Permanent pacemaker implantation techniques. In P Samet, N El-Sherif (Eds): *Cardiac Pacing*. 2nd ed. Grune & Stratton, New York, 1980, pp 229–253.

Fox S, Toonder FG: Simplified technique for permanent atrioventricular pacing via a single venipuncture. *Chest* 1981; 80:745–747.

Furman S: Venous cutdown for pacemaker implantation. *Ann Thorac Surg* 1986; 41(4):438–9.

Furman S, Fisher JD: Cardiac pacing and pacemakers. V. Technical aspects of implantation and equipment. *Am Heart J* 1977; 94:250–259.

Furman S, Hurzeler P, DeCaprio V: The ventricular endocardial electrogram and pacemaker sensing. *J Thorac Cardiovasc Surg* 1977; 73:258–266.

Gillette PC, Shannon C, Blair H, et al: Transvenous pacing in pediatric patients. *Am Heart J* 1983; 105:843–847.

Gillette PC, Wampler DG, Shannon C, Ott D: Use of cardiac pacing after the Mustard operation for transposition of the great arteries. *JACC* 1986; 7(1):138–41.

Hanley PC, Vlietstra RE, Merideth J, et al: Two decades of cardiac pacing at the Mayo Clinic (1961 through 1981). *Mayo Clin Proc* 1984; 59:268–274.

Hayes DL, Furman S: Atrio-ventricular and ventriculo-atrial conduction times in patients undergoing pacemaker implant. *PACE* 1983; 6:38–46.

Hayes DL, Holmes DR Jr, Maloney JD, et al: Permanent endocardial pacing in pediatric patients. *J Thorac Cardiovasc Surg* 1983; 85:618–624.

Hayes DL, Holmes DR Jr, Merideth J, et al: Bipolar tined polyurethane ventricular lead: A four-year experience. *PACE* 1985; 8:192–196.

Hickey M, Duff D, Neligan MC: Intrapleural permanent pacemakers in infancy. *Arch Dis Child* 1982; 57:521–522.

Kertes P, Mond H, Sloman G, et al: Comparison of lead complications with polyurethane tined, silicone rubber tined, and wedge tip leads: Clinical experience with 822 ventricular endocardial leads. *PACE* 1983; 6:957–962.

Lawrie GM, Seale JP, Morris GC Jr, et al: Results of epicardial pacing by the left subcostal approach. *Ann Thorac Surg* 1979; 28:561–566.

Littleford PO, Spector SD: Device for the rapid insertion of a permanent endocardial pacing electrode through the subclavian vein: Preliminary report. *Ann Thorac Surg* 1979; 27:265–269.

Martinis AJ: Pacemaker insertion. In DH Dillard, DW Miller Jr (Eds): *Atlas of Cardiac Surgery*. Macmillan Publishing Company, New York, 1983; pp 156–163.

McGoon MD, Maloney JD, McGoon DC, et al: Long-term endocardial atrial pacing in children with postoperative bradycardia-tachycardia syndrome and limited ventricular access. *Am J Cardiol* 1982; 49:1750–1757.

Messenger JC, Castellanet MJ, Stephenson NL: New permanent endocardial atrial J lead: Implantation techniques and clinical performance. *PACE* 1982; 5:767–772.

Miller FA Jr, Holmes DR Jr, Gersh BJ, et al: Permanent transvenous pacemaker implantation via the subclavian vein. *Mayo Clin Proc* 1980; 55:309–314.

Mond HG: *The Cardiac Pacemaker: Function and Malfunction.* Grune & Stratton, New York; 1983; pp 191–232.

Moss AJ, Rivers RJ Jr: Atrial pacing from the coronary vein: Ten-year experience in 50 patients with implanted pervenous pacemakers. *Circulation* 1978; 57:103–106.

Naclerio EA, Varriale P: Surgical techniques for permanent ventricular pacing. In P Varriale, EA Naclerio (Eds): *Cardiac Pacing: A Concise Guide to Clinical Practice.* Lea & Febiger, Philadelphia; 1979; pp 145–168.

Ong LS, Barold SS, Lederman M, Falkoff MD, Heinle RA: Cephalic vein guide wire technique for implantation of permanent pacemakers. *Am Heart J* 1987; 114(4 Part 1):753–6.

Parsonnet V: A stretch fabric pouch for implanted pacemakers. *Arch Surg* 1972; 105:654–656.

Parsonnet V, Crawford CC, Bernstein AD: The 1981 United States survey of cardiac pacing practices. *J Am Coll Cardiol* 1984; 3:1321–1332.

Parsonnet V, Furman S, Smyth NPD, et al: Optimal resources for implantable cardiac pacemakers. *Circulation* 1983; 68:226A–244A.

Parsonnet V, Werres R, Atherley T: Transvenous insertion of double sets of permanent electrodes: Atraumatic technique for atrial synchronous and atrioventricular sequential pacemakers. *JAMA* 1980; 243:62–64.

Smyth NPD: Pacemaker implantation: Surgical techniques. *Cardiovasc Clin* 1983; 14(no. 2):31–44.

Smyth NPD: Techniques of implantation: Atrial and ventricular thoracotomy and transvenous. *Prog Cardiovasc Dis* 1981; 23:435–450.

Stewart S: Placement of the sutureless epicardial pacemaker lead by the subxiphoid approach. *Ann Thorac Surg* 1974; 18:308–313.

Walls JT, Maloney JD, Pluth JR: Clinical evaluation of a sutureless cardiac pacing lead: Chronic threshold changes and lead durability. *Ann Thorac Surg* 1983; 36:328–331.

Ward DE, Jones S, Shinebourne EA: Long-term transvenous pacing in children weighing 10 kg or less. *Int J Cardiol* 1987; 15(1):112–5.

Chapter 9

PACEMAKER ELECTROCARDIOGRAPHY

David L. Hayes

An understanding of "Basic Concepts" of cardiac pacing and "Timing Cycles" of cardiac pacing (Chapters 2 and 4) is fundamental before approaching the paced electrocardiogram. The paced electro-cardiogram must be approached in a systematic fashion, much as a nonpaced electrocardiogram, chest x-ray, or other diagnostic proce-dure. Knowing the type of pacemaker, the programmed parameters, and the underlying rhythm necessitating pacing are important factors in interpreting the paced electrocardiogram. Obviously, this informa-tion makes the interpretation much easier, but it is frequently not available.

INITIAL ECG INTERPRETATION

In reviewing an electrocardiogram with an implanted pacemaker, one should carefully assess the underlying rhythm as well as its rela-tionship to the pacemaker artifact(s). The first step is to find any portion of the electrocardiogram during which the heart is unpaced, i.e., showing the intrinsic cardiac rhythm. That portion of the electrocardiogram should be interpreted as any electrocardiogram: PR, QRS, and QT intervals; rate; axis; voltage, etc. If no intrinsic rhythm is apparent, then the patient may be pacemaker-dependent or the pace-maker may be programmed to stimulate faster (i.e., at a shorter cycle length) than the intrinsic rhythm. After determining both the sponta-neous atrial and ventricular rhythms, one should look for any relation-ship between the two, i.e.,does a P wave result in a QRS complex indicating intact AV conduction?

After the intrinsic rhythm has been carefully scrutinized, pace-maker activity should be assessed. If pacemaker activity is present, is there one stimulus or two (Figures 1, 2)? If only one stimulus is present, does it result in atrial (Figure 3) or ventricular depolarization (Figure 1)? Is there an apparent relationship between pacemaker activity and atrial

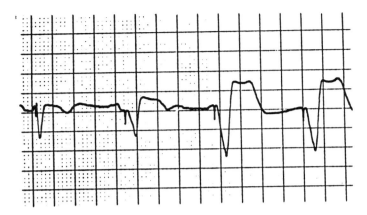

Figure 1.   *Normal ventricular demand pacing (VVI) in which the intrinsic rate is close to the programmed pacing rate. The first two beats of the ECG strip show varying degrees of fusion between the intrinsic QRS complexes and the paced beat; the third and fourth beats are totally paced.*

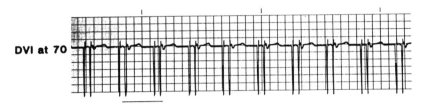

Figure 2.   *AV sequential pacing (DVI) at a rate of 70 bpm. No intrinsic P or QRS activity occurs. It is impossible to distinguish whether the patient is pacing in the DVI, DDD, or DOO mode.*

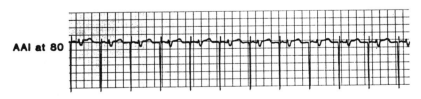

Figure 3.   *Normal AAI pacing in which no intrinsic P wave activity is seen. The pacemaker is set at a rate of 80. The paced atrial depolarization is followed by a conducted QRS complex. From this illustration alone, without any intrinsic P wave activity, it is impossible to distinguish between AAI, DVI noncommitted, or DDD modes of pacing.*

activity, ventricular activity, or both? If there is no relationship between the pacemaker stimulus and a preceding P wave and the pacemaker stimulus follows the intrinsic QRS complex at a consistent cycle length, then ventricular sensing as part of ventricular inhibited (VVI) pacing is present (Figure 1). If the same situation occurs but with a pacemaker artifact consistently found within intrinsic P or QRS complexes, then a triggered pacing mode (AAT or VVT) exists (Figures 4, 5).

In the initial evaluation of the paced electrocardiogram, it also may be possible to determine whether the pacemaker is of a unipolar or bipolar configuration by assessing the height of the pacemaker stimulus in standard lead 2. The ability to make this determination depends on the monitoring system used. With some systems, if the pacemaker artifact is large, then it is most likely of the unipolar configuration (Figure 6). If a very small pacemaker artifact is present in standard lead 2, it is most likely of the bipolar configuration (Figure 7). In monitoring or ECG systems, such as the digital electrocardiograph, which artifically simulate the pacemaker artifact, this analysis cannot be used.

RESPONSE TO MAGNET APPLICATION

The magnet mode should be activated for interpretation of the pacemaker electrocardiogram. It is helpful in identification of the pacing mode and often the specific pulse generator. It is equally useful for

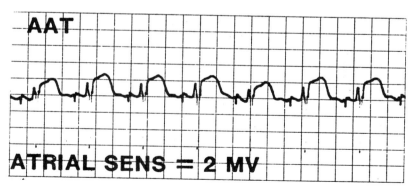

Figure 4.   *Normal atrial triggered pacing with the pacemaker programmed at a rate of 60 and atrial sensitivity of 2 mV. A pacemaker artifact can be seen within each intrinsic P wave. The intrinsic sinus rate is approximately 94 bpm. AV conduction is present.*

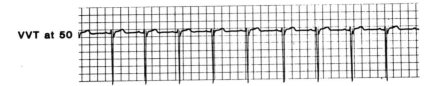

Figure 5.   *An example of normal ventricular triggered pacing. This pacemaker was set at a rate of 50 bpm. The intrinsic rate is approximately 75 bpm so that pacemaker is triggered and a stimulus artifact can be seen during the terminal portion of each QRS complex. If ventricular activity had not been sensed within 1200 ms (50 bpm) following a previous ventricular depolarization, a stimulus would have been emitted.*

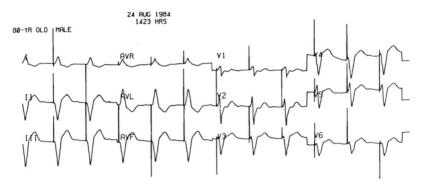

Figure 6.   *A 12-lead electrocardiogram from a patient with a VVI pacemaker. Note the large pacemaker artifacts. Large artifacts are typical of unipolar pacing as contrasted to the smaller artifacts usually seen in patients with bipolar pacing systems.*

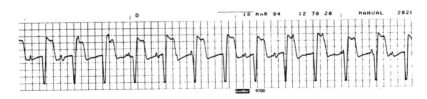

Figure 7.   *Lead II ECG of bipolar ventricular pacing. The pacemaker artifact is very small and not easily identified on this ECG. However, each QRS complex present is paced, and because there is no intrinsic activity, it is impossible to know whether the patient is being paced in the asynchronous (VOO) or demand (VVI) mode. Clearly, the P waves bear no relationship to the QRS complex.*

single- and dual-chamber pacing and can be particularly helpful for determining proper pacing and sensing.

Application of a magnet to a single-chamber pacemaker always results in asynchronous pacing. In dual-chamber pacemakers, magnet application usually but not always results in asynchronous pacing in both the atrial and ventricular chambers. Exceptions do exist. At least one model of a dual-chamber pulse generator does not have a magnet mode. The absence of one or more stimuli in the magnet mode, following apparently normal function is a strong indicator of lead fracture.

While in the magnet mode, the paced rate should be determined. Is the magnet rate faster or slower or the same as the programmed pacemaker rate (Figure 8). If the pacemaker is known to be a single-chamber pacemaker, does it result in atrial or ventricular depolarization? Having determined what chamber is being paced, one can assess the pacemaker artifact and subsequent depolarization to assure proper capture. Once magnet rate and cardiac capture have been determined, the magnet can be removed in order to assess proper sensing. It should be remembered that pacemakers of different manufacturers respond differently to magnet application. Some will continue to pace asynchronously for a specific number of beats following magnet removal and may do so at more than one rate. This should not be interpreted as sensing failure (Figure 8). The individual specifics of magnet application must be known for each pacemaker in order to determine that behavior is normal during magnet application and following removal. When a single chamber is being paced, the effect of the paced chamber on the remaining chamber should be ascertained. If an atrial pacemaker is present, does atrial depolarization result in AV conduction and an intrinsic QRS complex, demonstrating intact AV conduction (Figure 3)? Alternatively, if a ventricular pacemaker is present, is there retrograde activation of the atrium, resulting in retrograde P wave activity following the paced ventricular complex (Figure 9)?

The occurrence of a pacemaker artifact at an unexpected time, especially after magnet application has demonstrated normal function, may indicate abnormal sensing. Once the chamber a single-chamber pacemaker is to sense has been determined and a stimulus cannot be timed from the preceding event, abnormal sensing may be present. Prolonged intervals may result from inapparant pathological events, such as electromagnetic (EMI) or electromyographic interference or physiological events, such as P waves and QRS complexes isoelectric in the lead being analyzed. Multiple, simultaneous ECG leads are useful. Abbreviated intervals may result from unsensed events, EMI

MAGNET APPLICATION

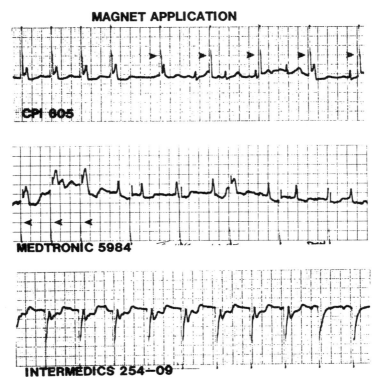

Figure 8.   *Magnet application to three different VVI pacemakers from three different manufacturers results in different responses. In the upper panel, magnet application to a CPI 605 pulse generator results in asynchronous pacing at a rate of 100 bpm. When the magnet is removed, the pacemaker stimulates asynchronously for five beats at the programmed rate (arrows). In the middle panel, magnet application to a Medtronic 5984 results in three paced beats at a rate of 100 per minute (arrows) followed by asynchronous pacing at the programmed rate. In the lower panel, an Intermedics 254-09 results in asynchronous pacing at a fixed asynchronous rate of 85 bpm.*

forcing the noise mode, a premature event falling into the noise sampling interval forcing the next stimulus, and a ventricular event during dual-chamber pacing, which falls into either the blanking interval or the safety pacing interval following an atrial stimulus.

If two stimuli appear when the magnet is applied to the pacemaker, a dual-chamber pacemaker is present. With both artifacts present, the AV interval should be measured and recorded. In most circumstances, application of a magnet to a dual-chamber pacemaker will result in asynchronous pacing in both the atrial and ventricular cham-

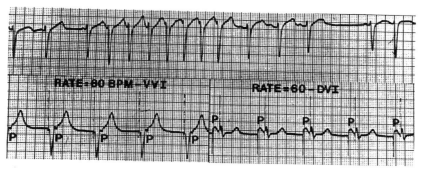

Figure 9. *Retrograde atrial activation can occur readily. A patient with nodal tachycardia with a committed DVI pacemaker programmed first to the VVI mode (below left) with retrograde P waves readily seen and then to the DVI mode, which positions the P wave before each QRS complex. The QRS complexes are fusion beats (below right).*

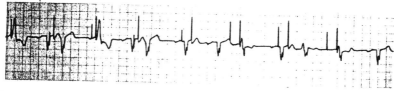

Figure 10. *Electrocardiographic recording from a patient with a Pacesetter-AFP DDD pacemaker programmed to a lower rate of 50 bpm. At the beginning of the ECG, both atrial and ventricular pacing artifacts occur asynchronously at a rate of 57 bpm and an AV delay of 101 ms. This is the normal magnet response (AV interval of 101 ms and a rate of 14% above the programmed lower rate). After the first four sets of atrial and ventricular pacing artifacts, the AV delay increases to 240 ms. When the magnet is removed, the pacemaker beats asynchronously for four additional cycles at the preset AV delay, the normal response for this pacemaker. At the end of the four asychronous beats, an intrinsic P and QRS occur without pacing artifact.*

bers (DOO mode) (Figure 10). There are dual-chamber pacemakers available in which magnet application will result in atrial asynchronous pacing but with retention of ventricular sensing (Figure 11). It is important that the physician make few assumptions concerning the details of the magnet mode of operation and be aware of the specifics of the magnet response in a particular unit or an erroneous interpretation of inappropriate operation may be made. The magnet mode is usually (but not always) free of sensing any events, and is often at a specific rate independent of the programmed rate and sensitivity settings. It allows determination, in the presence of a puzzling or unusual ECG, of whether the pulse generator is capable of operating normally.

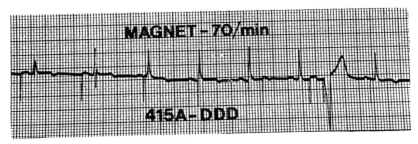

Figure 11.   *Magnet application to the Cordis 415A pacemaker results in asynchronous pacing from the atrial channel. Ventricular activity can be sensed following the atrial depolarization, and no ventricular output need occur even during magnet application. This is seen with the third and fourth pacing artifacts as well as the last pacing artifact in this example. In contrast to most DDD pacemakers that pace asynchronously in both channels, ventricular sensing is retained during magnet application.*

DETERMINATION OF PACING MODE

Single-Chamber Pacemakers

By following the preceding steps, determination will have been made as to whether a single- or dual-chamber pacemaker is present. If a single-chamber atrial pacemaker is present, stimulation produces atrial capture, and the pacemaker artifact is inhibited by intrinsic P waves, the pacemaker is in the atrial inhibited (AAI) mode (Figure 3). Paced ventricular activity will never be seen, with or without magnet application, and a pacer artifact will never occur within the intrinsic P waves.

If one stimulus is seen that results in ventricular capture with inhibition by QRS complexes, the pacemaker is in the ventricular inhibited mode (VVI) (Figure 1).

If the pacemaker is pacing asynchronously without sensing or capture of either the atrium or the ventricle, the mode cannot be determined. Similarly, with either a single-chamber atrial or ventricular pacer, if intrinsic activity is never seen and every complex is paced, the patient is either pacemaker-dependent or the pacemaker has been programmed faster than the intrinsic cardiac rate.

If a single stimulus falls consistently into the spontaneous P wave or QRS complex, then the mode is of the triggered variety (AAT/VVT) (Figures 4, 5). Although this mode of pacing is available in some multimodal programmable pacemakers, it rarely is utilized. Programming a pacemaker to the triggered mode is sometimes helpful to determine exactly where on the surface electrocardiogram sensing occurs (Figure 12).

An exception to the rule of the timing cycles in AAI and VVI pacing and a source of frequent confusion is hysteresis. This programmable feature allows the escape interval for the initial paced beat to be at a longer cycle length than subsequent paced intervals. For example, if a patient has sinus node dysfunction with episodes of sinus bradycardia or sinus arrest, the pacemaker can be programmed to pace continuously at an interval of 1,000 ms (rate of 60), but hysteresis takes place at a rate of 40, i.e., allow 1,500 ms without a paced event before initiating pacing. If it is unknown that hysteresis is present, it may appear that there are two different functioning intervals. If these

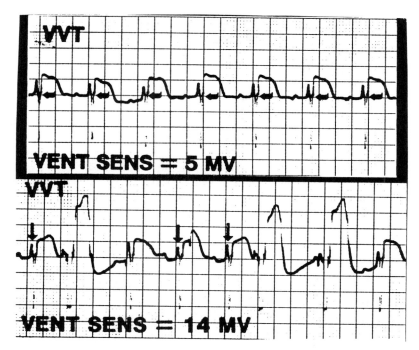

Figure 12. *Electrocardiogram demonstrating the VVT mode used to determine the ventricular sensing threshold. At a programmed rate of 75 bpm and a sensitivity of 5 mV, (upper strip) a pacing artifact can be seen within each intrinsic QRS complex. This documents normal sensing at a sensitivity level of 5 mV. In the lower strip with the pacemaker programmed to a sensitivity of 14 mV, QRS complexes are no longer being sensed, and pacing occurs at the programmed rate of 75 bpm. At a sensitivity level of 14 mV, there is failure to sense in the ventricle. (Arrows denote intrinsic QRS complexes that are not sensed.)*

intervals are seen to be repetitive, hysteresis is the most likely explanation (Figure 13).

Abnormalities of Single-Chamber Pacing

If each pacemaker stimulus is not followed by a QRS or P wave complex, failure to capture may exist (Figure 14). Failure to capture may be caused by a variety of factors, including, most commonly, lead dislodgment and stimulation thresholds above the output of the pulse generator.

The occurrence of pacemaker artifacts at an unexplained time suggests abnormal sensing (Figure 15). If the interval between the preceding QRS complex and the paced beat is shorter than the programmed paced cycle length, undersensing may be present. Failure to sense is often seen in combination with failure to capture (Figure 16) but the functions are separate and malfunctions may occur independently.

The pacemaker senses intracardiac electrograms referred to in Chapter 4, "Comprehension of Timing Cycles." It is not possible to know from the surface ECG exactly where in relation to the ECG the intrinsic deflection exists, and thus where sensing occurs. The pacemaker artifact may fall within the QRS complex (Figure 17). This does not necessarily represent failure to sense but, instead, an electrogram that occurs after the onset of the QRS as noted on the surface electrocardiogram. The stimulus may appear to be late when analyzed from the surface electrocardiogram, but reflects only pacemaker sensing

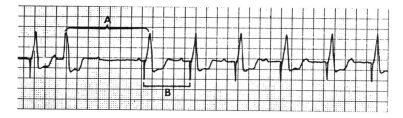

Figure 13.   *Ventricular demand (VVI) pacing at a programmed rate of 72 bpm (833 ms, interval B). The preceding interval (interval A) is approximately 1550 ms in duration and represents normal VVI pacing with hysteresis. This prolonged cycle following a sensed ventricular event allows a longer period for the patient's intrinsic conduction system to escape before pacing at the programmed rate. A pacemaker with hysteresis can be inhibited by a slower rate than it will pace.*

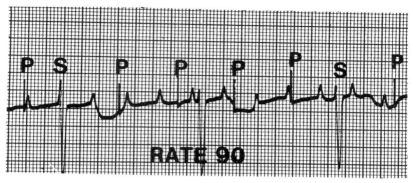

Figure 14.   *The pacemaker stimuli are below threshold and do not capture the ventricle. Sensing remains intact. The first and last spontaneous QRS complexes inhibit and recycle the pacemaker. The second falls during the refractory period after a stimulus and is unsensed. P = pacer stimulus; S = sensed QRS.*

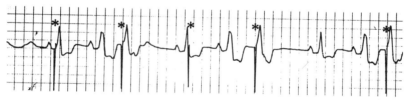

Figure 15.   *Ventricular inhibited pacing (VVI) with intermittent failure to sense but normal ventricular capture. Failure to sense is evidenced by the second, fourth, and fifth pacemaker artifacts. The pacemaker is set at a cycle length of 1500 ms (40 bpm), but the stimuli occur 600 to 700 ms following the previous intrinsic QRS complex. The third pacemaker artifact does not represent failure to capture as it occurs at a time when the ventricle is refractory.*

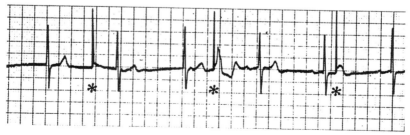

Figure 16.   *Ventricular inhibited pacing (VVI) with failure to sense and intermittent failure to capture. Of the three pacemaker stimuli, ventricular depolarization occurs only after the second, the third probably falls during partial ventricular refractoriness.*

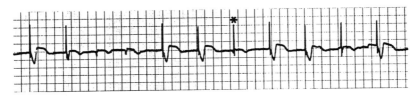

Figure 17. *Ventricular inhibited pacing (VVI) in which the fifth and eighth stimuli fall within the QRS complex (the fifth artifact appearing later in the QRS complex than the eighth). This does not represent failure to sense. The surface electrocardiographic finding reflects a difference in actual electrogram sensing and sensing apparent on the electrocardiogram. This may be particularly apparent in patients with right bundle branch block. The second pacemaker artifact results in a fusion beat.*

after the onset of the surface QRS complex or P wave. If the surface QRS represents elements of two depolarizations, it is a fusion beat, if of a single depolarization with a superimposed stimulus, it is a pseudofusion beat. Oversensing also may occur. The pacemaker interval is then reset by inappropriate sensed events so that the interval between the pacemaker stimulus or intrinsic QRS activity and the subsequent paced beat is greater than the programmed pacemaker cycle. T waves, P waves (Figure 18), afterpotentials from pacemaker discharge (Figure 19), muscle activity (Figure 20), and electromagnetic interference may result in oversensing.

Ventricular activity may arise from different foci within the ventricle and will appear with different configurations or even appear isoelectric on the surface electrocardiogram. An isoelectric QRS complex can cause an apparent "pause" that gives the impression of oversensing. Multichannel electrocardiograms are helpful in evaluating that possibility as it is unlikely that a QRS will be isoelectric in all leads (Figure 21). Alternatively, if an isoelectric event occurs at the time of paced artifact and a fusion beat results, it may appear as failure to capture. Pacemaker capture can be confirmed by noting the T wave or repolarization activity that follows the pacing artifact (Figure 17).

Dual-Chamber Pacemakers

If it has been ascertained that a dual-chamber pacemaker is present, the steps above should be followed with determination of the AV interval and the status of AV and VA conduction.

During the free-running (nonmagnet) pacemaker mode it should be determined whether P waves consistently are unsensed, i.e., does

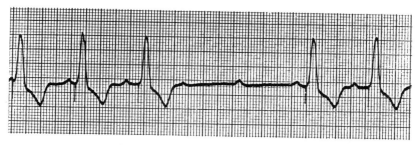

Figure 18. *Ventricular inhibited (VVI) pacing with a delay between the third and fourth paced complexes caused by P wave sensing and recycle. Note the paced rate with calipers and measure back from the fourth paced complex. The escape interval falls within the P wave, which is sensed by the pacemaker. P wave oversensing is uncommon but can occur in a bipolar lead as illustrated.*

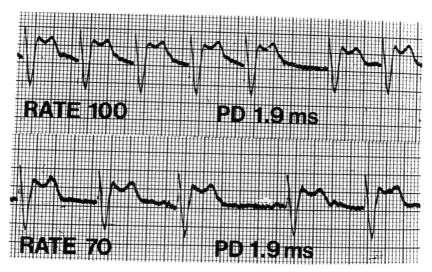

Figure 19. *Ventricular inhibited (VVI) pacing with a pause longer than the programmed cycle length in both the upper and lower panels. This prolonged cycle is caused by sensing of the afterpotential following a high output stimulus, i.e., a pulse duration of 1.9 ms. Note the escape cycle length and measure backward from the QRS complex following the prolonged cycle. It will be noted that the event sensed is the afterpotential. Decreasing the pulse duration corrects this problem. If the pulse duration cannot be safely decreased, then prolonging the refractory period or making the ventricular channel less sensitive may correct the problem (though this option is not possible with the pulse generator illustrated).*

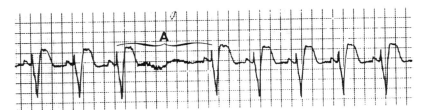

Figure 20. *An electrocardiogram of atrial synchronous (VDD) pacing with electro-myographic interference. During the interference (irregular baseline) the ventricular channel senses muscle activity and inhibits ventricular output.*

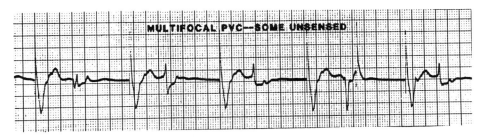

Figure 21. *Ventricular inhibited pacing (VVI) at a programmed rate of 75 bpm (800 ms cycle length) and multifocal PVCs in a bigeminal pattern. The first, second, and third PVCs are sensed appropriately. Sensing of the fifth PVC is uncertain because the tracing ends. The fourth PVC is not sensed. A paced ventricular beat follows 800 ms after the previous paced beat. The amplitude and frequency content of each ventricular focus differs, and all possible foci may not be sensed by the pacemaker. A retrograde P wave follows each ventricular contraction.*

the pacemaker always recycle from the ventricular stimulus? If so, the pacer may be in the DVI mode (ventricular sensing only) (Figure 22) or there may be atrial failure to sense in the DDD mode. If in the DVI mode, QRS complexes that occur during the AV interval may be sensed or unsensed. A QRS complex that occurs following an atrial stimulus may inhibit the pacemaker ventricular channel. If the ventricular channel is inhibited, then the pacemaker is of the DVI noncommitted variety (Figures 23, 24). If following paced atrial activity, unpaced QRS activity occurs but a ventricular artifact follows the atrial pacing artifact at the present AV delay, falling during or after the intrinsic QRS complex, the pacemaker is of the DVI committed variety (Figures 25, 26). Alternatively, the DVI pacemaker may be noncommitted but with failure of ventricular sensing.

If P wave activity is being sensed, does each P wave begin a pacemaker cycle? If each spontaneous P wave results in a paced ven-

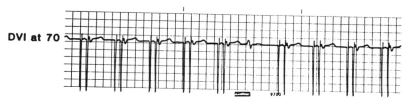

DVI at 70

Figure 22. *Continous AV sequential (DVI) pacing in which the atrium and the ventricle are stimulated with an AV delay. Recycle occurs from a spontaneous QRS complex.*

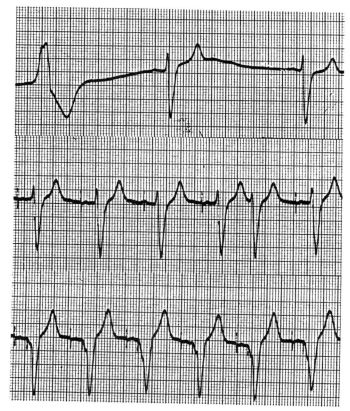

Figure 23. **ABOVE:** *Sinus bradycardia.* **MIDDLE:** *Atrial stimulation with the QRS complexes produced by AV conduction and recycle from a VPC.* **BELOW:** *Pacing of atrium and ventricle at a shortened AV interval during magnet application.*

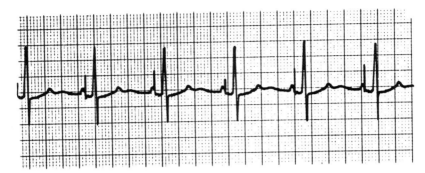

Figure 24.   *Normal noncommitted DVI pacing in which the lower rate limit is 70 bpm (850 ms). The intrinsic sinus rate also is approximately 70 bpm, and there is competition between the atrial stimuli and intrinsic P wave activity. As this is a noncommitted unit, QRS activity occurs following the atrial stimulus and inhibits the ventricular channel.*

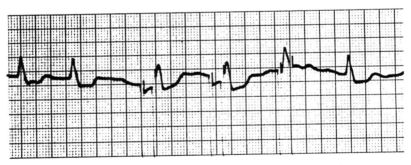

Figure 25.   *A DVI committed pacemaker with an AV interval of 155 ms programmed to a stimulation interval of 923 ms (i.e., 65 bpm). Two intrinsic QRS complexes during the VA interval inhibit atrial and ventricular output. With a delay following the second complex, an atrial stimulus, probably simultaneous with a P wave, occurs and is obligatorily followed by a ventricular stimulus that produces a paced ventricular event. The next complex is identical. The fifth complex begins with a spontaneous P wave (unsensed by the insensitive atrial channel). A conducted QRS follows after the atrial stimulus during the AV interval (the ventricular channel of a committed DVI pacemaker is insensitive during the AV interval). The QRS is followed by a ventricular stimulus. The last spontaneous QRS complex occurs sufficiently early to be sensed and inhibit both atrial and ventricular stimuli.*

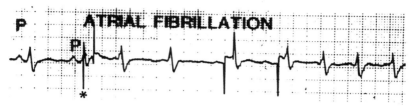

Figure 26. *A committed DVI pacemaker is inhibited by intrinsic activity during the first P-QRS complex. A normally unsensed P wave occurs, and the atrial stimulus is emitted during the vulnerable period of atrial depolarization and causes atrial fibrillation.*

tricular complex at a consistent preset AV delay, the pacemaker is P synchronous and may be in the DDD or VDD mode (Figures 27, 28). Most pacemakers today are of the DDD variety, but VDD pacemakers are still manufactured and many remain implanted. One can distinguish VDD from DDD pacing only if intermittent atrial pacing is present (Figure 29) or in the magnet test mode.

An additional but now obsolete means of P synchronous pacing is the VAT mode. In this mode, the ventricle is paced after sensing P waves but without ventricular sensing. The lack of ventricular sensing can cause competition with intrinsic ventricular activity and ventricular dysrhythmias (Figure 30).

If each sensed P wave inhibits pacemaker output but does not start a pacemaker cycle, the pacemaker is in the DDI mode (Figure 31). Sensed atrial activity inhibits atrial output but does not result in a ventricular stimulus following the AV delay. This is a refinement of the DVI mode that prevents competitive atrial pacing caused by a lack of

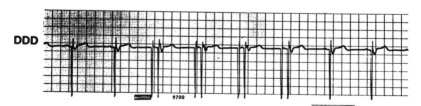

Figure 27. *Normal DDD pacing. In this example, the first, second, seventh, and eighth complexes show atrial sensing with ventricular pacing following a preset AV delay. In the second, third, fourth, and fifth paced complexes, atrial activity does not occur before the atrial escape limit is reached, and paced atrial activity and paced ventricular activity occur. Because atrial pacing and sensing exist as well as ventricular pacing, the most likely pacing modality is DDD.*

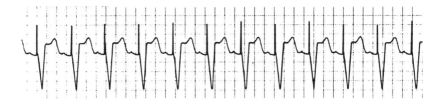

Figure 28. *Normal P synchronous or VDD pacing. Following each intrinsic atrial depolarization, the ventricle is paced at a preset AV delay. In this example, spontaneous ventricular activity does not occur. Without additional information, it is impossible to know whether the pacemaker is of the VDD, VAT, or DDD variety. One can only conclude that atrial sensing and ventricular pacing exist.*

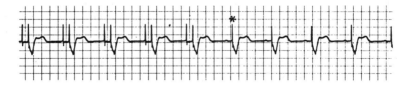

Figure 29. *DDD pacing in which the first five complexes are of continuous pacing of atrium and ventricle. From this portion of the ECG, DVI pacing cannot be distinguished from DDD. There is sensing of the intrinsic atrial activity with the sixth beat, and paced ventricular activity follows after the preset AV delay. This P synchronous pattern continues throughout the remainder of the strip. Thus, there is pacing of both chambers, and sensing of the atrium. The likely pacing modality is DDD.*

atrial sensing. As with the DVI mode, AV sequential pacing at the programmed rate will be provided in the absence of intrinsic activity. Intrinsic ventricular activity occurring during the atrial escape interval or AV delay will inhibit the pacer and reset the timing cycle.

Abnormalities of Dual-Chamber Pacing

Failure to capture and sense in the atrium and/or ventricle can occur with dual-chamber pacing as with single-chamber pacing (Figures 32, 33, 34, 35). Atrial and ventricular capture and sensing should be separately assessed to be certain that normal function exist. It must be remembered that failure to capture or sense in one chamber will most likely affect the function of the other chamber. Because of the complexity of the timing cycles of dual-chamber devices, it sometimes

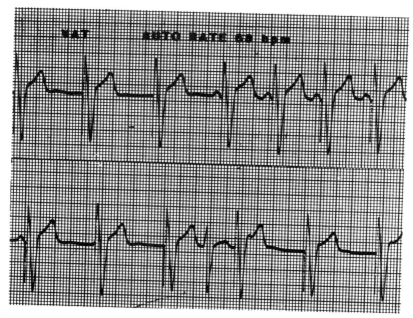

Figure 30. *Normal VAT pacing. In the upper panel, P wave activity does not drive the second and third paced complexes. The pacemaker ventricular escape is at a rate of 68 bpm (882 ms). When intrinsic P wave activity resumes, the ventricle is paced after the present AV delay. In the lower ECG, sinus bradycardia occurs again, and only the first ventricular stimulus may be a response to a sensed P wave. Each of the remainder is at the ventricular escape rate. A VPC occurs following the third paced QRS complex in the lower panel. As a VAT pacemaker is insensitive in the ventricle, another stimulus occurs at the escape interval from the previous paced stimulus.*

can be difficult to determine from the surface electrocardiogram whether normal sensing and pacing are present (Figure 36).

AV INTERVAL

This interval will have been measured earlier when it has been determined that dual-chamber pacing is present. In presently available DDD generators, the programmed AV delay is fixed and does not vary as a function of rate, although shortening of the AV interval at higher sensed atrial rates will be introduced in future DDD models. Nonetheless, the paced AV interval may not be consistent throughout the ECG.

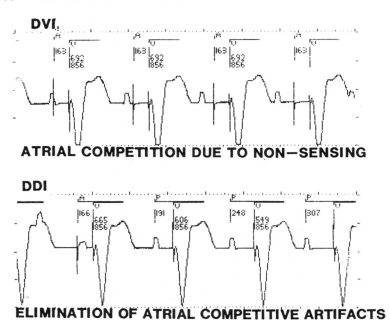

Figure 31. *Telemetered electrocardiograms with ECG interpretation channels from a patient with a Pacesetter-AFP pacemaker. In the upper panel, the patient is programmed to a noncommitted DVI mode. Atrial competition is caused by atrial insensitivity. In the lower panel, the same patient has been programmed to the DDI mode with resultant elimination of atrial competition. Variation in the AV interval occurs because the atrial and ventricular events are no longer separated by a fixed AV interval.*

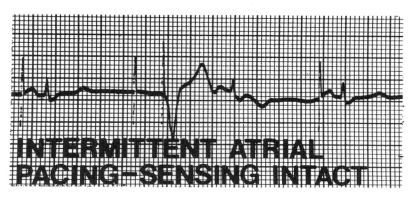

Figure 32. *DDD pacing with intermittent atrial capture. The first stimulus depolarizes the atrium and this results in a conducted QRS complex. The second atrial stimulus is ineffective, and the ventricular stimulus 250 ms later produces a paced complex. The next PQRS complex inhibits both channels, and the last demonstrates atrial capture with AV conduction.*

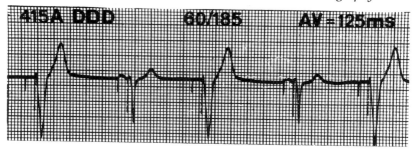

Figure 33. *DDD pacing with intermittent failure to capture the atrium in the first, third, and fifth paced complexes. The ventricle is paced in each. The second and fourth ventricular depolarizations represent fusion complexes between conducted intrinsic QRS activity and the pacemaker stimulus.*

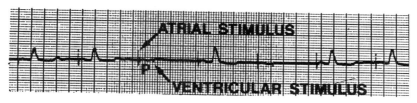

Figure 34. *DDD pacing in which the first, second, fourth, sixth, and seventh atrial stimuli are followed by atrial depolarizations and intrinsic ventricular activity. The third and fifth atrial pacing artifacts are followed by paced P waves without AV conduction and a ventricular stimulus without ventricular capture.*

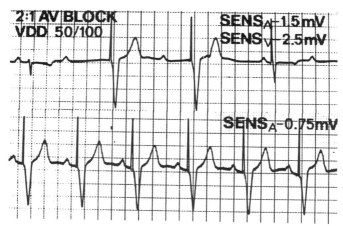

Figure 35. *VDD or P synchronous pacing at an atrial sensitivity of 1.5 mV with failure to sense atrial activity. Ventricular escape or VVI pacing results at a preset rate of 50 bpm (1200 ms, cycle length). With atrial sensitivity increased to 0.75 mV, normal P synchronous pacing is restored, and paced ventricular activity follows each intrinsic atrial depolarization at a preset AV delay.*

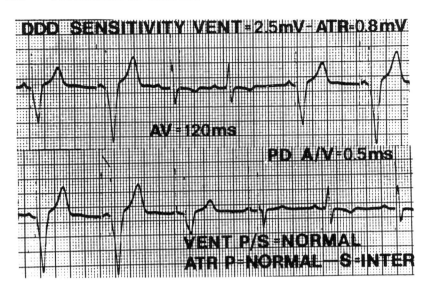

Figure 36.   ABOVE: *DDD pacing with programmed parameters as indicated. The first complex is started by an intrinsic atrial depolarization with paced ventricular activity following a preset AV delay of 120 ms. The second complex demonstrates pacing of atrium and ventricle when atrial activity fails to appear before the end of the lower rate limit followed by ventricular pacing at the preset AV delay. The third QRS complex is of a P wave followed by a normal QRS fused with two pacer artifacts. This represents failure to sense atrial activity followed by an unsensed QRS that falls into the ventricular blanking period. This is followed by an intrinsic P QRS complex that is sensed. The fifth P wave is sensed properly.* **BELOW:** *The first complex is started by normal atrial sensing, the second complex by atrial pacing. The third and fourth complexes are fused in atrium and ventricle, and determination of whether these complexes would have been sensed properly is impossible. The fifth and sixth complexes show atrial undersensing, but QRS occurs after the blanking period and inhibits the ventricular channel.*

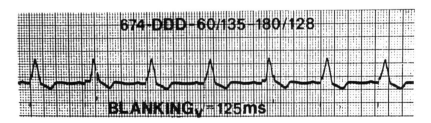

Figure 37.   *The second and fifth P waves are unsensed, and the atrial stimulus (the first of the pair) falls during the AV interval. The blanking period in the ventricular channel begins with the atrial stimulus and extends 125 ms. As the intrinsic deflection of the ventricular depolarization occurs during the blanking period, it is unsensed and the ventricular stimulus is emitted.*

The paced, or apparent, AV interval may be shorter or longer than programmed.

Shorter AV Interval

1. A P Wave Unused as a Timing Mechanism—

In atrial synchronous pacemakers still in use, the lower rate (escape) limit is between ventricular events. The programmed AV interval exists only when a sensed P wave causes the ventricular stimulus to fall at or before the elapse of the lower rate interval. If a P wave falls so late that the lower rate interval and the programmed AV interval cannot both be preserved, then the lower rate (or ventricular escape) interval will be preserved and the programmed duration of the AV interval will be sacrificed.

2. Safety Pacing—

AV interval inconsistencies can occur in the presence of crosstalk or in an attempt at prevention of crosstalk. Crosstalk is the sensing of the output of one pacemaker channel in the other. The major concern is the sensing of an atrial stimulus in the ventricular channel. To prevent crosstalk ventricular inhibition a blanking (or insensitive) period begins simultaneously in the ventricular channel with the atrial stimulus (Figure 35). This interval is of 12–50 ms duration, depending on the pulse generator, and it is programmable in some pulse generators. If the blanking period is too long, a spontaneous R wave, occurring soon after the atrial stimulus, will be unsensed and a competitive ventricular stimulus will be emitted. This situation is of greater concern the longer the blanking period. Any blanking period in excess of 100 ms duration is likely to compete with some VPC and to exaggerate ventricular competition in the presence of episodic atrial undersensing (Figure 36). If the blanking period is too short, the possibility exists that crosstalk and ventricular inhibition may result (Figure 37). Crosstalk occurs more frequently as the pulse duration increases, or, more likely, as the voltage output of the atrial stimulus increases. If higher than normal outputs are to be used in the atrial channel, crosstalk should be carefully evaluated and the blanking period appropriately lengthened.

In an effort to create the safest situation possible while retaining a relatively short blanking period, it is followed in some pacemakers by another portion of the AV interval during which activity sensed in the ventricular channel results in ventricular pacing. This has been referred to as ventricular safety pacing or the nonphysiological AV delay. Both terms are descriptive, as the paced interval is often shorter than the programmed AV interval and is present to assure ventricular pacing when crosstalk or other "noise" is sensed early in the AV interval. As the "safety" stimulus occurs at a fixed delay after the beginning of the "safety pacing" interval, the total AV interval is likely to be abbreviated. Because several early pulse generators had a ventricular safety pacing interval of 110 ms, this has been referred to as the "110 ms phenomenon," (Figure 38).

3. AV Interval Hysteresis—

Several pulse generators have two AV intervals, the shorter following a sensed atrial event and the longer following an atrial stimulus. This is an attempt to provide a PR interval, i.e., the hemodynamic interval, which is of equal duration whether the atrial contraction is paced or sensed. Therefore, two AV intervals will be seen on ECG.

Longer AV Interval

1. Operation at the Upper Rate Limit—

a. Pseudo-Wenckebach upper rate limitation is commonly the mode used. In this instance, the programmed upper rate limit is at a longer interval (i.e., a lower rate) than the total atrial refractory interval. The time difference between the two can be added to the AV interval. During Wenckebach operation, in which the atrial rate is at a shorter coupling interval (higher rate) than the upper rate limit, the AV interval will gradually prolong until one P wave is unsensed (Figure 39). If "endless loop" tachycardia occurs the AV interval will be prolonged continuously.

b. Rate Smoothing/Fallback. While operating in the basic pseudo-Wenckebach or AV block upper rate mechanism, some DDD generators avoid marked variation in the RR interval during sinus or atrial tachycardia by using a rate-smoothing or gradual fallback method (Figure 40). Instead of blocking the atrial event or prolonging the AV interval, rate fallback involves decoupling of atrial and ventricular events at the upper rate limit. The ventricular inhibited pacing rate is then gradually decremented to a programmed lower or fallback rate over a programmable duration. When the fallback rate is reached,

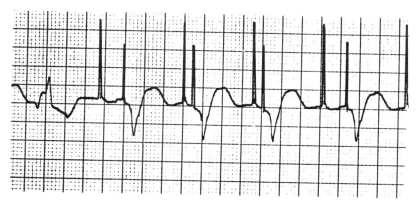

Figure 38. *Crosstalk is the sensing of the output of one channel in the other. "Safety pacing" is one means of dealing with crosstalk. In this instance, the atrial stimulus has been sensed in the ventricular channel after the end of the blanking period. The ventricular channel response is not inhibition but emission of a ventricular stimulus at a short AV interval. The first and fourth paced pairs are at the programmed AV interval. The second and third are at a short AV interval as a result of the safety pacing response to crosstalk.*

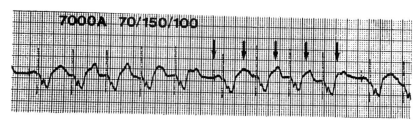

Figure 39. *An example of pseudo-Wenckebach activity occurring when the upper rate limit has been exceeded in a DDD pacemaker. The sensed atrial depolarizations are noted by the arrows. The AV interval progressively prolongs, one P wave falls in the atrial refractory interval and is unsensed and the cycle starts again.*

atrial synchrony is resumed. Although AV synchrony is lost temporarily, the gradual transition to a lower pacing rate may moderate the hemodynamic consequences of sudden shifts in RR intervals, which can occur with the AV block mechanism (Figure 41). Some models provide rate smoothing during fallback from a high rate as well as during return to the higher rate when atrial triggered pacing is resumed. As some models of DDD pacemaker can provide fallback and/or rate smoothing during pseudo-Wenckebach and AV block upper rate management, all as programmable options, the programmed settings must be known when the ECG is interpreted.

6 minutes – Postexercise

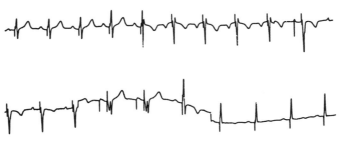

Continuous strip

Figure 40. *A continuous ECG strip (changing leads) taken six minutes postexercise from a patient with a CPI 0925 DDD pacing device. The pacemaker was programmed with "rate smoothing" at 3%. All ventricular activity is paced. In an effort to "smooth" the decrease in heart rate, an atrial stimulus can be seen to occur on three occasions to prevent the RR interval from slowing by more than allowed of the previous RR cycle.*

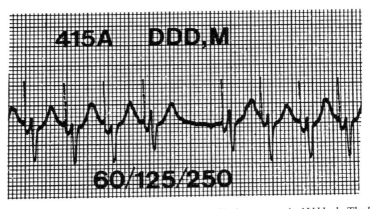

Figure 41. *DDD pacing in which the upper rate limit response is AV block. The lower rate limit is set at 60 and the upper rate limit at 125 with an AV delay of 250 ms. When the upper rate limit has been exceeded after the first four complexes, a P wave falls in the atrial refractory interval, and AV block occurs, with a pause of 760 ms until the next P wave starts a new cycle.*

DDDR ELECTROCARDIOGRAPHY

DDDR pacing is designed to allow restoration of rate responsiveness while maintaining atrioventricular (AV) synchrony for the paced patient. "DDDR" by definition indicates that there are pacing and sensing in both the atrial and ventricular chambers, that the response to sensing includes both triggered pacing and inhibition by intrinsic activity in each chamber, and that the device has rate modulated capability. As with any DDD pacing device, a DDDR pacemaker must have a programmed base or lower programmed pacing rate as well as a maximum atrial tracking rate. Because the upper rate limit of a pacemaker may be determined by sensor activity in a rate modulated pacemaker, a maximum sensor rate may need to be programmed separately in some DDDR pacemakers. Sensor function and programmability of the sensor obviously depend on the type of sensor incorporated in the pacemaker. In the future it will also depend on whether or not one or more sensors are incorporated. The electrocardiograms presented here are from a DDDR pacemaker that uses a piezoelectric crystal to sense activity and drive the pacing rate. Because future DDDR pacemakers will incorporate a variety of sensors, the electrocardiographic manifestations most likely will vary from pacemaker to pacemaker given the peculiarities and complexities of any one pacemaker.

When electrocardiograms from DDDR pacemakers are interpreted, it is also important to know the AV delay operation for the pacemaker. If there is AV hysteresis, the AV delay may be different after a sensed than after a paced atrial event, or the AV delay may shorten as the R-R cycle length decreases, i.e., the pacing rate increases. In the presence of the patient's intrinsic atrial rhythm while the patient is at rest or is active below the threshold of the sensor, normal P synchronous pacing will occur (Figure 28).

When activity occurs and the patient's intrinsic sinus rate is unable to respond, the patient is paced at an incremental rate based on the programmed values of the rate modulated indicators (Figure 42). (If antegrade conduction occcurs before the end of the programmed AV delay, the ventricular output will be inhibited. If not, AV sequential pacing will occur.)

As the patient continues to become more active, the pacemaker increases the rate in response to activity until the maximum programmed sensor rate is reached. Throughout this incremental period the intrinsic atrial rhythm may be intermittently evident and result in intermittent P wave tracking. In Figure 43 the sensor indicates that the paced rate should be at the maximum sensor rate, which is pro-

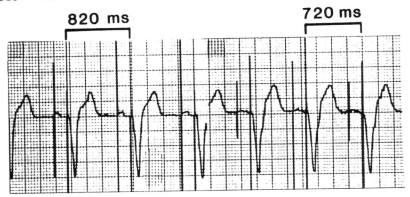

Figure 42. *Electrocardiogram obtained during exercise. The patient was exercising at 1.5 mph, 6% grade. At the beginning of the tracing, the paced R-R cycle length is 820 ms; at the end of the tracing, the cycle length has shortened to 720 ms.*

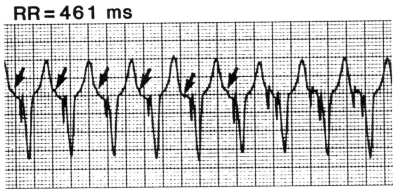

Figure 43. *Electrocardiogram demonstrating intermittent P synchronous pacing at 130 ppm with intermittent sensor driven AV sequential pacing at the same rate. The sensor indicated rate is 130 ppm. Sensor driven atrial pacing occurs if the intrinsic atrial rate falls below the sensor indicated rate or if the intrinsic atrial beat falls into the atrial refractory period and is not sensed. P waves are noted with arrows.*

grammed to 130 ppm. Sensor driven atrial pacing occurs if the intrinsic atrial rate falls below the sensor indicated rate or if the intrinsic atrial beat falls into the atrial refractory period and is not sensed.

DDDR pacing can alter the electrocardiogram when the maximum tracking rate is achieved. In the electrocardiogram shown in Figure 44A the patient's intrinsic atrial rate exceeds the programmed maximum atrial tracking rate, and a Wenckebach effect occurs during

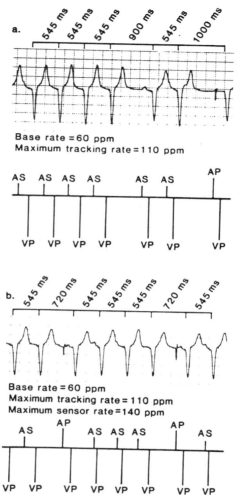

Figure 44. *A. Electrocardiogram showing DDD pacing (sensor is programmed "passive") with Wenckebach-type block at the maximum tracking rate of 110 ppm. R-R cycle length alternates from 545 to 1,000 ms. Under the electrocardiogram is a diagram done in "ECG Marker Channel" (Medtronic, Inc.) fashion. Normal DDD function is represented by an atrial sensed event (AS) followed by a ventricular paced event (VP) in the absence of a sensed ventricular event. In the absence of an atrial sensed event, an atrial pacing stimuli (AP) is emitted, followed by VP. In this tracing, it is difficult to be certain that AP stimuli result in atrial depolarization. B. Electrocardiogram showing DDDR pacing in the same patient with the same maximum tracking rate (110 ppm) and a maximum sensor rate of 140 ppm. With the sensor "on," there is less variation in cycle length, 545–720 ms. In the diagram under the tracing, it can be seen that an AP is emitted twice even though the escape interval is less than the programmed base rate. The decrease in cycle length variation occurs because the sensor level at that point in exercise indicates that the pacing rate should be 83 ppm (720 ms cycle length).*

DDD pacing. In contrast, Figure 44B demonstrates DDDR pacing when the maximum tracking rate is exceeded. In the latter example, the Wenckebach interval is shortened on the basis of sensor driven pacing. In contrast to standard upper rate function with a DDD pacemaker, which most commonly results in a Wenckebach-type behavior, there is actually very little change in the paced R-R interval in this electrocardiogram, hence a sensor driven rate-smoothing effect. This phenomenon can also affect the interval following ectopic beats that occur during activity with sensor driven pacing (Figure 45). When the

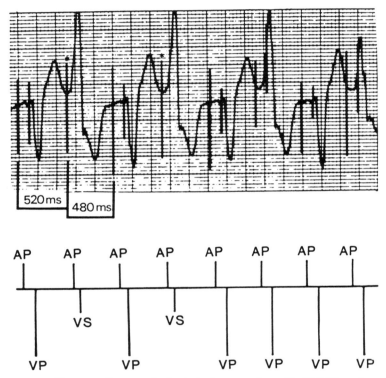

Figure 45. *Electrocardiogram obtained during exercise with DDDR pacing. The pacemaker is programmed to a base rate of 60 ppm, maximum tracking rate of 155, and maximum sensor rate of 150. Ventricular ectopy in a bigeminal pattern occurs during exercise. At times, the ventricular ectopic beat occurs early enough after the atrial pacing stimulus to inhibit ventricular output (asterisks), and at times the ventricular stimulus occurs during the early portion of the ectopic beat. Despite the ectopic beats, there is very little variation in cycle length, approximately 480–520 ms (measurements are made from atrial pacing stimulus to atrial pacing stimulus). A diagram in "ECG Marker Channel" (Medtronic, Inc.) fashion is used to further illustrate this electrocardiogram. AP, atrial paced event; VP, ventricular paced event; VS, ventricular sensed event.*

maximum sensor rate is reached and the patient is still exercising at that level, AV synchronous pacing at the programmed maximum sensor rate is seen (Figure 46).

When exercise is stopped, the R-R cycle will lengthen, i.e., the pacing rate will slow. In some pacemakers the decrement in pacing rate may be dependent on a programmed recovery time. This value would determine the miminum time required for a decrease in pacing rate from the programmed maximum rate to the programmed base rate, if the patient remains dependent on the sensor throughout that decrement (Figure 47).

In addition, some DDDR pacemakers may have the capability of AV delay hysteresis in both P synchronous pacing and AV sequential sensor driven pacing. AV hysteresis is intended to optimize the cardiac output by mimicking the normal physiologic decrease in P-R interval that occurs in the normal heart as the atrial rate increases (Figure 48). The AV delay hystersis may also improve atrial sensing by shortening the total atrial refractory period and thereby giving more time for the atrial sensing window.

The analysis of a paced electrocardiogram using these guidelines should allow one to determine if pacemaker function is normal. As variations are certain to occur, the electrocardiographic reader must be aware of the specifics of the operation of each pulse generator.

RR = 400 ms
AV delay = 100 ms

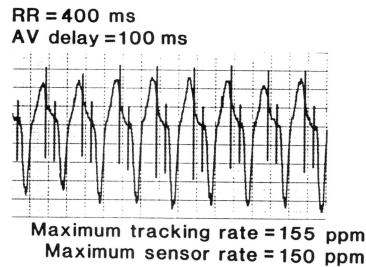

Maximum tracking rate = 155 ppm
Maximum sensor rate = 150 ppm

Figure 46. *Electrocardiogram showing DDDR pacing during exercise when the maximum sensor rate of 150 ppm has been reached.*

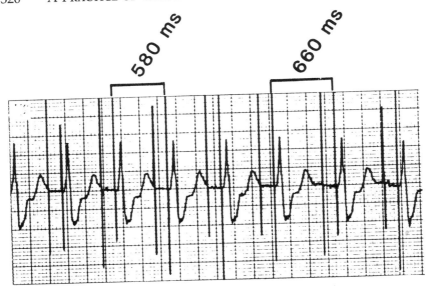

Figure 47. *Electrocardiogram obtained during the postexercise period with the pacemaker programmed to the DDDR mode. A slowing of the pacing rate can be seen: the R-R cycle length at the beginning of the tracing is 580 ms, and cycle length at the end of the strip is increasing to 660 ms. This gradual slowing would continue until the base pacing rate was achieved or the patient's intrinsic rate inhibited the pacemaker.*

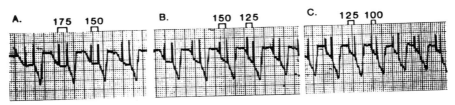

Figure 48. *Electrocardiogram demonstrating progressive AV delay shortening as the pacing rates exceed 90, 110, and 130 ppm. The AV delay was programmed to 175 ms and progressively shortened to 150 ms (A), to 125 ms (B), and to 100 ms (C) during exercise.*

BIBLIOGRAPHY

Barold SS: Fusion, pseudo-fusion and confusion beats. *Impulse,* Cardiac Pacemakers, Inc., St. Paul, Minnesota, 1977; pp. 1–6.

Barold SS, Falkoff MD, Ong LS, et al: Electrocardiographic analysis of normal and abnormal pacemaker function. *Cardiovasc Clin* 1983; 14:97–134.

Barold SS, Falkoff MD, Ong LS, et al: Characterization of pacemaker arrhythmias due to normally functioning AV demand (DVI) pulse generators. *PACE* 1980; 3:712–723.

Benditt DG, Tuna N, Benson DW Jr, et al: An approach to electrocardiographic interpretation in patients who have dual-chamber cardiac pacemakers. *Medtronic News* 1984; pp. 3–13.

Berger R, Jacobs W: Myopotential inhibition of demand pacemakers: Etiologic, diagnostic, and therapeutic considerations. *PACE* 1979; 2:596–602.

Berman ND: T wave sensing with a programmable pacemaker. *PACE* 1980; 3:656–659.

Calfee RV: Dual-chamber committed mode pacing. *PACE* 1983; 6:387–391.

Furman S, Cooper JA: Atrial fibrillation during A-V sequential pacing. *PACE* 1982; 5:133–135.

Furman S, Huang WM: Pacemaker recycle from repolarization artifact. *PACE* 1982; 5:927–928.

Goldschlager N: Pacemaker rhythms. *PACE* 1981; 4:317–320.

Goldschlager N: Pacer rhythms. *PACE 1981; 4:75–77.*

Hauser RG: The electrocardiography of AV universal DDD pacemakers. *PACE* 1983; 6:399–409.

Hayes DL, Higano ST, Eisinger G: Electrocardiographic manifestations of a dual-chamber, rate modulated (DDDR) pacemaker. PACE 1989; 12:555–562.

Higano ST, Hayes DL, Eisinger G: Advantage of discrepant upper rate limit in a DDDR pacemaker. *Mayo Clin Proc* in press.

Levine PA: Pacemaker pseudomalfunction. *PACE* 1981; 4:563–565.

Levine PA, Pirzada FA: Pacemaker oversensing: A possible example of concealed ventricular extrasystoles. *PACE* 1981; 4:199–203.

Levine PA, Sholder J, Duncan JL: Clinical benefits of telemetered electrograms in assessment of DDD function. *PACE* 1984; 7:1170–1177.

Luceri RM, Castellanos A, Zaman L, et al: The arrhythmias of dual-chamber cardiac pacemakers and their management. *Ann Intern Med* 1983; 99:354–359.

Marriott HJ, Gozensky C: Electrocardiogram problems created by pacemakers. *Cardiovasc News* 1976; 12:1–6.

Parsonnet V, Bernstein AD: Pseudomalfunctions of dual-chamber pacemakers. *PACE* 1983; 6:376–381.

Perrins EJ, Sutton R: Arrhythmias in pacing. *Med Clin North Am* 1984; 68(5): 1111–1138.

Rosenqvist M, Vallin HO, Edhag KO: Rate hysteresis pacing: How valuable is it? A comparison of the stimulation rates of 70 and 50 beats per minute and rate hysteresis in patients with sinus node disease. *PACE* 1984; 7:332–340.

Secemsky SI, Hauser RG, Denes P, et al: Unipolar sensing abnormalities: Incidence and clinical significance of skeletal muscle interference and undersensing in 228 patients. *PACE* 1982; 5:10–19.

Sutton R, Perrins EJ, Duffin E: Interpretation of dual chamber pacemaker electrocardiograms. *PACE* 1985; 8:6–16.

Yokoyama M, Wada J, Barold SS: Transient early T wave sensing by implanted programmable demand pulse generator. *PACE* 1981; 4:68–74.

Yokoyama M, Wada J, Hirosawa K: Unusual demand pacemaker arrhythmia due to partial recycling in the relative refractory period. *PACE* 1979; 2:225–229.

Chapter 10

PACEMAKER RADIOGRAPHY

David L. Hayes

PACING SYSTEM RADIOGRAPHIC INSPECTION

Radiographic inspection of a pacing system should be performed in an organized manner, much as a routine chest x-ray. Without such an organized approach, essential information may go unobserved. The posteroanterior (PA) and lateral chest x-rays of any patient with a permanent pacemaker should be obtained and reviewed by the implanting or follow-up physician. Both views are essential, a single PA projection is inadequate. Oblique views do not commonly provide additional data. As lead systems often are faintly visible, use of the thoracic spine rather than the lung technique may be helpful. One systematic approach is to interpret the radiograph's components in the following order:

1. bony structures,
2. aorta,
3. cardiac shadow,
4. trachea,
5. diaphragm,
6. lung,
7. other.

Inspection of the pacing system falls into the final category. It can then be further subdivided into the categories that follow.

I. Overall View

A radiographically normal pacing system will be reviewed in its entirety for reference throughout the remainder of this chapter. Posteroanterior (PA) and lateral views of a well-positioned dual-chamber pacing system show the pulse generator in the subcutaneous pectoral region. It is not adjacent to any bony structures except the underlying ribs and is clearly away from the axilla. The specific transvenous route may be difficult to determine. If lead placement is via subclavian puncture, on x-ray it is difficult to differentiate from the cephalic venous route. If leads enter the venous system superior to the clavicle, a jugular venous cutdown approach has most likely been used. If the lead enters above the clavicle and is relatively close to the trachea, then an internal jugular was likely used.

Ventricular Lead

The ventricular lead should be positioned in the right ventricular apex. Radiographically, the end of the ventricular lead appears on the PA projection to be between the left border of the vertebral column and the cardiac apex. The position of the heart, vertical or relatively more horizontal, largely determines the position of the lead in relation to the cardiac apex and varies among patients. The lateral view is necessary to distinguish between an apical position in which the lead tip is anterior and caudally directed, directed posteriorly in the right ventricle, or on the posterior surface of the heart, i.e., within the coronary sinus. The ventricular lead should have a gentle curve along the lateral wall of the right atrium and cross the tricuspid valve to the ventricular apex. Redundancy of the lead within the cardiac chambers, which normally should be avoided, may be visible (Figure 1).

Atrial Lead

The atrial lead is most commonly positioned in the right atrial appendage (other positions are considered later in this chapter). The "J" portion of the lead is slightly medial on the anteroposterior projection and anterior on the lateral projection. Optimally, the limits of the "J" should be no greater than approximately 80° apart. Redundancy proximal to the "J" within the atruim or superior vena cava should not be seen.

If pacing leads are present on the standard chest x-ray and no pulse generator is seen (and the full chest is included on the chest radiograph), a flat film of the abdomen may verify pulse generator type and placement in the subcutaneous tissue of the abdominal wall (Figure 2). The other possibility is that a temporary pacemaker is being used, and the lead can be traced as it exits the body.

Anatomical Variations

Several anatomical variations exist. In the presence of persistent left superior vena cava (Figure 3), the lead in the PA projection de-

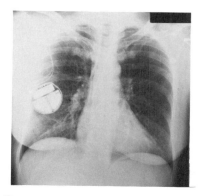
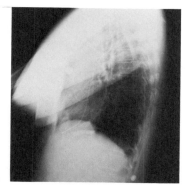

1B.

Figure 1. *An implanted dual-chamber pacing system. The atrial lead is well positioned in the right atrial appendage, slightly medially directed on the PA projection and anteriorly on the lateral projection. The ventricular electrode lies well to the left of the vertebral column in the ventricular apex on the PA projection and anterior on the lateral projection.*

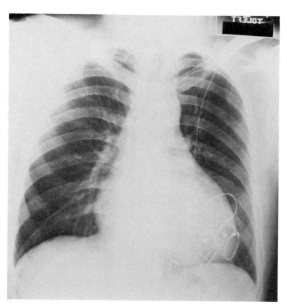

Figure 2. *Posteroanterior chest x-ray shows both transvenous, right ventricular (one) and epicardial (four) permanent pacing leads. No pulse generator is seen.* **A.** *The transvenous lead has been tunneled to an abdominal site.*

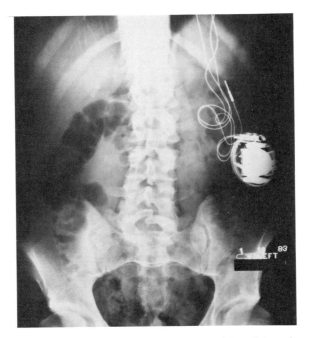

Figure 2B.   *Flat film of the abdomen documents the position of the pulse generator in the left upper quadrant. Two epicardial leads have been transsected.*

scends within the left side of the cardiac shadow and enters the atrium and then the ventricle via communication of the left superior vena cava and the coronary sinus. On the lateral projection, the ventricular lead will then be seen on the posterior cardiac wall within the coronary sinus. The right superior vena cava is also present. It is possible to have a temporary lead in one superior vena cava and the implanted lead in the other (Figure 4). Transposition of the great vessels can be diagnosed when the lead enters the superior vena cava, the right atrium, and the left or venous ventricle. In this instance, the lateral projection will show the lead anterior, and the PA projection will show it almost directly below the superior vena cava (Figure 5).

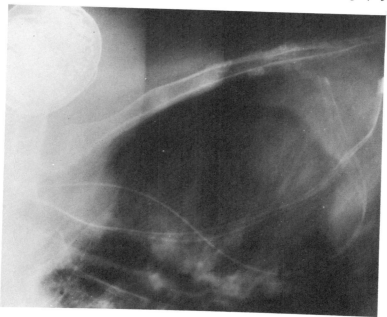

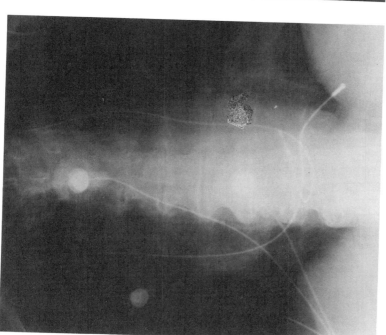

Figure 3.   *Persistent left superior vena cava can cause unusual radiographic lead positions. The permanent lead descends on the right and assumes a conventional position. The temporary lead from the left traverses the left superior vena cava and enters the ventricle via the communication of the left superior vena cava and the coronary sinus. On the lateral projection, the temporary lead (within the coronary sinus) is on the posterior wall of the heart.*

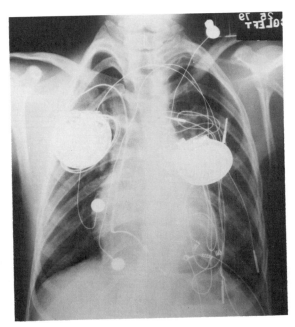

Figure 4. A PA chest x-ray in a patient with multiple leads and two permanent pacemakers. It is impossible to determine from this x-ray whether one or both pulse generators are functional and which of the various leads are intact, functional, or abandoned.

II. Pulse Generator Position

For most transvenous implants, the pulse generator is visible on the chest radiograph and most are high in the pectoral region, away from the axilla, well inferior to the clavicle, and relatively medial (Figure 6). Other chest positions may be lower in the retromammary space (Figure 7) or intrapleural (Figure 8).

In many myocardial implantations, especially those performed a decade or more ago, the pulse generator is placed in a superficial position in the upper abdomen (Figure 9). Nevertheless, myocardial implantation may be associated with pulse generator placement in either the right or left pectoral regions. This approach is more common at present (Figure 2).

In assessing pulse generator position, malposition may be readily noted. A pulse generator adjacent to or within the axilla is too far lateral, and placement within an excessively large pocket may allow its

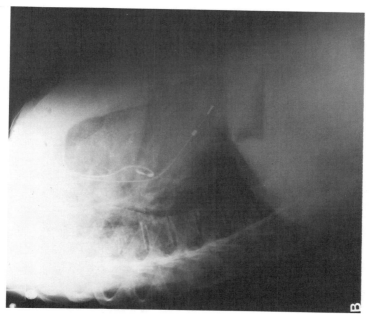

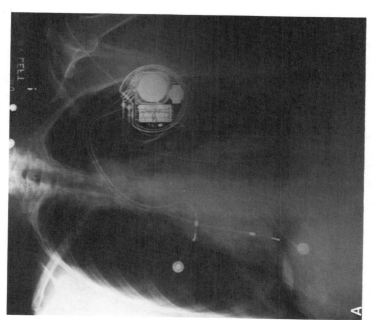

Figure 5. PA (**A**) and lateral (**B**) chest x-rays in a patient with corrected transposition of the great vessels and dextrocardia. An AV sequential pacemaker is in the pectoral region, and the leads were placed via the subclavian vein. The atrial lead lies in the lateral aspect of the right atrium, and the ventricular lead lies in the apex of the venous ventricle, the morphological left ventricle. The lateral projection seems less bizarre than the PA projection with the ventricular lead will positioned in the apex of the left ventricle.

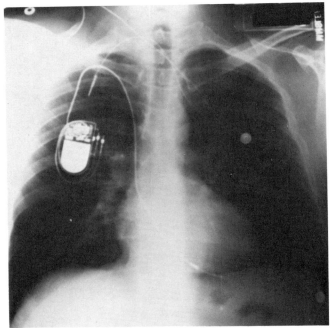

Figure 6.   *Typical right pectoral placement of a bipolar lead and pulse generator. The lead is positioned in the right ventricular apex (several monitoring leads are projected onto the chest).*

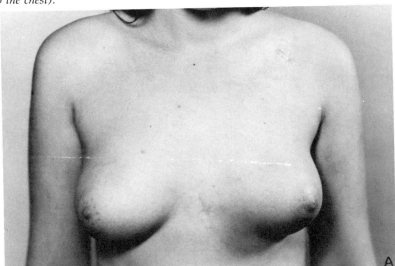

Figure 7A.   *For cosmetic reasons, the pulse generator may be placed in a retromammary position.*

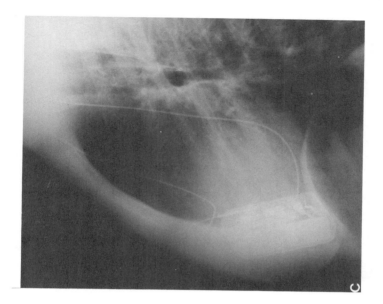

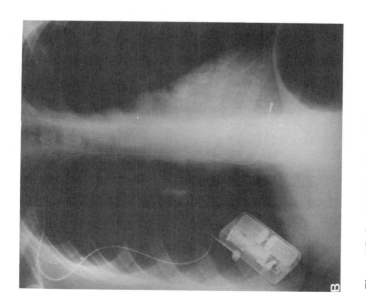

Figure 7B, C. *PA (B) and lateral (C) projections in the same patient show the retromammary placement, which is directly behind the breast and is therefore inferior to the usual higher pectoral position.*

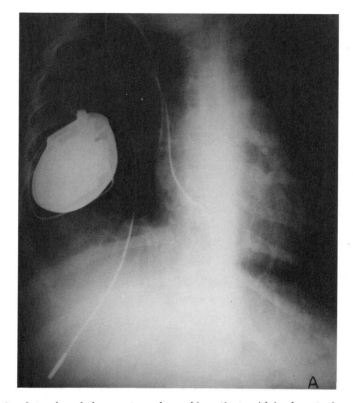

Figure 8.   *Intrapleural placement may be used in patients with inadequate tissue for a pectoral or retromammary position. In this child a single chamber ventricular pacemaker was placed in a dacron pouch and attached to the lateral pleura of the right pleural space. An atrial lead was implanted but unused and is seen in the right costophrenic sulcus unattached to a pulse generator. The generator size is substantially magnified. **A.** oblique.*

rotation with twisting or coiling of the lead (Figure 10), which may be spontaneous or result from patient manipulation (Twiddler's syndrome—Figure 11).

III. Pulse Generator Identification

All pulse generators can be identified by their x-ray appearance. As the position of the cell or battery and the position of the radio-

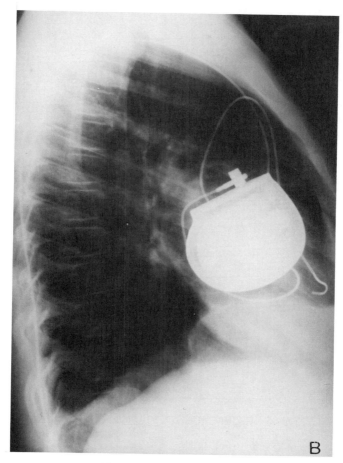

Figure 8B.   *lateral projection.*

opaque circuit components is unique to each model, identification of the individual model is possible. All new pulse generators contain some variety of radiographic identification code visible on x-ray within the generator shadow (Figure 12). These codes are unique to each manufacturer.

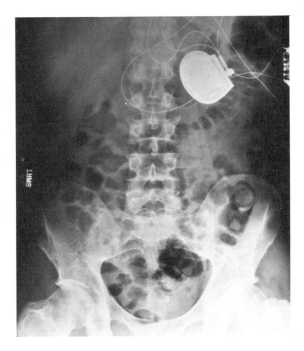

Figure 9. *A typical myocardial lead placement with a redundant lead. The pulse generator is positioned in the left upper quadrant in the anterior abdominal wall.*

RADIOGRAPHIC IDENTIFICATION CODES

1. Manufacturer's name or initials and model number
2. Model number only
3. Manufacturer's name and letter code for model number
4. Letter code for manufacturer and model
5. Manufacturer's logo and letter code for model

All manufacturers and several independent sources provide tables, charts, and other printed material to assist in radiographic identification. Data for x-ray identification is published periodically in *PACE* and in a number of books.

For older devices still implanted that do not have a specific x-ray identification code, the overall shape of the pulse generator, its electronics, and battery, provide an excellent identification, especially

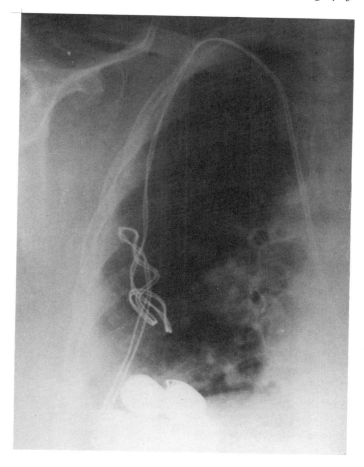

Figure 10.   *Continuous torsion on the pacing lead, either by spontaneous twisting of the pulse generator in the subcutaneous pocket or by patient manipulation, has withdrawn the electrode from the right ventricular apex.*

when compared to x-rays previously published for the purposes of such identification.

IV. Polarity

The polarity of the pulse generator can be determined from the pacemaker profile and the number and type of connector pins. Unipo-

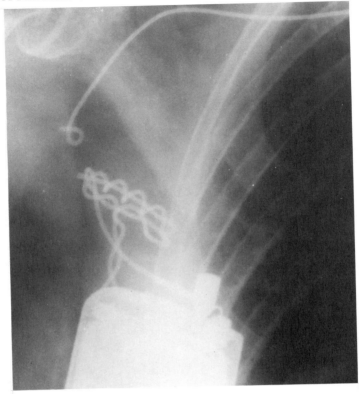

Figure 11.   *Patient manipulation of a pulse generator (Twiddler's syndrome) resulted in sufficient tension to cause lead fracture.*

lar, bifurcated bipolar, and coaxial (in-line) bipolar pulse generators can be distinguished. Several coaxial bipolar pacemakers may be programmable for polarity, so that a coaxial bipolar lead connector does not imply bipolar pacemaker function. Other bipolar generators may accept either a bipolar in-line or a unipolar lead. The connector assembly should be carefully scrutinized to ascertain which variety of lead is in use (Figure 13). A bifurcated bipolar lead may be unipolarized and connected to a unipolar pulse generator. The abandoned terminal usually can be found to be unattached to the pulse generator, lying free in the immediately adjacent subcutaneous tissue. Alternatively, a bipolar pulse generator can be connected to a unipolar lead, and an indifferent electrode connected to its positive terminal (Figure 14).

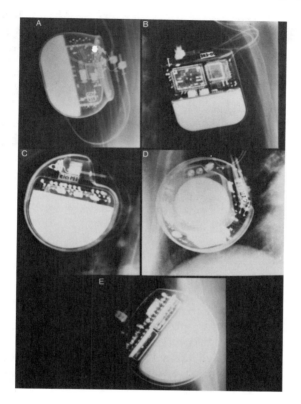

Figure 12. *Radiographic identification of pulse generators.* **A.** *Manufacturer's name and model number (CPI pulse generator, Model 630).* **B.** *Model number without manufacturer's name (Intermedics 283-01).* **C.** *Manufacturer's name and letter designation for model (ELA Pacemaker, model M1).* **D.** *Logo and letters (Medtronic).* **E.** *Letters only (Cordis).*

V. Connector Block

When the pulse generator has been located and identified, the connector block should be inspected to determine that connector and pin are firmly in contact. In a patient with intermittent complete pacemaker failure, an insecure connection may be diagnosed. Incomplete advancement of the pin into the connector receptacle or incomplete tightening of the screw, which also may be diagnosed radiographically, can produce similar findings (Figure 15).

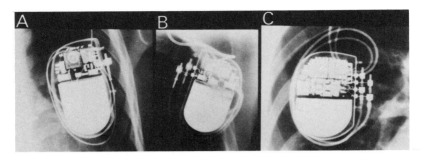

Figure 13. *Polarity of a pulse generator can be distinguished at the connector.* **A.** *Unipolar single-chamber pulse generator with a single connector;* **B.** *Dual-chamber unipolar pulse generator with two unipolar connectors;* **C.** *Bipolar dual-chamber generator with a bipolar, coaxial in-line connector block accepting two bipolar leads.*

VI. Lead Placement

Transvenous

The lead(s) may be transvenous or myocardial. If the lead is outside the cardiac shadow until the electrode enters the cardiac silhouette, then it is myocardial. If it courses within the heart, especially from the area of the neck or pectoral region, then it is transvenous. The vein of entry should be determined because different stresses on the lead system exist at different sites. The most frequently used sites, cephalic and subclavian, cannot be distinguished radiographically, both enter below the clavicle. If entry is above the clavicle, then it is via the external or internal jugular vein, the internal more medial than the external (Figures 16, 17, 18).

Intracardiac Position

1. Ventricular.   The transvenous ventricular lead is almost universally placed in the right ventricular apex. An active fixation (i.e. screw-in) lead is readily recognized on x-ray and may be placed elsewhere. Other active fixation leads with fine wires projecting from the electrode or with a jawlike assembly may also be recognized radiographically. If a passive fixation lead is not in the right ventricular apex, comparison with earlier films is important to determine whether the lead has been displaced or was initially placed elsewhere. The active fixation lead may be anywhere within the right ventricle, i.e., in the

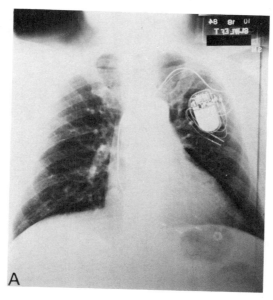

Figure 14. *A bipolar single-chamber pacing system. Because of rising thresholds the system had been unipolarized with placement of an indifferent electrode and abandonment of the original bipolar lead. Its connector pins are seen lying adjacent to the pulse generator and unconnected to it.* **A.** *PA projection.*

ventricular septum or the pulmonary outflow tract (Figure 19). Any lead may perforate the ventricular apex (Figure 20) or lie in the coronary sinus or the posterior coronary vein (Figure 21). Posteroanterior and lateral projections are required to distinguish the various sites of perforation.

2. Atrial. An atrial lead is most commonly placed in the right atrial appendage (Figure 22), less commonly in the lateral atrial wall (Figure 23), and infrequently in the coronary sinus (Figure 24). In patients with transposition of the great vessels, transvenous left atrial pacing is rarely possible (Figure 25). The lateral projection is especially useful to discern the coronary sinus position, which is on the posterior cardiac wall, while the PA view alone may not allow distinction between the coronary sinus and a right ventricular position.

3. Myocardial. The location and type of the leads also should be identified in the presence of a myocardial pacing system. Myocardial

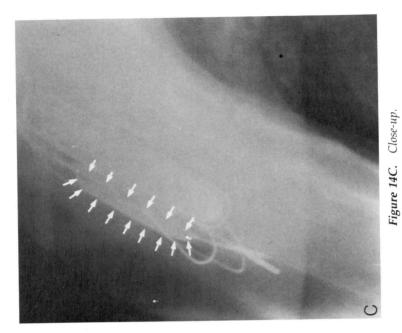

Figure 14C.   Close-up.

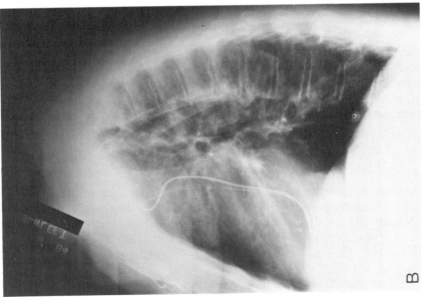

Figure 14B.   lateral projection.

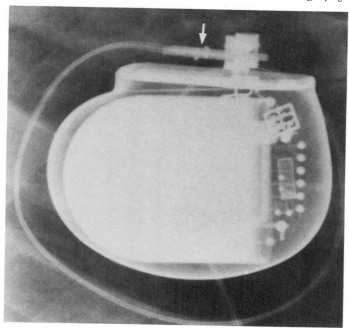

Figure 15.   *X-ray evidence of a disparity in alignment of the connector pins in a patient with intermittent failure to pace and a bipolar pulse generator. At operation, one pin was loose because a set screw had not been tightened adequately.*

ventricular pacing is usually accomplished from one of three positions. The right ventricle is usually paced from the diaphragmatic cardiac surface (Figure 26). The left ventricle is commonly paced from the free wall via left anterolateral thoracotomy or the subcostal route. Atrial myocardial leads may be present on either the right or the left atrial appendage (Figure 27). Identification of the specific lead type is important as different electrode configurations have different reliability characteristics (Figure 28).

VII. Lead Polarity

The lead may be radiographically identified as unipolar or bipolar. The cathode is always within the heart, and in the unipolar system, the anode is the metallic housing of the pulse generator; only the radio-

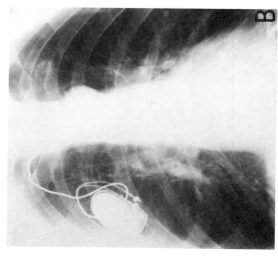

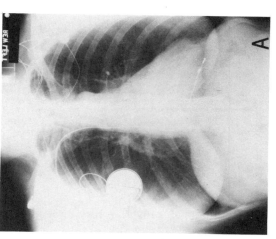

Figure 16. Differentiating a cephalic placement from a subclavian placement is very difficult radiographically. **Figure 16A.** A permanent pacing lead in the cephalic vein. **Figure 16B.** A permanent pacing lead in the subclavian vein.

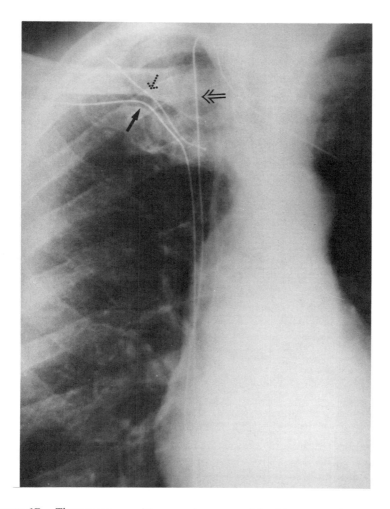

Figure 17. *Three venous positions can be compared in this x-ray with permanent pacing leads in: the right cephalic vein (closed arrow); right external jugular vein (dotted arrow); the internal jugular vein (open arrow). Jugular leads can be placed either deep or superficial to the clavicle.*

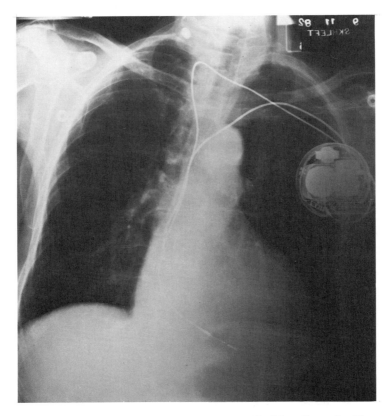

Figure 18. *Jugular and subclavian positions are seen in this radiograph with permanent pacing leads in the left subclavian vein and the right internal jugular vein.*

paque catheter electrode is seen. In a bipolar system, both the radiographic electrode at the lead tip and a more proximal ring electrode can be seen (Figure 13). On occasion, a bipolar lead has been unipolarized to accommodate a unipolar pulse generator or to take advantage of superior unipolar sensing or pacing. The positive terminal of the lead is insulated by placing a radiolucent rubber cap over the lead connector pin (Figure 14).

VIII. Lead Type

Although the specific type of transvenous lead often cannot be identified an attempt should be made. It can be determined whether

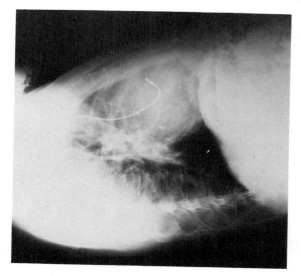

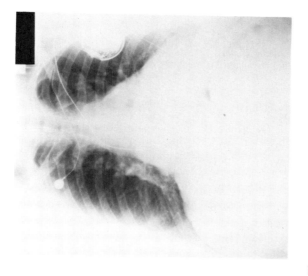

Figure 19. PA (A) and lateral (B) x-ray projections in a patient in whom the best stimulation and sensing thresholds were found in the right ventricular free wall adjacent to the outflow tract. The lead is far removed from the right ventricular apex.

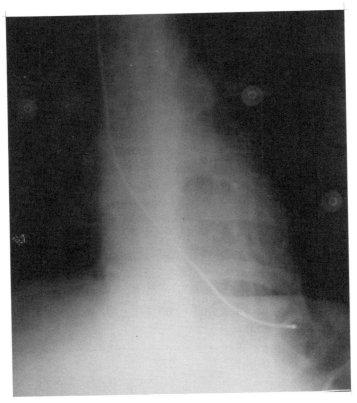

Figure 20.   *A rigid temporary pacemaker lead which has perforated the right ventricle and lies with a gentle curve within the pericardium.* **A**—*PA projection.*

lead fixation is active or passive. Active fixation leads can be differentiated from passive fixation leads with certainty only if an active fixation device can be seen to penetrate the endocardium (Figure 25) or the epicardium–myocardium (Figure 26). A variety of epicardial active fixation devices are available. In each instance the radiographic appearance of the active fixation mechanism will be different.

Four different myocardial leads account for the vast majority of all epicardial–myocardial pacing leads. These are the Medtronic 6917 (three-turn) and 6917A (two-turn) sutureless "screw-in" leads, the old "cobra head" (Medtronic 6913), and the Medtronic 4951 stab-in lead (Figure 26, 28, 29).

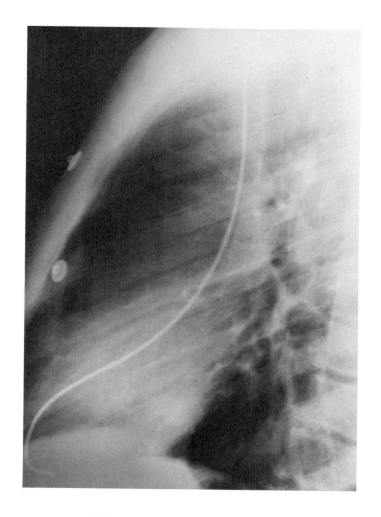

Figure 20B. *Lateral projection.*

IX. Lead Integrity

The lead should be inspected for integrity. An insulation break usually cannot be identified radiographically, but a lead fracture almost always can be identified (Figure 30). Fractures often occur at positions where strain is applied to the lead and, therefore, within the subcutaneous tissue at the point of fastening of the lead to the vein of entry or within the vein near the point of entry (Figure 31). A fracture may occur near the pulse generator at the connector block (Figure 32) or (infrequently) within the central vein itself. In the first two instances, repair may be possible and easy; in the third instance repair may not be possible.

"Pseudofractures" are radiographic findings only. The term has been applied to two entirely different circumstances. It applies most aptly to the indentations caused by ligatures compressing the insulating material of a rubber or, more recently, polyurethane lead. Such a finding is of special concern because it has been associated with polyurethane deterioration. Use of a nonopaque rubber "sleeve" may avoid both the radiographic finding and its actual consequences (Figure 33). The term "pseudofracture" has also been applied, incorrectly, to the normal radiographic appearance of some bipolar leads at the point of bifurcation. Discontinuity may be misinterpreted as a fracture, it is only a fine wire connection, which may not be recognized unless one anticipates its presence (Figure 34).

Lead integrity of myocardial systems may be easier to evaluate. Earlier designs (e.g., Medtronic model #6913) resulted in an incidence of fracture that is greater than in modern leads and which usually occurred at the site of higher stress (Figure 35).

LEAD POSITIONING

Adequate placement for all the atrial or ventricular, transvenous, and myocardial lead positions has been demonstrated radiographically. Lead dislodgment may occur and is a common cause of failure to pace. Dislodgment may be identifiable (macrodislodgment) or non-identifiable radiographically. The latter has been labeled "microdislodgment" but, in the absence of x-ray proof, there is no evidence of its presence. It is, therefore, a diagnosis by exclusion. A "macrodislodged" lead can be anywhere other than its original position, i.e., the pulmonary artery, coronary sinus, ventricular cavity, or superior or inferior vena cava. It is imperative that when lead malposition or

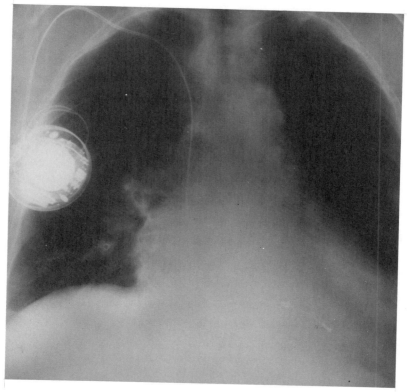

Figure 21. *A pacing lead inadvertently placed into a tributary of the coronary sinus.* **A.** *On the PA projection, the position appears to be satisfactory with the lead within the right ventricle.*

dislodgment is considered, the chest film be compared with previous radiographs (Figure 36, 37).

X. Multiple Leads

When multiple leads or, uncommonly, multiple pacemakers are visible on the chest radiograph, an attempt should be made to trace each lead from its origin in the pacemaker to its intracardiac or intravascular position. An abandoned lead should be traced on the x-ray to prove that it is free-standing and not connected to the pulse generator. With multiple leads present, the radiographic appearance can become confusing and individual leads can be difficult to trace (Figure 4).

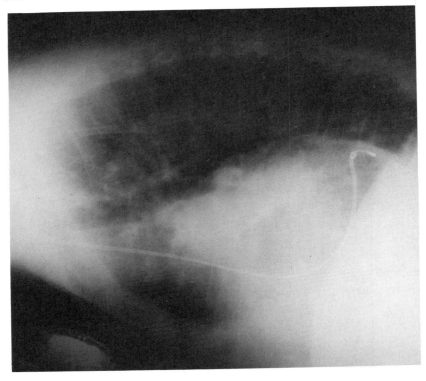

Figure 21B.   *On the lateral projection, the lead is clearly within the posterior cardiac surface.*

XI. Complications

Complications of the implant procedure itself (hemothorax, pneumothorax and hemo-pneumothorax) may be identified radiographically (Figures 1, 2 Chapter 9, Pacemaker Complications). Other complications, including lead perforation, malpositioned pulse generator, and displaced lead, have been discussed previously in this chapter or in chapter 9.

SUMMARY

A systematic approach to the interprétation of the radiographic appearance of the pacing system should follow a sequence.

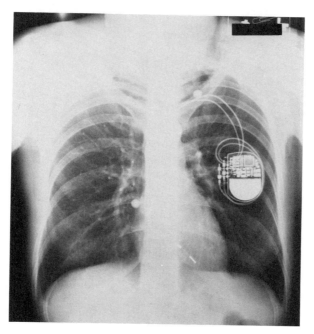

Figure 22.   *A dual-chamber bipolar pacing system with leads positioned in the right atrial appendage and right ventricular apex.*

INTERPRETATION OF RADIOGRAPHIC APPEARANCE OF THE PACING SYSTEM

1. Inspect the routine chest PA and lateral x-rays, ignoring the pacing system. Obtain over-penetrated, i.e., thoracic spine films if necessary.
2. Identify the pulse generator location.
3. Identify the pulse generator model and polarity.
4. Inspect the connector block.
5. Determine the lead position.
   a. transvenous or epicardial — myocardial
   b. atrial or ventricular, or both
   c. if transvenous, its location within a cardiac chamber or the coronary sinus
6. Determine lead polarity and type of fixation.
7. Evaluate lead integrity.
8. Look for other specific complications.

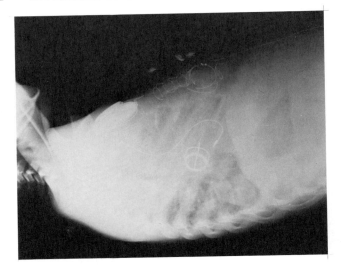

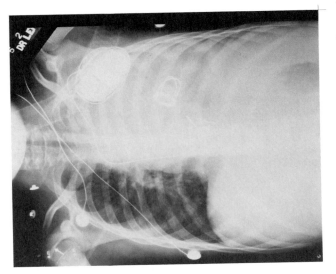

Figure 23.   PA (A) and lateral (B) chest x-rays in a patient in whom the right atrial appendage had been amputated at the time of open heart surgery. An active fixation pacing lead had been positioned in the right atrial septum.

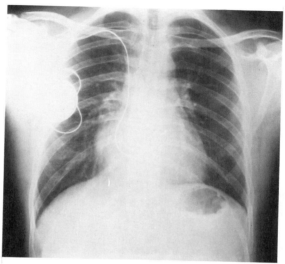

Figure 24.   *A pacing lead positioned in the coronary sinus for atrial pacing. Previous amputation of the right atrial appendage precluded the usual atrial position.* **A.** *PA projection in which the lead seems to be in the outflow tract of the right ventricle.*

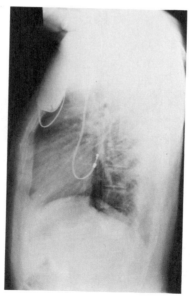

Figure 24B.   *Lateral projection which shows the lead to be on the posterior cardiac wall and not in the right ventricle.*

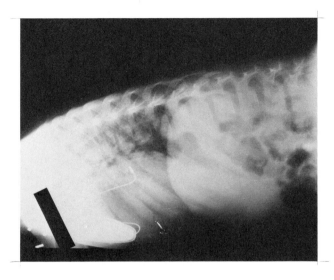

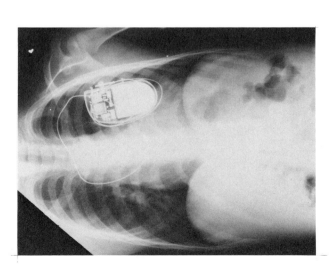

Figure 25.   *A patient with transposition of the great vessels and an active fixation lead in the left atrium.* **A.** *PA projection.* **B.** *lateral projection.*

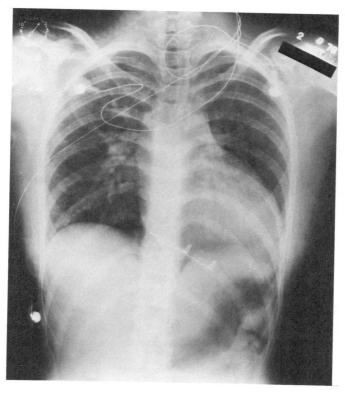

Figure 26.   *A bipolar right ventricular myocardial lead system. The sutureless myocardial lead is of the three-turn "screw-in" configuration. The leads have been placed on the diaphragmatic surface of the right ventricle.*

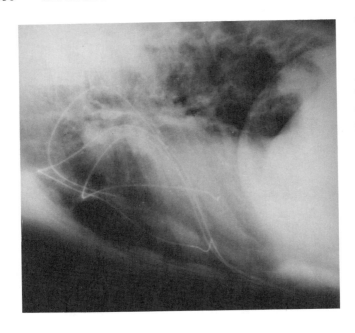

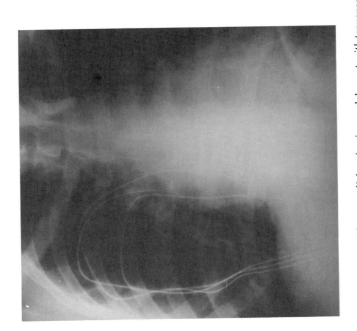

Figure 27. *Atrial myocardial pacing in an adolescent with transposition of the great vessels. The atrial myocardial lead ends in an open coil. The two myocardial leads are sutured into the right or systemic ventricle. The pulse generator is in the right upper quadrant of the abdomen.* **A.** *PA projection.* **B.** *Lateral projection.*

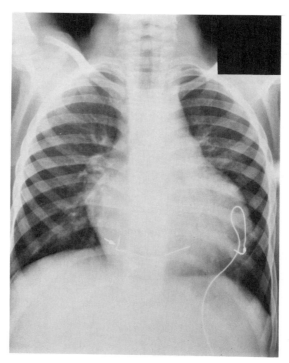

Figure 28. *PA (A) and lateral (B) chest x-rays in a child who had undergone multiple myocardial lead placements. Three different myocardial leads are seen: a fractured Medtronic 6913, of which only an abandoned remnant remains, the lead had been placed on the right ventricular wall; a Medtronic 5815 stab-in epicardial lead placed on the wall of the left ventricle; a Medtronic sutureless 6917 three-turn electrode placed on the diaphragmatic surface of the right ventricle between the fractured 6913 lead and the right ventricular apex.*

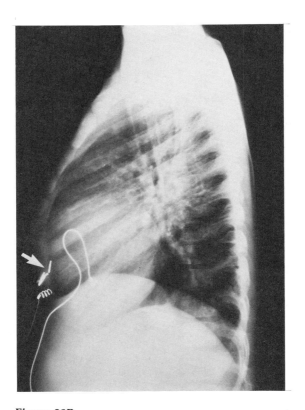

Figure 28B.

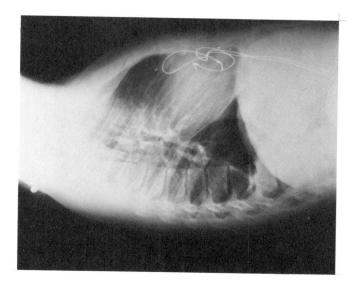

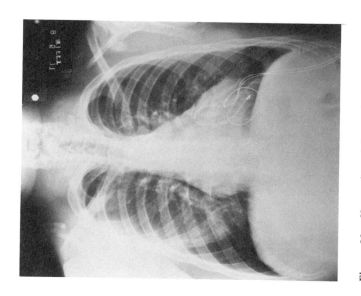

Figure 29.   X-ray of two left ventricular Medtronic 6913 myocardial electrodes. A. PA projection. B. lateral projection.

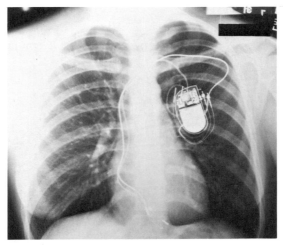

Figure 30.   *Two bipolar leads entering the left subclavian vein. A. PA projection showing the two leads.*

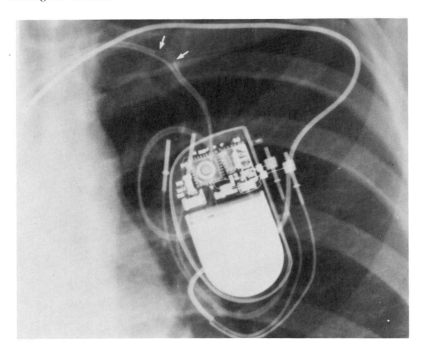

Figure 30B.   *A close-up of the pulse generator and leads as they enter the subclavian vein shows one lead to have a fracture of one of the conductors at the entry to the subclavian vein. The intact lead shows "pseudo-fracture" at the point of bifurcation.*

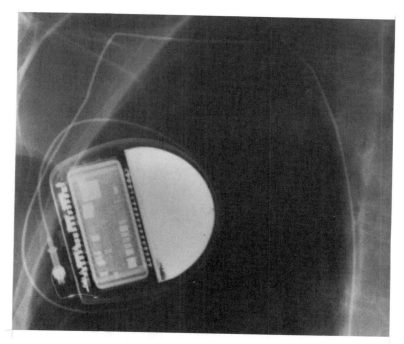

Figure 31. *X-ray of a patient in whom a stylet was left within a permanent pacing lead at the time of initial placement. A fracture occurred in both the lead and the stylet. A. PA projection of the pulse generator and the adjacent lead showing a sharp angulation.*

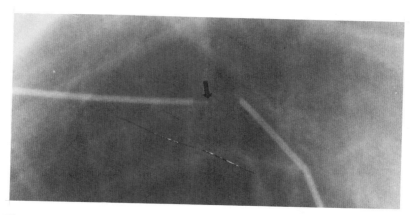

Figure 31B. *A close-up of the lead shows the fractured stylet within the coil of the lead.*

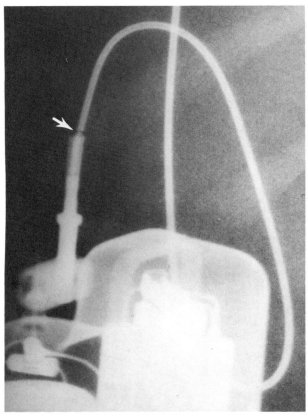

Figure 32.   Close-up of a PA projection of a lead fracture just beyond the connection of the lead and the connector pin.

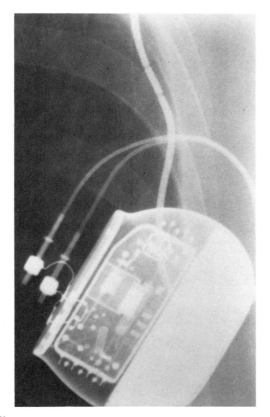

Figure 33. *Close-up of a PA projection of a pulse generator and a proximal portion of the implanted lead. Inspection of the lead clearly shows two areas of indentation caused by ligature compression of the lead unprotected by a rubber sleeve.*

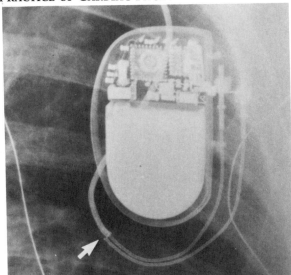

Figure 34.   Close-up of a bifurcated bipolar pulse generator and lead system demonstrating typical "pseudo-fracture." The arrow denotes the position of the lead where there appears to be discontinuity. This is not a fracture but normal x-ray appearance of this lead.

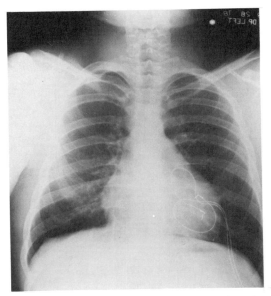

Figure 35.   PA (A), lateral (B), and close-up (C) chest x-rays of a patient with multiple myocardial electrodes. An arrow indicates a typical fracture of a stab-in myocardial electrode. The fracture occurs at the point of maximum stress.

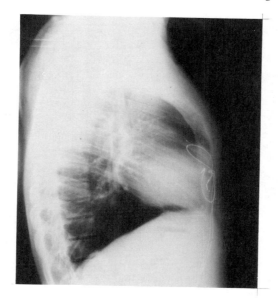

Figure 35B.

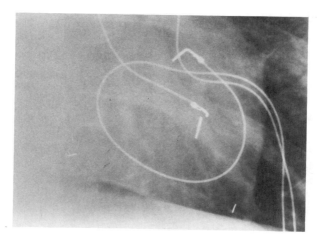

Figure 35C.

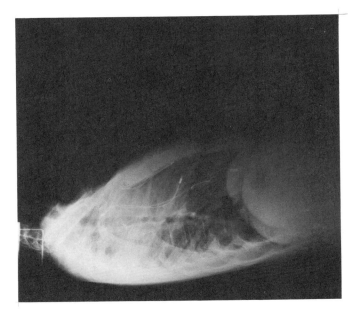

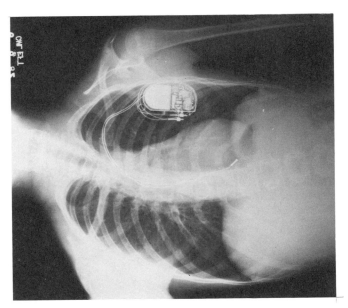

Figure 36.   PA (A) and lateral (B) chest x-rays of a patient with ventricular lead dislodgment. A large loop of the ventricular lead is coiled in the right atrium.

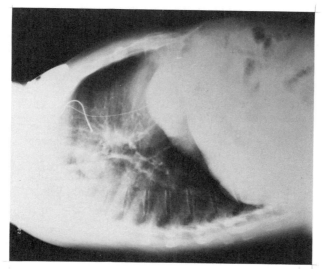

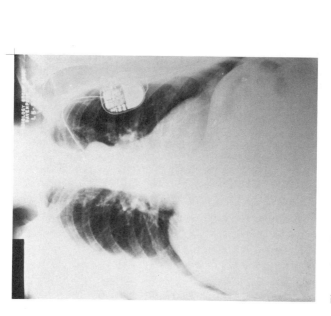

Figure 37. *PA (A) and lateral (B) chest x-rays of a patient in whom the atrial lead is dislodged and is now lying in the superior vena cava.*

BIBLIOGRAPHY

Branson JA: Radiology of cardiac pacemakers and their complications with three cases of superior vena caval obstruction. *Australas Radiol* 1978; 22: 125–131.

Chun PKC: Characteristics of commonly utilized permanent endocardial and epicardial pacemaker electrode systems: Method of radiologic identification. *Am Heart J* 1981; 102:404–414.

Dunlap TE, Popat KD, Sorkin RP: Radiographic pseudofracture of the Medtronic bipolar polyurethane pacing lead. *Am Heart J* 1983; 106:167–168.

Filice R, Hutton L, Klein G: Cardiac pacemaker leads: A radiographic perspective. *J Can Assoc Radiol* 1984; 35:20–23.

Gyarmati J, Worum F, Barnak G, et al: Radiological diagnosis of complications in pacemaker treatments. *Radiol Diagn* (Berl) 1979; 20:666–675.

Hall WM, Rosenbaum HD: The radiology of cardiac pacemakers. *Radiol Clin North Am* 1971; 9(2):343–353.

Helland J: Pacemaker lead complications: Clinical significance and patient management. *Medtronic News* 1983; pp. 8–14.

Kaul TK, Bain WH: Radiographic appearance of implanted transvenous endocardial pacing electrodes. *Chest* 1977; 72:323–326.

McHenry MM, Grayson CE: Roentgenographic diagnosis of pacemaker failure. *Am J Roentgenol* 1970; 109:94–100.

Ragaza EP, Shapiro R: Radiologic recognition of unusual sites of a transvenous catheter pacemaker. *J Can Assoc Radiol* 1970; 21:214–216.

Sorkin RP, Schuurmann BJ, Simon AB: Radiographic aspects of permanent cardiac pacemakers. *Radiology* 1976; 119:281–286.

Steiner RM: Radiology of cardiac pacemakers. In EK Chung (Ed.): *Artificial Cardiac Pacing: Practical Approach.* 2nd ed. Williams & Wilkins Company, Baltimore, 1984, pp. 43–61.

Steiner RM, Morse DP, Tegtmeyer CJ: Pacemaker lead psuedo-fracture. *Radiology* 1982; 143:793.

Steiner RM, Tegtmeyer CJ: The radiology of cardiac pacemakers. In D Morse, M Steiner, V Parsonnet (Eds): *A Guide to Cardiac Pacemakers.* F. A. Davis Company, Philadelphia, 1983, pp. 27–70.

Steiner RM, Tegtmeyer CJ: The radiology of cardiac pacemakers. *Cardiovasc Clin* 1983; 14(2):63–95.

Tegtmeyer CJ: Roentgenographic assessment of causes of cardiac pacemaker failure and complications. *CRC Crit Rev Diagn Imaging* 1977; 9:1–50.

Walter WH III, Wenger NK: Radiographic identification of commonly used implanted pacemakers. *N Engl J Med* 1969; 281:1230–1231.

Chapter 11

RATE MODULATED PACING

Seymour Furman

The initial approach to implanted ventricular pacing was to provide a stable, regular, reliably paced ventricular rate and rhythm more rapid than the idioventricular rate, which would eliminate the lethal episodes of ventricular asystole and escape tachycardias that characterized the unprotected, atrially dissociated idioventricular rate characteristic of complete heart block. It was recognized within several years that increased cardiac output resulted from an increase in the ventricular rate. Pacemakers responding to the atrial rate and producing atrial synchrony were evaluated as were ventricular asynchronous pacemakers with external rate control, manually set to be slower at rest and more rapid for activity. What seemed to be less well understood was that some level of physiological need, usually exercise, was necessary to increase cardiac output further, as a result of a greater increase in rate. Many studies demonstrated that during a rise in paced ventricular rate, the absence of physiological need produced a brief increase in cardiac output, which soon returned (at the higher rate) to the cardiac output at the lower rate (resulting, of course, from a decrease in stroke volume). As the increase in rate with constant cardiac output required a commensurate decrease in stroke volume, it was then speculated that such a decrease in stroke volume always occurred when rate was increased. The need for the critical element, physiological requirement or exercise, was not clearly understood (Figure 1).

The past decade has demonstrated the central role that ventricular rate plays in cardiac output. The role of the atrial contraction, ventricular preload or the "atrial kick," and of AV synchrony remains controversial as it has been for the past several hundred years. Present data seems to indicate that atrial synchrony may be more important at the lower end of the "normal" rate range, i.e., between 50 bpm and perhaps 90–100 bpm. At more rapid ventricular rates, i.e., 120–180 bpm, rate alone seems more important and AV synchrony less so. The normal atrium provides two functions, contraction to empty into and preload the ventricle for its contraction, and the provision of a cardiac rate derived from the sensitivity of the sinoatrial node to body metabolic changes, including changes in

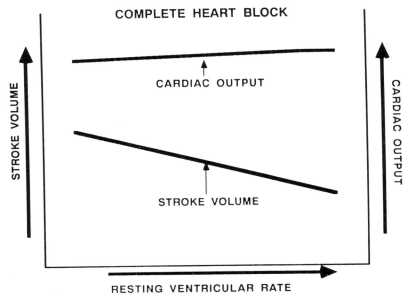

Figure 1. *An increase of resting cardiac rate increases cardiac output very little as stroke volume undergoes corresponding decrease. To increase cardiac output by rate increase, a physiological need must exist.*

blood pH, intra-atrial pressure, oxygen and carbon dioxide tension temperature, reflex signals from the carotid body and circulating catecholamines.

The four atrial functions relative to cardiac hemodynamics are, therefore, to:

1. propel blood into the ventricle;
2. set the ventricular rate appropriate for need;
3. separate the atrial and ventricular contractions by the most efficient AV interval;
4. avoid ventriculoatrial conduction.

As time has passed it has become progressively clearer that the AV interval itself has a relatively small hemodynamic importance between about 50 and 250 ms duration (Figure 2). Ventriculoatrial conduction can be of very great importance in some patients, and in the absence of such VA conduction, the ventricular rate is a major determinant of cardiac output (see Chapter 5). Specifically, body compensatory mechanisms reduce stroke volume at increased rates in the absence of need so that simply increasing rate, at rest, to determine the effect on cardiac output gives a result which, if incorrectly extrapolated, is erroneous.

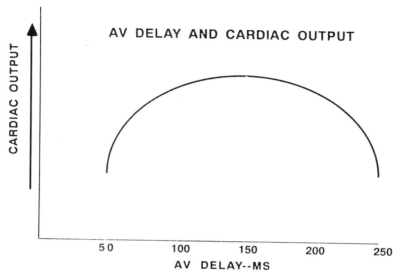

Figure 2. *The electronic analogue of the PR interval, the AV delay, affects cardiac output especially at the lower range of atrial rates. While the exact change depends on many factors, maximum output seems to be at about 150 ms from the beginning of atrial depolarization. Efficiency falls at shorter and longer interval durations.*

The effect of rate modulated ventricular pacing differs, depending on the rhythm being paced. Pacing complete heart block may provide one result while ventricular pacing in the presence of sinus bradycardia with retained retrograde conduction may produce retrograde atrial capture and the pacemaker syndrome. The consequences of making the right ventricular apex the most rapid "pacemaker" of the heart and the potential reversal of the cardiac contraction sequence remains uncertain. It is important to note that the incidence of retrograde conduction decreases with increases in ventricular rate. Further development in the area of rate modulated pacing is in the direction of dual-chamber pacing, which will, of course, retain the normal AV sequence. Each circumstance, whether atrial, ventricular or dual-chamber pacing, each rhythm, AV nodal or SA nodal disease, or combinations of both in the presence or absence of retrograde conduction, should be judged as pacemaker implantation, and the selection of a pacing mode is made. It should also be remembered that comparisons should be cautious between single- and dual-chamber pacing whether rate modulated or not. The comparison between atrial driven ventricular pacing (VDD or DDD) and rate modulated ventricular pacing (VVIR) should be made especially cautiously.

With the passage of a quarter of a century, the issues of the existence and duration of an AV delay, extensively discussed during the initial evaluation of atrioventricular sequential (DVI) pacing, have become better understood. The provision of an AV delay of physiological duration is important, and the avoidance of retrograde conduction is critical in some patients, but a cardiac rate responsive to activity is probably the single most important factor for increase of cardiac output.

It has also been demonstrated that in the presence of complete heart block with fixed antegrade and retrograde block, cardiac output during exercise is similar during atrial synchrony with a normal chronotropic response and ventricular pacing alone at a rate matched to the atrial rate but without atrial synchrony (Figure 3).

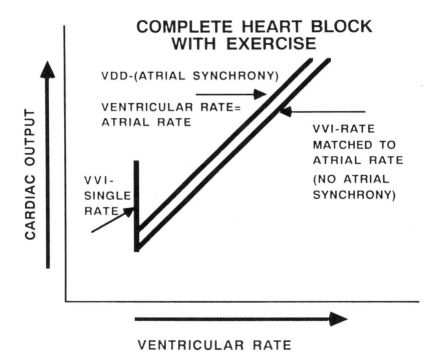

Figure 3.   *In patients with fixed antegrade and retrograde heart block, rate increase, with a normal AV delay, can occur during exercise by pacing with atrial synchrony (VDD), producing a ventricular rate equal to the atrial rate. The ventricular rate can also be paced at the atrial rate but without atrial synchrony. The cardiac output achieved will be similar for both. This realization is the basis for the use of single-chamber (VVI,R) rate modulated pacemakers. At a single rate, (VVI) exercise increases cardiac output far less.*

With the recognition of the importance of rate, several simultaneous approaches were undertaken. The one earliest to fruition was the development of a device that would sense the atrium to drive the ventricle and sense the ventricle to avoid competition. VDD and DDD pacemakers provided this capability. In 1976, Cammilli implanted a pacemaker that drove only the ventricle but its rate was set, independently of the atrial rate, by the pH of the central venous blood. This device, which never achieved widespread acceptance, demonstrated the feasibility of sensing a function other than the atrial depolarization to set the ventricular rate.

The increase in cardiac output follows the formula:

$$\text{Cardiac Output} = \text{Rate} \times \text{Stroke Volume}$$

In the normal, increase in cardiac output bears a linear relationship to oxygen consumption, which can be increased in three ways. The cardiac rate may be increased, in normals rate can increase about three times between rest and maximal activity. The stroke volume may increase by some 50%, and the AV oxygen difference broadens. Oxygen consumption thus depends on Rate × Stroke Volume × AV Oxygen difference. Other consequences, such as changes in peripheral and central arterial pressures and in blood pH follow.

PHYSIOLOGICAL RATIONALE

Several changes occur during exercise as the metabolic rate increases:

1. Arterial-venous oxygen difference is broadened, i. e., venous oxygen saturation decreases;
2. anaerobic metabolism can occur;
3. venous blood pH is reduced;
4. right-sided cardiac pressures are increased;
5. left-sided cardiac pressures are increased;
6. myocardial contractility is increased;
7. stroke volume increases;
8. body temperature rises;
9. pre-ejection interval changes;
10. changes occur in cardiac muscle electrophysiology.

With these mechanisms, cardiac output can be increased several fold at a fixed ventricular rate in a patient with relatively normal myocardial function. In the normal, without SA or AV nodal or myocardial disease, stroke volume can be increased with exercise by

50%, and rate increase can be 3–4 times. Even those with congenital complete heart block can achieve relatively normal cardiac output by the ability to increase stroke volume, associated with the modest rate increase of which congenitals are capable.

But increase of cardiac output by anaerobic metabolism and broadening of the arterio-venous oxygen difference causes oxygen debt which, when sufficiently severe, is always symptomatic producing: (a) breathlessness, and at still more severe levels; (b) chest pain; (c) lightheadedness; (d) muscle cramps; and (e) ventricular ectopy. Reduction of anaerobic metabolism during exercise is desirable.

Sensors of physiological function, whether directly measuring metabolic effect such as central venous pH or oxygen consumption, or indirectly by measuring activity can substitute for the normal atrial sensitivity to physiological need. The results of this measurement can then be used to trigger a pacemaker without sensing the atrium. Conditions for which sensor driven single-chamber ventricular pacing is useful include:

1. large silent atrium;
2. fixed sinus bradycardia with or without nodal rhythm;
3. fixed atrial fibrillation or flutter with AV block;
4. post ablation AV block with residual atrial arrhythmias
5. frequent atrial arrhythmias with AV block;
6. chronotropic incompetence, in which the responsiveness of the atrium is not proportional to activity needs, and in the absence of retrograde conduction;
7. atrial rate modulated pacing is useful in the presence of fixed sinus bradycardia or chronotropic incompetence with intact AV conduction.

Despite the more clear cut indications listed above, implantation of a rate modulated single-chamber pacemaker may be used in the presence of intermittent, partial or complete AV block and sinus node dysfunction to produce a rate variable ventricular pacemaker with a single ventricular lead. In the atrium, with satisfactory AV conduction, such a pacemaker can produce a variable ventricular rate by atrial drive. In the later instance both the normal AV sequence and rate response will result. A DVI or DDD pacemaker in a patient with atrial chronotropic incompetence restores the normal AV sequence but not the cardiac rate response. Dual-chamber rate modulated pacemakers are now becoming available.

SENSOR REQUIREMENT

During exercise (i.e., muscle metabolism), various byproducts are emitted. These are:

1. heat, producing body temperature;
2. electricity, producing the ECG and EMG (electromyogram);
3. carbon dioxide;
4. lactic acid, i.e., the blood pH will be reduced;
5. intracardiac pressure;
6. movement.

Other electrophysiological changes occur including changes in the duration of the electrocardiographic QT interval, in the ventricular depolarization gradient, i.e., the area under the curve of depolarization beginning with a stimulus and ending as the depolarization returns to baseline. The duration of the pre-ejection interval (PEI) from a stimulus to the resulting ventricular mechanical contraction also changes.

The sinus node responds by changes in rate of its stimulation to variation in carbon dioxide and oxygen tension, temperature and intra-atrial pressure and hormonal stimuli. Some of these parameters can be measured directly to change pacemaker stimulation rate. Atrial sensing is the traditional measure of body need.

A sensor useful in cardiac pacing is a transducer which will measure one of the effects of byproducts of increased metabolism and exercise and produce a signal (usually electrical), which can be sensed by the pacemaker electronic circuit to change the pacemaker automatic interval and therefore the escape rate. The response of the pacemaker to what the sensor detects is referred to as "rate responsiveness," "rate modulation," or "adaptive rate" pacing.

The sensor must respond to physiological or near physiological body activities and be proportional to and capable of mimicking the normal body response. The rate of increase in cardiac rate should be similar to that of the normal human, as should the rate of cool-down. The sensor response should parallel the normal response, i.e., it should neither be delayed until well into exercise nor persist after exercise has ended (Figure 4). The onset should be as rapid as the normal atrium, should be free of idiosyncracies, i.e., smooth over the entire exercise range, stable over the decades and reproducible from one time to the next. It should be suitable or adjustable for a wide range of patients from young to old, and from cardiovascular health to fragility. It should respond to nonphysical activity demands such as emotion and mental work. Finally, it should respond appropriately to three different states:

(a) rest;
(b) mild to moderate activity, i.e., the usual submaximal activity of normal life;
(c) maximal activity.

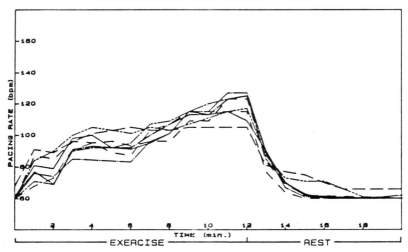

Figure 4. *A graph depicts the external Activitrax pacing rate responses, on a tread-mill, at setting MEDIUM 6, of each of 8 healthy volunteers.*

If response is not equal in all three states, the most important is to submaximal activity.

Development of a sensor based rate modulated pacing system requires at least four components:

1. Selection of a physiological indicator, changes of which are associated with metabolic need;
2. A sensor that will detect these changes and respond reliably and reproducibly;
3. An algorithm that will translate the changes in the physiological function, detected by the sensor, into a change in pacemaker stimulation rate;
4. A single- or dual-chamber cardiac stimulator (Figure 5).

The opportunity exists to improve upon the atrium, which responds to drugs, intercurrent illness, and to the development of arrhythmias. It is difficult to stop atrial control of ventricular response in the presence of AV conduction even in the presence of an arrhythmia. The artificial sensor should be self-monitoring, incapable of exceeding specific high and low rate limits, and should failure occur it must be in a safe manner. Its response should be similar to that of change in the physiological function, without non-linear response introduced by the sensor itself.

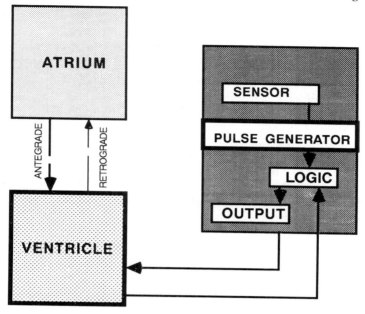

SINGLE CHAMBER-RATE MODULATED (VVIR)

Figure 5. *A diagrammatic representation of a single-chamber rate modulated pace-maker shows one ventricular input and output channel as in a conventional single-chamber pacemaker. In addition, a second input signal originates from the sensor and is directed to the logic system to achieve rate modulation.*

The algorithm is certainly a most important element. The algorithm absorbs the information generated by the sensor, and determines the response that will drive the impulse generator. An example of this effect is the pacemaker response in a temperature driven system. Blood warmed by lower extremity activity is driven into the central venous system, but is preceded by cool (unwarmed) blood. The first blood to reach an intracardiac thermister will reduce blood temperature. The algorithm should not reduce the cardiac rate in response to the flush of cool blood, rather in the usual algorithm, this flush will cause a step function INCREASE in cardiac pacing rate, perhaps by 15 bpm, i.e., from 70–85 bpm. If warm blood follows, the rate increase will be maintained and become proportional to temperature, if not, the rate will return to the preset level. The algorithm will determine the degree of rate change in response to a specific change in sensor activity. It will determine how long to consider a physiological function change as physiological or as artifactual.

New terminology is that of OPEN LOOP and CLOSED LOOP sensors. The OPEN LOOP sensor does not respond to a specifically physiological function. An example is the activity sensor that responds to imposed motion. It may increase rate in response to imposed extracorporeal movement such as vehicular motion, and will not respond to fever or mental stress, both of which are usually associated with increased metabolic needs. The CLOSED LOOP system responds to physiological change, and will increase or decrease rate as a response to such needs. For example, the stimulus-T sensor will increase cardiac rate as the stimulus-T interval is abbreviated, presumably in response to exercise. As the stimulus-T interval is prolonged the pacemaker-imposed cardiac rate will decline. The difference between the two is responsiveness to specific physiological function. In practice there may be little difference between the two approaches, and an open loop system may seem to function as well as or better than a closed loop system.

Sensor utility is based on its response to physiological need resulting from muscular and mental function, the rapidity of onset of response, its smoothness and flexibility, and physiological return to the resting setting. Some responses may be physiological but slow in onset. Central venous temperature, for example, follows muscular activity very well, but its responsiveness is slow, a brief burst of activity may be completed before a temperature response and a consequent cardiac rate response occurs. Imposed temperatures, such as the drinking of warm or cold liquids, will affect the central venous temperature and the pacemaker imposed cardiac rate. Neither activity, temperature, nor stimulus-T interval sensors respond proportionately to intellectual activity or to emotion.

Other idiosyncracies include unequal responsiveness to activity needs. The activity sensor responds to motion, not really to body needs. The response, for example, to movement of the arm on the side of the implanted activity sensor is much greater than to movement of the contralateral arm. Descending a staircase produces a similar or greater rate response to ascending the same staircase, though the metabolic needs are quite different.

The placement of two sensors in the same device is an approach being evaluated. The capabilities of both may be complementary, and the inadequacies of each can perhaps cancel. For the soon to be introduced dual-chamber rate modulated (DDDR) pacemaker, the atrial rate and another sensor, activity, temperature, pre-ejection interval, stroke volume or contractility, etc., will interact to produce a rate

Table I
Atrium and Artificial Sensor

Atrial Rate / Sensor Rate	Below LRL	Between LRL & URL	Above URL
Below LRL	Pace at lower rate limit	Track at atrial rate	Track atrial rate to URL
Between LRL & URL	Pace at sensor driven rate	Track or pace at higher rate- atrium/ sensor	Pace at maximum sensor rate
Above URL	Pace at maximum sensor rate	Track or pace at higher rate- atrium/ sensor	Pace at sensor rate

URL = upper rate limit for atrial tracking
LRL = lower rate limit for atrial tracking

determined to be most suitable. Another possibly useful combination for a single-chamber pacemaker is activity and temperature, which may provide a rapid onset of response to activity, and the longer term proportional response to central venous temperature (Table I).

PROGRAMMING

Programming the rate of a single-chamber, single-rate pacemaker is generally not difficult as the options are few and the indications for the proper rate under all conditions of activity are even fewer. It has been traditional, and probably correct, to program the rate of a patient in fixed or intermittent complete heart block at 70 bpm, while for those with sinus node dysfunction another rate may be selected. For the dual-chamber, atrial sensing pacemaker, the atrium itself sets the pacemaker rate. The person programming sets a lower rate limit, i.e., that rate below which the heart beat was not allowed, and an upper rate, that above which the pacemaker will not stimulate the ventricle (or track the atrium). Between the two limits the atrium controls the ventricular stimulation rate, the rate of increase or decrease, and the responsiveness to specific activities (Figure 6).

For a rate modulated pacemaker, the physician must set the lower and upper rates and the responsiveness of the pacing system, including the acceleration with which it increases and decreases rate, and the threshold of physiological or imposed change necessary to produce a change in pacing rate. While the setting of the non-sensor driven DDD pacemaker may be relatively simple because of the guide the atrium provides, that of the sensor driven single- or dual-chamber pulse generator may be much more difficult. Programming the DDD pacemaker may be far less labor-intensive than programming the rate modulated pacemaker. In the rate modulated device, the SENSITIVITY setting determines when response begins, and RESPONSIVENESS determines how much of a change will occur. Both settings are required. It is as yet unclear whether a stress or activity test will be routinely required. Should a stress test be performed, the most suitable is as yet unknown. The most widely used stress tests have been designed to evaluate coronary artery disease. It is likely that the majority of patients with implanted cardiac pacemakers have coronary artery disease, and testing them will only prove that that is so, but may not give an indication of how best to program the implanted pacemaker. The performance of a stress test is a labor-intensive effort. If the test is done at a single setting, which then proves to be "incorrect," one or more other tests must be done at other settings (Figure 7).

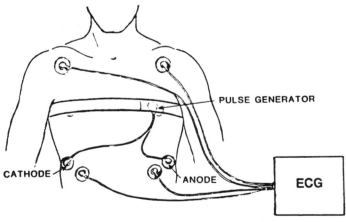

Figure 6.   *A bipolar rate modulated pulse generator is strapped to the chest wall and the two outputs are placed as indicated. Pacemaker output is programmed to maximum and produces stimuli, which can be detected on the ECG without being felt by the test subject. The response will mimic the implanted pulse generator response.*

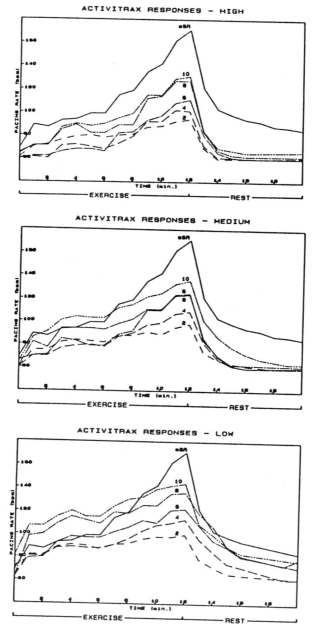

Figure 7. *This graphic display is of the pacemaker rate set at different levels of responsiveness at the three levels of sensitivity, in each instance compared to the mean sinus rate (mSR) of a group of normal subjects. An external Activitrax was used to determine its response.*

PROGRAMMING OF RATE MODULATED PACEMAKERS

Programming of the rate modulated parameters is essential to the pacemaker's proper function. Its sensitivity and responsiveness must be such that normal atrial function is approached. Upper and lower rates must also mimic the normal. Single-chamber, rate modulated pacing may be most useful in the child with congenital heart block in whom AV block is not associated with retrograde conduction. While implantation of a dual-chamber pacemaker can be successful, growth may cause difficulty with the lead system and few DDD pacemakers can readily accommodate the rapid atrial rates, of which a young person is capable, without developing AV block at the upper rate interval (URI). While a relatively prolonged Wenckebach interval can be programmed to ameliorate sudden onset of AV block, (see Comprehension of Pacemaker Timing Cycles) a single-chamber ventricular rate modulated device should be considered. A ventricular lead alone may give less long-term difficulty than both atrial and ventricular leads and when full growth has been reached, an atrial lead can be added during a pacemaker upgrade. A rate modulated upper rate of 150 bpm will allow vigorous physical activity.

Exercise testing and proper programming can set sensitivity, responsiveness, and upper and lower rates to be adequate to reproduce effective ventricular rate modulation. When such exercise programming is undertaken, an approximation of the normal atrial response to exercise should be reproduced (Figure 8). The normal atrial response to exercise is the standard that should be met by all rate modulated devices. If single-chamber, the modulation is based on the sensor alone, if dual-chamber, on the sensor and its interaction with the atrium.

Test of sensor function can be by specific exercise test, or formal stress test such as the Bruce, Naughton or the CAEP (see Table III). Probably, the Holter monitor is a more reliable means of assessing rate response than any specific test. Nevertheless, if the patient is inactive on the day of ambulatory monitoring little response may be seen. A small response may also not allow distinction between an inactive day and an underresponsive unit. In any event, it cannnot be assumed that programming to specific settings without exercise testing will be satisfactory for the individual patient (Figure 9). Several devices provide a sensor *Passive* mode in which the sensor will not drive the stimulation rate but in which a histogram can be printed to indicate what rates have been determined by the sensor to be appropriate for the patient's activity level. These can assist during evaluation of sensor programming in providing a rapid, numerical indication of the pacemaker sensor response.

The single-chamber rate modulated pacemaker should not be programmed to that rate modulated mode unless it is actually needed. In a person with episodic asystole, but who is largely in a normal spontaneous rhythm, it is unlikely that rate modulation programming will achieve exactly the *correct* rate modulation. Consequently, setting modulation to be excessively sensitive and/or responsive may cause ventricular stimulation when none is necessary. It is then probably wiser to provide a slower ventricular inhibited function merely to interrupt asystole, should it occur. Rate modulated atrial pacing should also be used when possible as it provides the equivalent of a dual-chamber rate modulated pacemaker. The status of AV conduction should be carefully assessed and the stimulation rate, in the modulated mode, should not be allowed to reach that rate at which onset of Wenckebach conduction occurs.

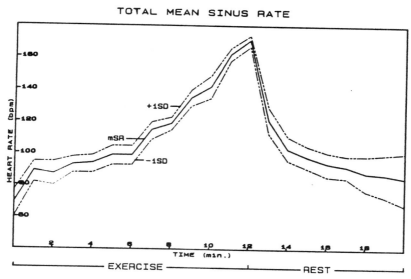

Figure 8. *This graphic display is of the overall mean sinus rate (mSR) ± one standard deviation of a group of normal volunteers of age 20 through age 70 during exercise testing.*

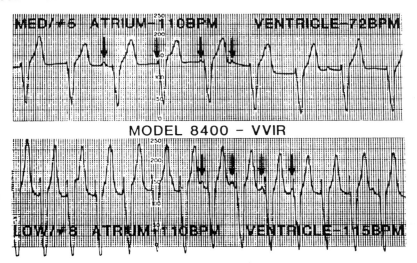

Figure 9. *Programming sensor sensitivity and responsiveness are essential to an appropriate response. In this analysis the atrial rate of approximately 110 per minute represents need, but the SENSITIVITY of MEDIUM and RESPONSIVENESS of level 5 do not produce a commensurate response. Programming to LOW (greater sensitivity to activity and 8 (greater responsiveness) yield a proportional response, i.e., equal to the atrial rate.*

CARDIAC RHYTHMS SUBJECTED TO PACING

There are two broad rhythm categories that are subjected to cardiac pacing. One is that of disturbance of AV conduction, often referred to as AV nodal dysfunction; the second is sinus (SA) node dysfunction or sick sinus syndrome. Some patients have both AV and SA nodal (binodal) dysfunction. The characteristics of the two conditions are different. While ventricular bradycardia and asystole are indications for cardiac pacing common to both conditions, several modifying circumstances exist. Those with sinus node dysfunction usually are characterized by the presence of antegrade conduction, and two-thirds of them have retrograde conduction at some rate. Those with AV block, whether intermittent or fixed, have retrograde conduction less frequently, about one-third of the time, at some paced rate (Chapter 2). Sinus node dysfunction is not progressive. Implant may be performed when arrhythmias and symptoms are most severe and both may recur, remain at the same level of severity or be ameliorated over the long term. In AV block, the severity of the conduction is likely to be progressive. Both antegrade and retrograde conduction deteriorate over time. The effect of ventricular stimulation, especially at different rates, is quite different. Pacemaker syndrome, which results, in part, from the effects of retrograde conduction, occurs more frequently in sinus node dysfunction than AV node dysfunction. Ventricular pacing in sinus node dysfunction is more likely to be associated with echo beating and with pacemaker syndrome.

Retrograde conduction after ventricular stimulation occurs, at some rate, in about 45% of patients who require pacemaker implantation, but that incidence includes ventricular rates of 60–80 bpm. The effects of retrograde (VA) conduction producing decreases in peripheral arterial pressure and cardiac output occur either with single-rate ventricular pacing, or with small increases in paced ventricular rate when that rate does not exceed the lower physiological range. At a rate of 100 bpm, only 25% of patients have 1:1 retrograde conduction, and at 120 bpm and above, fewer than 10% of patients will have retrograde conduction. As the main cause of pacemaker syndrome is retrograde conduction, it is possible that absence of VA conduction will allow decoupling of the atrium and ventricle at more rapid ventricular rates without deleterious effects. If so, some of the potential timing problems caused by dual-chamber pacemaker atrial and ventricular channel refractoriness and blanking, which occur at rapid paced atrial rates, may be avoided by a strategy of retaining atrial synchrony at slower rates and abandoning it at more rapid paced rates i.e., allowing sensor driven ventricular rates at the upper end of the physiological range. However, the issue of single- and dual-chamber pacing is resolved, rate modulation is certain to become a standard and programmable mode of operation of a cardiac pacemaker.

SENSORS FOR CLINICAL PACING

The Atrium

The atrium has been the traditional sensor of body need. In patients with congenital heart block, the ventricles may be moderately responsive in rate, and the overall result may be relatively normal cardiac output without AV synchrony or atrial drive of ventricular rate. Such ventricular responsiveness does not occur with postoperative heart block in the patient with congenital heart disease, or with acquired heart block occurring later in life. In both instances, ventricular rate is fixed (except that the idioventricular rate may slow or stop), and is unresponsive to body needs.

The atrium is a reliable sensor of body need for most people, but it may be dissociated from the ventricle via AV nodal disease, and it may suffer its own disabilities caused by sinus node dysfunction, atrial fibrillation, flutter and other supraventricular arrhythmias. In the presence of such dysfunction, the atrium becomes an unreliable sensor of body needs. An even more significant technical impediment to the atrium as a sensor of body needs is the present requirement of a lead specifically to sense the atrium. The placement of two leads, one for the ventricle and the other for the atrium, has never achieved popularity beyond about one-third of implants in the United States and even less in other countries. This problem has persisted despite the widespread availability of leads deemed to be reliable and readily implanted. Three ways of sensing atrial activity have been available:

a. The conventional lead which makes contact, either by active or passive fixation, with the atrial wall. This lead may sense or pace the atrium or do both;
b. A lead which senses atrial activity without direct contact with the atrium, i. e., is part of the ventricular lead, and therefore does not contact the atrial wall. This lead may sense atrial activity sufficiently discrete so that atrial synchrony can be provided for VDD pacing. Several such leads and pulse generators are available. One is named "orthogonal" (see Chapter 3).
c. The same lead may sense atrial activity, but less reliably, so that the generator must have a slow response time and avoid falling back to the lower rate escape interval when a P wave is unsensed. The pacemaker rate then rises slowly to approximate the atrial rate, and descends slowly. It never provides atrial synchrony, rather a ventricular rate, which approximates the atrial rate. One such lead and pulse generator system had been in clinical evaluation but are no longer available.

All of these techniques are prey to the problems of atrial arrhythmia, and in the event of its persistence the only effective resolution may be return to single-rate ventricular pacing. The first system (above) involves a second lead (clearly a less popular route), while the latter two involve a single lead only, in which atrial sensing occurs via an electrode that is part of the ventricular lead.

Activity

During the early 1980s, atrial synchronous (VDD) pacemakers were introduced that sensed atrial activity using a specific atrial lead (above) without the capability of pacing the atrium. With the advent of DDD generators, which are also capable of VDD pacing, most VDD generators fell from use. In one design the atrial channel input was replaced by input from a piezo electric crystal that was part of the pulse generator case (Activitrax[1]). This device was programmable, as was the original VDD generator, to three levels of sensitivity, corresponding to the three programmable levels of atrial electrogram amplitude, and to ten levels of responsiveness, which corresponded to programmable AV interval. In a single-chamber version, it has become the most successful of rate modulated pacing systems, and has been used in the atrium and in the ventricle. As presently available for ventricular use, it is programmable to three levels of sensitivity, the least sensitive referred to as HIGH, then MEDIUM and the most sensitive, LOW. There are also ten levels of responsiveness, numbered from 1, the least responsive, to 10, the most responsive.

The voltage developed by the crystal upon the pacemaker case may be 5–50 mV at rest and as much as 200 mV during running or other vigorous activity. The most sensitive responsiveness, i.e., number 10, corresponds to an AV interval of 25 ms, and the least sensitive, number 1, corresponds to an AV interval of 250 ms.

The response of the piezo electric crystal results from episodic or continuous pressure. Most sensed events result from body movement, though imposed movement as from vehicular movement, sleeping face down, applying pressure to the device in its pectoral subcutaneous position and actual tapping of the device can increase its rate.

In practice, the response of the piezo electric crystal is among the most rapid of any of the sensors, and movement causes as prompt a response as the normal atrium (Figure 10). The device seems to be tuned to a lower frequency limit of 2 Hz and an upper frequency limit of 70 Hz. The maximum sensitivity seems to be in the middle of that range, i.e., about 10–50 Hz. The vibrational frequency of body motion is reported to be in the range of 10 Hz.

Activity crystal signals are emitted singly, and their frequency and amplitude are determined within the device. These individual "on-off" signals are then counted, and the pacemaker rate response is determined. Another use of the piezo electric crystal is tuned similarly but with a somewhat lower upper frequency limit (Sensolog[2]). The pacemaker rate is determined by integrating the vibrational forces to which the pulse generator is subjected. The former design

---

[1]Medtronic, Inc., Minneapolis, MN

[2]Siemens-Pacesetter, Sylmar, CA

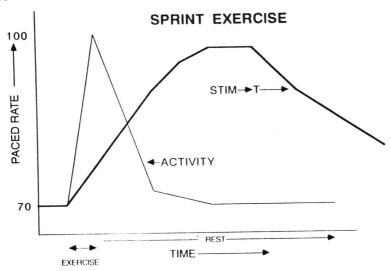

Figure 10. *The difference in onset of response of two different sensors, one rapid and the other relatively slower may be substantial. As a result of a short sprint exercise, the activity sensor increases its rate promptly and with rest returns to baseline. The stimulus to T sensor responds more slowly and, in this instance, the rate response occurs after the sprint has ended and persists during rest.*

sets the rate by detecting suprathreshold voltage emissions from the crystal which, in turn, is set by programming sensitivity. The later version integrates the electrical results of all vibrational forces. Clinical experience has suggested a somewhat smoother and more proportional response to workload, though the significance of the difference may not be great. Both approaches to the use of the piezo electric crystal sensor produce relatively similar responses. Both respond rapidly, Activitrax more rapidly on walking steps, Sensolog somewhat more proportionally. Both suffer from greater responsiveness to body vibration than to actual activity. Both respond to walking up and down stairs so that ventricular rate may not be proportional for the effort expended while walking up or down a staircase.

For activity sensitive units, other physical activities which have little vibrational effect produce little pacemaker response. Hand-grip, Valsalva maneuver and standing produce minimal response; jogging in place produces a prompt maximum response. Whether disproportionate response will occur with the other versions of piezo electric crystal, sensing remains to be determined. It must be emphasized that the idiosyncratic responses described remain relatively modest and have not limited the usefulness of the rate modulated approach. Activity sensing pacemakers are, by far, the most popular available. Indeed, the present field of rate modulated pacing, for single- and dual-chamber devices is based on activity sensing.

Endocardial Evoked Potential

QT Interval

It has been recognized since 1920 that the interval between the onset of the QRS complex and the end of repolarization, i.e., the T wave, varies as a function of cardiac rate. The QT interval duration and the variation of rate both result, at least in part, from the effect of circulating catecholamines and activity. In 1979, Rickards was able to demonstrate in the presence of complete AV block, that the interval between the stimulus beginning the ventricular depolarization and the end of repolarization, i.e., the T wave, was abbreviated during activity, even without change in the ventricular rate. Conversely, the duration of the stimulus-T (or QT) interval was prolonged at rest. The duration of the interval could then be considered an indicator of activity and of the need for an increased ventricular paced rate, could participate in an algorithm, and in turn, drive a pulse generator. Because of the absence of an easily discernible repolarization wave, the technique cannot be used for atrial pacing (Figure 11).

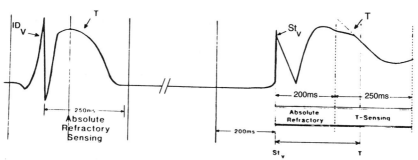

Figure 11. *The stimulus to T pacemaker sensor measures the interval following a pacemaker stimulus to the end of the repolarization (T) wave of the ventricular response. To the left is a spontaneous event, sensing of which is followed by a conventional 250 ms interval of ventricular refractoriness. The event to the right is a pacemaker induced contraction (ST$_v$) followed by 200 ms of absolute refractoriness then by another 250 ms during which the T wave is sensed to set the stimulus to T interval.*

A single unipolar ventricular lead can sense the stimulus-T interval. The principle operates by pacemaker emission of a stimulus to drive the ventricle and sensing of the end of the resultant T wave. In the absence of a paced ventricular event the stimulus-T interval cannot be determined so that should the patient, during rest or activity, assume a ventricular rate more rapid than the pacemaker lower rate limit, no rate modulation sensing mechanism exists (Figure 12).

In the presence of ventricular pacing, the emission of a stimulus causes the beginning of a 200 ms pacemaker absolute refractory period. No event can be sensed, particularly the depolarization of the ventricle. At the conclusion of 200 ms, a new window for sensing begins. This window is specifically designed to sense the T wave. During this interval, the pulse generator can be programmed for sen-

DETERMINATION OF STIMULUS TO T INTERVAL
AND PACING RATE DURING EVOKED POTENTIAL
⟶   PACING

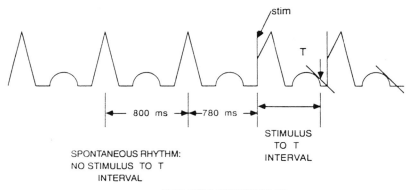

Figure 12. During use of any evoked response as the sensor of pacer rate the determination can only be made following a pacemaker stimulus. As long as the spontaneous ventricular rate is above (i.e., at a shorter coupling interval) than the lower rate limit (i.e., the escape rate), no rate modulation occurs. Periodically the pacemaker "tests" the rate by emitting a stimulus at a shorter coupling interval than the existing cardiac rate so that a ventricular capture beat occurs and the Stimulus to T interval can be determined.

sitivity to the T wave and for the duration of sensing. The interval between the stimulus and the sensed T wave can then be determined and the rate accordingly modified. Following the T wave sensing interval, the pacemaker becomes conventionally sensitive to ventricular activity until the end of the lower rate limit.

Should the coupling interval of the spontaneous ventricular rate be shorter (i.e., a more rapid rate) than the pacemaker lower rate limit, a QRS complex will fall during the conventional sensing interval that follows the absolute refractory period and the T sensing window. This will start another variety of cycle. In this instance, the absolute refractory period is 250 ms in duration and is followed by normal ventricular sensitivity. Each such cycle will be abbreviated by 6.4 ms in duration so that eventually the abbreviated cycle will be shorter than the patient's spontaneous ventricular cycle length and a stimulus will be emitted. Once that stimulus is emitted, the stimulus to T interval can be retested and the appropriate rate determined once again.

Because the T wave is of low amplitude and frequency content, maximum sensitivity must be available. High impedance leads generally attenuate the ventricular depolarization and repolarization electrograms and are therefore unsuitable for use with the stimulus-T pacemaker. Electrodes of generally low impedance such as large surface area, platinum-iridium, and porous and carbon tip electrodes seem better suited. Earlier, 8 mm^2 electrodes such as the continuous (or ball-tip) lead, which had very low and satisfactory pacing thresholds, seem unsuited for sensing the T wave.

The operation of the device as described may be problematic during alternation between paced and spontaneous ventricular activity. Two operating modes are therefore, available. The first is an operating mode in which it is assumed that there will be continuous pacing as exists during complete antegrade atrioventricular block. If this is not the case, then another mode referred to as "tracking" is useful. The tracking mode operates by the abbreviation of the interval by 6.4 ms as described above. A difficulty with this approach is the assumption that the change in duration of the stimulus-T interval is linear between the lower and the upper rate limit. The interval is not linear, and the algorithm that determines the change in rate as a function of the change in stimulus-T interval has been reworked to avoid the presumption of linearity, and to provide a dynamic change in slope so that the response as a change in rate is different at different ventricular rates. Other difficulties with this device have been the absence of response in some patients who, for reasons as yet unclear, do not develop the same degree of abbreviation of the QT interval either during exercise or during emotion as is anticipated. Some investigations have suggested that the duration of the stimulus-T interval is independently influenced by changes in sympathetic tone as well as heart rate and that in some patients, these influences may be in opposing directions. The stimulus-T interval is also affected by drugs such as beta-blockers, which will then modify the exercise response.

Another approach is based on the concept of the "ventricular gradient." If the endocardial electrogram voltages are integrated over a cardiac cycle, electrophysiological dispersion may be determined. Such dispersion may be measured via a right ventricular pacing electrode. This measurement, as the measurement of stimulus-T duration, depends on instantaneous recovery from post stimulus polarization. The area of the post stimulus ventricular depolarization gradient depends on the activity status of the myocardium. At implant, the desirable gradient is set at a specific level of rest or activity and the pacemaker attempts to adjust the cardiac rate to retain the "normal" depolarization gradient area. The cardiac rate is thus adjusted with need. Both this technique and the stimulus-T measure the cardiac evoked potential and as such, can determine whether a depolarization occurs after a stimulus. It is possible to increase stimulus energy if no depolarization follows a stimulus and consequently, a technique of automatic threshold determination to provide safety by automatic increase in output as necessary.

Body Temperature

In 1951 Bazett, who in 1920 described variation in duration of ventricular systole (QT interval) as a function of activity, described a change in central body temperature as a result of the metabolism resulting from increased muscular activity. Skeletal muscular contraction is about 20% efficient; that energy not expended in actual movement is converted into heat, which increases the local blood temperature. With maximum activity it is possible to increase central venous temperature from 37°C (98.6°F) to 38.5°C (101.3°F). A thermister in the central venous system, i.e., the right ventricle, can detect the change and increase the ventricular rate in response. The measurement of central venous temperature is thus a sensitive and reliable indicator of the metabolic state. Nevertheless, deficiencies exist. The increase in temperature is not linear with activity; and interrupted activity must be carefully assessed. In the absence of a linear relationship between temperature and cardiac rate, each algorithm defines activity as a deviation in temperature from the immediately preceding level. Brief activity will result in a temperature and cardiac rate change. If the subject rests briefly and then resumes activity, the calculation of the temperature change begins at the new, and higher temperature level, which resulted from the first activity. The repeat activity may then raise the temperature proportionately less. Careful preparation of the algorithm to which this data is provided is therefore required (Figure 13).

The algorithm must account for multiple factors. These include a slow temperature rise because of two characteristics. The first is that an increase in central venous temperature is a relatively slow response to activity. Brief activity, such as a sprint to catch a bus may not produce a sufficient temperature change to increase the cardiac rate or, if it does, may have ended before the central temperature has risen, so that the physiological tachycardia will occur after the end of the activity. Another difficulty is the response to fever. While tachycardia normally is associated with hyperthermia, the device is unable to distinguish between a physiological increase in body temperature and an imposed hyperthermia and so, after a variable interval following the increase in temperature, rate will return to the lower setting, in effect disregarding the fever. Some modest changes in core temperature result from the ingestion of very warm or very cold foods. These too, can inappropriately affect the pacemaker perception of body temperature

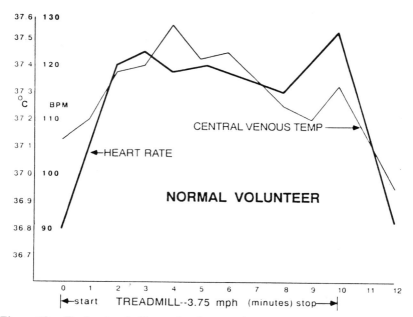

Figure 13. *During treadmill exercise the central venous temperature, measured by a thermistor in the right ventricle, correlates well with the cardiac rate in a normal volunteer. This correlation allows the change in temperature to be used as an indicator of physiologic need.*

and the cardiac rate. The biggest problem may be the difficulty in set-ting the device perception of the resting body temperature so that the baseline from which rate increases are calculated is properly leveled.

Still another problem is that of the site of the development of heat. The major site is the muscular mass of the lower extremities. With the onset of activity, local blood is warmed and muscular move-ment propels the blood toward the central system. The initial blood arriving in the heart is at a lower temperature than the blood already there as blood from the extremities is normally cooler than central blood. The initial flush of blood, therefore, reduces the temperature and may falsely slow the cardiac rate when an increase is required. The algorithm must be sensitive to this change and must be able to correct the rate should the flush of cool blood not be followed by warmer blood. A comnon resolution for the problem is an increase in pacemaker rate to result from the temperature reduction, with a con-tinued increase from the subsequent warm blood or a return to the lower rate if warm blood does not follow (Figure 14).

Still, with these difficulties, implantable temperature regulated single-chamber pacemakers have provided useful service and are now available for general use.

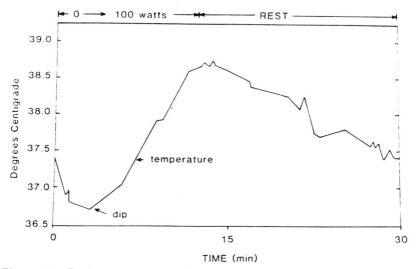

Figure 14. *During measurement of central venous temperature the first flush of returning blood after the beginning of lower extremity activity is relatively cool, producing the centrally measured temperature dip. Warm blood follows, in this in-stance, producing a temperature increase of over 1.5°C. This response is sufficient to drive a rate modulated pacemaker. Rest allows core temperature to decline.*

Respiration

The linkage of respiration and heart rate is conceptually relatively recent. An almost linear relationship exists between minute ventilation and cardiac rate during exercise. While there is individual variation from person to person, the correlation is close. Two factors that require measurement are the respiratory rate and the tidal volume. These can be measured in one of two ways, both of which are now in clinical evaluation. The basis for this variety of measurement is that oxygen consumption may be the single most physiological determinant of metabolic need. One technique of determining the respiratory rate is by impedance variations between the pacemaker case and a second lead implanted subcutaneously in the chest wall. The interelectrode impedance can be measured by placing current impulses between the electrode tip and the pulse generator. By maintaining a pulse repetition rate (125 ms per cycle) and a brief pulse duration and low intensity, no adjacent muscle stimulation occurs, and the current consumption from the pulse generator battery is sufficiently small so that there will be little effect on device longevity (Figure 15).

An alternative approach calculates minute ventilation by impedance measurements made between a bipolar pacemaker lead and the pulse generator case. As above, short duration, low amplitude constant current pulses one-tenth to one-hundredth of the level required either to stimulate the heart or to produce ventricular arrhythmias are delivered through the ring electrode and detected by the tip. The impedance of the system increases during inhalation and decreases during exhalation. The amplitude of these impedance changes is proportional to the tidal volume. Calculation of minute ventilation can readily be made as it is the product of frequency of respiration (breaths per minute) and tidal volume. Repetitive minute ventilation calculations continually update a timing mechanism which establishes the cardiac pacing rate. This respiratory pacemaker changes the cardiac stimulation rate in response both to the rate of respiration and to the tidal volume, both of which make up minute ventilation, a value that has been demonstrated to correlate well with exercise. Upper and lower rate limits for the cardiac rate are established and are independent of the respiratory rate. Respirations greater than 60 breaths per minute will not increase the cardiac pacemaker rate but will trigger a return toward the lower rate limit. A lower rate limit is established as well. The constant current pulses can be detected by the conventional sensing circuit of the pulse generator, and reduction of sensitivity may be required to allow unimpeded pacing (Figure 16).

RESPIRATORY SENSING PACEMAKER

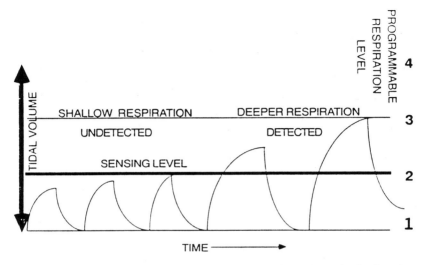

Figure 15. In the respiratory sensing pacemaker, which measures the depth and rate of respiration with a lead in the subcutaneous tissue, a sensing level and a resting cardiac rate are programmed. Should depth of respiration exceed the sensing level, stimulation rate increases. If the depth of respiration is adequate to be sensed and the rate increases, the cardiac rate increases further.

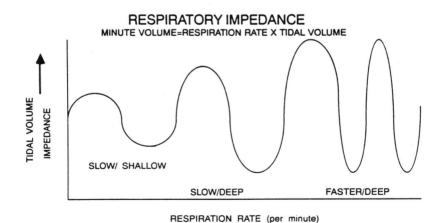

Figure 16. The sensor of intrathoracic impedance to determine minute ventilation senses the depth and rapidity of respiration by changes in impendace. Increase in respiratory rate and/or depth produce increases in the cardiac paced rate.

Pre-Ejection Interval

The interval between the beginning of electrical and mechanical systole in either the right or left ventricle has been referred to as the pre-ejection period or interval. This interval is mediated by autonomic influences, which normally increase cardiac rate, and the force and speed of contraction with metabolic need. The pre-ejection interval should then shorten with each of these stresses. This is, of course, a wholly physiological combination of events and varies with change in

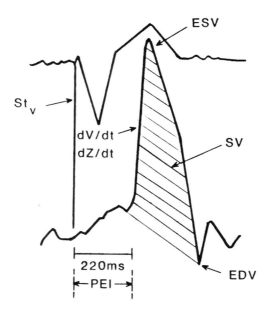

Figure 17. *The measurement of myocardial mechanics following a pacemaker stimulus (ST$_v$) allows determination of the interval between the stimulus and beginning of the ventricular response. The pre-ejection interval (PEI), and the rate of development of the myocardial contraction, i.e., the dV/dt of the upstroke velocity and the impedance of the system, dZ/dt, all change with contractility, which in turn changes with exercise. This system allows calculation of end-systolic volume (ESV), and end-diastolic volume (EDV), and stroke volume (SV), all of which also change with physiological need.*

metabolic state. Active exercise involving movement or isometric exercise such as hand grip, emotion and increase in circulating cathecolamines and sympathetic tone all abbreviate the pre-ejection interval to a degree well-correlated with atrial rate. In practice, the potentially measured pre-ejection interval during cardiac pacing will be between the ventricular pacemaker stimulus and the beginning of ventricular systole. The interval will be very different measured from the intrinsic deflection of a spontaneous beat to the beginning of mechanical systole.

It remains important to correlate the pre-ejection interval of the right ventricle (which is measured by a pacemaker lead) with that of the left ventricle, and to determine whether responsiveness, degree of response and its variation in duration are similar to that of the better known left ventricle. Presumably, measurement of electrical (depolarization) and mechanical events can be accomplished by a specialized right ventricular electrode. This parameter is better recorded during complete heart block, without spontaneous ventricular activity, as are other evoked potential measurements. To determine the appropriate cardiac rate when the spontaneous rate is more rapid than the lower rate limit, episodic cardiac stimulation will be required (Figure 17). Atrial pacing alone will probably not be possible, though for a dual-chamber mode, the atrial rate may be driven by the ventricular response.

pH

The initial effort at use of a sensor other than the atrium was that of Cammilli in 1977 in which he demonstrated that the pH of the mixed venous blood decreased (became more acidotic) during activity. This effect is mediated by the production of lactic acid during anaerobic metabolism. pH decreased by as much as 0.06 during activity. The pacemaker rate was correlated with pH, to increase with reduction in pH, and return to normal as pH rose.

The measurement of pH was by iridium/iridium oxide electrode positioned in the right atrium, upon the pacemaker lead and a reference electrode of silver/silver chloride on the pacemaker case. The system was not sufficiently stable to function permanently so that despite a satisfactory initial response it soon became unresponsive (Figure 18).

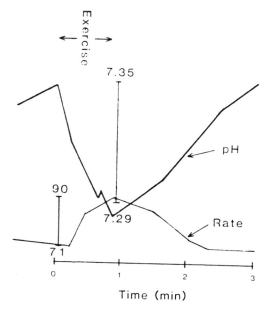

Redrawn from Cammilll,et al: PACE 1978:1:448-457

Figure 18. Measurement of blood pH beginning with rest, continuing for one minute, then returning to rest is demonstrated graphically. The resting pH is 7.35. With the onset of activity it descends to 7.29 and the pacemaker rate increases from 72 bpm to 90 bpm. With rest, pH rises and rate decreases.

Oxygen Saturation

During rest some 27% of oxyhemoglobin is reduced to hemoglobin with loss of oxygen to cells. During maximum activity some 80% of oxygen may be lost. Normal arterial oxygen saturation approximates 95–98%, and normal mixed venous oxygen approximates 75% while breathing ordinary air. A drop of one-third in mixed venous oxygen saturation to about 50% at maximum activity can occur. This can be measured with an optical oximeter and correlated with pacemaker rate (Figure 19).

Stroke Volume

The autonomic and humoral effects of exercise (as noted above) increase the cardiac rate and the force and speed of ventricular contraction. Because of increased contractile force and increased ven-

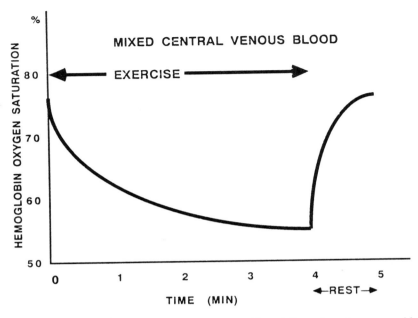

Figure 19. *Venous oxygen saturation declines with activity and can be measured by an intravascular oximeter on a pacemaker lead. During vigorous exercise central oxygen saturation may decline to 40–60%, a level which can be detected and used to set the stimulation rate.*

tricular filling resulting from increases in venous return, the Frank-Starling law mandates an increase in stroke volume. Variation in intracardiac impedance result from changes in stroke volume. Impedance can be measured through high frequency impulses well below stimulation threshold between two electrodes in the right ventricle and placed on the pacing electrode. Right ventricular impedance is higher during contraction as the blood being ejected has a higher resistivity than the blood arriving in the ventricle.

RATE MODULATED PACEMAKER LONGEVITY

The sensors for rate modulation can be defined in many ways, one of which is the current drain required to operate the sensor. These drains must be considered in the context of the actual operation of the sensor device. In actual practice, some of the sensors will draw less (or more) current than might be considered the theoretic drain.

In the non-rate modulated mode pacing is at a single rate and

pulse generator operation is entirely conventional with programmability in rate, output, sensitivity and possibly other functions. Only
the drain for sensing cardiac function, and the logic and output circuits exists. Each sensor requires some current drain; some drain
little, others much more. If the pulse generator is kept out of the
rate modulation mode much of the time its longevity may be the same
as that of other similar models. If the sensor is active, longevity will
decrease because of:

1. The increase in average rate of stimulation;
2. The operation of the sensor and the logic microprocessor.

The piezo electric sensors, as used in activity sensing pacemakers, drain little. The drain for sensing electrocardiographical changes,
such as that for the stimulus to T sensor, is also, relatively small. A
change in stimulation rate drains relatively little. The circuit for sensing the output of the special sensor should be equivalent in drain to
the atrial sensing circuit in a modern dual-chamber pacemaker, i.e.,
usually efficient but not always so. The drain for a special sensor for
impedance measurements, as used in measurement of respiratory
rate by impedance or the measurement of cardiac mechanics, consumes more energy. The longevity of a single-chamber pacemaker
with a piezo-electric sensor is likely to be similar to the longevity of a
dual-chamber pacemaker operating in the VDD mode from the same
manufacturer. The longevity of an impedance sensor single-chamber
device is likely to be substantially reduced compared to that in the
non-rate modulated mode. Other sensors are likely to fall between
the two limits (Figure 20).

LEAD SYSTEMS FOR RATE MODULATED PACING

Leads used with rate modulated pacemakers are either specialized or generally suitable for any pacing system. The difference is
based on whether the sensor for rate modulation is within the pulse
generator and whether the sensor is based on electrocardiographical
data.

Conventional Unipolar and Bipolar Leads

Piezo-electric sensors (activity) are within the pulse generator,
which may be either unipolar or bipolar and may be used with any
lead that can be physically connected. The electrocardiographical sen-

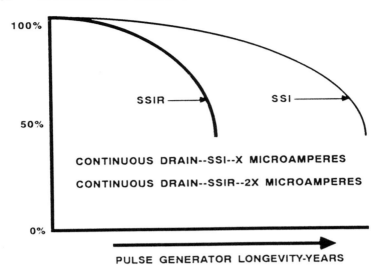

RATE MODULATED PULSE GENERATOR
LONGEVITY

Figure 20.   *Some sensors require no battery drain for their operation, the only drain is for the logic system to handle the data received, much as in a dual-chamber pacemaker. This graph demonstrates the relative longevities of the same pulse generator in the rate modulated mode (SSIR) with a sensor that requires relatively large amounts of current drain for its operation and with the sensor OFF (SSI). Differential longevities are based on the continuous battery drain for sensor operation.*

sor of stimulus to T requires a relatively normal to low impedance (by modern standards) unipolar lead. Some older unipolar leads were of very high impedance and attenuated the electrogram sufficiently so that satisfactory stimulus to T interval measurement could not be achieved.

Bipolar Leads

Impedance measurements must be made between two intracardiac electrodes. Consequently, thoracic impedance sensors require a bipolar lead as does the sensor of the evoked ventricular response. The lead may be a wholly conventional bipolar lead, but a unipolar lead is not suitable.

Specialized Leads

All of the other sensors that require an intravascular measurement also require a specialized lead. Measurement of intracardiac mechanics, temperature sensing with a thermister, oxygen tension and pH sensing all use an intravascular transducer and, therefore, need a specialized lead.

The major issue involved in the different leads to be used with different sensors is the possibility of pulse generator interchangeability at the time of pulse generator replacement. In the recent past, virtually all lead and pulse generator systems have been interchangeable. New connectors (e.g., VS-1) have caused some difficulty with adapters, but aside from that, virtually any pulse generator could be, somehow, connected to any lead. Obviously this will no longer be the case. Many patients now require pulse generator replacement after years of device service. Those sensors that are compatible with older leads can be used to upgrade to a rate modulated system. Pulse generators with sensors requiring a special lead will therefore be unsuitable or, alternatively, will require abandonment of an otherwise functional lead and placement of a new lead system.

SENSOR DRIVEN IDIOSYNCRACIES

Problems can exist with the operation of the various sensors and their delivery of reliable signals to the pulse generator. The idiosyncracy may be physiological or relate to the oversensing of some kinds of activity, the undersensing of others, and the lack of linearity in still others. For example, the stimulus to T sensor is quite nonlinear with the reduction of interval duration relatively large at the beginning of effort and much less so later as effort continues. The algorithm must be adjusted to accommodate differing intervals at different times of effort. Further, the stimulus to T interval seems to lose its flexibility with increasing patient age so that just when normal body mechanisms have lost their responsiveness so also may the stimulus to T interval.

The respiratory sensor using an accessory lead is quite sensitive to arm motion on the side of the pulse generator and such movement, in the absence of an increase in respiratory rate, will increase the stimulation rate. The respiratory sensor based on intracardiac impedance measurement is readily affected by speaking and respiratory rate so that a more appropriate rate response occurs with an increase in respiratory rate while silent than occurs when speaking. During speech the pacemaker rate will be slower and irregular. The temperature sensing pacemakers begin with a fall in central venous temperature and are slow to respond. Brief activity may be over before the cardiac rate increases. The activity, i.e., piezo-electric sensors, respond to what has been called the "heel strike" rate. In a simple way the "heel strike" rate, and consequently the pacemaker rate, is higher walking down steps than walking up steps though the effort expended is substantially greater. Bicycle riding, a vigorous activity, produces a modest sensor response. Direct pressure on the case of the piezo-electric sensor pulse generator will increase its rate as will gently tapping the case. Such tapping will drive the rate rapidly and promptly.

Electromyographic interference (EMI) also, can affect rate modulated pacemaker function. Despite the operation of the rate modulation sensor, output inhibition of unipolar systems can occur so that the sensor rate may increase, but actual output may cease or the device may revert to the noise mode. Some devices are more sensitive to such effects than others and relate to the effectiveness of conventional interference rejection rather than the operation of the sensor.

ASSESSMENT OF PACEMAKER PROGRAMMING AND EXERCISE RESPONSE

All dual- and single-chamber rate modulated pacemakers can be operated in the modulation insensitive mode. The single-chamber units can be programmed to SSI, and the dual to DDD and even lesser modes. The single-chamber inhibited (VVI) mode of operation is especially useful when a patient is deemed to have, for example, early AV block, requires a pacemaker to guard against episodic asystole, but does not yet require continual pacing. Later, when fixed block occurs and continuous pacing is required, the rate modulated mode can be activated.

Programming the implanted rate modulated device when it is in the modulation insensitive mode is identical to conventional multi-programmable pulse generators of single- or dual-chamber mode. In the rate modulated mode, output and conventional sensitivity to cardiac function is set as in the insensitive mode; but in addition, rate modulation settings are now required. Each device has settings specific to its own technology, but in general, there are four categories of setting.

1. The sensitivity of the sensor to the physiological (or non-physiological) event, which is to set the rate;
2. The responsiveness of the sensor to physiological change;
3. The rate at which the cardiac rate will be increased by the sensor response;

4. The maximum and minimum rates that are to be achieved, one at rest and the other with maximum activity.

Each device is delivered with a default setting for the rate modulated mode, i. e., one which is deemed to be safe and effective in producing modulation during exercise. It is frequently unclear how programming should be accomplished and what parameters should be sought. In setting a single-chamber pacemaker an escape rate is set, usually a conventional rate of 60–70 bpm, and no upper rate is required. In the patient capable of atrial synchronous pacing the atrium sets the rate. The lower rate may be set to allow atrial sensing at all times i.e., at a rate of 40–50 bpm. Atrial sensitivity and refractoriness are then set so that the pacemaker will respond to each P wave in a 1:1 fashion until a specific upper rate is achieved, commonly between 100 and 175 bpm. Then a mechanism of upper rate limitation is established (discussed elsewhere). The fact of atrial synchrony sets the responsiveness of the pulse generator in stimulating the ventricle (and sometimes the atrium). It is immediately apparent whether atrial synchrony is occurring and how the pacemaker is responding, even at absolute rest during a programming sequence. For the rate modulated device, the setting of the lower rate limit is about the same as for a single- or dual-chamber unit. Responsiveness and upper rate are different matters. A careful determination must be made in three ways:

1. That the device is neither too responsive nor underresponsive. Proper response mimics the responsiveness of the normal SA node. While it may be found that a different level or response is superior to that of the normal SA node, no such evidence now exists.
2. The device may surely be underresponsive. At the usual default settings the increase in cardiac rate with modest and even severe exercise may be very blunted and be unrelated to the atrial response (Figure 21).
3. That determination can only be made by some controlled challenge or formal exercise test protocol. Often the patient with the rate modulated pacemaker will not be able to use the upper rate that is programmable, and a lesser maximum rate will be required. All of this can be ascertained by stress evaluation and the pacemaker response. The stress should be carefully selected to mimic reasonably normal activity. Those stress tests that evaluate the presence and severity of coronary artery disease may be excessively strenuous for the setting of sensor sensitivity and responsiveness and, further, may not even give a result compatible with patient needs. As the activity sensor is by far the most widely used at present, and that situation is likely to be so for a very prolonged period, the quirks of that sensor should be considered. A formal stress test is labor intensive and is likely not to be used at all while an evaluation, which can be easily accomplished may, as a practical matter, provide significantly greater information.

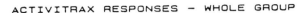

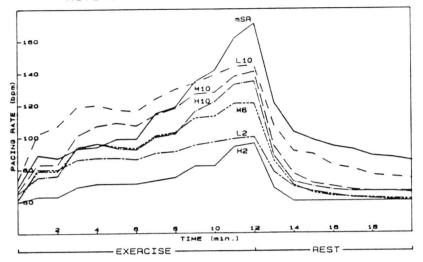

Figure 21. *The responsiveness of an activity sensing rate modulated system at various levels of SENSITIVITY AND RESPONSIVENESS is compared to the mean sinus rate (mSR) under similar test conditions. The pacemaker lower rate limit was set to 60 per minute, the upper rate limit to 150 per minute. The least RESPONSIVE AND SENSITIVE setting (H2) produces barely a response. The most (L10) produced an earlier and greater response than the atrium. Return to the lower rate limit with rest approximates the atrium. Even at maximum RESPONSIVENESS the pacemaker rate does not reach the atrial rate or the upper rate limit.*

EXERCISE TESTING AFTER PACEMAKER IMPLANT

During evaluation of the settings of a rate modulated pacemaker the lower limit of the modulation response is determined. In general, an attempt to mimic the sinus rate should be made. If the atrium is in a persistent arrhythmia such as atrial fibrillation, flutter, supraventricular tachycardia, or if AV block has been accomplished by interruption of the AV conduction system, the atrial rate cannot be a satisfactory guide to the ventricular rate and an assessment will be required of the lower rate, upper rate, and the rate of increase.

1. The pacemaker is programmed to the settings to be tested;
2. The pacemaker rate is determined with the patient at rest. Fifteen minutes of supine, sitting or standing rest are adequate to establish the lower sensor rate
3. An exercise protocol is followed and the pacemaker response is recorded on the ECG. In some pacemakers a histogram of rates achieved can be read directly from the device (Figure 22). In a patient

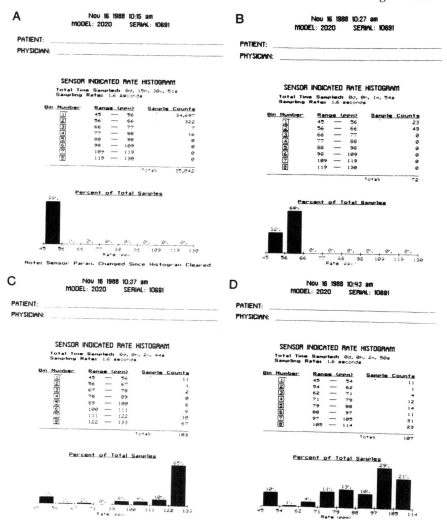

Figure 22. *A rate histogram is available in several pulse generators and is useful in programming the best level of sensitivity and responsiveness.* **A.** *In a patient with chronotropic incompetence, a fifteen hour recording shows that the pacemaker rate has not varied from a range of 45–56 when the lower rate setting had been at 50 bpm.* **B.** *During walking evaluation, with programming to modest sensitivity and responsiveness, and with recordings made for several minutes only a slight increase in responsiveness occurs, this time largely to 56–66 bpm.* **C.** *With the pacemaker programmed to be much more sensitive and responsive, similar activity produces an excessive response near the programmed maximum.* **D.** *A more moderate programmed setting produces a response across the range of possible rates.*

with a temporary pacemaker in place, especially if in sinus rhythm at the time of test, an activity sensitive pacemaker can be strapped to the chest and its response determined prior to implant. Sensors depend on measurement of some body function, i. e., temperature, stroke volume, etc., and cannot be tested in this way.

4. Care must be taken with activity sensing pacemakers to remember that cardiac demand and activity are independent, and that the activity sensing pacemaker responds to activity rather than to workload. Consequently, responsiveness may be greater to lesser activity, and tempered with greater workload requirements. The protocol selected may influence apparent pacemaker responsiveness.

5. Different exercise protocols exist. Most are based on the traditional Bruce and Naughton protocols, but as these are based on testing for coronary artery disease and not for setting of pacemaker responsiveness, they may be less useful (Table II).

As in all protocols, the patient is continuously monitored by ECG and with attendance by a knowledgeable technician. The goal is the establishment of a pacemaker rate similar to the spontaneous atrial rate or of a known rate response. This protocol can be compared to a widely used CAEP protocol developed by Wilkoff, Harvey, and Blackburn, and to the Bruce Protocol (Table III).

Still, alternative approaches can be used without a treadmill but still requiring an ECG, Holter monitor or telemetry ECG. Satisfactory setting can be made using a level walking protocol and a stairwell protocol. (Ferroconcrete building stairwells are reasonably standardized worldwide). Effort is controlled by time restraint using an electronic metronome, which the patient wears.

Level Walk Testing

Slow walk—two minutes.   Each metronome beat is one step. Rates of 55–72 steps per minute are comfortable for most patients on a

Table II

Stage	Speed (mph)	Grade (%)	Duration (mins)	Approx. Workload (METS)
Rest	Lying	Supine	1	0
I	1	0	2	1.9
II	2	0	2	2.6
III	2	3.5	2	3.4
IV	3	5.5	2	5.0
V	4	5.5	2	8.0
VI	5	5.5	2	12.0
Rest	Sitting		8	0

Table III
Comparison of Treadmill Exercise Protocols

TIME	MMC McAlister Soberman Furman (modified Naughton) Speed/Grade/Mets (mph)/ (%)	CAEP Wilkoff Harvey Blackburn Speed/Grade/Mets (mph)/ (%)	Bruce Speed/Grade/Mets (mph)/ (%)
1 2	STAGE 1 1.0 / 0 / 1.9	STAGE 1 1.0 / 2 / 2.0	STAGE 1 1.7 / 10 / 5
3 4	STAGE 2 2.0 / 0 / 2.6	STAGE 2 1.5 / 3 / 2.8	STAGE 2 2.5 / 12 / 7
5 6	STAGE 3 2.0 / 3.5 / 3.4	STAGE 3 2.0 / 4 / 3.6	
7 8	STAGE 4 3.0 / 5.5 / 5.0	STAGE 4 2.5 / 5 / 4.6	STAGE 3 3.4 / 14 / 9.5
9 10	STAGE 5 4.0 / 5.5 / 8.0	STAGE 5 3.0 / 6 / 5.8	STAGE 4 4.2 / 16 / 13
11 12	STAGE 6 5.0 / 5.5 / 12.0	STAGE 6 3.5 / 8 / 7.5	
13 14		STAGE 7 4.0 / 10 / 9.6	STAGE 5 5.0 / 18 / 16
15 16		STAGE 8 5.0 / 10 / 12.1	
17 18		STAGE 9 6.0 / 10 / 14.3	
19 20		STAGE 10 7.0 / 10 / 16.5	
21		STAGE 11 7.0 / 15 / 19.0	

straight level course such as a hospital corridor. Walk is in one direction for one minute and then the reverse for another.

Rapid walk—two minutes.   As above, but the metronome is set for 100–120 steps per minute.

Stairway Response

Once again, the metronome sets the rate for the "standardized" stairwell. Three rates can be used, approximating 30 steps per minute as the slow rate, 60 steps as the moderate rate, and 90 steps per minute as the rapid rate. Record the ascending rates and the descending rates (Figure 23).

TOTAL WORK = VERTICAL WORK + HORIZONTAL WORK

The workload descending is about one-third of that ascending the staircase (Figure 24) (Table IV).

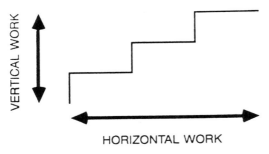

CALCULATION OF WORKLOAD
STAIRWELL PROTOCOL

VERTICAL WORK-ASCENT
VO_2 (ml/kg·min) = height(m/lift) x rate(lifts/min) x 1.8 ml/kg
DESCENT = ONE THIRD ASCENT

SOBERMAN ET AL-1988

Figure 23.   A staircase is an especially good place to test rate modulation. The two means of stress, ascending and descending, are identical except that the work of ascending is three times that of descending. Regulation of the degree and variety of stress can further be modified by changing the rate of ascent and descent and whether that rate is equal, ascending and descending.

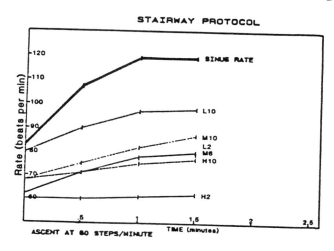

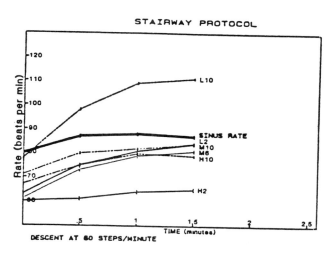

Figure 24. *These graphs represent a comparison of activity response to staircase ascent and descent. A paradoxical response is produced because of variation in "heel strike" vigor even when the rate of ascent and descent is controlled, in this instance at 60 steps/minute. The activity sensing rate modulated unit was strapped to the chest of a person with a normal cardiovascular system and programmed through six settings. The pacemaker lower rate limit was set a 60 bpm, the upper rate limit at 150 bpm. The sinus rate and the pacemaker stimulus rate were read from the ECG. **ASCENT:** The sinus rate reaches 120 bpm one minute after onset. Even maximum pacemaker sensitivity and responsiveness (L10) only produces a rate of 95 bpm. Three conventional settings are well below the sinus node in rate response. **DESCENT:** The sinus rate reaches 85 bpm at about 1 minute after onset of exercise and then declines slightly. Three conventionally programmed settings follow the sinus rate as well.*

Table IV
Maximum Workloads Achieved
(Approximate)

Ascent		Descent	
Rate (Steps/min)	Workload (METS*)	Rate (Steps/min)	(Workload) (METS*)
30	3.5	30	2.0
60	6.5	60	3.0
90	9.0	90	4.0

*MET = 3.5 ml/kg.min

ELECTROCARDIOGRAPHY OF RATE MODULATED PACEMAKERS

Single-Chamber

Electrocardiography is relatively simple. As in any electrocardiographical interpretation, it must be remembered that the interval between one stimulus and the next varies, and that the stimulation rate is a result of these individual variations. A smooth rate of acceleration or deceleration with continuous pacing provides a small variation from one stimulus to the next (Figure 25). If the sensor modifies its rate but spontaneous events occur simultaneously and inhibit and recycle pacemaker output, then the interval between a sensed spontaneous event and the next pacemaker stimulus will vary depending on the sensor imposed escape interval. Interpretation of the ECG should consider the absence of a fixed pacemaker stimulus escape interval during sensor operation (Figures 26, 27, 28).

While the action of some sensors is electrocardiographically invisible except for changes in the escape interval, others produce an ECG mark. The two respiratory impedance sensor pacemaker models continually emit rapid small amplitude stimuli, which can be seen readily on the ECG. These should be recognized as representing normal pacemaker function. In the absence of these stimuli, the pulse generator is in the "sensor off" mode and no modulation of rate or escape interval can be anticipated. In the presence of these stimuli, rate and escape interval modulation can be anticipated.

The stimulus to T wave sensor and the evoked potential sensor can only make a rate determination following a paced event. During pacemaker inhibition, i.e., with the sensor determining a rate that is

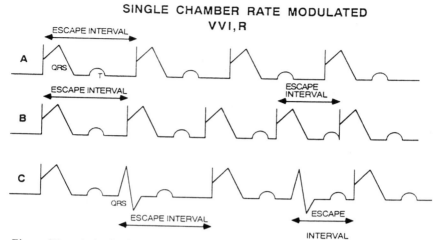

Figure 25. *A single-chamber rate modulated (SSI,R, VVI,R or AAI,R) unit differs from a single rate (SSI) unit as the escape (lower rate) interval can change because of the operation of the rate modulating sensor. In this diagram, a VVI,R, unit is illustrated. In (A) operation is at or near the lower rate interval with a prolonged escape interval. In (B) the sensor progressively abbreviates the escape interval between stimuli. In (C) the escape interval between spontaneous beats and the succeeding stimulus is also abbreviated.*

less than the spontaneous rate, the sensor "tests" the cardiac status, i.e., the stimulus to T wave interval or the area under the curve of the evoked potential, by determining the actual rate (i.e., spontaneous QRS coupling interval), and emitting stimuli at a briefer coupling interval, stimulating the ventricle and determining what the pacemaker rate should be. Two possibilities then exist. The appropriate rate will be determined to be less than the spontaneous rate, and the pacemaker will return to its inhibited state and soon emit three test stimuli again; or the appropriate rate will be determined to be more rapid than the spontaneous rate and pacing will continue. During continuous pacing each QRS interval will be evaluated to determine an increase or decrease in rate.

Stimulation threshold can be determined by those pacemakers which test the response evoked by the ventricular stimulus. The two such devices are the stimulus-T device and the evoked ventricular response device. Possibly other devices will have similar capabilities. In each instance, the measurement of a ventricular response to the pacemaker stimulus is part of sensor operation. In both instances, the

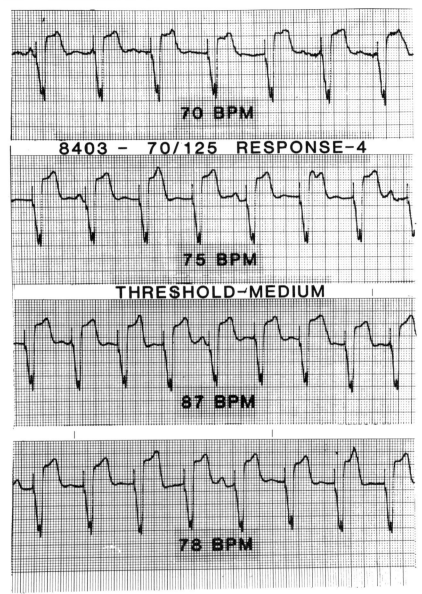

Figure 26. This elderly patient, with long standing complete heart block and normal atrial activity, underwent replacement of a single-rate single-chamber pacemaker by a single-chamber rate modulated unit. Despite relatively unresponsive settings, the rate increase of only 17 bpm with activity produced a dramatic improvement in exercise tolerance.

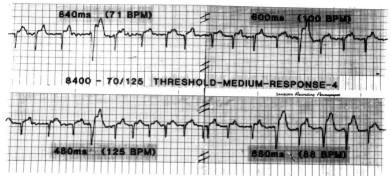

Figure 27. *In addition to changing the interval between pacemaker stimuli, the rate modulating sensor changes the escape interval between a spontaneous event and the next paced event. In this instance, during atrial fibrillation with episodically slow ventricular response, the change in escape interval results from sensor operation. The escape varies between 840 ms (71 bpm) and 480 ms (125 bpm) depending on the sensor's state of activity response.*

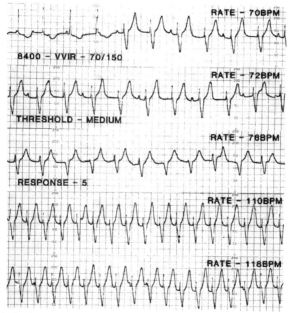

Figure 28. *A single-chamber rate modulated unit may be especially useful in a young patient with congenital heart block, allowing avoidance of an atrial lead. This five-year old who had had a syncopal episode had also been fixed in ventricular rate at about 70 bpm and had been markedly restricted in exercise tolerance. Following implantation of an activity responsive unit, even at modestly sensitive and responsive settings, she readily developed exercise rates as high as 118 bpm with marked improvement in exercise capacity.*

absence of a response, the T wave (Figure 29) in one and ventricular depolarization in the other, (Figure 30) is interpreted as an ineffective stimulus, and the pacemaker response can be an increase in stimulus amplitude.

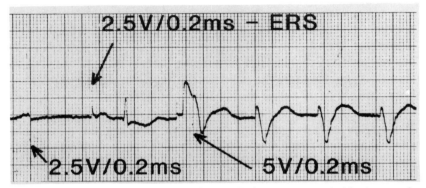

Figure 29. *Pacemakers which sense the ventricular response evoked by a pacemaker stimulus can determine whether one has, indeed, occurred. The first stimulus (left) is without ERS (evoked response sensing), and is below capture threshold. When ERS function is activited, the second stimulus, also without a ventricular response, is followed 170 ms later by a stimulus of double amplitude, i.e., from 2.5 Volts to 5.0 Volts and consequent ventricular capture.*

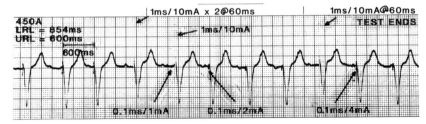

Figure 30. *A pacemaker that senses the ventricular evoked response can determine whether capture has occurred. This threshold tracking sequence begins with two pulses of 1 ms duration and 10 mA output separated by 60 ms, followed by a pulse of 0.1 ms duration and 1 mA amplitude, which does not capture and is followed 60 ms later by a rescue pulse of 1 ms/10mA. Next 0.1 ms/.2 mA is tested and does capture. The pacemaker output is then stabilized at 0.1 ms/4 mA. Capture is determined at each stimulus and threshold is actively determined twice daily. The margin of output above threshold is kept small to conserve energy.*

Dual-Chamber

As a single timing interval exists in a single-chamber pacemaker, several exist in a dual-chamber device. The lower rate limit is set by atrial and then ventricular pacing rate at rest. The AV delay is also set and can be of fixed or modulated duration (Figure 31). The fixed AV delay will be of the same duration at the lower rate limit, i.e., when both atrium and ventricle are being paced and the upper rate limit or the maximum atrial tracking limit. A modulated AV delay will be set to be abbreviated at higher rates whether sensor driven or spontaneous.

The upper rate limit, as determined by atrial tracking, is determined as in other DDD modes of operation (see Chapter 4) by the duration of atrial refractoriness. But, in the rate modulated (i.e., DDDR unit) a second and independent, i.e., sensor driven upper rate limit, can exist. There can, therefore, be three different upper rate limits (the first two exist in most conventional DDD models):

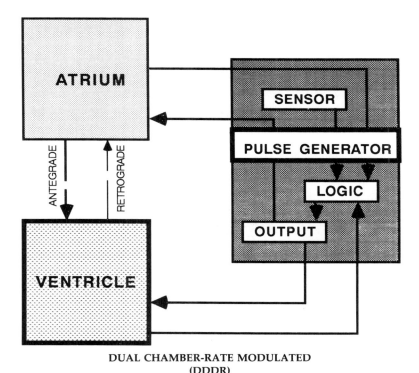

DUAL CHAMBER-RATE MODULATED
(DDDR)

Figure 31. *A diagrammatic representation of a dual-chamber rate modulated pacemaker shows inputs and outputs from atrium and ventricle. There are three signals which affect function of the logic system: that from the atrium, from the ventricle (both as in a conventional DDD pacemaker), and from the sensor. Each plays a role in setting the stimulation rate and, in some units, the rate-modulated AV interval.*

1. That determined by atrial refractoriness alone;
2. That set independently of atrial refractoriness, as in the conventional DDD pacemaker. It is always lower (i.e., at a longer R-R interval than that set by the duration of atrial refractoriness;

   Both of these exist in most conventional DDD models.

3. An upper rate limit based on the maximum sensor rate.

As in the conventional DDD mode, the atrial refractory determined upper rate limit and that independently programmed may be similar or not. Different upper rate mechanisms will result. In the DDDR all three upper rate limits may be the same, or all three may be different, resulting in markedly different pacemaker operation and ECG manifestation (Figure 32).

DUAL CHAMBER RATE MODULATED
DDD,R

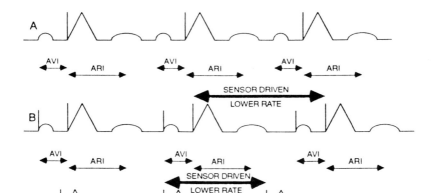

AVI=ATRIO-VENTRICULAR INTERVAL
ARI=ATRIAL REFRACTORY INTERVAL,
AFTER THE VENTRICULAR EVENT
(PVARP)

Figure 32. This is a diagrammatic representation of some of the operation of a DDDR pacemaker with AV interval modulation. For diagrammatic purposes the P wave is sensed at its beginning. The total atrial refractory interval is as usual, the sum of the AVI and ARI. The upper rate for atrial tracking is determined by atrial refractoriness. With the decrease in AV interval, total atrial refractoriness decreases and the upper tracking rate increases.

If all three are the same then, as the atrial rate rises, the atrium will be driven or sensed to drive the ventricle depending on which is at a shorter coupling interval.

If the independently set upper rate limit is lower than that based on atrial refractoriness, and the maximum sensor rate is equally low, then the upper rate will be manifested by conventional pseudo-Wenckebach operation. If the upper rate limit based on atrial refractoriness is lower than the maximum sensor driven rate, then P waves may fall into the atrial refractory period after the ventricular event and be unsensed. Each will be followed thereafter by an atrial channel stimulus that may be:

1. Competitive with the earlier unsensed P wave;
2. May produce a second P wave or a competitive atrial arrhythmia;
3. May fall into atrial refractoriness and be ineffective.

The electrocardiography of dual-chamber rate modulated pacemakers (see Chapter 9) can be extremely complex as the sensor setting, providing a third source of pacing interval setting (atrium, ventricle and sensor) within the device, changes the conventional rules of pacemaker ECG interpretation (Figure 33). A device may be so set that AV block or pseudo-Wenckebach operation occurs or does not

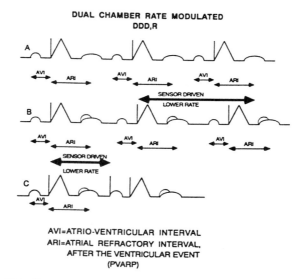

DUAL CHAMBER RATE MODULATED DDD,R

AVI=ATRIO-VENTRICULAR INTERVAL
ARI=ATRIAL REFRACTORY INTERVAL,
AFTER THE VENTRICULAR EVENT
(PVARP)

Figure 33. This diagram is a representation of the difference between a sensor driven upper rate and that based on response to atrial activity. As in the conventional DDD pacemaker the duration of total atrial refractoriness determines the upper rate of atrial tracking. But, as there is another determinant of upper rate in operation, the two may result in different upper rates. For example, in diagram B. the atrial rate and atrial refractoriness are such that the pacemaker is operating in the 2:1 AV block *(continued)*

Figure 33. (cont.)   *mode. As the sensor does not require a pacemaker rate more rapid, i.e., a ventricular coupling interval shorter than half the atrial rate, the pacemaker will stimulate the ventricle at half the atrial rate. In diagram C. the pacemaker is still operating in the 2:1 AV block mode based on atrial refractoriness. However, sensor operation now indicates a rate higher than, i.e., a coupling interval briefer than half the atrial rate. In this instance, despite the alternate blocked P waves, the atrium will be driven at a more rapid rate.*

occur at the upper rate limit. AV intervals that are set to be reduced in duration at increasing atrial and sensor rates may be both reduced and simultaneously prolonged as the upper rate limit is approached, and as Wenckebach operation is progressively invoked. Careful evaluation of each ECG, knowledge of operation of the device and of its specific settings is mandatory (Figure 34).

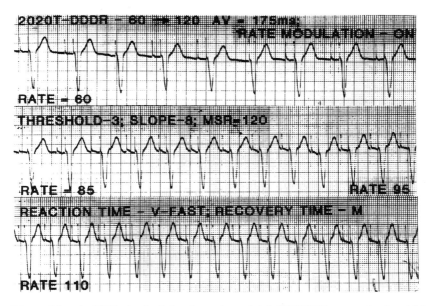

Figure 34.   *An ECG of a dual-chamber rate modulated (DDDR) pacemaker in which the atrium is less responsive than the sensor to activity shows, at rest, (upper line) atrium and ventricle are paced at a rate of 60 bpm (1,000 ms). The AV interval has been programmed to 175 ms, other rate and sensor functions (i.e., sensitivity and responsiveness) are shown. The rate increases progressively (middle line), and the AV interval is modulated and abbreviated with the increase in rate.*

Acknowledgment: Thanks should be given to the efforts of Drs. Hugh McAlister and Judith Soberman, whose work forms a partial basis for this text.

BIBLIOGRAPHY

Alicandria C. Fouad FM, Tarazi RC, Castle L, Morant V: Three cases of hypotension and syncope with ventricular pacing: Possible role of atrial reflexes. *Am J Cardiol* 1978; 42:137–142.

Alt E, Hirgstetter C, Heinz M, Blomer H: Rate control of physiologic pacemakers by central venous blood temperature. *Circulation* 1986; 73:1206–1212.

Alt E, Hirgstetter C, Heinz M, Theres H: Measurement of right ventricular blood temperature during exercise as a means of rate control in phsyiological pacemakers. *PACE* 1986; 9:970–977.

Alt E, Theres H, Heinz M, Matula M, Thilo R, Blomer H: A new rate-modulated pacemaker system optimized by combination of two sensors. *PACE* 1988; 11:1119–1129.

Anderson KM, Moore AA: Sensors in pacing. *PACE* 1986; 9:954–959.

Auerbach AA. Furman S: The autodiagnostic pacemaker. *PACE* 1979; 2:58–68.

Ausubel K, Furman S: The pacemaker syndrome. *Ann Int Med* 1985; 103:420–429.

Balke B, Ware R: An experimental study of physical fitness of Air Force personnel. *US Armed Forces Med J* 1959; 10:675–688.

Bazett HC: An analysis of the time relationship of electrocardiograms. *Heart* 1920; 7:353–370.

Bazett HC: Theory of reflex controls to explain regulation of body temperature at rest and during exercise. *J Appl Phys* 1951; 4:245–262.

Benditt DG, Mianulli M, Fetter J, et al: Single chamber cardiac pacing with activity-initiated chronotropic response: Evaluation by cardiopulmonary exercise testing. *Circulation* 1987; 75:184–189.

Benditt DG, Milstein S, Buetikofer J, Gornick CC, Mianulli M, Fetter J: Sensor-triggered, rate-variable cardiac pacing. Current technologies and clinical implications. *Ann Int Med* 1987; 107:714–724.

Bevegard S, Jonsson B, Karlof I, Lagergren H, Sowton E: Effect of changes in ventricular rate on cardiac output and central pressures at rest and during exercise in patients with artificial pacemakers. *Cardiovasc Res* 1967; 1:21–33.

Bruce RA, Kusumi F, Hosmer D: Maximal oxygen intake and nomographic assessment of functional aerobic impairment in cardiovascular disease. *Am Heart J* 1973; 85:546–562.

Brundin T: Temperature of mixed venous blood during exercise. *Scand J Clin Lab Invest* 1975; 35:539–543.

Cammilli L, Alcidi L, Papeschi G: A new pacemaker autoregulating the rate of pacing in relation to metabolic needs. In Y Watanabe (ed): Cardiac Pacing. Proc Vth Internatl Symposium, Amsterdam, *Excerpta Medica*, 1977; 414.

Cammilli L, Alcidi L, Papeschi G, Wiechmann V, Padeletti L, Grassi G: Preliminary experience with the pH-triggered pacemaker. *PACE* 1978; 1:448–457.

Chin C-F, Messenger JC, Greenberg PS, Ellestad MH: Chronotropic incompetence in exercise testing. *Clin Cardiol* 1979; 2:12–18.

Chirife R: Physiological principles of a new method for rate responsive pacing using the pre-ejection interval. *PACE* 1988; 11:1545–1554.

Chirife R, Spiodick DH: Densitography: A new method for evaluation of cardiac performance at rest and during exercise. *Am Heart J* 1972; 83:493–503.

Cohen TJ: A theoretical right atrial pressure feedback heart rate control system to restore physiologic control to the rate-limited heart. *PACE* 1984; 7:671–677.

den Dulk K, Bouwels L, Lindemans F, Rankin I, Brugada P, Wellens HJJ: The Activitrax rate responsive pacemaker system. *Am J Cardiol* 1988; 61:107–112.

Donaldson RM, Fox K, Richards AF: Initial experience with a physiological rate responsive pacemaker. *Br Med J* 1983; 286:667–671.

Donaldson RM, Rickards AF: Rate responsive pacing using the evoked QT principle. A physiological alternative to atrial synchronous pacemakers. *PACE* 1983; 6:1344–1349.

Donaldson RM, Rickards AF: The ventricular endocardial paced evoked response. *PACE* 1983; 6:253–259.

Economides AP, Walton C, Gergely S: The ventricular intracardiac unipolar paced-evoked potential in an isolated animal heart. *PACE* 1988; 11:203–213.

Ellestad MH, Allen W, Wan MCK, Kemp GL: Maximal treadmill stress testing for cardiovascular evaluation. *Circulation* 1969; 39:517–522.

Epstein SE, Beiser GD, Stampfer M, Robinson BF, Braunwald E: Characterization of the circulatory response to maximal upright exercise in normal subjects and patients with heart disease. *Circulation* 1967; 35:1049–1062.

Faerestrand S, Breivik K, Ohm O-J: Assessment of the work capacity and relationship between rate response and exercise tolerance associated with activity-sensing rate-responsive ventricular pacing. *PACE* 1987; 10:1277–1290.

Faerestrand S, Ohm OJ: A time-related study by Doppler and M-mode echocardiography of hemodynamics, heart size, and AV valvular function during activity-sensing rate-responsive ventricular pacing. *PACE* 1987; 10:507–518.

Fananapazir L, Bennett DH, Monks P: Atrial synchronized ventricular pacing: Contribution of the chronotropic response to improved exercise performance. *PACE* 1983; 6:601–608.

Fearnot NE, Jolgren DL, Nelson JP, et al: Increasing cardiac rate by measurement of right ventricular temperature. *PACE* 1984; 7:1240–1245.

Fearnot NE, Smith HJ, Geddes LA: A review of pacemakers that physiologically increase rate: The DDD and rate-responsive pacemakers. *Prog Cardiovasc Dis* 1986; 29(2):145–164.

French WJ, Haskell RJ, Wesley GW, Florio J: Physiological benefits of a pacemaker with dual chamber pacing at low heart rates and single chamber rate responsive pacing during exercise. *PACE* 1988; 11:1840–1845.

Gesell RA: Auricular systole and its relation to ventricular output. *Am J Phys* 1911; 29:32–63.

Gillette P: Critical analysis of sensors for physiological responsive pacing. *PACE* 1984; 7:1263–1266.

Goicolea de Oro A, Ayza MW, de la Llana R, Morales JA, Diez JRG, Alvarez JG: Rate-responsive pacing: Clinical experience. *PACE* 1985; 8:322–328.

Griffin JC, Jutzy KR, Claude JP, Knutti JW: Central body temperature as a guide to optimal heart rate. *PACE* 1983; 6:498–501.

Hanich RF, Midei MG, McElroy BP, Brinker JA: Circumvention of maximum tracking limitations with a rate modulated dual chamber pacemaker. *PACE* 1989; 12:392–397.

Hayes DL, Higano ST, Eisinger G: Electrocardiographic manifestations of a dual chamber, rate-modulated (DDDR) pacemaker. *PACE;* April 1989; 12:555–562.

Heiman DF, Helwig J: Suppression of ventricular arrhythmias by transvenous intracardiac pacing. *JAMA* 1966; 195:1150–1153.

Hermansen L, Ekblom B, Saltin B: Cardiac output during submaximal and maximal treadmill and bicycle exercise. *J Appl Physiol* 1973; 29:82.

Humen DP, Anderson K, Brumwell D, Huntley S, Klein GJ: A pacemaker which automatically increases its rate with physical activity. In: K Steinbach, et al. (eds): *Cardiac Pacing.* Darmstadt, Steinkopff Verlag, 1983, p 259–264.

Janicki JS, Weber KT: Equipment and protocols to evaluate the exercise response. In: KT Weber, JS Janicki (eds): *Cardiopulmonary Exercise Testing: Physiologic Principles and Clinical Applications.* Phila, WB Saunders, 1986, p 138–150.

Jolgren D, Fearnot N, Geddes L: A rate-responsive pacemaker controlled by right ventricular blood temperature. *PACE* 1984; 7:794–801.

Judge RD, Wilson WS, Siegel JH: Hemodynamic studies in patients with implanted cardiac pacemakers. *N Engl J Med* 1964; 270:1391–1395.

Kappenberger LJ, Herpers L: Rate responsive dual chamber pacing. *PACE* 1986; 9:987–991.

Karlof I: Haemodynamic effect of atrial triggered versus fixed rate pacing at rest and during exercise in complete heart block. *Acta Med Scand* 1975; 197:195–206.

Karlof I: Haemodynamic studies at rest and during exercises in patients treated with artificial pacemaker. *Acta Med Scand* 1975; 3:195–206.

Kristensson BE, Arnman K, Ryden L: The hemodynamic importance of atrioventricular synchrony and rate increase at rest and during exercise. *Eur Heart J* 1985; 6:773–778.

Kristensson BE, Arnman K, Smedgard P, Ryden L: Physiological versus single-rate ventricular pacing: A double-blind cross-over study. *PACE* 1985; 8:73–84.

Kruse I, Ryden L: Comparison of physical work capacity and systolic time intervals with ventricular inhibited and atrial synchronous ventricular inhibited pacing. *Br Heart J* 1981; 46:129–136.

Kruse I, Ryden L, Duffin E: Clinical evaluation of atrial synchronous ventricular inhibited pacemakers. *PACE* 1980; 3:641–650.

Laczkovics A: The central venous blood temperature as a guide for rate control in pacemaker therapy. *PACE* 1984; 7:822–830.

Lau CP, Antoniou A, Ward DE, Camm AJ: Initial clinical experience with a minute ventilation sensing rate modulated pacemaker: Improvements in exercise capacity and symptomatology. *PACE* 1988; 11:1815–1822.

Lau CP, Mehta D, Toff WD, Stott RJ, Ward DE, Camm AJ: Limitations of rate response of an activity-sensing rate-responsive pacemaker to different forms of activity. *PACE* 1988; 11:141–150.

Lau CP, Ritche D, Butrous GS, Ward DE, Camm AJ: Rate modulation by arm movements of the respiratory dependent rate responsive pacemaker. *PACE* 1988; 11:744–752.

Lau CP, Stott JRR, Toff WD, Zetlein MB, Ward DE, Camm AJ: Selective vibration sensing: A new concept for activity-sensing rate-responsive pacing. *PACE* 1988; 11:1299–1309.

Lau CP, Tse WS, Camm AJ: Clinical experience with Sensolog 703: A new activity sensing rate responsive pacemaker. *PACE* 1988; 11:1444–1455.

Lillehei CW, Varco RL, Ferlic RM, Sellers RD: Results of the first 2,500 patients undergoing open-heart surgery at the University of Minnesota Medical Center. *Surgery* 1967; 62:819–832.

Lindemans FW, Rankin IR, Murtaugh R, Chevalier PA: Clinical experience with an activity sensing pacemaker. *PACE* 1986; 9:978–986.

Maisch B, Langenfeld H: Rate adaptive pacing—Clinical experience with three different pacing systems. *PACE* 1986; 9:997–1004.

Maksud MG, Coutts KD, Hamilton LH: Time course of heart rate, ventilation and VO2 during laboratory and field exercise. *J Appl Physiol* 1971; 30:536–539.

McAlister HF, Soberman J, Klementowicz P, Andrews C, Furman S: Treadmill assessment of activity modulated pacemaker. *PACE*; 1989; 12:486–501.

McElroy PA, Janicki JS, Weber KT: Physiologic correlates of the heart rate response to upright isotonic exercise: Relevance to rate-responsive pacemakers. *JACC* 1988; 11:94–99.

Moura PJ, Gessman LJ, Lai T, Gallagher JD, White M, Morse DP: Chronotropic response of an activity detecting pacemaker compared with the normal sinus node. *PACE* 1987; 10:78–86.

Muller OF, Bellet S: Treatment of intractable heart failure in the presence of complete atrio-ventricular heart block by the use of internal cardiac pacemaker: Report of 2 cases. *N Engl J Med* 1961; 265:768–772.

Murtaugh RA, Rueter JC, Watson WS: *Activitrax clinical study report.* Minneapolis, Medtronic Inc, October 1986.

Nappholtz T, Valenta H, Maloney J, Simmons T: Electrode configurations for a respiratory impedance measurement suitable for rate responsive pacing. *PACE* 1986; 9:960–964.

Nordlander R, Hedman A, Pehrsson SK: Rate responsive pacing and exercise capacity. *PACE*; May 1989; 749–741.

Oetgen WJ, Tibbits PA, Abt MEO, Goldstein RE: Clinical and electrophysiologic assessment of oral flecainide acetate for recurrent ventricular tachycardia: Evidence for excerbation of electrical Instability. *Am J Cardiol* 1983; 52:746–750.

Patterson JA, Naughton J, Pietras RJ, Gunnar RM: Treadmill exercise in assessment of the functional capacity of patients with cardiac disease. *Am J Cardiol* 1972; 30:757–762.

Pehrsson SK: Influence of heart rate and atrioventricular synchronization on maximal work tolerance in patients treated with artificial pacemakers. *Acta Med Scand* 1983; 214:311–315.

Penton GB, Miller H, Levine SA: Some clinical features of complete heart block. *Circulation* 1956; 13:801–824.

Pinsky WW, Gillette PC, Garson A Jr, McNamara DG: Diagnosis, management, and long-term results of patients with congenital complete atrioventricular block. *Pediatrics* 1982; 69:728–733.

Rickards AF, Donaldson RM: Rate responsive pacing. *CPPE* 1983; 1:12–19.

Rickards AF, Norman J: Relation between QT interval and heart rate. New design of physiologically adaptive cardiac pacemaker. *Br Heart J* 1981; 45:56–61.

Ross J Jr, Linhart JW, Braunwald E: Effects of changing heart rate in man by electrical stimulation of the right atrium. Studies at rest, during exercise, and with isoproterenol. *Circulation* 1965; 32:549–558.

Rossi P: Rate-responsive pacing: Biosensor reliability and physiological sensitivity. *PACE* 1987; 10:454–466.

Rossi P, Aina F, Rognoni G, Occhetta E, Plicchi G, Prando MD: Increasing cardiac rate by tracking the respiratory rate. *PACE* 1984; 7:1246–1256.

Rossi P, Plicchi G, Canducci G, Rognoni G, Aina F: Respiration as a reliable physiological sensor for controlling cardiac pacing rate. *Br Heart J* 1984; 51:7–14.

Rossi P, Rognoni G, Occhetta E, et al: Respiration-dependent ventricular pacing compared with fixed ventricular and atrial-ventricular synchronous pacing: Aerobic and hemodynamic variables. *JACC* 1985; 6:646–652.

Ryden L: Atrial inhibited pacing—An underused mode of cardiac stimulation. *PACE* 1988; 11:1375–1379.

Salo RW, Pederson BD, Olive AL, Lincoln WC, Wallner TG: Continuous ventricular volume assessment for diagnosis and pacemaker control. *PACE* 1984; 7:1267–1272.

Samet P, Bernstein WH, Medow A, Nathan DA: Effect of alterations in ventricular rate upon cardiac output in complete heart block. *Am J Cardiol* 1964; 14:477–482.

Samet P, Castillo C, Bernstein WH: Hemodynamic consequences of sequential atrioventricular pacing. *Am J Cardiol* 1968; 21:207–212.

Sellers TD, Fearnot NE, Smith HJ, DiLorenzo DM, Knight JA, Schmaltz MJ: Right ventricular blood temperature profiles for rate responsive pacing. *PACE* 1987; 10:467–479.

Singer E, Gooch AS, Morse DP: Exercise induced arrhythmias in patients with pacemakers. *JAMA* 1973; 224:1515–1518.

Smedgard P, Kristensson B-E, Kruse I, Ryden L: Rate-responsive pacing by means of activity sensing vs single rate ventricular pacing: A double-blind cross-over study. *PACE* 1987; 10:902–915.

Stangl K, Wirtzfeld A, Heinze R, Laule M: First clinical experience with an oxygen saturation controlled pacemaker in man. *PACE* 1988; 11:1882–1887.

Stephenson SE Jr, Brockman SK: P wave synchrony. *Ann NY Acad Sci* 1964; 111:907–914.

Sugiura T, Kimura M, Mizushina S, Yoshimura K, Harada Y: Cardiac pacemaker regulated by respiratory rate and blood temperature. *PACE* 1988; 11:1077–1085.

Webb SC, Lewis LM, Morris-Thurgood JA, Palmer RG, Sanderson JE: Respiratory-dependent pacing: A dual response from a single sensor. *PACE* 1988; 111:730–735.

Weber KT, Kinasewitz GT, West JS, Janicki JS, Reichek N, Fishman AP: Long-term vasodilatory therapy with trimazosin in chronic cardiac failure. *N Engl J Med* 1980; 303:242–250.

Wiens RD, Lafia P, Marder CM, Evans RG, Kennedy HL: Chronotropic incompetence in clinical exercise testing. *Am J Cardiol* 1984; 54:74–78.

Wilson FN, Macleod AG, Barker PS, Johnston FD: The determination and the significance of the areas of the ventricular deflections of the electrocardiogram. *Am Heart J* 1934; 10:46–61.

Wilson JH, Lattner S: Apparent undersensing due to oversensing of low amplitude pulses in a thoracic impedance-sensing, rate-responsive pacemaker. *PACE* 1988; 11:1479–1481.

Wirtzfeld A, Heinze R, Stanzl K, Hoekstein K, Alt E, Liess HD: Regulation of pacing rate by variations of mixed venous oxygen saturation. *PACE* 1984; 7:1257–1262.

Zegelman M, Beyersdorf F, Kreuzer J, Cieslinski G: Rate responsive pacemakers: Assessment after two years. *PACE* 1986; 9:1005–1009.

Chapter 12

AUTOMATIC IMPLANTABLE CARDIOVERTER DEFIBRILLATOR

David R. Holmes, Jr.

INTRODUCTION

The introduction of the automatic implantable defibrillator, and subsequently the cardioverter/defibrillator has had a significant impact on the mortality and morbidity from recurrent ventricular tachycardia and fibrillation. The systems used have evolved rapidly since their introduction in 1980. This evolution has been mandated by clinical problems associated with the initial units, and facilitated by technological advances. Problems remain with unit size, longevity (which averages approximately 20 months), detection algorithms, and discrimination between pathological and physiological tachycardias. Improvements continue and incorporate better detection, low energy cardioversion, higher energy defibrillation, backup pacing, and easier implantation.

CURRENT SYSTEM

The only currently-approved device (Ventak CPI AICD) is rather large (11.2 x 7.11 x 2.54 cm), and heavy at 290 grams (Figure 1). It consists of a sensing device, batteries, and energy storage capacitor. The lithium power source has a projected life of approximately one to two years irrespective of whether shocks are given or not. The average is approximately 20 months (Figure 2). Once the device detects an arrhythmia (vide infra), a capacitor charging cycle is initiated, following which a truncated exponential pulse averaging 25 J is delivered. Higher output devices can be specially ordered that can deliver 40–45 J for patients with high defibrillation thresholds. Ten to 35 seconds elapse between arrhythmia detection and energy delivery. If the detected arrhythmia is ventricular tachycardia, the initial shock is synchronized to the R wave. If baseline rhythm is not restored, the sequence is repeated up to three additional times after recharging. These subsequent shocks deliver 10–15 J more energy than the initial

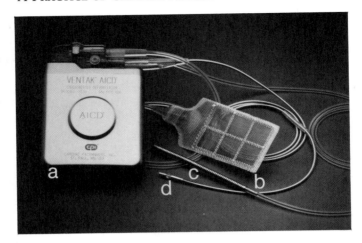

Figure 1. AICD. External appearance of pulse generator (A) connected to epicardial patch electrode (B), superior vena cava spring electrode (C), and intravascular bipolar sensing electrode catheter (D). (Courtesy of Cardiac Pacemakers, Inc., St. Paul, Minnesota.)

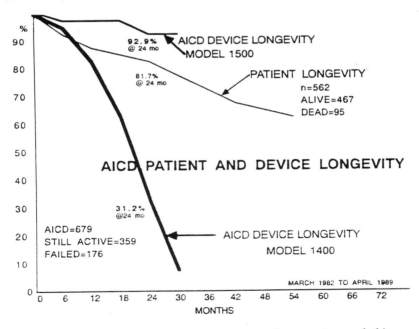

Figure 2. AICD patient and device longevity curves demonstrate a marked improvement in the longevity of the more recent model 1500 compared to previous model 1500. Patient survival is 63.1% ± 9.5% 54 months after implant. (Data from Bilitch Report).

shock. If baseline or sinus rhythm is not detected after four shocks, the device will not discharge again until a new episode has been detected.

Sensing continues to be a problem despite current algorithms for arrhythmia detection. To optimize accurate and reproducible sensing, two criteria have been used.

Probability Density Function (PDF)

The PDF was developed as a morphology criterion. The concept underlying this algorithm is that different rhythms have different characteristic waveform profiles (Figure 3). During sinus rhythm or supraventricular tachycardia, a large portion of the transcardiac electrogram is isoelectric. This is different than ventricular tachycardia or ventricular fibrillation in which there is a relative absence of isoelectric potentials on the electrocardiogram. Narrow complex well-organized

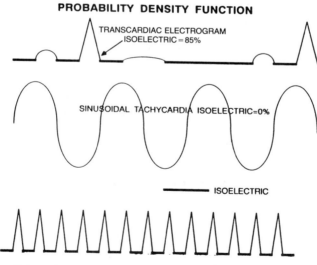

PROBABILITY DENSITY FUNCTION

TRANSCARDIAC ELECTROGRAM
ISOELECTRIC = 85%

SINUSOIDAL TACHYCARDIA ISOELECTRIC=0%

ISOELECTRIC

Figure 3. *Schematic diagram of the probability density function. During sinus rhythm (TOP), the majority of the transcardiac electrogram is isoelectric. During wide complex ventricular tachycardia or ventricular fibrillation, there is marked absence in isoelectric potentials (MIDDLE). During narrow complex tachycardia (BOTTOM), the amount of isoelectric intracardiac electrogram is in between. As can be imagined, narrow complex ventricular tachycardia, i.e., fascicular tachycardia may not meet PDF criteria.*

ventricular tachycardia, such as fascicular tachycardia, may not meet PDF criteria. Conversely, supraventricular tachycardia with a marked intraventricular conduction delay may satisfy the PDF criteria.

Preset Heart Rate Cutoff

A second algorithm uses rate criteria alone. This rate is preset by the manufacturer. A variety of special order rates are available, ranging from 120–200 bpm. The most common rate cutoff is approximately 150 bpm. If the ventricular arrhythmia is slower than the rate cutoff, detection will not occur. To ensure accurate sensing, it has been recommended that the rate cutoff be 10 bpm less than the rate of spontaneous monomorphic ventricular tachycardia. If polymorphic ventricular tachycardia is present, the rate cutoff of the device should be lower, because not all ventricular depolarizations may reach the gain setting required for sensing.

Two types of devices are currently available. The most common device requires both rate cutoff and PDF criteria for detection. These devices may decrease false detection and mistaken labeling of supraventriclar tachycardia as a ventricular arrhythmia. Such devices with combined detection criteria, however, may fail to recognize fascicular tachycardia because the PDF may not be met. In this setting, a rate alone cutoff device is useful. Rate cutoff devices alone, however, do not distinguish supraventricular tachycardia from ventricular tachycardia.

Either type of device usually requires 5–20 seconds for arrhythmia detection. The detection time is usually shorter for ventricular fibrillation (2.5–5.0 seconds average) compared to ventricular tachycardia (average 5.0–20.0 seconds).

LEAD SYSTEMS

The lead systems used have changed considerably. Currently there are three types of leads: ventricular patch leads, which are either 20 cm^2 or 10 cm^2; conventional epimyocardial screw-in or "harpoon-like" electrodes; and endocardial leads (Figure 4).

Transcardiac Patch Electrodes

The titanium mesh ventricular patch electrodes monitor the electrical waveforms for the PDF circuit in addition to delivering the

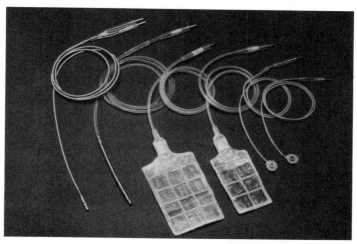

Figure 4. *Lead systems currently used for AICD implantation. From left to right, transvenous right ventricular endocardial lead; superior vena cava spring lead; 20 cm² patch, 10 cm² patch; and conventional epimyocardial electrodes.*

cardioverting/defibrillating energy. The standard patch has a 10 cm² surface area while the larger patch is 20 cm². Defibrillation thresholds are lowest with the largest electrode surface area. The decision to use a specific patch configuration, for example, a large and a small patch, depends on the cardiac anatomy, the need to perform other procedures such as bypass grafting, and the defibrillation thresholds. The patches are usually fixed to the parietal pericardium with synthetic, nonabsorbable suture material to prevent migration. Typically, a 20 cm² patch is placed on the posterolateral left ventricle, and the other patch (another 20 cm² size) is placed over the anterior left ventricular surface or the right ventricle (Figures 5A, 5B, 5C, 5D).

Endocardial Electrodes

A superior vena cava spring lead may be used instead of one of the patches for monitoring PDF function, and serves as the anode. This lead is 100 cm long and has a 10 cm² surface area. It is placed in the venous system near the junction of the right atrium and the superior vena cava. When the spring lead and a left ventricular patch are utilized, the threshold may be higher than when two patches are used. Another potential disadvantage, although rare, is that there may be dislodgement of the spring lead.

A transvenous right ventricular endocardial lead is also available. This bipolar lead is placed in the right ventricular apex for rate sensing and R wave synchronizing.

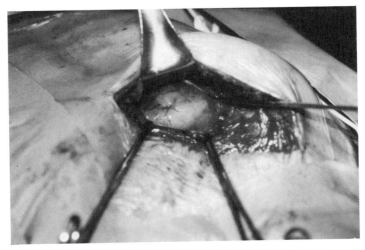

Figure 5A.   *AICD implantation may be accomplished via a left subcostal incision. The chest is rotated approximately 30° with the left side up, and the lower portion of the left chest is further elevated with a sand bag. The pericardium is approached extrapleurally. The pericardium is opened to expose the cardiac apex.*

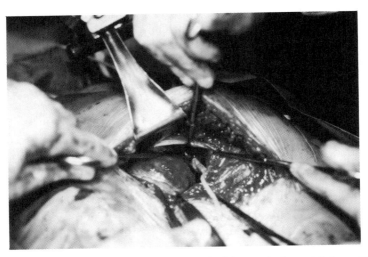

Figure 5B.   *With the pericardium retracted, the left ventricular patch is positioned and sutured, at its corners, to the epicardium.*

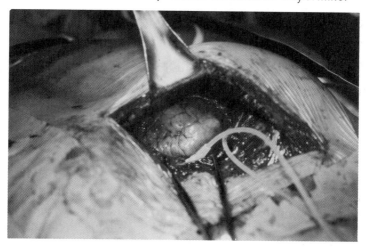

Figure 5C. *The right ventricular patch is then placed and also sutured to the epicardium.*

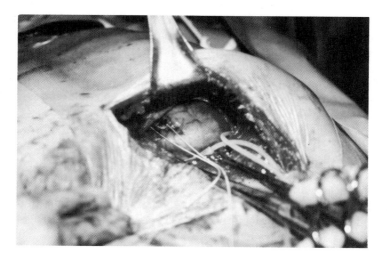

Figure 5D. *The two 4951 epimyocardial leads for sensing a tachyarrhythmia are placed between the two patches. The four leads are tunneled to the subcutaneous tissue of the left upper quadrant and are attached to the AICD pulse generator. The entire procedure is accomplished via a single incision with general, endotracheal anesthesia.*

Epimyocardial Electrodes

Conventional epimyocardial electrodes can also be used in place of the endocardial lead for rate sensing and R wave synchronizing. These should be placed within 1–2 cm of each other on either the right or left ventricle.

Given the number of electrodes available, several implant combinations are possible: (1) epimyocardial systems, (2) combined epimyocardial and endocardial systems, (3) transvenous systems.

Epimyocardial System

If only epimyocardial systems are used, two patch electrodes are placed for PDF analysis and defibrillation, and two epimyocardial electrodes are used for rate sensing and R wave synchronizing. Selection of the patch size will depend upon what other procedures are planned, and the details of the cardiac anatomy and size. As mentioned before, larger patch sizes usually are associated with improved lower defibrillation thresholds.

Combined Epimyocardial and Endocardial Systems

A variety of options are available at this time. At least one patch electrode must be used. This patch electrode can be used with either a second patch electrode, or in combination with the superior vena cava spring lead as the anode. In combined systems, the transvenous bipolar endocardial lead can be used for rate sensing and R wave synchronization. In one of our institutions, a single left ventricular patch lead is placed during thoracotomy, and then combined with the spring lead and a transvenous lead.

Transvenous Systems

All but a few automatic implantable cardioverter defibrillators have been implanted by one transthoracic technique or another. As mentioned, some have had all leads—sensing and defibrillating—implanted via thoracotomy. Others have been a mixed approach with sensing via a transvenous lead in the right ventricular apex and one of the two defibrillating leads in the lower superior vena cava near the junction with the right atrium with the other an epicardial patch. Development of a complete transvenous system could have major advantages and if reliable, could be expected to become the dominant approach for AICD implantation, analogous to the shift from epimyocardial permanent cardiac pacing to transvenous permanent pacing. Recently it has become apparent that in at least some patients, the left ventricular patch need not be on the epicardial surface of the heart;

instead, it can be somewhat remote and even against the subcutaneous rib surface, for example, outside of the pleural space (Figure 6).

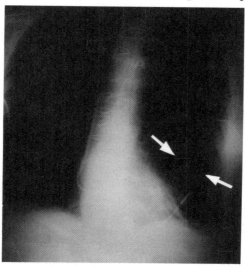

Figure 6A.   *PA chest X-ray of a nonthoracotomy lead system with an Endotak C and SQ lead (Cardiac Pacemakers, Inc., St. Paul, Minnesota). Arrows indicate the patch electrode in the subcutaneous tissue.*

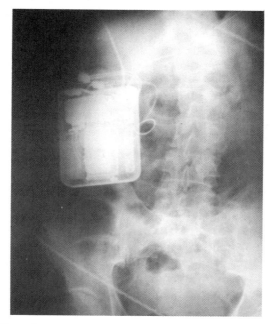

Figure 6B.   *The pulse generator is placed in an upper abdominal pocket on the right side.*

A new endocardial lead has been developed encompassing both sensing and defibrillating electrodes. This ENDOTAK^{tm} system uses a 100 cm long, tripolar silicone rubber endocardial lead, 3.95 mm (12 F) in diameter, which is implanted via a cutdown on the cephalic vein, the external jugular vein, or by conventional subclavian puncture. The lead tip is a sensing electrode adjacent to four silicone rubber tines, which is placed in the right ventricular apex. There are two additional electrodes, one immediately proximal to the tip electrode, and the second more proximal, separated by a variable distance (10, 13, or 16 cm) from the first.

These two electrodes may be connected in one of various configurations determined to be the best during the implant procedure. One or both of the two endocardial defibrillating electrodes may be used as the cathode of the system. A subcutaneous or submuscular (but extrathoracic) silicone rubber insulated patch lead is placed within the left lateral chest wall and always acts as the anode. A "Y" adapter connects the endocardial and the subcutaneous leads with the defibrillator. Because of the chest wall incision, the placement of a large defibrillator device in the subcutaneous tissue of the abdomen, and the need to induce and terminate ventricular fibrillation via the implanted leads or by higher outputs across the intact chest, general endotracheal anesthesia is used. The duration of ventricular fibrillation and consequent circulatory arrest is likely to be longer during defibrillator implant and testing than during programmed electrical stimulation since initial test defibrillating shocks are more likely to be at, below, or just above defibrillation threshold. During the final defibrillation shock, given by the implanted AICD, ventricular fibrillation is induced and detected by the device, which then charges and then discharges itself, a process that may occupy as much as 20 seconds. Should that shock be unsuccessful, the arrhythmia and circulatory arrest will be even longer as the device recycles through subsequent shocks.

During implantation, one or both of the two electrodes of the endocardial lead are connected to the Y connector. The single limb of the Y connects to the cathode of the AICD. The patch lead is connected to the anode. Alternate connections are possible. Overall, there are four options (Figure 7) that may all be explored to find the one with the lowest defibrillation threshold. (1) The distal coil ENDOTAK electrode may be connected directly to the cathodal AICD output, and the patch to the anode, without the Y connector. (2) A second alternative is that the two endocardial electrode coils may be connected together at the Y so that two intracardiac cathodes exist. (3) A third alternative is that the proximal endocardial coil is made the

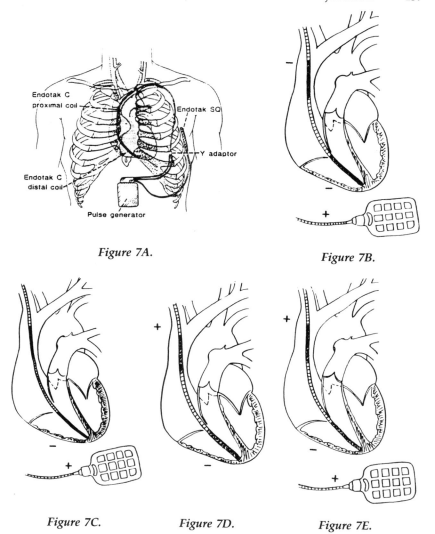

Figure 7A.

Figure 7B.

Figure 7C.

Figure 7D.

Figure 7E.

Figure 7. (A) An Endotak system involves pulse generator, tripolar tined tranvenous catheter with a proximal and distal coil, and a subcutaneous patch (Endotak SQ). The Y adaptor is used for various lead connections. (B) One option involves use of both the proximal and distal coils of the transvenous lead system as the common cathode (-) with the subcutaneous patch as the anode (+). (C) A second option uses the distal coil as cathode (-) and the subcutaneous patch as the anode (+). (D) A third option uses the proximal coil as the anode (+) and the distal coil as the cathode (-) without a patch. (E) A fourth option uses the distal coil as the cathode (-) and both the proximal coil and subcutaneous patch as the anode (+).

anode as is the extracardiac patch, and both are connected to the Y. (4) The final alternative is that the proximal coil electrode is connected to the anode, the distal to the cathode, and no patch electrode is used.

The position of the two intracardiac coil electrodes and the patch electrode is critical to the success of the defibrillating system. Consequently, the endocardial lead should be positioned in the right ventricular apex. More or less pressure should be applied to vary the relative positions of the two coil electrodes relative to the right ventricle and to each other. Similarly, the position of the patch is important, and it should be moved about until the optimal position is found.

The process of positioning the endocardial lead and the patch, and selecting the best of the four configurations may make this process extremely time consuming. Preliminary data indicates that the implant works best in smaller people. In taller or larger individuals (as distinguished from those who are obese), a lower success rate has been achieved. The configuration and endocardial approach are still in clinical evaluation, and data is necessarily incomplete. Nevertheless, completely successful implantation in each patient has not been achieved. Further refinement is likely.

PATIENT SELECTION

As the experience with AICD devices has increased, and the devices themselves have become more available and reliable, the indications have broadened. The indications, however, do vary among institutions depending upon the availability of other options, for example, electrophysiological surgery, catheter ablation, antitachycardia pacing, and investigational drug use. In some institutions, an AICD is only considered when drugs have failed and ablation or electrophysiological surgery is not possible. In other institutions, an AICD may be used earlier in the patient's course. This has important implications in assessing the results from different centers. Long-term survival will be affected by patient selection as well as by device performance. If the AICD is only implanted after every other option has failed, the results will be poorer than if the AICD is implanted as the first line of treatment.

Theoretically, any patient with ventricular fibrillation or hemodynamically unstable ventricular tachycardia that is not the result of acute myocardial infarction or a reversible cause such as an electrolyte disturbance or drug toxicity, is a potential candidate. There are a few generally accepted indications.

Resuscitated Cardiac Arrest

Patients with cardiac arrest not associated with acute myocardial infarction have an increased incidence of recurrent arrhythmic events, and increased one year mortality. In these patients, if an inducible arrhythmia cannot be controlled or prevented with medications or with a surgical procedure, an AICD should be considered. In patients in whom no arrhythmia is inducible, if significant heart disease is present and recurrent cardiac arrest has occurred, an AICD can also be considered. As mentioned before, as experience with AICD increases, they may become the treatment of choice. In some institutions an AICD is implanted in all patients with resuscitated cardiac arrest, and then the decision whether to use antiarrhythmic drugs is considered.

Sustained Ventricular Tachycardia with Hemodynamic Instability

In patients with inducible sustained ventricular tachycardia who fail drug therapy, or in patients who are not candidates for ablation or surgery, an AICD should be considered. As mentioned, in some institutions an AICD is saved as a last resort while in others, it may be used as a first line of therapy because of considerations of drug failure and potential side effects.

There are other indications for implantation. In patients undergoing electrophysiological surgery for ventricular arrhythmias, the ventricular defibrillation patches and epimyocardial sensing leads may be placed without the generator. In these patients, should an arrhythmia recur or still be inducible postoperatively, the generator can be easily placed without the need for repeat thoracotomy. An alternative approach is to implant a single left ventricular patch to be used later with a spring lead and a transvenous lead if needed.

Several specific clinical situations are contraindications to the use of the AICD. These include: (1) slow ventricular tachycardia, which is well tolerated. In these patients, the arrhythmia may either not be detected or the patient may receive a discharge while awake. This may cause severe distress and limits the use; (2) Recurrent nonsustained ventricular tachycardia, which cannot be controlled pharmacologically, but which is of sufficient duration to initiate a discharge. In these patients, the nonsustained ventricular tachycardia will initiate discharges; (3) Recurrent supraventricular tachycardia, including atrial flutter or fibrillation, particularly in patients with bundle branch block, which cannot be controlled pharmacologically, but which may be sufficient to trigger a discharge; (4) Patients with such severe underlying cardiac disease or extracardiac disease, which will limit survival to <6 to 12 months; (5) AICD implantation is contraindicated in centers without experienced personnel including electrophysiologists, cardiovascular surgeons, and nursing personnel needed for initial implantation, screening, and follow-up of these patients; (6) Patients who are unwilling to or cannot accept the limitations of the device.

PATIENT EVALUATION

Preoperative

In all patients in whom an AICD is contemplated, a baseline electrophysiological study is required to document the underlying ventricular arrhythmia. Drug testing is performed in all patients to determine if a successful drug regimen can be identified, whereby an AICD may not be needed. The effect of drugs on the rate and duration of tachycardia should also be assessed. If drug therapy slows the tachycardia and makes it nonsustained or very well tolerated, the device may also discharge while the patient is awake. The use of amiodarone is important in this regard since this drug may change defibrillation thresholds as well as inducibility. If amiodarone is to be used, a steady state should be reached, if possible, before AICD testing, and the drug continued during testing and surgery.

Prior to electrophysiological evaluation or implantation, thorough evaluation should be given to exclude any remediable cause for the ventricular arrhythmia, e.g., electrolyte disturbances or uncontrolled congestive heart failure. These should be corrected before baseline evaluation.

It is also important to thoroughly evaluate the underlying heart disease with left ventricular angiography and coronary angiography. This is essential in planning operative interventions such as coronary artery bypass graft surgery, or electrophysiologically guided surgery.

The preoperative assessment also includes evaluation of the need for permanent pacing. Unipolar pacemakers are contraindicated because of the potential for sensing of the stimulus artifact, thus resulting in spurious discharges. Patients with unipolar pacemakers must have these pulse generators replaced with bipolar systems.

A final evaluation is psychosocial. The patients and their families must be able to understand and accept potential complications with the device, and the follow-up requirements.

Operative Technique

Testing and implantation of the AICD requires expertise as well as a considerable amount of equipment (Tables I–V). A variety of operative approaches are used. If other cardiac surgery, for example, aneurysmectomy or coronary artery bypass graft surgery is planned, a median sternotomy is used. A median sternotomy may also provide the best exposure for biventricular patches and placement of the epicardial sensing leads. Other approaches are also used. When only an AICD placement is to be performed, a left lateral thoracotomy, subxiphoid or subcostal approach may be used (Figures 5A–D). Of these three, the left lateral thoractomy is most common because it provides the best exposure for placement of left ventricular patches.

As mentioned before, two patches are most commonly used although a patch and a spring lead can also be placed. The selection of patch size (10 cm^2 or 20 cm^2) depends upon the size of the heart, the need to perform other procedures, for example, coronary grafting, and surgeon preference. Thresholds are lowest with the largest surface area patches. In patients undergoing surgery aimed at abolishing tachycardia, for example, endocardial resection, leads are placed alone. The sensing screw-in or "harpoon-like" epimyocardial electrodes are also positioned; alternatively, but less commonly, a bipolar endocardial lead may be used.

With the nonthoracotomy approach, the defibrillation catheter is inserted transvenously and placed in the right ventricular apex. The second defibrillation lead is placed subcutaneously via a submammary incision on the left side of the chest over the cardiac apex. The latter lead is placed so that the largest mass of the heart is between the patch lead and the transvenous lead.

After placement of the leads, the ventricular arrhythmia is reinduced by programmed ventricular stimulation or rapid ventricular pacing. Details of specific stimulation sequence used for induction during the preoperative electrophysiological study should be available to decrease the time needed during operation. After induction of

---

Table I
Equipment for AICD Implant

Physiological recorder
Stimulator for tachycardia induction
Pacing analyzer
External Cardioverter/Defibrillator (ECD)
ECD cables
    one high voltage for patches
    one monitoring cable for epicardial pacing leads

---

ventricular tachycardia or ventricular fibrillation, the defibrillation threshold (DFT) is measured by using an externally, manually operated cardioverter/defibrillator (ECD) to terminate the arrhythmia (Figure 8). The ECD must be tested before use (Table II). Low energy

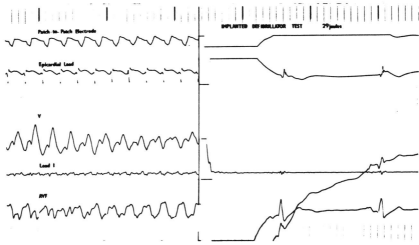

Figure 8. Intraoperative testing in a patient during implantation of an automatic implantable cardioverter-defibrillator. Patch electrodes are placed on the left ventricle. Additional electrodes are placed either on the epicardium or via transvenous route. Rapid ventricular tachycardia or ventricular fibrillation is automatically detected and converted to sinus rhythm with 29 J.

Table II
To Test ECD

1. Place ECD in "SAFE" position.
2. Turn on power.
3. Connect a 50-ohm dummy load to the high voltage pulse jacks.
4. Place a short circuit jumper cable across the bipolar and pacer input jacks.
5. Turn on 40 Joules.
6. Turn to "ENABLE."
7. Place in "ASYNC" mode.
8. Press the charge button.
9. Wait seven seconds and depress the trigger button.
10. The "CHARGING" and "READY" lights should extinguish.
11. Now place ECD in "SYNC" mode.
12. Press charge button.
13. Depress trigger button–the "CHARGING" and "READY" lights should remain unchanged.
14. With the trigger button still depressed, press the 5 millivolt calibration button on the BIPOLAR channel.
15. "CHARGING" and "READY" lights should extinguish.

levels are used initially. If these fail, a shock of 25 J is used as quickly as possible. If this fails to terminate the arrhythmia, conventional cardioversion is used. It must be remembered that these studies are carried out in a patient who is not on bypass. Sufficient time must be made available for hemodynamics to return to baseline between tests. If the DFT is <15 J, the AICD can be implanted. A 10 J safety margin is desirable. If possible, both ventricular tachycardia and ventricular fibrillation are induced to check DFT's with both arrhythmias.

Occasionally, defibrillation thresholds are excessively high. This may be the result of poor epicardial contact or too small a surface area. In this setting, if small 10 cm^2 patches had been used initially, these may need to be replaced with the larger patches, the lead polarity may be reversed, or the configuration may need to be changed, for example, to go from a patch and spring superior vena cava electrode to two patches. Care should be taken to separate the patches, and cover the largest amount of ventricular myocardium. If despite these maneuvers DFT remains borderline or high (>20 J), a high energy unit is required. In this case, two large patches are used and the lead is tunneled to the abdominal wound. When the high energy unit becomes available from the manufacturer, it can be implanted. At the time of subsequent unit placement, general anesthesia usually is used because implantation involves induction of ventricular tachycardia/ventricular fibrillation.

If the DFT's are within acceptable range (<15 J), the AICD unit is checked (Table III). If the generator function is normal, it is then

---

Table III
To Test Generator (Before Opening onto Sterile Field)

1. AICD comes deactivated (will hear a steady tone when magnet is placed over).
2. To re-activate, place magnet over generator for 30 seconds. You should first hear a constant tone, then a few random tones, and then no tone.
3. Remove magnet–WAIT ONE MINUTE.
4. Place the AIDCHECK probe near the upper left corner of the device (do not move).
   Place magnet over upper right corner for three to five seconds, then remove it.
5. The charge time on the display will begin advancing and a continuous charging tone will be heard.
6. Check to make sure charge time is the same as on AICD package. If the charge time is not within one second of nominal, wait ten minutes and then perform a second magnet test. Up to three magnet tests may be needed.
7. Check to make sure patient pulse count matches the value on AICD package.
8. If AIDCHECK flashed "7," telemetry is transmitted incorrectly. REPEAT PROCEDURE without moving AIDCHECK probe from upper left corner of device.

connected to the lead system. After placing the pulse generator in the pocket, testing is repeated with the AICD by tachycardia induction, and then allowing the pulse generator to sense and terminate the tachycardia. The pulse generator is then left in an inactive mode to reduce or decrease the chance that cautery, or supraventricular or ventricular arrhythmias occurring immediately postoperatively may trigger the device. It is then activated in the first 24–48 hours.

It must be remembered that the pulse generator is large and bulky (290 grams; 11.2 x 7.1 x 2.5 cm) (Figure 1). Construction of an adequate pocket is important to avoid problems with migration or erosion. This may be a particular concern in smaller or thinner patients.

Knowledge of the sequence for activation or inactivation of the AICD is essential. As new units become available, the sequences will undoubtedly change. To inactivate the current unit, a magnet is placed over the pulse generator. The inactive state is signaled by a continuous audio tone. Removal of the magnet while the steady tone is present will leave the pulse generator in its inactive state. To acti-

---

Table IV
To Test Patch and Epicardial Lead Thresholds

1. Epi leads–need bipolar R wave and pacing threshold.
2. Patch electrodes–R wave.

To Test Cardioversion Thresholds

1. After patches are sewn on, connect large white cable to patch electrodes—LV Patch to Red, RV Patch to Black; then connect cable to ECD in the Spring-Patch Input.
2. Epicardial leads—use blue cable, connect leads bipolar with lead adaptors, and connect to the bipolar input of ECD.
3. Black recording cables are used to record event on paper.
   Top Channel–epicardial leads; connect from input channel of physiological recorder to bipolar output of ECD.
   Bottom Channel–patch electrodes; connect from input channel of physiological recorder to Spring-Patch Output of ECD.
4. Now you are ready to induce tachycardia.
5. Turn ECD to SAFE.
6. Turn on power.
7. Set energy level desired.
8. Turn ECD to ENABLE.
9. Press "CHARGE"–charge light will come on.
10. Press "TRIGGER" when ready to cardiovert.

   (Steps 1–8 can be done before or after tachycardia is induced depending upon how well the patient tolerates rhythm. The test can be repeated at lower energy levels.)

vate the unit, the magnet is once again placed over the pulse generator. The continuous audio tone will then change to a random intermittent tone, and then a regular tone synchronous with the heart beat. Removal of the magnet at that time leaves the unit activated.

Prior to hospital dismissal, a repeat electrophysiological study is performed. The patient is returned to the electrophysiological laboratory, and a single transvenous catheter placed for ventricular stimulation. The unit is inactivated while the ventricular arrhythmia is reinduced by programmed ventricular stimulation or rapid ventricular pacing. This step eliminates the potential of the device sensing the sequence of beats in the stimulation protocol and identifying it as ventricular tachycardia (Table IV). After tachycardia induction, the unit is activated. The charge time of the unit is recorded. An external defibrillator must be available should the device fail to operate normally. If the device senses nonsustained ventricular tachycardia during this time and initiates capacitor charging while the patient is awake, a magnet is used to shunt the pulse to the AICD internal test load and thereby avoid shocking the patient.

FOLLOW-UP

The patient is scheduled for follow-up visits every two months. At each visit, the pulse generator is tested noninvasively by discharging the defibrillator energy to an internal test load. An external defibrillator must be available for these checks in the event of a circuit failure, which may cause the electrical charge to be delivered to the heart, inducing an arrhythmia.

Noninvasive testing is accomplished with the use of an Aidcheck (Figure 9). The Aidcheck probe is placed over the upper end of the implanted AICD. A donut magnet is then applied under the Aidcheck probe. With newer generation devices, the placement of the probe and donut magnet is the right upper pole and left upper pole of the pulse generator respectively. Once this is applied, a regular intermittent tone synchronous with the patient's QRS complex will identify proper positioning. The magnet is then removed in a vertical motion, perpendicular to the face of the pulse generator. Removal of the magnet begins a charging cycle. The end point of this charging cycle is that the energy that would have been delivered to the patient is instead channeled to the internal test load resistor.

The Aidcheck will display the charge time (the time required to charge the capacitor), and the total number of times a shock has been

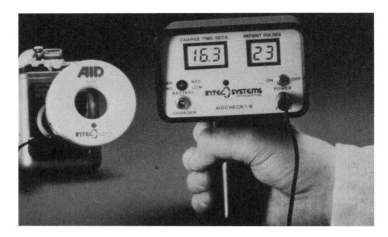

Figure 9.   *Aidcheck used to noninvasively test AICD (Cardiac Pacemakers, Inc., St. Paul, Minnesota). This measures the charge time and number of discharges.*

Table V
After Generator is Reactivated, Final Test Defibrillation Can Be Made

1. Leave magnet over generator.
2. Place probe over generator.
3. Induce tachycardia.
4. Take magnet off and leave probe on.
5. It will take from 10 to 30 seconds for the AICD to cardiovert. (If unsuccessful, generator will recharge and cardiovert again—AICD will shock 3 times at lower Joule setting and once at the upper Joule setting).
6. If AICD is unsuccessful, external paddles can be used.
7. If the arrhythmia is reversed with the 1st, 2nd or 3rd pulse, a 35 second recycle time is required.
8. If the rhythm is stopped but recurs within 35 seconds, the second pulse of the 4-pulse sequence will be delivered.
9. However, if the tachycardia recurs more than 35 seconds after the first pulse, the next pulse delivered would be the first of a new sequence.
10. After the 4th pulse is delivered, the AICD will not pulse again if the arrhythmia continues.

delivered to the patient (Figure 9). After the test charge is dumped internally into the device, the total number of charges available is decreased by 1. The magnet test charge is not included in the number of patient pulses displayed on the Aidcheck, and each magnet test charge must be recorded to make it possible to identify the total number of times the device has charged and delivered a shock. A second magnet test is performed after waiting 10 minutes. This second magnet test may be useful in attempting to identify an elective replacement time.

The charge time represents the time it takes for the batteries to charge the storage capacitor to the nominal 25–35 J. It has been suggested as an end-of-life indicator although its reliability has been questioned. The second magnet test charge time has been felt to be more reliable than the first. This is the basis for the recommendation that a second magnet test be performed 10 minutes after the first. The rationale for a second magnet test rests on the fact that capacitor deformation/reformation changes after the battery has been inactive. This results from the fact that there is reduction in the thickness of the aluminum oxide layer of the capacitor due to increased current leakage. The initial magnet test allows the aluminum oxide layer to reform. A shorter charge time is, therefore, seen during the second magnet test, which is felt to be a better indicator of remaining battery longevity. An elective replacement indicator (ERI) is given to each AICD unit by the manufacturer. It is based on experience with the performance, and longevity of the AICD circuits and pulse generator. It is obtained in each patient at the eighth month by multiplying the second magnet test charge time by 1.2. When this value is reached, there are approximately 200 seconds of remaining cumulative charging time left, or approximately three months of monitoring time. The use of ERI is a rough guide only. Although a two year survival of current AICD units has been projected, the average unit longevity is approximately 20 months (Figure 2).

COMPLICATIONS

Operative Complications

The incidence and specific type of complications are affected by the patient population undergoing implantation. In patients with very poor left ventricular function or severe extracardiac diseases, there may be substantial morbidity and even mortality. An overall 30-day operative mortality of 2–3% has been reported.

Infections have been reported usually in the early postoperative period. As has been true with all infections involving foreign bodies, successful treatment almost always requires removal of all the implanted hardware. Other complications include bleeding and lead fractures. Erosion may also occur, particularly in thin patients. Threatened erosion with thinning of the skin, pain, and erythema may be treated by pocket revision. Once actual erosion has occurred, replacement of the pulse generator may be necessary to prevent infection. If an endocardial lead has been used, it may migrate or cause superior vena cava thrombosis.

Pulmonary complications are perhaps the most frequent early postoperative problems and include atelectasis, infiltrates, pleural effusions, and pneumothorax.

Device Malfunction

Complications related to pulse generator fabrication include early battery depletion secondary to corrosion of the glass insulator, random component failure, and loss of the hermetic seal. The most common problem has been early battery depletion occurring in approximately 5–10% of devices.

Spurious Discharges

Spurious discharges are considered to be discharges of the device in the absence of symptoms consistent with sustained ventricular tachycardia or ventricular fibrillation. Unless the patient is being monitored, it is impossible to identify the exact cause of the discharge, which may range from device malfunction to sensing atrial fibrillation or other types of supraventricular tachycardia, sinus tachycardia, nonsustained ventricular tachycardia, myopotentials, or electrocautery devices. Spurious discharges may be difficult to evaluate and prevent. They are also very bothersome for the patient and may result in psychological disability. Careful patient selection and treatment of other types of tachycardia are important to limit the frequency of spurious discharges. They may be frequent, however, and have been documented in up to 40% of patients in some series. Patients are instructed to report any device discharges. This is important for monitoring device performance and efficacy as well as for ensuring optimal patient care. If frequent discharges are reported, ambulatory monitoring or exercise testing may be helpful in identifying the cause.

The presence of a pacemaker and an AICD in the same patient poses some unique interactions (Figures 10, 11). As has been men-

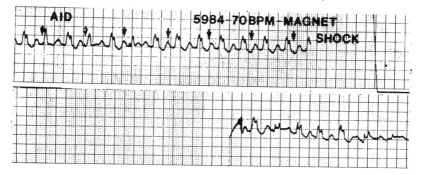

Figure 10. *The interaction of a pacemaker and an implanted defibrillator must be carefully monitored. It is possible that pacemaker stimuli will be sensed and treated as ventricular contractions. In this ECG, each stimulus was treated as a ventricular event, each paced QRS and each spontaneous QRS added to the count. As the total exceeded the tachycardia criterion, the AICD was discharged.*

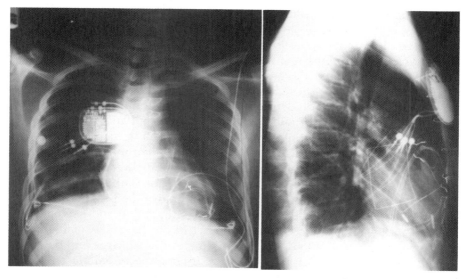

Figure 11. *PA (left), and lateral (right) chest X-ray of a 16-year old patient with a pacemaker and an AICD.*

tioned, unipolar pacemakers can result in device discharge from double sensing of the unipolar stimulus artifact and the QRS electrogram. Alternatively, the presence of a unipolar stimulus during ventricular fibrillation may delay sensing of the arrhythmia. The use of bipolar pacemakers avoids some of these problems. There are, however, other interactions. Programming the pacemaker can result in AICD discharge. This interaction is complex and depends upon whether the programmer uses an electomagnetic or radiofrequency signal, as well as the specific AICD used. For this reason, it has been recommended that the AICD be transiently inactivated during pacemaker programming. In addition, magnet application should be avoided during routine transtelephonic monitoring of the permanent pacemaker.

FUTURE DEVELOPMENTS

Current devices already have a proven record of safety and efficacy. Future developments should improve upon that record. These developments will facilitate broader use of the devices. Improvements should come in several areas. (1) Tachycardia detection—improved algorithms will allow more reliable detection of ventricular tachycardia and ventricular fibrillation. This function will be programmable so that changes in arrhythmia over time can be detected and treated effectively. These improvements should decrease the frequency of spurious discharges. (2) Expanded termination parameters—an ideal device would allow a range of termination parameters ranging from treatment of ventricular tachycardia by single or paired extrastimuli or burst pacing to low energy synchronized cardioversion to high output defibrillating discharge. In addition, backup bradycardia pacing will become available for rate support following cardioversion. Ideally all of these parameters will be programmable. (3) Improved battery life—continued miniaturization and use of hybrid circuits should increase the number of discharges available. (4) Transvenous application—currently, the devices are large and bulky, and require a major surgical procedure for epimyocardial placement. (5) Telemetry functions—these will allow review of the event that triggered the discharge.

Several new devices are being developed and tested clinically (Figure 12). These will be increasingly complex but should allow more flexibility, and widen the applicability of these devices as well as decrease the problems associated with their use.

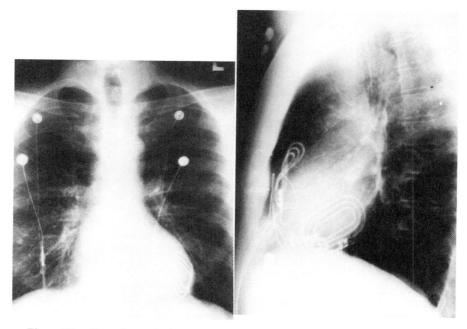

Figure 12. *Several new devices are being developed and tested. PA (left), and lateral X-ray (right) demonstrating Medtronic device (courtesy of Dr. R. Yee; London, Ontario).*

BIBLIOGRAPHY

Bach SM: *Aid-B cardioverter-defibrillator: Possible interactions with pacemakers.* Intec Systems Technical Communication, August 1983.

Bilitch M, Hauser RG, Goldman BS, Furman S, Parsonnet V: Performance of implantable cardiac rhythm management devices. *PACE* 1986; 9:256–267.Bilitch M, Hauser RG, Goldman BS, Maloney JD, Harthorne JW, Furman S, Parsonnet V: Performance of implantable cardiac rhythm management devices. *PACE* 1987; 10:389–398.

Brodman R, Fisher JD, Furman S, Johnston DR, Kim SG, Matos JA, Waspe LE: Implantation of automatic cardioverter-defibrillators via median sternotomy. *PACE* 1984; 7:1363–1369.

Brodman R, Fisher JD, Johnston DR, et al: Results of electrophysiologically guided operations for drug-resistant recurrent VT and ventricular fibrillation due to coronary artery disease. *J Thorac Cardiovasc Surg* 1984; 87: 431–438.

Cannom DS, Winkle RA: Implantation of the automatic implantable cardioverter defibrillator (AICD): Practical aspects. *PACE* 1986; 9:793–809.

Chilson DA, Heger JJ, Zipes DP, Browne KF, Prystowsky EN: Electrophysiologic effects and clinical efficacy of oral propafenone therapy in patients with ventricular tachycardia. *JACC* 1985; 5:1407–1413.

Cohen AI, Wish MH, Fletcher RD, et al: The use and interaction of permanent pacemakers and the automatic implantable cardioverter defibrillator. *PACE* 1988; 11:704–11.

Cox JL: Temporary cardiac pacing following cardiac surgery. In: Barold SS (ed), *Modern Cardiac Pacing*, Futura Publishing Co, New York, 1985, p. 495–510.

Deeb GM, Griffith BP, Thompson ME, Langer A, Heilman S, Hardesty RL: Lead systems for internal ventricular fibrillation. *Circulation* 1981; 64:242–245.

Deeb GM, Hardesty RL, Griffith BP, et al: The effects of cardiovascular drugs on the defibrillation threshold and the pathological effects on the heart using an automatic implantable defibrillator. *Ann Thorac Surg* 1983; 35:361–364.

Denes P, Gabster AL, Huang SK: Clinical, electrocardiographic and follow-up observations in patients having ventricular fibrillation during Holter monitoring. *Am J Cardiol* 1981; 48:9–16.

Echt DS: Potential hazards of implanted devices for the electrical control of tachyarrhythmias. *PACE* 1984; 7:580–587.

Echt DS, Armstrong K, Schmidt P, et al: Clinical experience, complications, and survival in 70 patients with the automatic implantable cardioverter/defibrillator. *Circulation* 1985; 71:289–296.

Echt DS, Winkle RA: Management of patients with the automatic implantable cardioverter/defibrillator. *CPPE* 1985; 3:4–16.

Epstein AE, Kay GN, Plumb VJ, Shepard RB, Kirklin JK: Combined automatic implantable cardioverter-defibrillator and pacemaker systems: Implantation techniques and follow-up. *JACC* 1989; 13:121–131.

Fain ES, Lee JT, Winkle RA: Effects of acute intravenous and chronic oral amiodarone on defibrillation energy requirements. *Am Heart J* 1987; 114:8–17.

FDA Drug Bulletin, December 1985; 15(4):39.

Fisher JD, Kim SG, Waspe LE, Johnston D: Amiodarone: Value of programmed electrical stimulation and Holter monitoring. *PACE* 1986; 9:422–435.

Furman S: AICD benefit. *PACE* 1989; 12:399–400 (editorial).

Furman S: Combined automatic implantable cardioverter-defibrillator and pacemaker systems. *JACC* 1989; 13:132–133 (Editorial comment).

Furman S: Venous cutdown for pacemaker implantation. *Ann Thorac Surg* 1986; 41:438–442.

Furman S, Brodman R, Pannizzo F, Fisher J: Implantation techniques of antitachycardia devices. *PACE* 1984; 7:572–579.

Gabry MD, Brodman R, Johnston D, et al: Automatic implantable cardioverter-defibrillator: Patient survival, battery longevity and shock delivery analysis. *JACC* 1987; 9:1349–1356.

Goodman LR, Almassi GH, Troup PJ, et al: Complications of automatic implantable cardioverter defibrillators: Radiographic, computed tomographic and echocardiographic evaluation. *Radiol* 1989; 170:447.

Graboys TB, Lown B, Podrid PJ, DeSilva R: Long term survival of patients with malignant ventricular arrhythmias treated with antiarrhythmic drugs. *Am J Cardiol* 1982; 50:437–443.

Guarnieri T, Levine JH, Velti EP, et al: Success of chronic defibrillation and the role of antiarrhythmic drugs with the automatic implantable cardioverter/defibrillator. *Am J Cardiol* 1987; 60:1061–64.

Hamer A, Vohra J, Hunt D, Sloman G: Prediction of sudden death by electrophysiologic studies in high risk patients surviving acute myocardial infarction. *Am J Cardiol* 1982; 50:223–229.

Intec Systems, Inc: *Final report of IDE G800033 for the AICD System—Investigational period from Feb 4, 1980 to Sept 15, 1985.* Submitted to FDA by Intec Systems, Inc, and Cardiac Pacemakers, Inc, Jan 10, 1986.

Intec Systems, Inc: *Report of the clinical investigation: Automatic implantable cardioverter-defibrillator.* Intec Systems, Inc, Pittsburgh, November 9, 1984.

Kelly PA, Cannom DS, Garan H, et al: The automatic implantable cardioverter-defibrillator: Efficacy, complications and survival in patients with malignant ventricular arrhythmias. *J Am Coll Cardiol* 1988; 11:1278–86.

Kempf FC, Josephson ME: Cardiac arrest recorded on ambulatory electrocardiograms. *Am J Cardiol* 1984; 53:1577–1582.

Kim SG, Furman S, Matos JA, Waspe LE, Brodman R, Fisher JD: Automatic implantable cardioverter/defibrillator: Inadvertent discharges during permanent pacemaker magnet tests. *PACE* 1987; 10:579–582.

Kim SG, Furman S, Waspe LE, et al: Unipolar pacer artifacts: Induced failure of an automatic implantable cardioverter/defibrillator to detect ventricular fibrillation. *Am J Cardiol* 1986; 57:880–881.

Lawrie GM, Griffin JC, Wyndham CRC: Epicardial implantation of the automatic implantable defibrillator by left subcostal thoracotomy. *PACE* 1984; 7:1370–1374.

Luceri RM, Thurer RJ, Castellanos A, et al: Initial experience with automatic defibrillator-implanted pacemaker interactions. *PACE* 1985; 8:296 (abstract).

Marchlinski FE, Flores BT, Buxton AE, et al: The automatic implantable cardioverter-defibrillator: Efficacy, complications, and device failures. *Ann Intern Med* 1986; 104:481–488.

Mirowski M: The automatic implantable cardioverter-defibrillator: An overview. *JACC* 1985; 6:461–466.

Mirowski M, Mower M, Reid PR, et al: The automatic implantable defibrillator. New modality for treatment of life-threatening ventricular arrhythmias. *PACE* 1982; 5:384–401.

Mirowski M, Reid PR, Mower MM, Watkins L, Platia E, Griffith L, Prystowsky E: The automatic implantable cardioverter-defibrillator. *PACE* 1984; 7:534–540.

Mirowski M, Reid PR, Mower MM, et al: Clinical performance of the implantable cardioverter-defibrillator. *PACE* 1984; 7:1345–1350.

Mirowski M, Reid PR, Watkins L, et al: Clinical treatment of life-threatening ventricular arrhythmia with the automatic implantable defibrillator. *Am Heart J* 1981; 102:265–270.

Mirowski M, Reid PR, Winkle RA, et al: Mortality in patients with implanted automatic defbrillators. *Ann Intern Med* 1983; 98:585–588.

Pannizzo F, Mercando AD, Fisher JD, Furman S: Automatic methods for detection of tachyarrhythmias by antitachycardia devices. *JACC* 1988; 11:308–316.

Platia EV, Griffith LSC, Watkins L Jr, Mower MM, et al: Treatment of malignant ventricular arrhythmias with endocardial resection and implantation of the automatic cardioverter-defibrillator. *N Engl J Med* 1986; 314:213–216.

Reid PR, Griffith L, Mower MM, Platia EV, Watkins L Jr, Juanteguy J, Mirowski M: Implantable cardioverter-defibrillator: Patient selection and implantation protocol. *PACE* 1984; 7:1338–1344.

Reid PR, Mirowski M, Mower MM, Platia EV, Griffith LSC, et al: Clinical evaluation of the internal automatic cardioverter-defibrillator in survivors of sudden cardiac death. *Am J Cardiol* 1983; 51:1608–1613.

Reid PR, Mower M, Mirowski M: Pathophysiology of ventricular tachyarrhythmias amenable to electrical control. *PACE* 1984; 7:505–513.

Ruffy R, Smith P, Laseter M, Lal R, Kim SS: Out-of-hospital automatic cardioversion of ventricular tachycardia. *JACC* 1985; 6:482–485.

Saksena S, Lindsay BD, Parsonnet V: Developments for future implantable cardioverters and defibrillators. *PACE* 1987; 10:1342–58.

Schaffer WS, Cobb LA: Recurrent ventricular fibrillation and modes of death in survivors of out-of-hopsital ventricular fibrillation. *N Engl J Med* 1975; 293:259–262.

Swerdlow CD, Winkle RA, Mason JW: Determinants of survival in patients with ventricular tachyarrhythmias. *N Engl J Med* 1983; 308:1436–1442.

Tchou PJ, Kadri N, Anderson J, et al: Automatic implantable cardioverter defibrillators and survival of patients with left ventricular dysfunction and malignant ventricular arrhythmias. *Ann Int Med* 1988; 109:529–534.

Thurer RJ, Luceri RM, Bolooki H: Automatic implantable cardioverter-defibrillator: Techniques of implantation and results. *Ann Thorac Surg* 1986; 42:143–47.

Troup PJ: Lessons learned from the automatic implantable cardioverter-defibrillator: Past, present and future. *J Am Coll Cardiol* 1988; 11:1287–89.

Troup PJ, Chapman PD, Olinger GN, Kleinman LH: The implanted defibrillator: Relation of defibrillating lead configuration and clinical variables to defibrillation threshold. *JACC* 1985; 6:1315–1321.

Waspe LE, Brodman R, Kim SG, et al: Activation mapping in patients with coronary artery disease with multiple ventricular tachycardia configurations. *JACC* 1985; 5:1075–1086.

Watkins L Jr, Mirowski M, Mower MM, Reid PR, Freund P, Thomas A, Weisfeldt ML, Gott VL: Implantation of the automatic defibrillator: The subxiphoid approach. *Ann Thorac Surg* 1982; 34:515–520.

Watkins L Jr, Mirowski M, Mower MM, et al: Automatic defibrillation in man. The initial surgical experience. *J Thorac Cardiovasc Surg* 1981; 82:492–500.

Watkins L Jr, Mower MM, Reid PR, Platia EV, Griffith L, Mirowski M: Surgical techniques for implanting the automatic implantable defibrillator. *PACE* 1984; 7:1357–1362.

Watkins L Jr, Platia EV, Mower MM, et al: The treatment of malignant ventricular arrhythmias with combined endocardial resection and implantation of the automatic defibrillator: Preliminary report. *Ann Thorac Surg* 1984; 37:60–66.

Winkle RA: Editorial comment: Amiodarone and the American way. *JACC* 1985; 6:822–824.

Winkle RA, Bach S, Echt D, Swerdlow C, Imran M, Mason J, Oyer P, Stinson E: The automatic implantable defibrillator: Local ventricular bipolar sensing to detect ventricular tachycardia and fibrillation. *Am J Cardiol* 1983; 52:265–270.

Winkle RA, Stinson EB, Echt DS, et al: Practical aspects of automatic cardioverter/defibrillator implantation. *Am Heart J* 1984; 108:1335–1346.

Chapter 13

Pacing for Tachycardia

David R. Holmes Jr.

The application of pacing for the treatment or prevention of tachycardia is not new, but it is increasing in frequency. This increase is the result of widespread use of electrophysiological evaluation, improved knowledge about the mechanism of arrhythmias, and changes in pacing technology. These developments should allow for even greater utilization of pacing for tachycardia in the future.

There are two basic approaches to pacing for tachycardia: (1) pacing for prevention, and (2) pacing for termination. A third approach, which is only rarely utilized, is to alter the rate of tachycardia without terminating it in an attempt to improve the patient's physiological tolerance of the tachycardia. Before these approaches are used, it is necessary to identify the specific arrhythmia, its anatomical/physiological substrate, and the setting in which it occurs. In the majority of patients, detailed electrophysiological assessment is required; in some patients, analysis of ambulatory monitoring data can supply all of the information required.

PACING FOR PREVENTION OF TACHYCARDIA

Elimination of Bradycardia

The most common reason for pacing to prevent tachycardia is to eliminate bradycardia. The typical sequence is bradycardia followed by escape supraventricular or ventricular arrhythmias, some of which may be sustained (Figure 1, 2). In this setting, the tachycardia is usually the result of bradycardia; the bradycardia is often symptomatic and would require pacing in any event. Pacing acts to prevent arrhythmias by one of several mechanisms including: (a) shortening diastole and providing less opportunity for ectopic escape beats; (b) decreasing the variability in the rate of recovery of excitability, and (c) decreasing the dispersion of refractoriness, which is aggravated by bradycardia (thus reducing the likelihood of re-entrant arrhythmias).

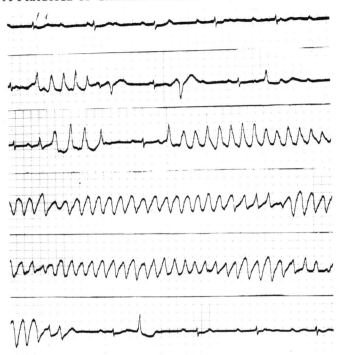

Figure 1.   *Electrocardiogram documenting complete heart block. Escape ventricular ectopy results in nonsustained ventricular tachycardia and torsades de pointes. Permanent pacing may suppress ventricular ectopy and prevent ventricular tachycardia.*

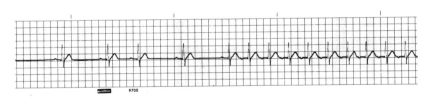

Figure 2.   *Underlying sinus bradycardia with atrial premature contractions that result in supraventricular tachycardia.*

In addition to providing a physiological support of the cardiac rate, permanent pacing may improve hemodynamics in patients with organic heart disease, and may decrease atrial and ventricular ectopy, thus decreasing the precipitating or triggering events for tachycardia.

Bradycardia followed by an escape arrhythmia is relatively common in patients with sinus node dysfunction, and may result in recurrent tachycardia. Support of the base rate, and avoidance of atrial bradycardia may prevent or reduce episodes of tachycardia without the need for antiarrhythmic agents. Bradycardia-dependent ventricular arrhythmias, either in the setting of sinus node dysfunction or atrioventricular (AV) block, may also be improved or even eliminated by providing a physiological base rate support. It must be emphasized that identification of bradycardia followed by tachycardia is essential to improve the likelihood that pacing may prevent tachycardia in these patients. Ambulatory or in-hospital monitoring is necessary to document the typical sequence of bradycardia, then tachycardia. Detailed invasive electrophysiological assessment may not be required in this setting.

Overdrive Suppression

Arrhythmias may also be prevented by overdrive suppression, particularly in patients with ventricular ectopy. In patients with ventricular arrhythmias, suppression by atrial overdrive pacing may even be more effective than ventricular overdrive pacing, particularly if there is hemodynamic benefit achieved by maintaining AV synchrony. Increasing the paced rate results in suppression of both atrial and ventricular ectopy, and thereby, decreases the precipitating triggering event for tachycardia. This technique has its widest application as a temporary treatment, for example, in the postoperative setting, following myocardial infarction, or in the patient with drug or metabolic induced arrhythmias. In this setting, while treatment of either the underlying cardiac disease or the cause of the arrhythmias is being undertaken, temporary overdrive pacing may be useful. In those patients with symptomatic, drug resistant arrhythmias, permanent overdrive pacing also may be helpful.

Ventricular arrhythmias associated with QT prolongation syndromes are particularly well suited for overdrive pacing. The QT prolongation may be drug related in which case the accompanying ventricular arrhythmia can be managed by temporary atrial pacing until the offending drug has been withdrawn, or may be idiopathic or congenital. In the latter, if temporary pacing is effective, a permanent overdrive unit may be implanted.

The pacing rates chosen for overdrive suppression vary. The rate used may be significantly slower than the rate of tachycardia to be suppressed. If the patient is in tachycardia at the onset of pacing, tachycardia is terminated by overdrive suppression. The pacing rate needed for overdrive termination and suppression is then gradually decreased until the lowest rate that will prevent tachycardia from recurring. This rate then is continued. Alternatively, the pacing rate is initially set at 5 to 10 beats above the intrinsic normal rate, and then gradually increased until prevention of recurrent arrhythmias is achieved. The final rate should be the lowest rate that suppresses tachycardia. This concept is particularly important in the patient with arteriosclerotic heart disease or valvular heart disease in whom increasing the rate may aggravate hemodynamics or ischemia, and actually worsen the arrhythmia.

Tachycardia can also be prevented by eliminating the electrophysiological substrate for the arrhythmia. This approach received increased attention with the recognition of pacemaker-mediated tachycardia. In these patients, with intact ventriculoatrial (VA) conduction, ventricular pacing often resulted in recurrent tachycardias. Other pacemaker-induced arrhythmias include atrial fibrillation, for example, when DVI pacing was used or when intact VA conduction resulted in atrial stimulation during the atrial vunerable period. Recognition of the mechanisms of these arrhythmias has resulted in modifications in the devices available as well as changes in pacing modalities selected, which have been useful in preventing these pacemaker-mediated arrhythmias.

PACING FOR TERMINATION OF TACHYCARDIA

In addition to preventing tachycardia, pacing can be useful for terminating paroxysmal tachycardia. This application has achieved increasing clinical utility. Evaluation of the role of pacing in the termination of tachycardia is complex, and involves consideration of the two major mechanisms of tachycardia, re-entry and automaticity. Differentiation of these two mechanisms is based, in part, upon findings at the time of electrophysiological study. Supraventricular or ventricular arrhythmias that can be induced and terminated by single or multiple critically-timed premature extrastimuli or rapid stimulation are felt to be re-entrant. Automatic arrhythmias are those that cannot be reliably induced and terminated by stimulation techniques. This differentiation is arbitrary and overlap exists, particularly in triggered automatic arrhythmias. Even though the classification is arbitrary, it is very useful, particularly as it relates to pacing for tachycardia. It follows that pacing is more useful in arrhythmias that can be reliably induced, and then terminated by stimulation techniques (i.e., re-entrant arrhythmias).

Re-entry

Re-entry is the most common mechanism of tachycardia. It may occur at any level within the conduction system, and requires three conditions (Figure 3).

RE-ENTRY CONDITIONS

1. Two pathways connected proximally and distally, forming the limbs of the reentrant circuit.
   —The two limbs need not be anatomically distinct but only functionally different in terms of electrophysiological properties of impulse conduction and refractoriness.
2. Differential conduction of the impulse down the two limbs.
   —This differential conduction may be the result of autonomic tone, electrolyte changes, or anatomical abnormalities such as fibrosis, infarction, dilatation, or hypertrophy.
3. Unidirectional block in one pathway which allows antegrade conduction in one limb and retrograde conduction via the other limb.—It is dependent on the refractory periods of each limb and can be affected by drugs, metabolic changes, autonomic tone, and structural abnormalities.

In patients with re-entry arrhythmias, tachycardia can be initiated in the electrophysiological laboratory by single or multiple extrastimuli, or a train of premature impulses (Figure 4A, 4B). These impulses, if appropriately timed, change conduction or refractoriness (or both) in the re-entrant circuit, and can either start or terminate an existing tachycardia. During the tachycardia, premature impulses or a train of impulses (burst pacing) can invade one or both limbs of the re-entrant circuit and, by capturing the circuit or interrupting it, terminate the tachycardia (Figure 5).

Atrioventricular nodal tachycardia is one of the most common, and is the prototypical re-entrant arrhythmia. In patients with this electrophysiological substrate, there are two functional limbs within the AV node: (1) the alpha limb, characterized by slow conduction but rapid recovery (shorter refractoriness), and (2) the beta limb, characterized by faster conduction but slow recovery (longer refractoriness). A premature impulse (Figure 3) arriving at the AV node is conducted down the alpha pathway but is blocked in the beta pathway because of its slower recovery. When the impulse reaches the distal common

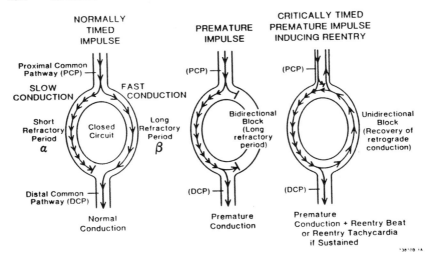

Figure 3. Schematic diagram of dual AV nodal pathways and AV nodal reentry. Proximal and distal common pathways are shown. The two limbs of the re-entrant circuit are characterized by different conduction and refractory properties. The slow-conducting pathway (α) has a short refractory period. During sinus rhythm, impulses are conducted down the fast pathway (β). A premature impulse (middle panel) is blocked in the fast pathway because of its long refractory period, and is conducted down the slow pathway. A critically timed premature impulse (right panel) can induce an atrial echo or re-entrant paroxysmal supraventricular tachycardia. (From Brandenburg RO, Fuster V, Giuliani ER, et al: Cardiology: Fundamentals and Practice. Yearbook Medical Publishers, Chicago, 1987. By permission of Mayo Foundation.)

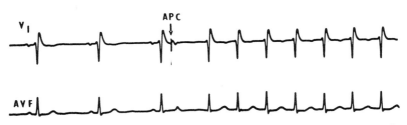

Figure 4A. Induction of supraventricular tachycardia by atrial premature complexes (APC). The prolonged PR interval following the APC is the result of block in the fast pathway and conduction down the slow pathway (see Figure 3).

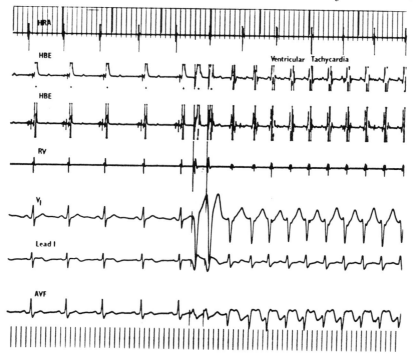

Figure 4B. *Induction of ventricular tachycardia by premature ventricular beats. After five sinus beats, two ventricular premature contractions (VPCs) are delivered, resulting in sustained ventricular tachycardia. HRA = high right atrium; HBE = His bundle electrogram; RV = right ventricular electrogram.*

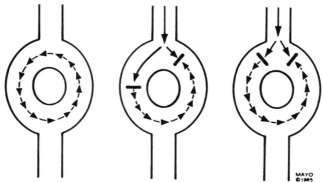

Figure 5. *Schematic of the effect of atrial stimulation on AV nodal re-entry tachycardia. Re-entrant arrhythmia circuit is shown on the left. An impulse may invade one limb of the circuit and block in the other limb (middle panel), or may block in each limb, interrupting the re-entrant circuit, and terminating tachycardia. (By permission of Mayo Foundation.)*

pathway, the beta pathway has recovered so that the impulse can travel in a retrograde direction and set the stage for AV nodal re-entry. All re-entrant arrhythmias share these common features, for example, two functional pathways connected proximally and distally with differential conduction and refractoriness in each limb, which allows for unidirectional block in one pathway. Electrophysiological assessment of the mechanisms is essential prior to consideration of pacing for termination of tachycardia.

Several factors affect the feasibility of terminating re-entrant arrhythmias by pacing. These include, (1) the site of stimulation. If the site of stimulation is remote to the re-entrant circuit, particularly if conduction to the re-entry circuit is delayed by associated conduction system disease, the ability to terminate tachycardia is decreased. Conversely, delivering single or multiple extrastimuli in close proximity to the re-entrant circuit increases the chance of termination. (2) Characteristics of the re-entrant circuit include cycle length and entrance and exit of cardiac impulses to and from the remainder of the heart. In general, if the tachycardia is fast and the circuit small and remote, termination will be more difficult, requiring rapid burst pacing as compared to single or double extrastimuli. In such circumstances, termination may not be possible. Conversely, with a slow tachycardia and large re-entrant circuit, for example, a slow atrioventricular re-entrant tachycardia, a single stimulus close to the site of re-entry may be very effective. The importance of these parameters can be assessed in the electrophysiological laboratory by determining how difficult it is to terminate tachycardia, and what stimulation protocol is needed, for example, single extrastimuli versus rapid cardiac pacing. Analysis of these factors is of utmost importance in evaluating a patient for pacing for tachycardia.

Automatic Arrhythmias

Automatic arrhythmias may occur at any level within the heart. These arrhythmias arise from disorders in impulse formation, compared to re-entry, which is related to impulse propagation. Automatic arrhythmias may arise in areas capable of spontaneous impulse formation, for example, the AV node, or may arise as the result of abnormalities, such as ischemia, which allows spontaneous depolarization of tissues that do not normally depolarize spontaneously, for example, ventricular muscle. Automatic arrhythmias usually cannot be terminated in the laboratory by electrical stimulation and therefore, pacing techniques for termination are not usually successful. However, if these automatic arrhythmias are bradycardia-dependent, then pacing to prevent tachycardia may be very successful.

CRITERIA FOR SELECTION OF PATIENTS

Pacing is only one of an expanding number of treatment options available for patients with recurrent tachycardia. These treatment methods are sometimes complementary and used in combination; at other times they are used alone. Drug therapy remains a standard treatment of choice. In some patients, drugs either do not work or are associated with significant cardiac or non-cardiac toxicity. This is particularly important in young patients who face a long duration of therapy for intermittent tachycardia. Current options to standard drugs include investigational agents, ablation of ventricular tachycardia foci, and ablation of re-entrant circuits such as anomalous atrioventricular pathways (either surgically or with catheter techniques), endocardial resection, left ventricular aneurysmectomy, electrophysiologically-guided endocardial resection, pacemakers, and implantable cardioverter/defibrillators. Selection of the most appropriate method of treatment depends on clinical factors, the availability of investigational drugs and devices, and the experience of the physician treating each patient.

Identification of patients who may be candidates for pacemaker termination of tachycardia follows electrophysiological assessment during which the tachycardia is induced by extrastimuli or rapid pacing. The mechanism is identified, for example, intra-atrial re-entry, AV nodal re-entry, or atrial flutter, and the stability and hemodynamic consequences of the arrhythmia are assessed. Once tachycardia is induced, a careful search for specific termination sequences is made. To consider permanent pacing for the treatment of paroxysmal tachycardia, one must repeatedly demonstrate its efficacy and safety. Efficacy and safety usually are documented for several days with temporary pacing, during which time the arrhythmia must be repeatedly induced, and safely and reliably terminated. One commonly used criterion involves 100 inductions of the arrhythmia with 100 successful terminations without its acceleration or its conversion to an unstable rhythm such as ventricular fibrillation. It is important to remember that changes in position, autonomic tone, and medications may all affect initiation and termination of tachycardia.

Patient selection criteria in antitachycardia pacing are evolving. The most important are documented efficacy, safety, and patient symptoms. If the patient's symptoms are very minimal and attacks can be easily self-terminated, for example, by vagal maneuvers, even though pacing is very effective and safe, it may not be warranted. The most suitable patients are those with infrequent but significantly symptomatic episodes, which cannot be self-terminated. Many of these patients have required repeated, urgent medical evaluations. Pacing may be an excellent alternative to long-term daily administration of medications to prevent infrequent attacks. In other patients, medications may be ineffective in preventing tachycardia, or may be associated with significant side effects, and pacing may be the treatment of choice. Many antiarrhythmic medications are especially unsuitable in young women who may become pregnant.

In patients with very frequent episodes of tachycardia, each of which could be terminated by pacing, the potential for rapid battery depletion exists. Concomitant antiarrhythmic therapy may need to be used to decrease the frequency of tachycardia in this situation.

Pacing is useful for a variety of supraventricular and ventricular arrhythmias (Table I), although it is more commonly used in patients with supraventricular tachycardia because of concerns about safety. In patients with ventricular tachycardia, these concerns are of greater importance because of the potentially severe or life-threatening consequences of deterioration to rapid ventricular tachycardia or ventricular fibrillation. In very carefully selected patients with stable ventricular tachycardia, long-term pacing can be safe and effective. In each patient, whether the arrhythmia is supraventricular or ventricular, these concerns must be addressed during evaluation, and prior to implantation of a permanent antitachycardia pacing system.

Table I
Rhythms Amenable to Pacing

Prevention of tachycardia	Termination of tachycardia
• Bradycardia-dependent	• Paroxysmal supraventricular tachycardia
Atrial flutter	Atrioventricular nodal re-entry
Atrial fibrillation	Atrioventricular re-entry
Supraventricular tachycardia	Intra-atrial re-entry
Ventricular ectopy	Atrial flutter
Ventricular tachycardia	• Paroxysmal ventricular tachycardia

PATIENT EVALUATION

Patient evaluation includes both invasive and noninvasive testing (Table II). The presence or absence of associated diseases, which may impact on the arrhythmia or its treatment, should be evaluated. The spontaneous characteristics of the arrhythmia should be studied to determine precipitating events. Careful invasive assessment is a cornerstone that defines the mechanism of tachycardia, and the underlying pathophysiologic substrate. During testing, tachycardia is induced, and its stability and hemodynamic consequences are assessed. With current devices, the tachycardia must be hemodynamically stable enough to allow for pacing termination. This is particularly true for the patient with ventricular tachycardia. In the future, combined devices with antitachycardia pacing capability but defibrillation back-up should have a major input. If the patient is a good candidate from a clinical treatment standpoint, then the baseline electrophysiological study is modified for extensive testing of tachycardia initiation and termination. In some patients this may be performed at the time of a second electrophysiological study. The effectiveness of different pacing sites and modes, the stability of the atrium or ventricle to the stimulation protocol during tachycardia, and the presence of associated electrophysiological abnormalities are assessed. Repeated testing is necessary to be certain that the stimulation protocol used does not result in acceleration of the tachycardia, conversion to another arrhythmia, for example, ventricular tachycardia to ventric-

---

Table II
Patient Evaluation

• Characterize Spontaneous Tachycardia
  Electrophysiological mechanism, rate, precipitating factors, frequency, response to medications, hemodynamic stability.
• Electrophysiological Assessment
  Characterize anatomical pathophysiological substrate, associated abnormalities, stability of tachycardia, identify optimal termination sequences, ascertain adverse effects of stimulation, evaluate effects of medication on rate and stimulation.
• Subsequent Testing
  Repeated induction and termination of tachycardia to document continued safety and efficacy of stimulation strategy using devices similar or identical to those to be implanted. Evaluate effects of time, changes in autonomic tone, and any antiarrhythmic medications to be used on initiation and termination.

---

ular fibrillation, or adverse hemodynamic effects. This is most important concerning patients in whom ventricular tachycardia is the arrhythmia to be treated. Ideally, a pulse generator similar to the one to be implanted should be used for termination testing. In addition to multiple attempts at termination in the laboratory, the patient is usually sent to the intensive care unit with a temporary pacemaker in place to allow for repeated testing over the next several days. If possible, this should be performed at rest, with changes in position, and even with limited exercise since all of these factors may impact on the ability to terminate spontaneous episodes. If antiarrhythmic drugs are to be used in conjunction with the pacemaker, the patient should be evaluated while on the specific drug regimen, prior to receiving the permanent pacemaker. This is important because antiarrhythmic drugs may affect tachycardia cycle length and termination parameters, which may require a change in the stimulation protocol. Increasing the number of attempts at tachycardia termination prior to implantation is optimal to try as to ensure continued efficacy of the device after permanent implantation.

SAFETY CONCERNS AND PACING

1. The potential for converting one arrhythmia, such as stable ventricular tachycardia to fibrillation.
2. The conversion of a stable ventricular tachycardia to one that is more malignant, cannot be terminated by the implanted device, or will convert to fibrillation either spontaneously or when termination is attempted automatically.
3. Rapid 1:1 AV conduction during high rate atrial pacing.
4. Accurate detection of the tachycardia, either automatically by the pulse generator or manually during a well-tolerated tachycardia by patients who have patient-activated units.
5. Prompt termination of the arrhythmia.
6. Maintenance of stimulation sequences that are stable over time and that will reliably terminate the tachycardia under a variety of clinical conditions.

Even with reliance on stringent criteria prior to implantation, during follow-up, in a sizable number of patients—up to 20–50%, the ease and ability of terminating tachycardia will change. Newer devices, which are programmable and adaptive, are helpful in this regard. The ability to use these implanted devices to initiate tachycardia and evaluate its termination noninvasively, following implantation, may also be helpful.

DEVICE DESIGN

There are two major device types: those that require patient interaction and those with automatic tachycardia detection and treatment.

Patient Interactive Devices

To use an interactive device, the patient must be able to detect tachycardia accurately, tolerate it until it is terminated, operate the pacemaker unit or device, and then recognize return to normal sinus rhythm. The device used for activation must always be available. These factors have limited the use of patient activated devices. The devices have the advantage that they allow patients to go to a medical facility, for example, an emergency room before activating the unit. In patients in whom pacing is used for the treatment of recurrent ventricular tachycardia, this ensures that resuscitation equipment is available if arrhythmia acceleration results.

There are two basic types of devices, one with an implanted power source, and the other with a power source supplied by an external electromagnetically-coupled unit.

Implanted Power Source

Devices with an implanted power source range from a conventional pacemaker to sophisticated antitachycardia pacing devices. For some patients in whom underdrive pacing is effective for termination, application of a conventional magnet, which converts the pulse generator to an asynchronous mode, is all that is needed (Figure 6). More sophisticated units now available can be programmed to deliver a variety of stimulation sequences, and can also be used for noninvasive initiation of tachycardia.

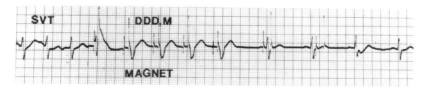

Figure 6. *Underdrive dual-chamber pacing in patient with supraventricular tachycardia (SVT). Application of magnet terminates tachycardia.*

External Power Source

Hand-held radiofrequency units have also been used. These units consist of a small implanted receiver (Figure 7). The hand-held portable transmitter activates the pacemaker to deliver preset stimulation sequences (Figure 8). The pulse frequency is adjustable in a wide range up to 400 pulses per minute. This device has the advan-

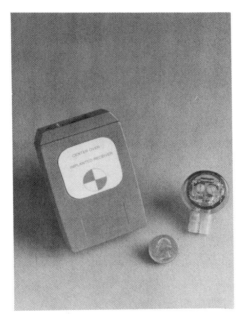

Figure 7.   *Hand held radiofrequency unit for stimulation. The hand-held portable transmitter (left) is centered over the implanted receiver (right). The device is of small size, as illustrated by the quarter.*

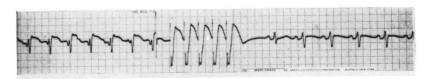

Figure 8.   *Stable recurrent ventricular tachycardia at 110 bpm. The patient recognizes the arrhythmia and terminates it by a short burst of pacing at 150 bpm from the radiofrequency pacemaker.*

tage of small size because it is a receiver only, and does not need sophisticated tachycardia detection systems. It has the disadvantage of limited flexibility in stimulation protocol. Another disadvantage is that the patient must be able to identify the pathological versus a physiological arrhythmia, such as sinus tachycardia.

AUTOMATIC DEVICES

Pulse generators capable of automatic detection and interruption of the tachycardia are being used with increasing frequency (Figure 9). These units do not depend on having the patient recognize the tachycardia. Instead, variable and often programmable criteria are used to detect a tachycardia. These criteria include absolute rate, number of impulses, percent change in cycle length compared to previous cycle lengths, and rate of change of cycle length over time. A programmable absolute rate and duration above which tachycardia is recognized is the simplest detection system. For example, the tachycardia detection criterion may be set at 187 beats per minute. The pulse generator treats any rate >187 bpm as tachycardia. The tachycardia detection mechanism is not activated by a lesser rate. A slower

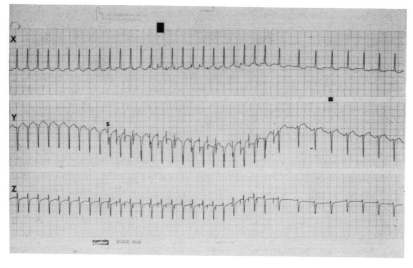

Figure 9. *Three lead electrocardiogram from a patient with recurrent supraventricular tachycardia. An implantable automatic overdrive pacemaker detects supraventricular tachycardia, and delivers a train of impulses (S) that terminates the arrhythmia, restoring sinus rhythm.*

tachycardia, for example with a longer cycle length, will not be detected as such, while a sinus (and therefore normal) tachycardia at a more rapid rate, i.e., a shorter cycle length, will be detected as pathologic.

Relying on rate alone does not provide the greatest flexibility. Tachycardia cycle length may vary over time, particularly with the addition of medications. Newer algorithms are being used and developed that recognize the suddenness of a rate of onset of tachycardia compared to the preceding normal beats. Other systems rely on biological and physiological sensors. These newer algorithms should make tachycardia detection more flexible and adaptive, and allow reliable differentiation of pathological from physiological arrhythmias.

For automatic devices, accurate sensing is essential. Because stimulation techniques can induce as well as terminate tachycardia, should abnormal sensing occur, for example, from electromyographic interference, and the pulse generator pace during normal sinus rhythm, it may initiate a tachycardia. It also is essential that the patient's spontaneous tachycardia rate be faster than the programmed detection rate criteria. For example, if the tachycardia rate is usually 175–180 bpm, the detection criteria must be <170 bpm or the pacemaker will not recognize the tachycardia. Difficulties may occur if the tachycardia rate detection criteria is less than the maximum sinus rhythm. This is of concern in several clinical circumstances, including:

1. slow tachycardia, for example, rates of 130–140 bpm;
2. a sinus rate faster than the tachycardia criterion, for example, sinus tachycardia during exercise;
3. more than one arrhythmia, for example, intermittent atrial flutter or fibrillation with rapid ventricular response, and also paroxysmal AV nodal re-entry. In this circumstance, depending on the rate of the two tachycardias, the pacemaker may only detect one. A variety of medications may be required in this situation, for example, beta blockers to reduce the maximum sinus rate, or other antiarrhythmic drugs to eliminate one tachycardia, leaving only one to be electrically terminated.

As mentioned before, new sensing algorithms should improve detection and facilitate correct treatment.

After recognition of tachycardia by the pulse generator, preset stimulation sequences (identified at the time of electrophysiological testing to be safe and effective) are automatically delivered to terminate a tachycardia. After each stimulation sequence, the pulse generator senses either return to sinus rhythm and is inhibited, or it senses tachycardia and repeats the stimulation sequence.

The management of tachyarrhythmias by implantable devices is a highly complex and rapidly evolving clinical effort requiring a high level of knowledge about the tachycardia as well the means of its termination. In addition to terminating tachycardia, current devices allow for performance of a limited electrophysiological study noninvasively by stimulation through the pulse generator. This may be of help in follow-up if the tachycardia changes or the device is not effective. Current devices also have counters that can document the frequency of tachycardia and the frequency of conversion sequences used for termination. Finally, adaptive devices are available that compile the most successful termination sequences. When tachycardia occurs, these successful sequences are initially tried before others are used.

STIMULATION STRATEGIES FOR TERMINATION OF TACHYCARDIA (Table III)

Underdrive Pacing

Underdrive pacing may be used in patients with either supraventricular or ventricular tachycardia (Figure 10). The ability to terminate tachycardia by one or more than one extrastimulus depends on the characteristics of the re-entrant circuit. During tachycardia, extrastimuli may be able to invade and capture a portion of the re-entrant circuit, thus disrupting the circling wave front. Underdrive pacing may be performed manually by magnet application, changing an implanted inhibited pacemaker to an asynchronous unit (Figure 6). The

---

Table III
Stimulation Strategies for Termination of Tachycardia

• Underdrive (Single-or Dual-Chamber)
   Asynchronous
   Scanning
      sequential, incremental, decremental, adaptive table
• Overdrive (Single-Chamber)
   Radiofrequency
   Automatic
• Combined Burst Pacing and Scanning
    Autodecremental, scanning burst, shifting burst, rapid burst

---

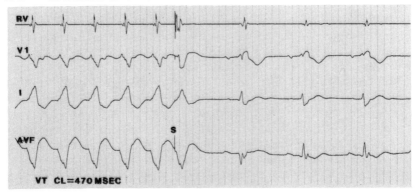

Figure 10. Underdrive pacing during ventricular tachycardia induced during elec-trophysiological testing. During VT (CL 470 msec), a single VPC (S) terminates tachycardia. RV = right ventricle, standard ECG leads V1, I, AVF.

pacemaker then stimulates asynchronously with stimuli falling at different times of the cardiac cycle. There is often a range of critical coupling intervals between the QRS complex and the extrastimulus. One, two, or more stimuli delivered during this "time window" can terminate the tachycardia by capturing and changing the re-entry circuit. If a single extrastimulus is not effective, adding additional extrastimuli may successfully terminate tachycardias. Both single-chamber atrial or ventricular, and dual-chamber pacemakers have been used.

Single-Chamber Pacemakers

Single-chamber pacemakers can be used for both atrial and ventricular arrhythmias. These are most effective in patients with slow tachycardia (usually <160 bpm), a large re-entrant circuit, a wide termination time window, and in patients in whom the single stimulus can be delivered in close proximity to the re-entrant circuit. This mode is not used frequently because if these criteria are not met, underdrive pacing is often not effective. In addition, unless the critical stimulation time window is wide, the time to termination is long. When found to be effective, however, underdrive pacing is a reasonable and quite safe option (Figure 10). It must be remembered that although uncommon, tachycardia acceleration can occur (Figure 11).

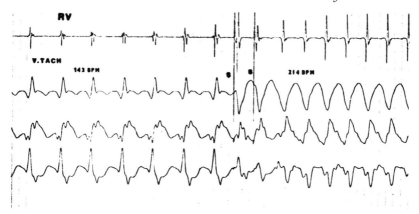

Figure 11. *Acceleration of ventricular tachycardia by two VPCs (S). Ventricular tachycardia (rate 143 bpm) induced during electrophysiological study. Two underdrive extrastimuli (S) are delivered, resulting in acceleration of VT to 214 bpm.*

Dual-Chamber Pacemakers

Dual-chamber pacemakers are particularly useful in patients with atrioventricular re-entry due to accessory pathways (Figure 12). The rationale is that nearly simultaneous capture of both atrium and ventricle may prevent continuation of the re-entry circuit. Underdrive dual-chamber pacing is again more effective in patients in whom there is a wide range of coupling intervals that can terminate tachycardia, and in patients with slower tachycardia rates. Because there is random stimulation during the cardiac cycle, termination of tachycardia may be delayed. Stimulation during the atrial vulnerable period may occur with the potential for inducing atrial fibrillation; this

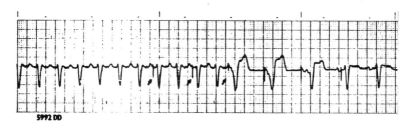

Figure 12. *Dual-demand pacemaker in patient with recurrent atrioventricular re-entry secondary to bypass tract. After detection of tachycardia, the pacemaker stimulates both atrium and ventricle (arrows), and terminates tachycardia.*

may promptly return to normal sinus rhythm or may be sustained. The potential for ventricular stimulation with induction of ventricular tachycardia or ventricular fibrillation must also be studied in the electrophysiological laboratory prior to implantation.

Scanning Pacemakers

Scanning is a type of underdrive pacing (Figure 13). As was true with conventional underdrive pacing, success with scanning strategies is increased with increasing cycle lengths (slower rate), a wider ter-

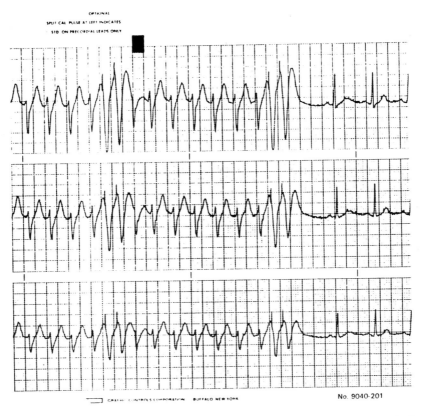

Figure 13.   *Three-channel electrocardiogram in a patient with recurrent ventricular tachycardia. An implantable patient-activated scanning pacemaker has been implanted. The first pair of coupled extrastimuli fail to terminate tachycardia, the second pair successfully return the patient to normal sinus rhythm.*

mination time window, and close proximity to the re-entrant circuit. Both patient-activated and automatic scanning devices are available. The automatic devices are extensively programmable (Figure 14).

TACHYCARDIA DETECTION

Select desired algorithm			1
1--high rate only			
Select criteria			
High rate	Rate, bpm	163	
	Interval, msec	369	
	Intervals, no.	10	
Sudden onset	Delta, msec	123	
Rate stability	Delta, msec	26	
	Intervals, no.	20	
Sus high rate	Intervals, no.	75	

Tach   Response   Return

CG114659B 4

Figure 14A. *Some devices currently used are extensively programmable. The tachycardia detection criteria can be modified according to, for example, rate, onset, rate stability, and sustained rate.*

TACHYCARDIA RESPONSE

Parameter	Primary	Secondary
Scanning	On	Off
Pulses, no.	10	
Delay, msec	5	
Burst cycle length	85%	
Attempts, no.		
Autodecrement		
Minimum cycle length, msec	20	

Scanning parameter   Return

CG114659B-1

Figure 14B. *The tachycardia response can be programmed for number of pulses delivered, delay, and burst cycle length.*

SCANNING PARAMETERS

		Primary burst cycle length	
Sequence		Dec	
Step Size, msec		10.2	
Dec = 0.5 inc		No	
Steps, no.		7	
Window duration		72	msec
Sequences, no.		5	
			Return

CG1146598 2

Figure 14C. *Finally, scanning parameters can also be programmed decremental scanning, sequence number, etc.*

After detection of tachycardia and activation, these units introduce an extrastimulus or multiple extrastimuli at progressively shorter coupling intervals during diastole. Scanning during diastole maximizes the chance of prompt stimulation during the range of coupling intervals in which the tachycardia can be terminated. In addition, it is adaptive. This is helpful in dealing with the problem of a variable termination zone. In some units, the coupling intervals can be programmed to a percentage of the tachycardia cycle length. This may help dealing with the variable tachycardia rates caused by changing autonomic tone or drug effects. It must be kept in mind that when more than one extrastimulus is delivered, the chance of acceleration is greater than when a single extrastimulus is used.

Several pacing modalities have been used including sequential and incremental or decremental scanning. Other forms incorporate a self-searching mode and adaptive table scanning (Figure 15). With decremental scanning, the initial extrastimulus is delivered at a slightly shorter interval than the tachycardia cycle length, and then progressively shorter coupling intervals are used until termination. If a single stimulus is ineffective, then two can be programmed. For incremental scanning, a similar sequence is performed in reverse beginning just beyond the refractory period determined at the time of electrophysiological study. Such units are extensively programmable. This is important because the tachycardia may vary under different circumstances. Even though scanning is effective, the mean duration

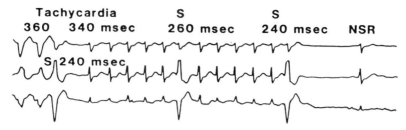

Figure 15. *Adaptive scanning. During a wide QRS complex tachycardia at CL 360 msec, the last beat of a scanning sequence (S) at 240 msec converts the wide QRS complex tachycardia to a narrow complex tachycardia at a faster rate of 340 msec. The pacing system senses the arrhythmia, and adapts the next extrastimulus to be delivered at 260 msec. The second extrastimulus is then delivered at 240 msec, and terminates tachycardia. (From Holmes DR Jr., Vlietstra RE:* Interventional Cardiology. *F. A. Davis Publishers, Philadelphia, in press.)*

of pacing prior to termination may be up to 1 to 1½ minutes. Therefore, it is important to select patients with well tolerated tachycardia.

Some new pacing systems include an adaptable table scanning. For this, the most successful stimulation protocols previously used are stored in the pacemaker and are used first, at the time of subsequent tachycardia. Self-searching modes are also available in which the stimulation protocol is adjusted automatically, depending upon the effect of stimulation on tachycardia.

Overdrive Pacing

Overdrive pacing has been a more widely used method of terminating tachycardia. It has the advantage that it is often more effective than underdrive pacing, and results in more prompt return to normal sinus rhythm. In fact, burst pacing may be effective when all other pacing sequences fail. It will potentially terminate all types of re-entrant arrhythmias. It also has the potential for accelerating arrhythmias or converting tachycardia to fibrillation (Figure 16). For this reason, it has been more commonly used in patients with supraventricular tachycardia; although, in some patients with slow stable ventricular tachycardia, it has been used after extensive testing. In patients with ventricular tachycardia, the development of a device with combined rapid pacing and defibrillation capability may be very useful.

The rate required for termination varies. In general, a rate ap-

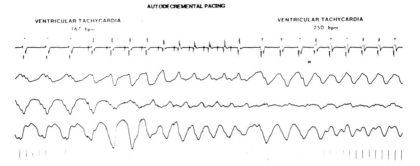

Figure 16. Autodecremental tachycardia acceleration. Autodecremental pacing during rapid ventricular tachycardia, resulting in tachycardia acceleration associated with hemodynamic compromise. bpm = beats per minute. (From Holmes DR Jr., Vlietstra RE: Interventional Cardiology. F. A. Davis Publishers, Philadelphia, in press.)

proximately 25% faster than the tachycardia rate is required for termination. Pacing at slower rates that are just slightly faster than the rate of tachycardia may entrain the arrhythmia without terminating it. Alternatively, with very fast stimulation rates, the arrhythmia may be changed from an organized tachycardia to fibrillation. With supraventricular tachycardia (SVT) and rapid pacing, atrial fibrillation may result; this is sometimes transient and then returns to normal sinus rhythm. In patients with enhanced AV nodal conduction or a rapidly conducting accessory pathway, the potential for rapid 1:1 conduction also exists. Stimulation sequences should be as short as possible, and limited to that required for termination. In general, 5–10 capture beats are sufficient. If that sequence is not effective, a slightly more rapid rate should be tested.

For ventricular arrhythmias, overdrive pacing is commonly used during electrophysiological testing. Similar concerns exist as for supraventricular tachycardia, namely that the more rapid the stimulation, the greater the chance of acceleration of the arrhythmia, or conversion to ventricular fibrillation. In addition, with more rapid pacing, the hemodynamics are further depressed. Attempts should be made to keep the burst rate as slow and short in duration as possible to minimize the potential for acceleration or adverse hemodynamic consequences. In some patients, identification of a drug that slows tachycardia rate but has failed to prevent it is useful so that the slowest pacing sequence for termination can be used. New devices with combined defibrillation capacity should make overdrive burst pacing for ventricular tachycardia more readily used.

Combined burst pacing/scanning devices have recently been developed that combine scanning and burst techniques. These include autodecremental burst pacing, scanning burst and shifting burst modes (Figure 17). With autodecremental pacing, after tachycardia detection, the first stimulus cycle length is delivered at a slightly shorter (programmable) cycle length. Each subsequent stimulus cycle length is decreased by similar degree. Shifting or scanning burst modes offer a different approach with the introduction of premature impulses at a specific delay following a tachycardia complex. A burst or multiple extrastimuli is then administered. The role that these combination devices will have for the treatment of ventricular arrhythmias remains unclear.

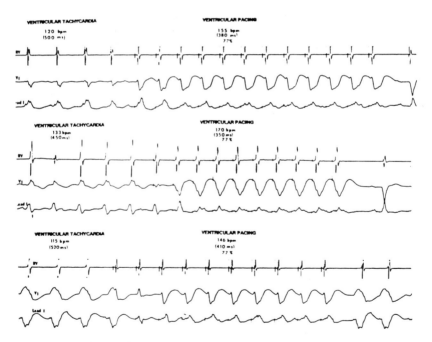

Figure 17. *Shifting (adaptive) burst pacing. Three morphologically different ventricular tachycardias in the same patient. Burst is synchronized to R wave during tachycardia, and burst rate is programmed to be 77% of the tachycardia cycle length. bpm = beats per minute; RV = right ventricular electrogram. Electrocardiographical leads: V_1, I. (From Holmes DR Jr., Vlietstra RE:* Interventional Cardiology. *F. A. Davis Publishers, Philadelphia, in press.)*

SUMMARY

The number of pacemakers available for the treatment of arrhythmias is increasing rapidly. The units are becoming more complex and sophisticated. Problems exist including optimal sensing algorhithms, backup pacing modes, lack of cardioversion and defibrillation capacity, and lack of enough flexibility to adapt to changing tachycardia characteristics over time. In many instances, the technology has gone beyond the ability of casual users to understand and manage the systems. This has important implications for the follow-up care and evaluation of these patients. At present, the decision to use any of these technology approaches must be made after the most careful analysis of the clinical setting and the specific arrhythmia. Electrophysiological testing, an essential part of this decision making, is required to document the mechanism of arrhythmia, and the safety and efficacy of the tachycardia termination technique. Careful follow-up is required to make sure that the devices perform in the manner for which they are intended. Repeated electrophysiological testing, either using the pacemaker itself for tachycardia induction, or using temporary transvenous pacemakers, may be required.

BIBLIOGRAPHY

Akhtar M, Gilbert CJ, Al-Nouri M, et al: Electrophysiologic mechanisms for modification and abolition of atrioventricular junctional tachycardia with simultaneous and sequential atrial and ventricular pacing. *Circulation* 1979; 60:1443–1454.

Bennett MA, Pentecost BL: Suppression of ventricular tachyarrhythmias by transvenous intracardiac pacing after acute myocardial infarction. *Br Med J [Clin Res]* 1970; 4:468–470.

Bertholet M, Demouilin JC, Waleffe A, et al: Pacing methods for the treatment of recurrent paroxysmal ventricular tachycardia. *Ann NY Acad Sci* 1984; 427:286–296.

Camm AJ, Davies DW, Ward DE: Tachycardia recognition by implantable electronic devices. *PACE* 1987; 10:1175–1190.

Castellanos A, Waxman HL, Berkovits BV, et al: Implantable pacemakers for cardiac tachyarrhythmias. *Cardiovasc Clin* 1980; 11(no. 1):159–173.

Cheng TO: Transvenous ventricular pacing in the treatment of paroxysmal atrial tachyarrhythmias alternating with sinus bradycardia and standstill. *Am J Cardiol* 1968; 22:874–879.

Critelli G, Grassi G, Chiarello M, et al: Automatic "scanning" by radiofrequency in the long-term electrical treatment of arrhythmias. *PACE* 1979; 2:289–296.

den Dulk K, Bertholet M, Brugada P, et al: Clinical experience with implantable devices for control of tachyarrhythmias. *PACE* 1984; 7:548–556.

DiSegni E, Klein HO, David D, et al: Overdrive pacing in quinidine syncope and other long QT-interval syndromes. *Arch Intern Med* 1980; 140:1036–1040.

Fisher JD: Role of electrophysiologic testing in the diagnosis and treatment of patients with known and suspected bradycardias and tachycardia. *Prog Cardiovasc Dis* 1981; 24:25–90.

Fisher JD, Cohen HL, Mehra R, et al: Cardiac pacing and pacemakers. II. Serial electrophysiologic-pharmacologic testing for control of recurrent tachyarrhythmias. *Am Heart J* 1977; 93:658–668.

Fisher JD, Johnston DR, Furman S, et al: Long-Term efficacy of antitachycardia pacing for supraventricular and ventricular tachycardias. *Am J Cardiol* 1987; 60:1311–1316.

Fisher JD, Kim SG, Furman S, et al: Role of implantable pacemakers in control of recurrent ventricular tachycardia. *Am J Cardiol* 1982; 49:194–206.

Fisher JD, Kim SG, Matos JA, et al: Comparative effectiveness of pacing techniques for termination of well-tolerated sustained ventricular tachycardia. *PACE* 1983; 6:915–922.

Fisher JD, Mehra R, Furman S: Termination of ventricular tachycardia with bursts of rapid ventricular pacing. *Am J Cardiol* 1978; 41:94–102.

Griffin JC, Mason JW, Ross DL, et al: The treatment of ventricular tachycardia using an automatic tachycardia terminating pacemaker. *PACE* 1981; 4:582–588.

Hartzler GO: Treatment of recurrent ventricular tachycardia by patient-activated radiofrequency ventricular stimulation. *Mayo Clin Proc* 1979; 54:75–82.

Hartzler GO, Holmes DR Jr, Osborn MJ: Patient-activated transvenous cardiac stimulation for the treatment of supraventricular and ventricular tachycardia. *Am J Cardiol* 1981; 47:903–909.

Holt P, Crick JCP, Sowton E: Antitachycardia pacing: A comparison of burst overdrive, self searching and adaptive table scanning programs. *PACE* 1986; 9:490–497.

Johnson RA, Hutter AM Jr, DeSanctis RW, et al: Chronic overdrive pacing in the control of refractory ventricular arrhythmias. *Ann Intern Med* 1974; 80:380–383.

Kastor JA, DeSanctis RW, Harthorne JW, et al: Transvenous atrial pacing in the treatment of refractory ventricular irritability. *Ann Intern Med* 1967; 66:939–945.

Medina-Ravell V, Maduro C, Mejias J, et al: Use of dual-demand AV sequential (DVI, MN) pacemakers in the management of supraventricular tachycardias. *Cardiovasc Clin* 1983; 14(no. 2): 227–238.

Mirowski M, Reid PR, Mower MN, et al: Termination of malignant ventricular arrhythmias with an implanted automatic defibrillator in human beings. *N Engl J Med* 1980; 303:322–324.

Mirowski M, Reid PR, Mower MM, et al: Clinical performance of the implantable cardioverter-defibrillator. *PACE* 1984; 7:1345–1350.

Moss AJ, Rivert RJ Jr, Griffith LSC, et al: Transvenous left atrial pacing for the control of recurrent ventricular fibrillation. *N Engl J Med* 1968; 278:928–931.

Osborn MJ, Holmes DR: Antitachycardia pacing. *Clin Prog Electrophysiol Pacing* 1985; 3:239–269.

Peters RW, Shafton E, Frank S, et al: Radiofrequency-triggered pacemakers: Uses and limitations. *Ann Intern Med* 1978; 88:17–22.

Preston TA, Haynes RE, Gavin WA, et al: Permanent rapid atrial pacing to control supraventricular tachycardia. *PACE* 1979; 2:331–334.

Ruskin JN, Garan H, Poulin F, et al: Permanent radiofrequency ventricular pacing for management of drug-resistant ventricular tachycardia. *Am J Cardiol* 1980; 46:317–321.

Saksena S, Camm AJ, Bilitch M, et al: Clinical investigation of implantable antitachycardia devices: Report of the policy conference of the North American Society of Pacing and Electrophysiology. *J Am Coll Cardiol* 1987; 10:225–229.

Spurrell RAJ, Sowton E: Pacing techniques in the management of supraventricular tachycardias. Part 2. An implanted atrial synchronous pacemaker with a short atrioventricular delay for the prevention of paroxysmal supraventricular tachycardias. *J Electrocardiol* 1976; 9:89–96.

Sugrue DD, McLaran C, Hammill SC, et al: Refractory supraventricular tachycardia in the neonate: Treatment with temporary antitachycardial pacing. *Mayo Clin Proc* 1985; 60:169–172.

Sung RJ, Styperek JL, Castellanos A: Complete abolition of the reentrant supraventricular tachycardia zone using a new modality of cardiac pacing with simultaneous atrioventricular stimulation. *Am J Cardiol* 1980; 45:72–78.

Waldo AL, MacLean WAH, Karp RB, et al: Continuous rapid atrial pacing to control recurrent or sustained supraventricular tachycardias following open heart surgery. *Circulation* 1976; 54:245–250.

Waldo AL, Wells JL Jr, Cooper TB, et al: Temporary cardiac pacing: Applications and techniques in the treatment of cardiac arrhythmias. *Prog Cardiovasc Dis* 1981; 23:451–474.

Watkins L Jr, Mower MM, Reid PR, et al: Surgical techniques for implanting the automatic implantable defibrillator. *PACE* 1984; 7:1357–1362.

Wellens HJJ: Value and limitations of programmed electrical stimulation of the heart in the study and treatment of tachycardia. *Circulation* 1978; 57:845–853.

Wellens HJJ, Bär FW, Gorgels AP, et al: Electrical management of arrhythmias with emphasis on the tachycardias. *Am J Cardiol* 1978; 41:1025–1034.

Wiener I: Pacing techniques in the treatment of tachycardias. *Ann Intern Med* 1980; 93:326–329.

Winkle RA: Electronic control of ventricular tachyarrhythmias: Overview and future directions. *PACE* 1984; 7:1375–1379.

Zipes DP: Electrical treatment of tachycardia *Circulation* 1987; 75(suppl III): III 190–193.

Zipes DP, Heger JJ, Miles WM, et al: Preliminary experience with the implantable transvenous cardioverter. *PACE* 1984; 7:1325–1330.

Chapter 14

PACEMAKER COMPLICATIONS

David L. Hayes

Pacemaker complications are relatively infrequent. They can occur intraoperatively, soon after implantation, or at a time distant from implantation (Table 1).

Table I
Pacemaker Complications

Early Complications	Late Complications	Early or Late Complications
Pneumothorax	Skin erosion	Lead dislodgment
Hematoma formation	Skin adherence	Arrhythmias
Lead perforation	Thrombosis	Tip extrasystoles
Lead damage	Radiation damage	Runaway pacemaker
	Pacemaker failure	Twiddler's syndrome
	Development of	Direct current countershock
	high threshold	Electrocautery induced
		abnormalities
		Pacemaker infection
		Pacemaker syndrome
		Pacemaker allergy

EARLY COMPLICATIONS

Most patients undergoing pacemaker implantation have some discomfort at the site of the incision in the early postoperative period. Although the incision is usually small, the operation is not different from any other surgical procedure, and mild analgesics (not aspirin, which can cause bleeding) may be required. Mild ecchymoses around the incision are not uncommon.

Pneumothorax

Access to the subclavian vein, commonly used for implantation of an endocardial pacemaker lead, is usually by subclavian vein puncture with a modified Seldinger technique. The vein usually is approached blindly. Because of the relationship of the subclavian vein to the apex of the lung, the possibility of lung injury and traumatic pneumothorax (Figure 1) or hemopneumothorax (Figure 2) is always

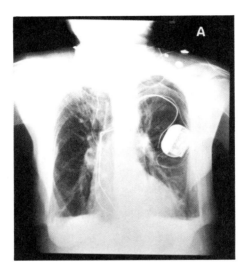

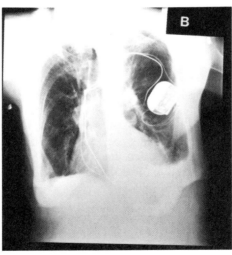

Figure 1. A.   *Left apical pneumothorax after pacemaker implantation.* ***B.*** *Two days later, there has been some resolution of pneumothorax.*

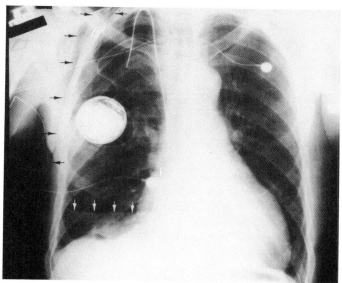

Figure 2. *Right apical pneumothorax after implantation of a transvenous pacemaker via the right subclavian vein. In addition, there is subcutaneous emphysema (black arrows). White arrows denote hemothorax.*

present. Hemothorax can be caused by laceration of the subclavian artery and hemopneumothorax by laceration of the lung and the subclavian artery. In a patient with unusual anatomy of the chest wall or clavicle, the subclavian vein can be displaced and the usual landmarks used for subclavian puncture can be altered. Anatomy must be taken into account before subclavian puncture is undertaken.

If pneumothorax occurs, it may be manifest during the pacemaker procedure or as late as 48 hours after implantation. Prompt chest x-ray after subclavian puncture is very useful. Indications that pneumothorax has occurred are as follows: (1) apiration of air during the subclavian puncture when the exploring needle is either introduced or removed; (2) unexplained hypotension; (3) chest pain; (4) respiratory embarrassment.

Following subclavian puncture, the lung fields should be visualized intraoperatively with fluoroscopy and postoperatively with a chest radiograph. A pneumothorax that brings the apex of the lung down to the second or third interspace or involves less than 10% of the pleural space probably can be observed without thoracic intubation. Surgical consultation should be considered if any of the following exist: (1) a pneumothorax of greater than 10%; (2) respiratory embarrassment; (3) hemopneumothorax.

Hematoma Formation (see also Chapter 5)

Because local ecchymoses (Figure 3) are common after pacemaker implantation, a small or large ecchymosis that is not expanding is treated by observation only. Discrete hematoma formation at the site must be dealt with on the basis of its secondary consequences (Figure 4). If there is continued bleeding or the hematoma is painful, it must be evacuated. If it does not compromise the suture line or skin integrity, it should be observed without intervention. Because of ineffectiveness and the risk of infection, early hematoma aspiration should not be attempted. Late aspiration may be attempted in a careful sterile procedure after the hematoma has liquified.

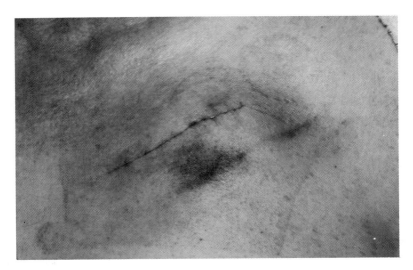

Figure 3.   *An incision shortly after placement of a permanent pacemaker with surrounding ecchymosis. This small amount of bruising is considered normal after pacemaker implantation.*

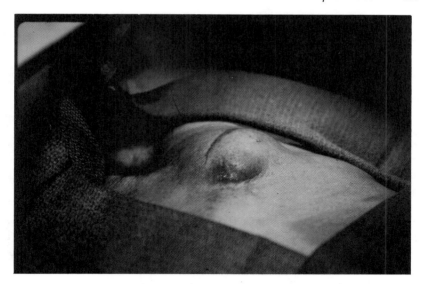

Figure 4. *Erythema at a margin of the pulse generator, even if the remainder of the overlying skin appears normal, is a frequent indication of low-grade, indolent infection. The wound should be cultured.*

To avoid hematoma formation, patients should have a normal prothrombin time before pacemaker implantation, and heparin administration should have been discontinued at least 6 hours before implantation. The patient should not have recently used aspirin or other platelet-inhibitory drugs. Antiplatelet drugs may be the most common cause of hematoma formation. In patients who have been receiving them, hemostasis during implantation often is quite difficult.

In patients who require therapeutic anticoagulation, a 48-hour delay after implantation is wise before resuming full heparinization. Warfarin (Coumadin) administration probably can begin at the patient's maintenance dose 24 hours after implantation, but the absolute timing varies from patient to patient. Anticoagulation at greater than therapeutic levels can result in late hematoma formation.

Arterial Lead Puncture and Cannulation

Subclavian artery puncture is a well recognized complication of subclavian vein puncture. It is usually easily recognized by the pulsating nature of the blood return and/or the aspirating syringe being filled under pressure. If this is recognized promptly and the needle removed and pressure held over the area for a short period of time, it is unlikely to result in any problem as a result of the arterial puncture. A hemothorax could occur if the artery is lacerated but this is an extremely rare complication.

There have been many anecdotal reports of an introducer and/or pacing lead being passed into the subclavian artery before it is realized that the arterial system has been cannulated. The most common reason for this mistake is that the systemic pressure is low and no pulsations are appreciated when the vessel is punctured. If arterial lead placement occurs, it is almost always recognized as the lead is passed and fluoroscopy reveals an unusual course of the lead. There have been anecdotal reports of this going unrecognized and the lead remaining in a left ventricular position. While the left ventricle can easily be stimulated, the concern is that of possible embolization into the arterial circulation. In the rare event that a patient presents with a permanent lead in the arterial circulation, it should be removed.

A pacing lead may also be placed in the left ventricle by passing it across an unsuspected ventricular septal defect. In a patient with a ventricular septal defect, endocardial pacing should be avoided. Even though symptomatic embolization is uncommon with right ventricular endocardial pacing, the potential exists for small emboli that are too small to cause clinical manifestations. Such small emboli could potentially cause symptoms in the arterial circulation.

Lead Perforation

Lack of symptoms after ventricular perforation by a lead is not uncommon. The only sign may be a rising stimulation threshold. In other patients, the signs may include:

1. right bundle block paced rhythm when the lead has been placed in the right ventricle;
2. intercostal muscle or diaphragmatic contraction;
3. friction rub after implantation;
4. pericarditis, pericardial effusion or cardiac tamponade (Figure 5).

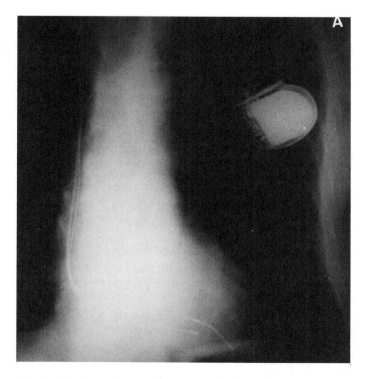

Figure 5.   *Ventricular perforation by a pacing lead.* **A.** *On a posteroanterior film, although the lead can be seen to cross the border of the diaphragm, perforation is difficult to diagnose.*

The diagnostic techniques used to identify ventricular perforation are chest radiography, electrocardiography, and two-dimensional echocardiography (Figure 6). Once the perforation has been identified, the lead must be withdrawn and repositioned. Lead withdrawal rarely results in pericardial bleeding or tamponade.

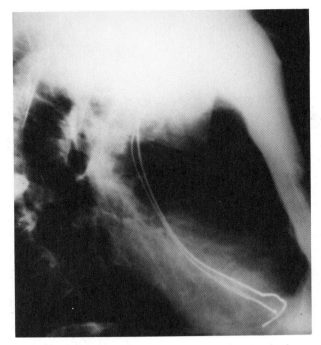

Figure 5B. *On a lateral projection, however, the perforating lead extends past the end of the pacing lead within the ventricle, enters the pericardium, and forms a curve in the pericardial space.*

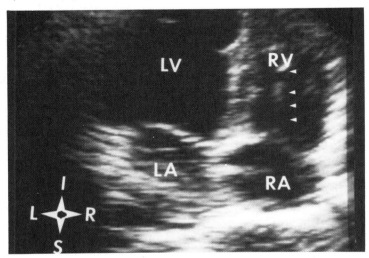

Figure 6. *An echocardiogram identifies a lead (arrowheads) in a correct ventricular apical position. I = Inferior; L = Left; LA = Left Atrium; LV = Left Ventricle; R = Right; RA = Right Atrium; RV = Right Ventricle; S = Superior.*

Lead Damage

Lead damage during pacemaker implantation may be more common than is recognized. Damage of silicone rubber leads seemed to occur less frequently in the past, but urethane leads are more vulnerable to mishandling during the operative procedure. Both types of leads are easily cut by scissors or scalpel, and repair is difficult. Polyurethane leads can be easily damaged by placement of a ligature directly around the lead itself (Figure 7). To secure the lead, the protector sleeve provided on many polyurethane leads or a "butterfly" sleeve that can be secured around the lead and then to the underlying support structures should be used.

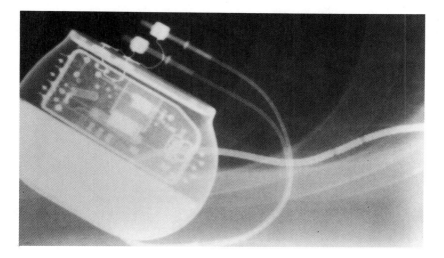

Figure 7. *Two indentations on the pacemaker lead are ligature compression of the insulating material. This anomaly has been referred to by some as "pseudofracture". Polyurethane leads can be easily damaged by tight ligatures.*

LATE COMPLICATIONS

The definition of the late postimplantation period varies, but generally begins one month after pacemaker implantation. The complications listed below usually are seen after one month, but there are exceptions to all cases.

Skin Erosion

Although erosion of the pulse generator through the skin usually occurs long after implantation, it is most often related to the implantation technique (Figure 8). Erosion is a rare complication that usually occurs in four situations.

CAUSES OF EROSION

1. The pacemaker pocket formed at the time of surgery is too small for the implanted pulse generator;
2. The pulse generator is implanted too superficially, as in children or small-framed adults in whom lack of adipose tis-

sue results in the pacemaker being "tight" despite adequate pocket size;
3. The generator is implanted too far laterally in the anterior axillary fold;
4. An indolent infection is present (see below).

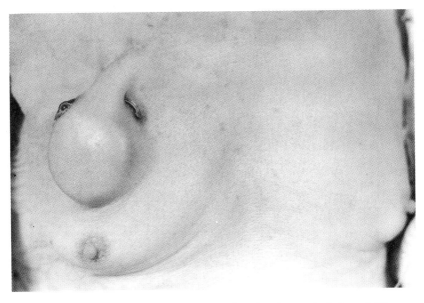

Figure 8. *Extrusion of an implanted pacemaker placed excessively lateral. The pacemaker is very adherent to the skin and the pocket is tight. Portions of the lead and pacemaker are exposed.*

When pacemaker erosion occurs, the only choice is surgical revision of the pacemaker site. If associated with infection, the entire system (both pulse generator and lead) must be removed and a completely new pacing system implanted at a clean site. In rare situations, in the proved absence of infection, it may be possible to revise the pacer site, enlarge the "pocket", and fashion a satisfactory skin flap.

Skin Adherence

Adherence of the pulse generator to the skin is a strong suggestion of infection (see Chapter 8), and salvage of the site may not be possible. Impending erosion, (skin thinned to the point of transparency) should be dealt with as an emergency. Once the skin is opened, infection is virtually certain—while it is still closed, the wound is protected. If revision is accomplished before the pacemaker has fully eroded and become contaminated, the original pacemaker can be reimplanted and, if uninfected, the original site can be successfully revised and reused. Cultures should be obtained in all such circumstances.

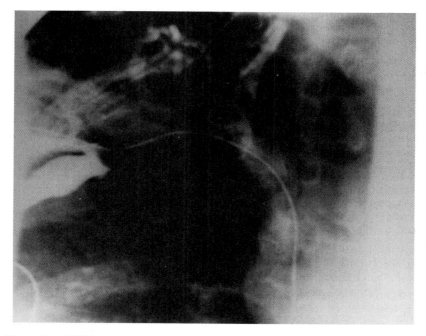

Figure 9.   *Still frame of a venogram of the right upper extremity shows occlusion of the subclavian vein. The patient had clinical venous insufficiency.*

Thrombosis

Thromboembolic complications after permanent pacemaker implantation are rare. If thrombosis involves the superior vena cava, axillary vein, or area around the pacemaker lead in the right atrium or right ventricle, several problems can develop.

1. Occlusion of the superior vena cava and superior vena caval syndrome.
2. Thrombosis of the superior vena cava, right atrium, or right ventricle, with hemodynamic compromise or pulmonary embolus.

Partial or silent inconsequential thrombosis is common and clinically insignificant (Figure 9).

Radiation Therapy

Implanted pacemakers should be shielded from the field of therapeutic radiation. Radiation damage can have unpredictable effects, and radiation dose to the pulse generator is cumulative.

Lung and breast carcinomas commonly present problems. If radiation therapy is to be administered at the site of the existing pacemaker, the pacemaker should be moved or adequately shielded before therapy begins (Figures 10A, 10B) (see also Chapter 10).

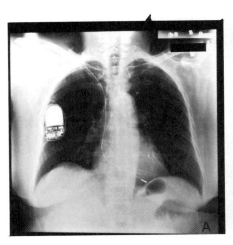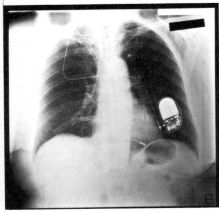

Figure 10. A. *A permanent pacemaker in the right pectoral position and the lead entering right external jugular vein.* *B.* *Carcinoma of the right breast developed and because the pacemaker would have been in the field of therapeutic radiation, the pacemaker was moved to the left chest wall. The lead was temporarily disconnected and tunneled subcutaneously to the left side of the chest where it was reconnected to the pulse generator.*

Pacemaker failure—and development of high threshold—are other complications that should be considered (see Chapter 10).

EARLY OR LATE COMPLICATIONS

Lead Dislodgement

Active and passive fixation mechanisms that are common to current pacing leads have significantly reduced the incidence of lead dislodgement. Secondary intervention rates for dislodgement should be well below 2% for ventricular leads and below 5% for atrial leads. Dislodgement has been classified by some as "macrodislodgement" and "microdislodgement". Macrodislodgement is radiographically evident and microdislodgement is not. Adequate lead position is assessed by posteroanterior and lateral chest x-ray (Figures 11-12). (see Chapter 10, Pacemaker Radiography).

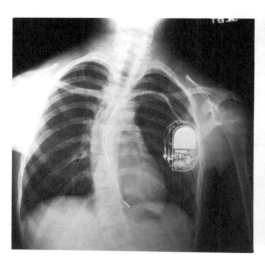 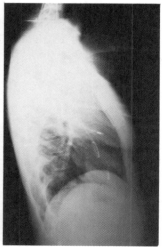

Figure 11A and B. Posterioanterior and lateral chest x-ray of a patient with dual-chamber pacemaker system. The ventricular lead has been dislodged and the lead is coiled in an intracardiac position. In addtion, the atrial lead appears to have been pulled back into a very shallow position. Clinically, the patient presented with normal atrial pacing and sensing but failure to capture and sense the ventricle.

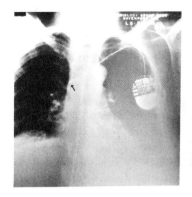
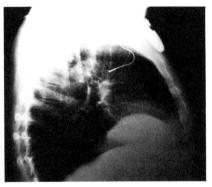

Figure 12A and B.   *PA and lateral chest x-ray of a patient with a dual-chamber pacing system. The atrial lead has been displaced into the superior vena cava. The arrow notes the tip of the atrial pacing lead.*

Arrhythmias

Supraventricular and ventricular arrhythmias are often encountered during pacemaker implantation. They are discussed in Chapter 8, "Permanent Pacemaker Implantation".

In the early postoperative period, "tip extrasystoles" frequently are seen (Figure 13). These are complexes of the same form and originate at the same site as the paced beats. They are not preceded by a

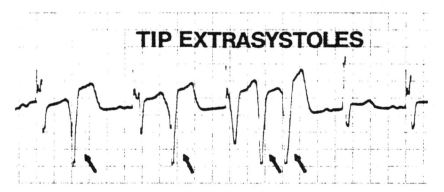

Figure 13.   *An electrocardiogram obtained during the first 24 hours after pacemaker implantation. A paced beat is followed by several spontaneous beats of similar morphology. These are tip extrasystoles.*

pacemaker stimulus. Tip extrasystoles most often occur during the first 24–48 hours after implantation and usually resolve spontaneously.

The "runaway pacemaker," a sudden increase in pacing rate caused by circuit malfunction, is rare with present-day pulse generators, but was more common with earlier pulse generators. Should runaway occur, the pulse generator must be disconnected. In an emergency, the lead may be cut and the transsected lead used with an external pulse generator. In other situations, prompt removal of the pulse generator is required, and, if possible, should be accomplished under sterile conditions (Figure 14). If the "runaway" spontaneously stops, the pulse generator should still be removed because the circuitry is unreliable, and it is likely that runaway will recur.

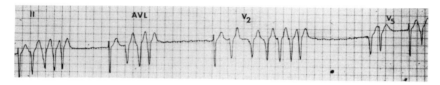

Figure 14. *An electrocardiogram of a runaway pacemaker. A pacemaker stimulus and the depolarization are followed by erratic pacing, which if sufficiently rapid and sustained may lead to ventricular fibrillation.*

Twiddler's Syndrome

Purposeful or absentminded "twiddling" or manipulation of the pulse generator by the patient has been named "twiddler's syndrome." Constant manipulation causes pacer axial rotation, twisting of the lead, and its eventual fracture or dislodgement. The pulse generator usually is not damaged. The syndrome commonly occurs when the pacemaker sits loosely in the pacemaker pocket (Figure 15) either because the pocket was too large or because the pacemaker migrated.

If the problem has occurred because of pacemaker migration or a poorly fashioned pacemaker pocket, the pocket should be revised (Figure 16). Routine use of a tightly fitting dacron pouch about the pulse generator will prevent such rotation.

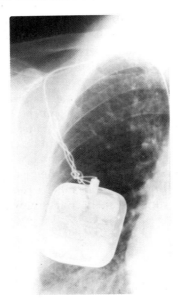

Figure 15. *Twiddler's Syndrome. The pacemaker was placed in a too large pocket and the patient was able to manipulate it. Manipulation caused lead twisting, which can cause fracture.*

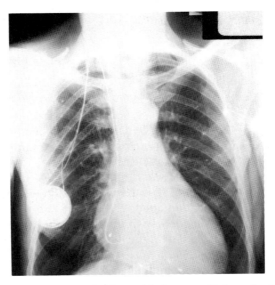

Figure 16. *A permanent pacemaker in an elderly man with lax subcutaneous tissue. With time, the pacemaker migrated inferiorly in the right anterior chest wall and was suspended by the lead.*

Direct Current Countershock

Direct current countershock in patients with implanted pacemakers may cause the pulse generator to malfunction. Although all modern pulse generators have protective shunting circuits, during defibrillation the paddles should be as far away from the pulse generator and electrode as possible. An anteroposterior paddle position is optimal.

EFFECTS OF ELECTROCAUTERY

1. Electromagnetic interference.
2. Reprogramming.
3. Permanent damage to the pulse generator.
4. Inhibition of the pulse generator.

5. Reversion to a fall-back mode. The characteristics of the fall-back mode should be known so that its presence is not confused with malfunction.

Electrocautery most likely will produce these effects if used in the vicinity of the pulse generator or lead. At times, however, abonormalities can occur even if the electrocautery is used at a distant site. It is recommended that after any surgical procedure in which electrocautery is used, the pacemaker be checked to be certain that the programmed setting is unchanged.

Local Muscle Stimulation

Pectoral muscle stimulation is unusual with bipolar pacemakers. When pectoral muscle stimulation occurs with unipolar devices, it is usually noted in the early post-implant period. Pectoral muscle stimulation occurring in the late post-implant period may be due to erosion of the pacemaker's protective coating (Figure 17). In this unusual situation, muscle stimulation will likely be present to some degree at even the lowest programmable pulse width and/or voltage.

Insulation defect, which is known to exist and be extremely troublesome in lead systems, can also exist on a pulse generator. Unipolar pulse generators are insulated on one side, generally that opposite to the side engraved with the pulse generator identification. The insulated side should be placed toward muscle and the uninsulated side toward the subcutaneous tissue. The insulation material can be removed, or, it seems, deteriorate with time, from the pulse generator.

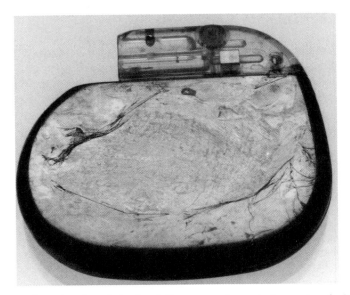

Figure 17. Deterioration of the insulating cover of a unipolar pacing device. The patient developed pectoral muscle stimulation when the insulating material was no longer intact.

Should that occur two circumstances may follow. The first is that electromyographic interference (EMI) may occur and inappropriately inhibit the pulse generator. Alternatively, a small area of defect may shunt a relatively high current density to the muscle causing a local twitch with each stimulus. This is especially true in the case of the atrial stimulus in a pulse generator with a superfast recharge circuit. It may not then be possible to program an atrial channel output sufficiently low to avoid local muscle stimulation. This may be especially true in a patient with chronotropic incompetence who requires continued atrial stimulation.

If the pacemaker can operate in the effective VDD mode, in which there is no atrial stimulation, this effect may be avoided. If there is no possibility of ending atrial channel stimulation, operative intervention will be required. Once the insulation defect is found, an accessory silicone rubber boot may be placed on the generator. Alternatively, the pulse generator may be replaced. This condition is unusual but has been seen by the authors on several occasions. It should be suspected when local muscle stimulation occurs. No detectable defect may be present during preoperative evaluation as the current leak is extremely close to that which occurs during normal unipolar DDD pulse generator function.

Pacemaker Infection

In published series, the incidence of infection after pacemaker implantation varies from 0–12.6%. Careful attention to surgical details and sterile procedures are of paramount importance in avoiding pacemaker site infection. The prophylactic use of antibiotics before implantation and in the immediate post-operative period remains controversial. Most studies do not show any significant difference in the rate of infection between patients who have had prophylactic administration of antibiotics and those who have not. Irrigation of the pacemaker pocket with an antibiotic solution at the time of pacemaker implantation may help to prevent infection.

Pacemaker infection must be recognized and be treated properly. It may appear as:

1. Local inflammation and abcess formation in the area of the pulse generator pocket.
2. Erosion of part of the pacing system through the skin and then secondary infection.
3. Fever associated with positive blood cultures with or without a focus of infection elsewhere.

The most common clinical presentation is an abscess around the generator; septicemia is an uncommon mode of presentation. Early infections usually are caused by *staphylococcus aureus,* are agressive, and are often associated with fever and systemic symptoms. Other organisms may be involved. Late infections commonly are caused by *staphylococcus epidermidis* and are more indolent—usually without fever or systemic manifestation. Treatment requires removal of the entire infected pacing system, pulse generator and leads. There is some controversy about how to proceed once the infected system has been removed. A one-stage surgical approach involves implantation of a new pacing system at a distant clean site after explantation of the infected pacing system. Others favor removal of the infected system, temporary pacing and antibiotic management in the interim, and implantation of a new system at a later date.

Retained Lead Fragments

Multiple leads can be left in place as long as none of the leads have been part of an infected system (see Chapter 10). If the pacing system is infected, it is essential that the entire lead be removed. Chronically implanted tined leads can be difficult, if not impossible,

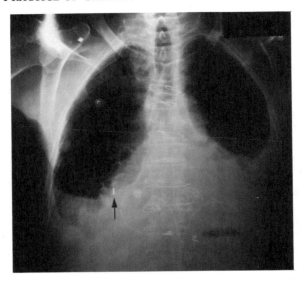

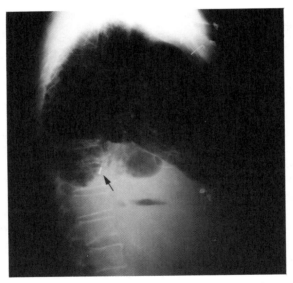

Figure 18A and B. *Posteroanterior and lateral chest x-ray of a patient with a retained lead fragment. This patient had undergone surgery for mitral valve replacement and at the time of surgery the previously implanted endocardial pacing system was removed. A portion of the transvenous ventricular lead was only partially removed because it could not be removed from the right ventricular wall despite considerable traction to the point of inversion of the free wall of the right ventricle. The lead was transsected and a portion of the lead left in place. On the postoperative chest x-ray this retained fragment is noted by the arrow.*

to remove. Several techniques have been described to remove chronically implanted leads. It is possible that a portion of the lead, specifically, portions of the "tines" may be left in an endocardial position. There have been no reports of complications as a result of a non-infected portion of a pacing lead being left embedded in the endocardium following attempted extraction. A mobile, or non-embedded, portion of the lead could embolize into the pulmonary circulation. Figure 18 demonstrates a chest x-ray where a portion of the pacing lead has been retained.

Pacemaker Syndrome

Pacemaker syndrome, which results from loss of atrioventricular synchrony and ventriculoatrial conduction, is described in Chapter 5, "Hemodynamics of Cardiac Pacing."

Pacemaker Allergy

Allergy to the pacemaker itself is a rare but reported complication. Usually, the allergy is to the pulse generator case. Proof of such an allergy requires sophisticated allergy testing, and correction of the problem may require changing to another type of system. Some of the cases of "allergy" are, in reality, low-grade *s.epidermidis* infections, which should be treated as infections rather than allergies. No diagnosis of allergy should be made until infection has been ruled out.

BIBLIOGRAPHY

Adamec R, Haefliger JM, Killisch JR, et al: Damaging effect of therapeutic radiation on programmable pacemakers. *PACE* 1982; 5:146–150.

Alferness CA: Pacemaker damage due to external countershock in patients with implanted cardiac pacemakers (letter to the editor). *PACE* 1982; 5:457–458.

Aylward P, Blood R, Tonkin A: Complications of defibrillation with permanent pacemaker in situ. *PACE* 1979; 2:462–464.

Barold SS, Center S: Electrographic diagnosis of perforation of the heart by pacing catheter electrode. *Am J Cardiol* 1969; 24:274–278.

Bassan MM, Merin G: Pericardial tamponade due to perforation with a permanent endocardial pacing catheter. *J Thorac Cardiovasc Surg* 1977; 74:51–54.

Bayliss CE, Beanlands DS, Baird RJ: The pacemaker-Twiddler's syndrome: A new complication of implantable transvenous pacemakers. *Can Med Assoc J* 1968; 99:371–373.

Belott PH, Sands S, Warren J: Resetting of DDD pacemakers due to EMI. *PACE* 1984; 7:169–172.

Blamires NG, Myatt J: X-ray effects on pacemaker type circuits. *PACE* 1982; 5:151–155.

Boughner DR, Gulamhusein S: Echocardiographic demonstration of a left ventricular endocardial pacemaker wire. *JCU* 1983; 11:240–243.

Bramowitz AD, Smith JW, Eber LM, et al: Runaway pacemaker: A persisting problem. *JAMA* 1974; 228:340–341.

Byrd CL, Schwartz SJ, Gonzales M, Byrd CB, Sivina M, Yahr WZ, Ciraldo RJ, Greenberg JJ: Pacemaker clinic evaluations: key to early identification of surgical problems. *PACE* 9(6 Part 2):1259–64, 1986.

Calfee RV: Therapeutic radiation and pacemakers. *PACE* 1982; 5:160–161. (editorial)

Castberg T: Complications from the pacemaker pocket: Prophylaxis, treatment and results. *Acta Med Scand* 1976; Suppl 596:51–54.

Chamorro H, Rao G, Wholey MH: Superior vena cava syndrome: A complication of transvenous pacemaker implantation. *Radiology* 1978; 126:377–378.

Choo MH, Holmes DR Jr, Gersh BJ, et al: Infected epicardial pacemaker systems: Partial versus total removal. *J Thorac Cardiovasc Surg* 1981; 82:794–796.

Choo MH, Holmes DR Jr, Gersh BJ, et al: Permanent pacemaker infections: Characterization and management. *Am J Cardiol* 1981; 48:559–564.

Das G, Eaton J: Pacemaker malfunction following transthoracic countershock. *PACE* 1981; 4:487–490.

Flaker GC, Mueller KJ, Salazar JR, et al: Total venous obstruction following atrioventricular sequential pacemaker implantation. *PACE* 1983; 6:815–817.

Furman S: Pacemaker emergencies. *Med Clin North Am* 1979; 63:113–126.

Furman S, Behrens M, Andrews C, Klementowicz P: Retained pacemaker leads. *J Thorac Cardiovasc Surg* 94(5):770–2, 1987.

Gothard JWW, Branthwaite MA: Cardiac pacemaker insertion: A study of the anaesthetic and postoperative complications. *Anaesthesia* 1979; 34:269–274.

Gould L, Patel S, Gomes GI, et al: Pacemaker failure following external defibrillation. *PACE* 1981; 4:575–577.

Iliceto S, Di Biase M, Antonelli G, et al: Two-dimensional echocardiographic recognition of a pacing catheter perforation of the interventricular septum. *PACE* 1982; 5:934–936.

Irnich W: Interference in pacemakers. *PACE* 1984; 7:1021–1048.

Katzenberg CA, Marcus FI, Heusinkveld RS, et al: Pacemaker failure due to radiation therapy. *PACE* 1982; 5:156–159.

Kostiainen S: Complications of transvenous and transthoracic electrodes. *Acta Med Scand* 1976; Suppl 596:40–43.

Krug H, Zerbe F: Major venous thrombosis: A complication of transvenous pacemaker electrodes. *Br Heart J* 1980; 44:158–161.

Lee ME, Chaux A: Unusual complications of endocardial pacing. *J Thorac Cardiovasc Surg* 1980; 80:934–940.

Markewitz A, Hemmer W, Weinhold C: Complications in dual chamber pacing: a six-year experience. *PACE* 9(6 Part 2):1014–8, 1986.

Mitrovic V, Thormann J, Schlepper M, et al: Thrombotic complications with pacemakers. *Int J Cardiol* 1983; 2:363–374.

Mond HG, Stuckey JG, Sloman G: The diagnosis of right ventricular perforation by an endocardial pacemaker electrode. *PACE* 1978; 1:62–67.

Nanda NC, Barold SS: Usefulness of echocardiography in cardiac pacing. *PACE* 1982; 5:222–237.

Pauletti M, Di Ricco G, Solfanelli S, et al: Venous obstruction in permanent pacemaker patients: An isotopic study. *PACE* 1981; 4:36–42.

Peters MS, Schroeter AL, van Hale HM, et al: Pacemaker contact sensitivity. *Contact Dermatitis* 1984; 11:214–218.

Phillips R, Frey M, Martin RO: Long-term performance of polyurethane pacing leads: mechanisms of design-related failures. *PACE* 9(6 Part 2): 1166–72, 1986.

Sinnaeva A, Piret J, Stroobandt R: Potential causes of spurious programming: Report of a case. *PACE* 1980; 3:541–547.

Stokes KG, Church T: Ten-year experience with implanted polyurethane lead insulation. *PACE* 9(6 Part 2):1160–5, 1986.

Stoney WS Addlestone RB, Aflord WC Jr, et al: The incidence of venous thrombosis following long-term transvenous pacing. *Ann Thorac Surg* 1976; 22:166–170.

Von-Mengden HJ, Mannweiler J, Stelzig HH, Kempf P: Clinical incidence of subclavian thromboses following pacemaker implantation. *Z-Kardiol* 75 (10):621–7, 1986.

PART III.

PRACTICAL MANAGEMENT

Chapter 15

PACEMAKER FOLLOW-UP

Seymour Furman

The function of implanted pacemaker systems is variable. Lead or generator failure and intercurrent medical events affect the interaction of pacemaker system and patient. Pacemaker systems with long-lived power sources and hermetically sealed complementary metal oxide semiconductor (CMOS) circuitry provide stability and longevity, but the interaction between the pacemaker and the patient has become correspondingly more complex. Patient welfare requires continued observation to reduce the incidence of sudden and unpredicted pacemaker system failure, detect substandard performance of some models, and produce maximum longevity of those units capable of prolonged operation. It should be remembered that for the patient's safety all failures to pace are equivalent, whether caused by lead or electronic failure or power source depletion. Approximatley 80% of lithium pulse generators remain capable of function eight years after implantation. Nevertheless, lead fractures and displacements, infections, and sudden "no output" electronic failure remain important considerations. They can be avoided in a variety of ways.

PACEMAKER FOLLOW-UP SYSTEMS CHECK LIST

All pacemaker follow-up systems should:

1. Predict impending pacemaker system failure before that patient is at risk;
2. Ascertain the nature of the malfunction when failure is about to occur or has occurred;
3. Record patient location should a pattern of systematic pulse generator or lead failure develop or recall occur;
4. Develop statistical data specific for one clinic or that is part of a much larger data base.

The pacemaker clinic analyzes the patient's pacemaker electrocardiography, stimulus waveform, the range of programmability, sensing and pacing thresholds, the stability of patient-pacemaker interaction, and physiological response to yield maximum rhythmic stability with-

511

out pacemaker syndrome. The wound is evaluated for comfort and freedom from infection.

Programming is important for single-chamber pacemakers. It is even more important for dual-chamber pacemakers where decisions concerning atrial pacing and sensing and ventricular pacing and sensing have significant impact on device longevity, whether the various chambers will be paced or sensed appropriately, and whether maximum hemodynamic and rhythmic benefit will occur.

ORGANIZATION OF A PACEMAKER CLINIC

PACEMAKER CLINIC ORGANIZATION

1. Patients should be seen on a consistent schedule, not solely when symptoms return. The early schedule should be based on electrode(s) stability so that patients are seen soon after implant of a new electrode and pulse generator. They need not be seen soon after pulse generator replacement.
2. Pacemaker records should be kept separate from the hospital record system, be immediately retrievable, and contain:
   a. patient data, i.e., name, age, identification number, address, and phone number;
   b. pacemaker data, i.e., model and serial number and updated records of rate, electrocardiogram, and other indicators of function.
3. Patients should be subjected to:
   a. x-ray annually or as necessary to note electrode and pacemaker position in a growing child;
   b. 12-lead ECG at each visit—both pacing and with the pacemaker inhibited;
   c. a rhythm strip in the free-running and magnet modes in a lead in which pacer artifacts and P and QRS complexes are readily discernible;
   d. recording of the pulse generator stimulus in the free-running and magnet modes and representative programmed functions;
   e. programming of programmable and dual-chamber pacemakers to a variety of functions with recording of representative waveforms, rates, and other significant programmable factors;
   f. evaluation of the stimulation and sensing thresholds of atrium and ventricle;
   g. measurement and recording of the pacemaker rate in the free-running and magnet modes;
   h. evaluation of the implant wound site.

It is probably not wise to provide general medical or cardiologic follow-up in the pacer clinic.

DEMOGRAPHIC PATIENT DATA

A major part of follow-up is having records available of patient location and all pacemaker related data. Each patient should be easily identifiable and his location known. Patients who have a pacemaker implanted sometimes improve, within a few minutes, from grave illness to lack of symptoms. However, symptoms can return as rapidly if the pacer system fails. After pacemaker implantation, such patients may forget that they are well managed but not cured. As the device has a finite longevity that depends on how frequently it stimulates the heart, how it is programmed, and whether it is single-or dual-chamber, no specific number can be placed on the longevity of any single device. Leads also have a finite longevity although it's far less certain how long that is. Apparently, random fractures continually occur, but at an apparently accelerating rate after about 10 years of implant (Figure 1).

Patients with implanted pacemakers, whether pacer-dependent or not, require follow-up. In preparation for a possible recall, it may be wise to determine which patients are to be considered "pacer-dependent" and require early intervention should system unreliability occur.

Recall, generated by manufacturer or government regulators or by the physician responsible for the clinic, may be required. It will be important to locate patients and to have further information, such as the degree of pacer dependency and the consequent potential for injury, should the pacemaker cease functioning suddenly. Computerized data bases are useful for this purpose. Most manufacturers maintain computer records of patients with pacemakers of their manufacture. It is helpful if the physician cooperates by providing registration of the pacemaker upon implant, returning the pulse generator on removal, and reporting a patient's death. These computerized reports can be very useful at the time of recall, should one occur. Data provided to the manufacturer is also available to another physician in the event of an emergency. Patients carry little information beyond a registration card, and often, even that is not available. As the manufacturer of most pacemakers can be identified on x-ray (Figure 2), manufacturer's records are often the best source of information about a patient who has developed an emergency away from his customary

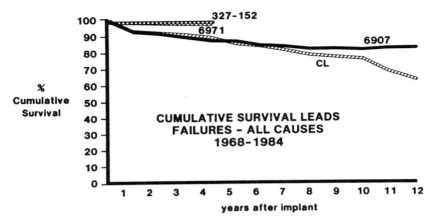

Figure 1. *Survival of individual leads is calculated on a time base of years similar to that of the longer lasting lithium anode powered pacemakers. Patterns of wear are readily apparent. Two older silicone rubber leads (CL and 6907) have had cumulative survivals at eleven years of over 70% and 80%, respectively. While some urethane leads have had very high failure rates, most have not. All urethane leads have had a far shorter exposure but models (Medtronic 6971 and Cordis 327-152) have had almost 100% survival four years after implant by which time the older leads had already shown a substantial failure incidence.*

medical attention. Even better than a manufacturer-generated list is one generated and maintained by the individual physician.

The twin bases of any pacemaker clinic are follow-up and the quality of record keeping. Follow-up should be organized, not haphazard. A schedule should be established with both patient and clinic staff so that there is little uncertainty concerning the constancy and schedule of follow-up. Records of each visit should be available for comparison with earlier visits. Rate changes and alterations in other functions, such as shape or amplitude of the oscilloscopic artifact, assume importance largely in comparison with previous data. The oscilloscopic photograph of an implanted polyurethane lead that shows a modest change may herald deterioration of the polyurethane. Such a visible change may occur before clinical manifestation and may be detectable only in comparison with an earlier, presumably "normal" finding. This is especially important as at least one implanted lead is in Class I or "danger to life and/or health" status.

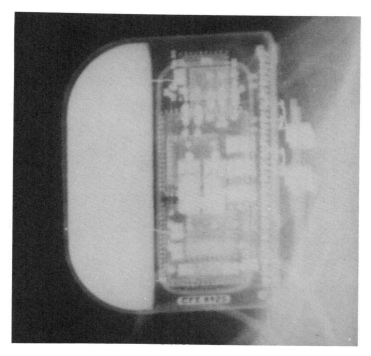

Figure 2.   *Pacemaker identification is readily possible with newer pulse generators—most contain written identification of the pulse generator model and manufacturer on a radiopaque label. In this unit the manufacturer and model are readily visible.*

PULSE GENERATOR END-OF-LIFE

A pulse generator has reached its end-of-life when the power source has been depleted to the point at which it cannot drive the circuit reliably or if failure is impending. Electronic circuit-caused end-of-life occurs when the pulse generator is no longer operating within its design specifications and has become unreliable, erratic, or unsafe but the cause is not battery failure or depletion. End-of-life is not necessarily associated with clinical manifestations. Indeed it is better to determine that end-of-life has been reached before clinical manifestations occur. The magnet pacemaker rate may be at battery depletion level while otherwise normal function exists. Nevertheless, the unit will be at end-of-life.

Determination of end-of-life may be difficult. A pulse generator that has begun to show change, for example, a shift in some, or all, programmed rates, but in which overall operation seems stable may still have years of satisfactory operation. Consultation with the manufacturer may be desirable, but it is the physician's responsibility to decide whether a pulse generator or any other device should be left in place. If a device is operating out of specification (accurate documentation is mandatory), its removal is the physician's option and decision.

Barring intercurrent events, all pulse generators will go to battery depletion end-of-life if they are left in service for a sufficient (but highly variable) period. Many lithium silver chromate powered pulse generators have gone to battery depletion in four to five years while some of the earliest lithium iodine cell models remain functioning ten years after implant with no clearly defined model longevity expectation. The lithium thionyl chloride cells with a high voltage and large energy capacity went from apparently normal function to depletion within days or weeks, too short a period to follow realistically. For them, end-of life was a statistically determined period. The longevity when the first of these units failed is the time to remove them all, electively. Some lithium cupric sulfide cell models have behaved in a similar manner, though less precipitously. Originally designed to indicate battery depletion by a 10% decline in rate, sudden failures appeared when a 3% rate change had occurred. Consequently this has become the indication of battery depletion, i.e., 3% (Figure 3).

Rate change has been the primary indication of battery depletion since manufacture of the first pacemakers. At present, all pulse generators decrease rate with battery depletion, but different pulse generators may have different criteria. Early lithium iodine generators relied on the increasing battery impedance to slow the rate of the circuit, and 6%−7% rate decrease was an indication of depletion with both the magnet and free-running rates in parallel. With a gradual shift to digital circuits, increasing battery impedance with depletion was not allowed to produce a gradual rate change in the free-running mode. Two different approaches were widely, but not universally, adopted. In one, the free-running rate is stable almost to impending battery exhaustion, and the magnetic rate (usually 90 or 100 bpm) is different from the usual programmed rate. Battery depletion indicators appear in the magnet rate only. In one series, a gradual rate decline occurs in the magnet mode with rate stability in the free-running mode. Battery depletion is indicated at 7% for some models and 16% for others. Another approach is stability of the programmed free-running rate

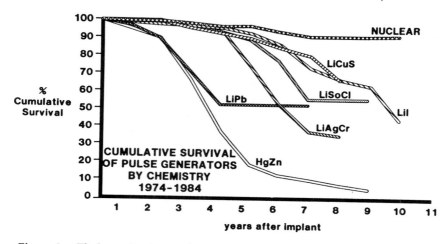

Figure 3.   *The longevity characteristics of various power sources are clearly different. Ten years of observed longevity data is now available. The nuclear pulse generators powered by plutonium have behaved best of all with a cumulative survival at ten years of over 90%; lithium cupric sulfide and lithium iodine have done well with over 60% cumulative survival at eight and nine years, respectively.Lithium thionyl chloride, lithium lead, and lithium silver chromate are intermediate in longevity. The 50% cumulative survival time for mercury-zinc generators was reached 3½ years after implantation.*

with a step function rate decline in the magnet rate with 15% decline indicating battery depletion. The characteristics of the pacer used must be known. Keeping the physician's manual packed with each pacemaker is wise.

RECALL

Recall of defective devices is important in the management of pacemaker patients. Follow-up will detect routine battery depletion well. It may not detect earlier than anticipated battery depletion, sudden electronic failure, and the two most dangerous but uncommon failure modes, sudden "no output" and "runaway", which are electronic in origin. A failure pattern, rather than random failure, in a pacemaker model population should be dealt with in a different fashion than continued routine follow-up. In the event the patient is believed to be at risk, the device should be electively replaced. The

individual physician should not be dissuaded from action by a manufacturer or by the absence of a formal recall by a governmental agency.
Industry may have inadequate data and government may be too slow
in reaching a judgment. For example, the physician may determine
that battery depletion is occurring in an orderly fashion but at a time
when it is unanticipated, and, therefore, follow-up should be at lesser
intervals. Follow-up intervals should then be adjusted. S/he may decide that end-of-life characteristics are not smooth, i.e., that sudden no
output failure may occur without detectable warning when the battery
is fully depleted, such pulse generators should be electively removed.

The "recall" mechanism, whether it involves more intense observation or actual replacement of a defective device, is an integral part of
follow-up. It should be used sparingly, but it should be used. If device
replacement is decided on, the patients who are at greater risk should
be operated on early, those at lesser risk, later. With the more formal
recognition of pacemaker recall, physicians will receive a manufacturer-
generated list of patients who require careful observation. These
manufacturer-generated lists are required by the government and
should be reviewed carefully. While manufacturers approach these
"advisory" notices with dread, the physician should consider them as
a means of assistance in patient management. The physician should
determine the accuracy of a manufacturer-generated list.

The need for elective replacement of a device may also be based on
the degree of follow-up required. While in some circumstances, a
patient can be monitored telephonically weekly, or more frequently,
the shortest realistic routine follow-up interval is one month. Patients
who require follow-up at lesser intervals probably should have elective
replacement. Therefore, as a general rule, if a device can go from
apparently normal function to gross malfunction or absence of function in less than a month, it should be electively replaced.

The problem of polyurethane lead deterioration is potentially of
greater magnitude. The number of leads at risk is greater than any
pacemaker model ever subjected to recall, and the incidence of failure
is now as high as 20%. It is likely that failure of these leads is time-
dependent, therefore, with the passage of more time, more leads will
fail. While a pulse generator can be removed cleanly, a lead cannot. A
polyurethane lead subjected to extraction may fragment and embolize.
A polyurethane lead undergoing deterioration in situ may deteriorate in
a way so far undetermined and cause a far greater problem. All of this
is, as yet, unknown, but these patients will receive observation despite
removal of such a lead from service.

PACEMAKER DEPENDENCY

The term pacemaker dependency has been used to indicate which patients are at substantial risk should a pacer fail. While widely used, the term is undefined, and different knowledgeable physicians use different criteria, often resulting in substantial confusion. The issue is especially important to regulators who will want to assess the overall risk to a patient population and to the physician who must assess intervention for his/her own patients. While there is no general agreement concerning the method of definition of pacemaker dependency, the authors suddenly inhibit pacemaker output during each clinic visit and assess the state of the underlying rhythm. This unpaced rhythm is a clue to the degree of risk. There is little doubt that patients may be at different levels of risk at different times. A patient with complete heart block will not have syncope each time sudden pacemaker failure occurs but, if restored to AV block from a paced rhythm, will certainly enter a category of increased risk. The estimates (all inaccurate rate to a lesser or greater degree) of patient pacer dependency range from 5% to 30%.

For practical purposes, a patient is pacer-dependent if the sudden (from one beat to the next) loss of pacing will result in a Stokes-Adams episode, serious injury, or death. Questions of definition and even more questions of how to make the clinical determination of potential sudden injury or death exist. During inhibition of the pacemaker, dependency is determined in the following way: If no escape rhythm occurs the patient is pacemaker-dependent (Class I). If the ventricular escape rhythm is complete AV block with atrial fibrillation or sinus rhythm, the patient is substantially pacemaker-dependent (Class II). If escape is by a lesser degree of AV block, an arrhythmia, or a sinus bradycardia of 30 bpm or less the patient is moderately dependent (Class III). If escape is by regular sinus rhythm of normal rate (50 or more bpm), the patient is not pacer-dependent (Class IV). Patients vary in pacer dependency from time to time and, of course, the worst assessment a patient *ever* has defines his status. In making these determinations, note that a patient who has had syncopal episodes because of infrequent *documented* asystole before pacemaker implant does requires pacing, but not for more than a few minutes each month. He will probably test as nondependent on each follow-up visit. The greatest caution and wisdom must be exercised during evaluation of pacer dependency (Figure 4).

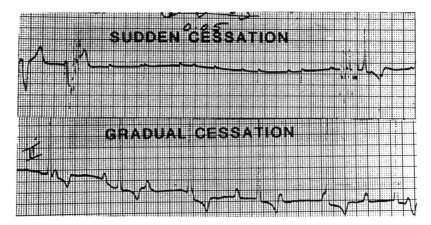

Figure 4. *Pacemaker dependency is a commonly used but not well understood term. Certainly the circumstance of failure to pace is a determinant of the cardiac response. In this patient, ECGs recorded several minutes apart show prolonged asystole following sudden cessation of pacing (above) and a satisfactory escape rhythm with complete AV block following gradual cessation of pacing (below).*

FOLLOW-UP SCHEDULES

The schedule for follow-up of implanted cardiac pacemakers in the United States is largely determined by that suggested by Medicare. A new schedule published during October 1984 revised the previously announced schedule.

The transtelephonic monitoring contact consists of a determination of the pacemaker rate in the free-running and magnet modes and ECGs in both the free-running and magnet modes. The free-running ECG and the magnet ECG should be of at least 30 seconds duration unless specifically contraindicated. Medicare assumes that these ECGs and rates will be part of a permanent record.

Different categories are now established for single- and dual-chamber pacemakers and for pacing systems of proven durability and for those of less well-known durability. The criteria for longevity are those that have been recommended by the Intersociety Commission for Heart Disease Resources. The data used to make the determinations are published periodically in *PACE*. Guideline I is for those pacemakers that have not yet developed sufficient experience to meet the ICHD criteria or have had sufficient exposure and have not met the criteria. Guideline II is for those pacemakers that have met the ICHD criteria. The two operative criteria for longevity and end-of-life decay are

1. 90% or better cumulative survival at five years following implant;
2. an end-of-life decay or less than a 50% drop of output voltage and less than 20% deviation of magnet rate, or a drop of 5 bpm or less, over a period of three months or more.

As two criteria are involved, it is possible for a pacemaker to meet one and not the other. For example, a model may meet the 90% survival criteria and yet, once end-of-life is reached, failure may be sudden. Alternatively, failure may be orderly but sooner than five years. The Medicare guidelines also recognize the influence of lead longevity on the longevity of the entire pacing system but do not clearly define the schedule alterations that will be based on lead requirements. Because of the various complexities related to the criteria for pacemaker system longevity and single- and dual-chamber pacemakers, follow-up schedules are likely to be variable and perhaps even the source of uncertainty (Table I).

Table I

GUIDELINE I. The majority of pacemakers.

SINGLE-CHAMBER PACEMAKERS

1st Mo.	2nd Mo.–36th Mo.	37th Mo.–Failure
Every 2 weeks	Every 8 weeks	Every 4 weeks

DUAL-CHAMBER PACEMAKERS

1st Mo.	2nd Mo.–6th Mo.	7th Mo.–36th Mo.	37th Mo.–Failure
Every 2 weeks	Every 4 weeks	Every 8 weeks	Every 4 weeks

GUIDELINE II. The minority of pacemaker systems (pacemaker and leads) for which sufficient long-term clinical information exists to assure that they meet the standards of the Inter-society Commission for Heart Disease Resources (ICHD) for longevity and end-of-life decay.

SINGLE-CHAMBER PACEMAKERS

1st Mo.	2nd Mo.–30th Mo.	31st–48th Mo.	Thereafter
Every 2 weeks	Every 12 weeks	Every 8 weeks	Every 4 weeks

DUAL-CHAMBER PACEMAKERS

1st Mo.	2nd Mo.–30th Mo.	31st–48th Mo.	Thereafter
Every 2 weeks	Every 12 weeks	Every 8 weeks	Every 4 weeks

TRANSTELEPHONIC MONITORING

Telephonic monitoring is the most useful technique available for the long-term observation of patients with implanted cardiac pacemakers. As the total number of these patients increases, face-to-face observation becomes relatively more difficult and cumbersome. As face-to-face follow-up in the pacemaker center becomes evermore complex, it should be preserved for the extensive work-up necessary to determine pacemaker function and establish proper pacemaker settings. Clinic monitoring on a frequent basis, for prolonged periods is burdensome for staff and patients and should be replaced by transtelephonic monitoring. Transtelephonic monitoring is very useful in overall follow-up of the paced patient.

Telephone monitoring with rate determination and an ECG can be used at frequent intervals following pacemaker implantation to ascertain electrode stability. Later, longer intervals between contacts will be appropriate and, as the unit ages, at shorter intervals.

The accuracy of telephone monitoring in detection of battery depletion is not matched by that of electronic monitoring because of the ease and frequency of the transmissions. The single area of failure has been the inability to detect impending lead fracture, which, unfortunately, is usually not detectable by any means in advance of the event itself.

PURPOSES OF TELEPHONIC MONITORING

1. Careful pacemaker follow-up to achieve maximum safety and longevity.
2. Careful and frequent observation of pulse generators and lead systems in models known to have a high incidence of electronic failure, lead fracture, or insulation deterioration, or observation of devices that are no longer operating normally but clear-cut malfunction has not been demonstrated.
3. Electrocardiographic monitoring for an intercurrent arrhythmia.
4. Follow-up as a laboratory resource for the physician in overall responsibility for a patient's welfare.
5. Provision of pacemaker follow-up to areas remote from a pacemaker clinic and for patients unable to travel.
6. Provision of technical expertise for facilities without that capability, such as the nursing home.

Rate and ECG

Transmission of rate and the ECG is now the standard of trans-telephonic monitoring, providing rate for determination of battery and electronic status and ECG to confirm cardiac capture and sensing. The ECG is the universally recognized indicator of cardiac activity and therefore is mandatory for any follow-up system, as normal or abnormal function is readily recognized. The ECG clearly demonstrates pacemaker malfunction early or late after implant and is invaluable for the detection of intercurrent arrhythmias that occur with pacemaker malfunction or despite normal pacemaker function. Even stimulation threshold can be determined if the unit implanted has a magnet-activated automatic threshold determination such as the Vario system provided by several manufacturers (Figure 5).

A wide variety of monitors for patient use exists. Some equipment has been carefully designed to be easy to use, with comfortable wrist or

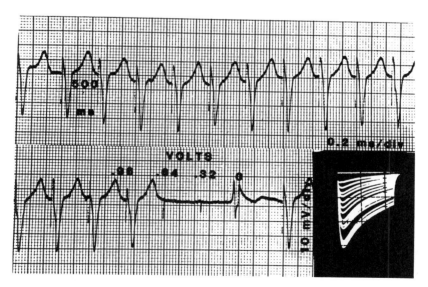

Figure 5. *Automatic test of threshold is an important capability, and if it can be magnetically activated as in the "Vario" system, threshold can be determined via the telephone. In this illustration each stimulus is ¹⁄₁₅ the voltage below each preceding stimulus. The inverted stimulus at the right is a zero voltage mark. The threshold is 0.96 V. Once the magnet is removed from the pacer, the output returns to its programmed setting.*

axillary electrodes, positive coupling between the telephone handset and monitor, and convenient hand application of the monitor. Other equipment is small and light but practically unusable. Some ECGs are easy to read, others, virtually impossible. In selection of equipment, the capabilities of the usual patient (average age 70 years) and the ease or complexity of use should be the primary consideration.

RECORD KEEPING

Records are of prime importance in knowledge of when failure will occur in an individual patient and for the collection of data concerning an entire model, to indicate when careful follow-up or elective replacement (see Recall) should be undertaken. As larger groups of patients are followed by a single facility, routine secretarial effort becomes inadequate to maintain satisfactory observation of the patient population. Under these circumstances, computer-generated record keeping facilities become mandatory. At Montefiore Medical Center the transtelephonic monitoring clinic is based on human interpretation and computerized record storage.

The computer provides the list of daily calls to be made and includes time, name, identification number (a four-digit number unique to our facility), and telephone number. Once the operator selects a patient on that list, the patient's previous data, including pacemaker model, date of the last telephone call, and free-running and magnet rates at that time are displayed on the screen. Additionally, the percent decline of magnetic rate since pacemaker implantation and the percent of magnetic rate decline, which is the indicator of elective replacement, are displayed. All of the specific data, including the quality of electrocardiographic capture and sensing and overall function for the last eight contacts are also displayed. The nurse then proceeds with the transmission of data and the interpretation of a telephonically transmitted ECG. With the transmission completed, the computer prompts the operator with requests for the free-running and magnetic rate to three significant figures. It then prompts the request concerning interpretation of the quality of capture and sensing, and the overall summary of the quality of pacing. When all of this has been entered, the computer will ask whether the next call is to be on a monthly or weekly schedule. Once one or the other is selected, it will recommend a date. Holidays and weekends are programmed into memory so that those dates are not selected. The operator can override the computer recommendation and assign another date. At the conclusion of the test procedure, a line printer provides a report with the free-running and magnet ECG as well as a full report of the transmission and appropriate interpretation. Each report is a history of the entire transtelephonic record and allows the physician who overreads the report to acquaint himself with all of the data specific to that patient. The paper report can serve as a backup for computer failure. It also can be mailed to other facilities or physicians (Figure 6).

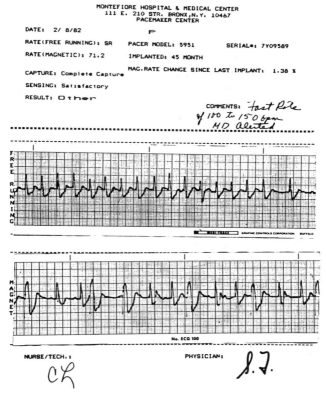

Figure 6. *Transtelephonic monitoring is useful for routine monitoring of pacemaker function. In addition, intercurrent arrhythmias can be detected. In this instance, an arrhythmia, possibly atrial fibrillation, was detected during normal pacemaker function. Only a 1.38% rate decline had occurred, and sensing and capture were documented. The free-running rhythm strip is shown above and the magnet strip below.*

ELECTROCARDIOGRAPHY IN TRANSTELEPHONE MONITORING

ECG transmission provides interpretive difficulties and artifacts that are similar to conventional electrocardiography and clearly indicate failure to capture, sense, or both. A few artifacts are unique to transtelephone monitoring. The most serious is that caused by the use of a single-lead rhythm strip, usually lead I (right arm, left arm) in which the QRS or the pacemaker artifact may be isoelectric or, for some other reason, insufficiently diagnostic. Another lead should be selected and transmission repeated. The diagnostic lead can be used thereafter. Telephone noise is frequently picked up from continuous interference and electrical transients. Both usually are readily detected. Reversal of the limb leads is easily detected and is of little consequence. Motion artifacts occur frequently. Troublesome 60 Hz interference can exist with all systems though the stimulus rate, and the ECG can usually be discriminated. Because the determination of rate in the magnet mode requires a magnet to be held over the pacemaker, its movement (as in a patient with Parkinson's disease) can cause a variety of artifacts including brief inhibition of the pacer. Respiratory movement is recognized, as on a conventional ECG, by a slow rhythmic oscillation of the baseline (Figure 7).

A wide variety of pathology may be detected with ECG monitoring. Included are the range of pacemaker malfunctions: rate change and loss of pacing or sensing, or both. Relatively common intercurrent findings are multifocal premature ventricular contractions, tachycardia, atrial fibrillation, and other arrhythmias.

The induction of a competitive, magnet-produced rhythm to detect pacemaker rate is without meaningful effect. Pacemaker-produced premature ventricular contractions (PVC) occur but are not sustained and only rarely do multiple PVCs require cessation of use of the magnet. No episode of competitively induced ventricular fibrillation or sustained tachycardia has occurred in our patients (Figure 8).

Dual-chamber transtelephonic monitoring represents additional problems and complexities. Some dual-chamber telephonically monitored ECGs are extremely difficult to read, and equipment for interpretation of the ECG and rate is not yet as widely available as it is for single-chamber pacemakers. The increasing use of dual-chamber pacemakers makes monitoring of those devices important despite the associated difficulties (Figure 9).

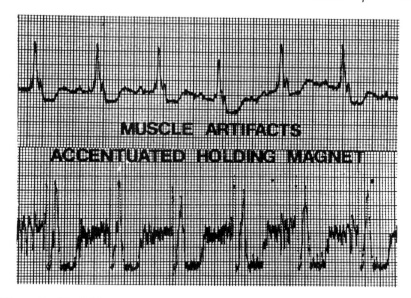

Figure 7. *The ECG is readily transmitted by telephone. A variety of artifacts also can be transmitted. In this instance, the muscle artifacts caused by magnet application are readily seen. The pacemaker is not inhibited or triggered.*

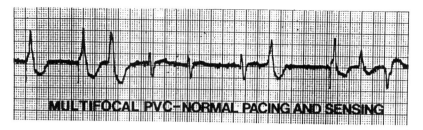

Figure 8. *Multifocal premature ventricular contractions can be detected as they are here. Ventricular capture and sensing of all of the foci are demonstrated.*

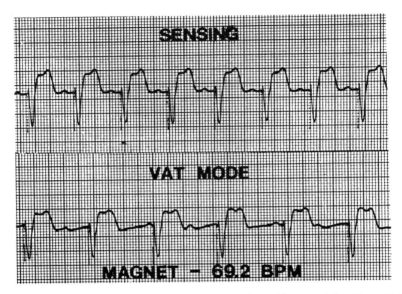

Figure 9. *An atrial synchronous (VAT) pacemaker with normal function. Atrial sensing and ventricular capture are demonstrated as is a "normal" magnet rate indicative of satisfactory function of the power source.*

RECURRENT SYMPTOMATOLOGY AFTER PACEMAKER IMPLANT

It is often assumed that once a pacemaker is implanted all symptoms vanish. Indeed, many patients make that assumption and refer all intercurrent illness or later symptoms to pacemaker malfunction. Some will even date remote symptoms such as those of the musculoskeletal system from the time of pacer implant. These are very dangerous miscalculations. Each patient who has an implanted pacemaker should have a general medical physician and/or a caridiologist who will care for all nonpacemaker related conditions.

Recurrent symptoms fall into the general categories of *noncardiac* symptoms, which are usually readily separated from the implanted pacemaker; *nonpacemaker cardiac* symptoms, such as those related to congestive heart failure, angina, or myocardial infarction; and those which *approximate the symptoms* that necessitated the pacemaker implant in the first instance. Some patients will have been implanted who had been relatively asymptomatic and may even be asymptomatic with lead or pacemaker failure. An increasing number of patients are being implanted for electrocardiographically detected arrhythmias, for example, AV block, sick sinus syndrome with long pauses but with minimal symptoms. Although this approach is controversial, it seems to be widely practiced.

In our own evaluation and that of others, some 8% to 10% of patients will complain of return of symptoms, such as dizziness, syncope, palpitations, shortness of breath, angina, or edema only some of which may be pacemaker related. About one-third of symptoms result from some pacemaker malfunction, the remainder will be of cardiovascular origin unrelated to the pacemaker. One of the recently recognized causes of recurrent symptomatology is the pacemaker syndrome. The pacemaker syndrome occurs in lesser or greater degree during single-chamber ventricular pacing and results from

1. Cyclic atrial and ventricular synchronization, which causes cyclic variation of cardiac output and of peripheral blood pressure;
2. Retrograde conduction and entrainment of the P wave. Such an event can cause a marked drop in cardiac output, a feeling of pressure in the precordium (sometimes analogous to angina), and pounding in the neck and chest resulting from cannon waves in the jugular venous system and the pulmonary vasculature.

The pacemaker syndrome can be very severe in some patients, although almost one-quarter of patients paced only from the ventricle have been estimated to have some level of severity. It can be diagnosed by noting fluctuation in peripheral blood pressure, by physical examination, and the finding of cannon waves in the neck. The diagnosis can be made by history alone. Management is by restoration of the normal AV sequence. If a patient with sinus bradycardia is paced at a more rapid rate from the ventricle, P waves may be entrained retrograde. Lowering the ventricular paced rate in order to prevent asystole but allow sinus bradycardia will restore the normal AV sequence. Atrial or dual-chamber pacing usually is preferred (Figure 10).

Symptoms may recur because of episodic pacemaker inhibition. Unfortunately, this is a common occurrence, occurring in almost one-third of patients with unipolar inhibitory pacemakers. About one-half of those affected will by symptomatic. Pacemaker inhibition by electromyographic inhibition (EMI) occurs almost exclusively in unipolar systems in which sensing is of the pectoral musculature adjacent to the pacemaker. If a pacemaker is inhibited, the patient will return briefly to the unprotected circumstance. If that is asystole, syncope may occur. In newer dual-chamber pacemakers, the devices are both inhibited and triggered. Unusual arrhythmias may occur, and an endless loop tachycardia can be started by EMI.

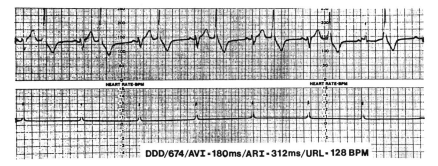

DDD/674/AVI-180ms/ARI-312ms/URL-128 BPM

Figure 10.   *Echo beating is readily determined on Holter monitoring. This recording, with a pacemaker channel (below), demonstrates echo beating following each ventricular stimulus. Atrial sensing, ventricular capture, coupled VPCs, and normal recycle are all demonstrated.*

The test for EMI pacemaker effect is the provocation of pectoral muscle activity by raising a weight or vigorously pressing the hands together during electrocardiographic monitoring. A very large number of unipolar pacemakers will be affected, but the incidence will be falsely positive. Ambulatory monitoring is a much more realistic approach that will detect EMI very well in daily usage (Figure 11).

Evaluation of returned symptoms can be a difficult undertaking. Pacemaker function should be carefully evaluated. Chest x-ray should be read for intermittent lead fracture and lead displacement. Fluoroscopy may be useful. Physiological evaluation and ambulatory monitoring is useful in any unusual situation. In the end, the 90% of patients who have returned symptoms for reasons other than the pacemaker will be treated for tachyarrhythmias, hypertension, angina, or primary neurological conditions, as necessary.

TELEMETRY

Pacemaker telemetry is noninvasive transmission of data from the implanted pulse generator to an external receiver. Both physiological and hardware data may be transmitted. Telemetry has been available in limited format for the past five years. It will become more complex and will assume progressively greater importance as electronic computer-based memory becomes available and as electronic capability for data analysis and processing becomes more sophisticated.

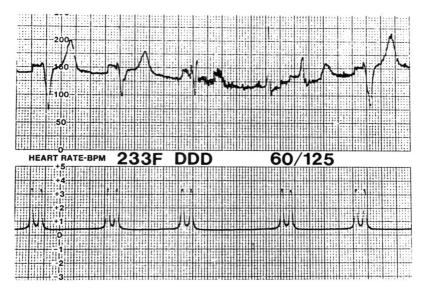

Figure 11.   *Holter monitoring is the best means of correlating symptoms with ECG findings. This is especially true for electromagnetic inhibition with pacemaker inhibition or false triggering. In this instance, the upper channel is a conventional ECG and the lower channel is that of the stimuli emitted by the pacemaker. Here, the EMI is seen clearly on the ECG, and inhibition of the pacemaker is clearly indicated.*

Telemetry was initially devised for the capability of transmitting hardware data such as the state of the pulse generator battery. Battery impedance, which rises progressively in a lithium iodine cell, corresponding to battery depletion is a good indication of the longevity remaining in a pulse generator. Lead impedance, also a measurable parameter, should lie within a narrow range, approximately that at implant. If impedance rises, lead fracture may have occurred. If it falls, insulation disruption or short circuit in a bipolar lead may have occurred. A low impedance will result in rapid depletion of a pulse generator, and reliable data of low impedance should be an indication for intervention or a resetting of the time of impending depletion and, therefore, the need for reschedule of follow-up.

More recently, additional hardware telemetry has become available including pulse duration, pulse amplitude in one or two channels, and the current drain from the battery and refractory intervals set for atrial and ventricular channels. Other telemetric capabilities include the display of upper and lower rates and the entire range of sensitive and refractory intervals after pacemaker programming.

Recently available telemetric capabilities involve transmission of memory data concerning the pacer use. Several pulse generators now have a memory for the number of stimuli emitted. If uncertainty exists concerning how frequently pacing is required, the counters can be reset to zero at each visit and read at a subsequent visit. If visits are sufficiently frequent and pacing sufficiently infrequent, the number of pacer stimuli can be counted. These memory banks are presently limited in capacity so that frequent pacing will overwhelm the data storage capability. With the impending development of high-density memory chips, it is likely that some variety of ambulatory ECG monitoring will be possible.

Despite all the hardware telemetry, this is of less present and potential utility than the availability of telemetry of physiological data. It is likely that some physiological functions will be telemetered in the near future. As physiological sensing pacemakers can set a stimulation rate based on pH, pCO_2, pO_2, or some other physiological parameter, that data can be telemetered out of the pulse generator for the physician's information.

Important present telemetry is that of the electrogram and of ECG interpretation channels. Electrogram telemetry can give an indication of the quality of the signal sensed by the pacemaker and which signal triggers its function. Telemetry can be of the atrial and/or the ventricular channels or both. Such telemetry indicates the quality of the EGM and can be invaluable in determining the nature of a malfunction caused by lead displacement, poor EGM amplitude, slew rate, or lead fracture. Atrial EGM telemetry can be useful in detecting a retrograde P wave and determine timing and existence of retrograde conduction. Not all EGM transmission is at an adequately high frequency to be valuable, some is not yet calibrated (Figures 12, 13).

ECG interpretation channels are at least equally important. The highly complex ECGs now being developed from dual-chamber pacemakers may not be capable of interpretation without assistance from pacemaker-generated markers. An EGM transmission is of a physiological signal, even when it may be of less than interpretable quality. A marker is an indication of how the pacemaker interprets a specific cardiac event. Simultaneous recording of marker information and a surface ECG can indicate what is being sensed and how the pacemaker deals with the sensed event. For example, a P wave that occurs too late in the lower rate interval cycle, which is always between ventricular

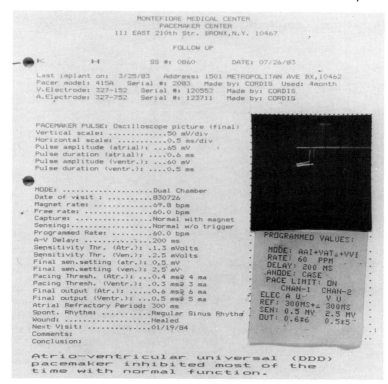

MONTEFIORE MEDICAL CENTER
PACEMAKER CENTER
111 EAST 210th Str. BRONX,N.Y. 10467

FOLLOW UP

K   H   SS #: 0860   DATE: 07/26/83

Last implant on: 3/25/83   Address: 1501 METROPOLITAN AVE BX,10462
Pacer model: 415A   Serial #: 2083   Made by: CORDIS Used: 4month
V.Electrode: 327-152   Serial #: 120552   Made by: CORDIS
A.Electrode: 327-752   Serial #: 123711   Made by: CORDIS

PACEMAKER PULSE: Oscilloscope picture (final)
Vertical scale: ....50 mV/div
Horizontal scale: ....0.5 ms/div
Pulse amplitude (atrial): ...65 mV
Pulse duration (atrial): ....0.6 ms
Pulse amplitude (ventr.): ...60 mV
Pulse duration (ventr.): ....0.5 ms

MODE: ....Dual Chamber
Date of visit : 830726
Magnet rate: ....69.8 bpm
Free rate: ....60.0 bpm
Capture: ....Normal with magnet
Sensing: ....Normal w/o trigger
Programmed Rate: ....60.0 bpm
A-V Delay: ....200 ms
Sensitivity Thr. (Atr.): .1.3 mVolts
Sensitivity Thr. (Ven.): .2.5 mVolts
Final sen.setting (atr.): 0.5 mV
Final sen.setting (ven.): 2.5 mV
Pacing Thresh. (Atr.): ...0.4 ms@ 4 ma
Pacing Thresh. (Ventr.): .0.3 ms@ 3 ma
Final output (Atr.): .....0.6 ms@ 6 ma
Final output (Ventr.): ...0.5 ms@ 5 ma
Atrial Refractory Period: 300 ms
Spont. Rhythm: ....Regular Sinus Rhythm
Wound: ....Healed
Next Visit: 01/19/84
Comments:
Conclusion:

PROGRAMMED VALUES:

MODE: AAI+VAT$_4$+VVI
RATE: 60 PPM
DELAY: 200 MS
-ANODE: CASE
PACE LIMIT: ON
CHAN-1   CHAN-2
ELEC A U-   V U
REF: 300MS+≜ 300MS
SEN: 0.5 MV 2.5 MV
OUT: 0.6*6   0.5*5

Atrio-ventricular universal (DDD)
pacemaker inhibited most of the
time with normal function.

Figure 12. *Telemetry may be of physiological data such as the electrogram or it may be of hardware data only. In this instance, hardware data only is transmitted and is provided on a paper tape printout. This provides information concerning sensitivity, output, rate, and refractory settings. The tape is attached to a site made available on the clinic visit form. The oscilloscopic photograph is also attached to the form. The remainder of the format, uniquely designed for each pulse generator, is computer-generated from patient data stored in the computer and information generated during the clinic visit.*

events, may be sensed but unused by a VDD pacemaker to begin an AV interval. An anomalously short AV interval is thus explained. The absence of ventricular sensing and ventricular pacer stimuli on ECG and the presence of atrial sense markers and markers of ventricular stimuli clearly indicate ventricular lead fracture. ECG interpretation channels are invaluable (Figures 14, 15).

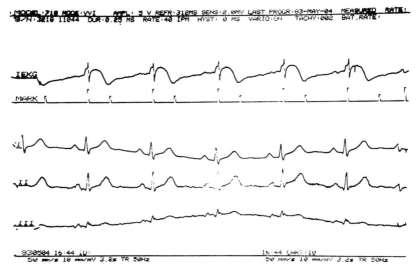

Figure 13.   *The use of a multichannel recorder with alphanumeric capabilities is invaluable. In the first channel telemetric text concerning model, mode, serial number, and date of last programming along with other data is recorded on paper from the programmer telemetry. Channel two is that of the telemetered intracardiac electrogram, and channel three is a marker indicating the instance of sensing and the duration of pacemaker refractoriness. Below are three ECG channels and then a "housekeeping" channel with date, time, paper speed, and patient identification.*

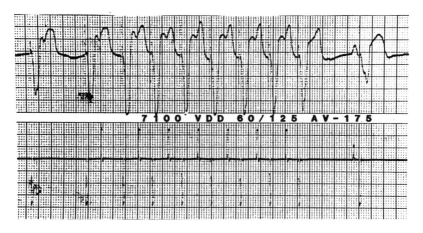

Figure 14.

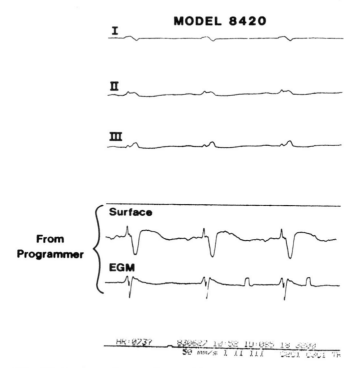

Figure 15. *Electrogram telemetry is especially valuable when compared to surface leads on a multichannel recorder. In this five-channel recording lead I, II, III are compared with both a telemetric transmission of the electrogram (surface) and a higher frequency direct telemetric recording (EGM). The timing and quality of the EGM can be determined readily via the telemetered EGM.*

Figure 14. *(Opposite) ECG interpretation channels are useful in indicating what a pacemaker senses and how it responds. Simultaneous ECG and ECG interpretation channels, with the ECG interpretation channel as the lower of the two, during endless loop tachycardia. The upward markers are atrial events, the taller indicating a sensed event that starts a timing cycle, the lower, a sensed but unused event. The downward markers are ventricular pace markers. The ventricular escape interval is 1,000 ms. The minimum interval between ventricular events is 480 ms. The retrograde P wave is sensed 260 ms after the ventricular event, and after a delay, readily measured as 220 ms, a ventricular stimulus is emitted. Bottom right, no retrograde P occurs. The next P wave appears too late to begin a full AV interval and is indicated by a lower mark.*

HOLTER MONITORING

Ambulatory ECG monitoring is a most effective means of determining satisfactory pacemaker function. In the presence of a malfunction that has occurred or has been provoked by daily activity, there is no technique that provides greater accuracy for determination of the state of the function of the pacemaker device and interaction with the patient. Passive ECG, even with provocative testing, can frequently detect malfunction of an implanted pacemaker and is, of course, the basic technique. However, it is often impossible to duplicate specific daily events and, certainly, it is impossible to record for a prolonged period. Ambulatory monitoring will frequently distinguish between false-negative results in the pacer center and false-positive results. False-positive results can be troublesome when pacer inhibition is found in the pacer center and its finding cannot be correlated with clinical findings.

Provocative tests of pacemaker function can detect failure to a substantial degree, but many episodes can only be detected by continuous ambulatory monitoring. Episodic events such as brief runs of endless loop tachycardia, which occur only during a brief return of retrograde conduction, can be detected as a source of symptoms by ambulatory monitoring and frequently not during passive ECG. Events related to daily activity, EMI, loss of capture in a specific body position, or activity and the effect of sleep or activity on patient-pacemaker interaction can be readily demonstrated.

PACEMAKER CLINIC

The pacemaker clinic represents an organized effort to detect abnormal pacemaker function. The overall management of the implanted patient or group of patients involves knowledge of the specific functional capabilities of the pacemaker system, i.e., the pulse generator and lead system and the anticipated variety of failure modes. If the lead system is known to have a proclivity for deterioration of the insulation material, such as has occurred in some models of polyurethane leads, then careful evaluation of sensing function loss of capture or high threshold and early battery depletion is to be anticipated as these can be the earliest manifestation of impending system failure. If a generator has a tendency toward sudden no output failure then that generator must be handled differently than those generators which experience has indicated will deplete slowly and in an orderly fashion. Once these considerations are understood and noted, it should be further understood that transtelephonic monitoring is an integral part of follow-up as clinic visits are time consuming and labor intensive. Large numbers of patients are best managed by transtelephonic monitoring punctuated by annual visits to the pacemaker center during which time more extensive investigation of the pacemaker status, including x-ray, programming, and determination of the underlying cardiac function, can be determined.

During a pacemaker center visit the patient is logged in on a schedule. The schedule for follow-up is the single most important consideration because it determines that follow-up will indeed occur (Table II). The patient should be connected to a multichannel ECG recorder in which at least three (or better six) channels simultaneously will be recorded. The pacer site is inspected. The wound should be clean and not tender. The pacemaker should be freely movable, and the overlying skin should be of normal color. If the skin is tight, tender, or erythematous, then infection may be present. If discomfort exists and infection is suspected, then the wound should be irrigated and cultures performed. For culture, the skin is carefully cleansed and painted with antiseptic solution (iodine is preferred) and a needle directed to the pulse generator. The passage of the needle will be stopped by the generator itself and will lie in a potential space around the generator. A syringe filled with isotonic saline from an intravenous infusion bottle rather than from solution used to dilute medication (such solutions contain bacteriostatic preservation and will defeat attempts at culture) should be used. The fluid irrigates the pacer site

---

Table II

Clinic visits may be mixed with transtelephonic monitoring but the schedule guideline is

SINGLE-CHAMBER PACEMAKERS
Twice-1st 6 months (following implant)

THEN

Once-Every 12 months

DUAL-CHAMBER PACEMAKERS
Twice-1st 6 months (following implant)

THEN

Once-Every 6 months

---

and is then placed in infusions for aerobic and anaerobic culture. A confirmed culture of a pathogen requires removal of the pacemaker hardware.

If the initial ECG demonstrates normal pacing with appropriate sensing and pacing in each channel, then the pacemaker should be inhibited to determine the underlying cardiac rhythm—a determination which is useful in following the progression or improvement in the rhythmic basis for original implantation and to determine whether pacemaker dependency exists (Figure 16).

If the pacemaker is entirely inhibited by spontaneous cardiac rhythm, then a magnet should be placed over the pulse generator. The (almost) universal response to placement of a magnet over the pulse generator is the asynchronous mode of operation during which capture in atrium and ventricle can be determined. The threshold of capture should then be tested to ascertain whether it is stable or even lower in relation to a previous determination or whether it has deterio-

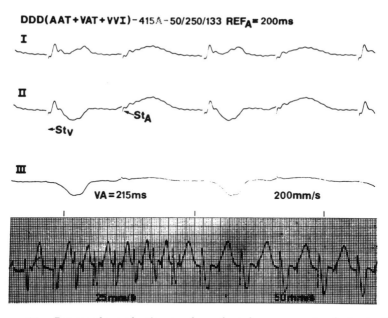

Figure 16.   *Retrograde conduction can be evaluated on an ongoing basis. In this instance, the DDD pacemaker is programmed to the atrial triggered mode so that the instant of sensing the P wave is marked by an emitted stimulus. In a multichannel recording (100 mm/s) the ventricular stimulus interval to the atrial "mark" stimulus is 215 ms. The same recording is possible with slightly less accuracy on a conventional electrocardiograph at 50 mm/s (below).*

rated (increased). All programmable pacemakers will allow such determination, and several have mechanisms that allow rapid, automatic determination of threshold operated either via the pulse generator or the programmer. If threshold is stable, no further intervention is required.

Check of sensing threshold can be accomplished by setting the dual-chamber pacemaker in the single-chamber ventricular then atrial or dual-chamber mode. If the unit is then set below the spontaneous cardiac rate, appropriate inhibition indicates satisfactory sensing of spontaneous cardiac activity. The sensitivity settings of the pacemaker can then be altered to determine the actual threshold and the sensitivity set appropriately. A major portion of the issue of sensitivity is the secondary effect of sensitivity to electromagnetic and electromyographic interference. If a higher output for cardiac stimulation is set than is necessary and if no adjacent structures (such as intercostal musculature or diaphragm) are stimulated, there are no secondary effects other than earlier battery depletion. The sensitivity setting, if higher than necessary, allows inappropriate sensing and, therefore, inappropriate response to noncardiac signals (Figure 17).

When all of the determinations and all of the appropriate settings have been made, the maintenance of records is the most important consideration. Thresholds of sensing and stimulation, the presence or absence of retrograde conduction and the possibility of endless loop tachycardia, final sensitivity settings, and final outputs should be recorded in a format that allows retention of all data and its ready access. This is especially important in modern multiprogrammable dual-chamber pacemakers in which contents of memory may contain additional information concerning the number of spontaneous and paced events and given some indication of the need of pacing. With such large volumes of information, only computer maintained data bases can process, retain, and generate a paper copy of the appropriate data (Figure 18).

SECONDARY INTERVENTION

The quality of the application of pacemaker therapy and effectiveness of follow-up is based on the stability of the lead system, quality of the electrodes, durability of the power source, and pulse generator programmability. Operator and follow-up capability is also intrinsic to the quality of the result. Unlike an operative procedure that does not involve the implantation of hardware, the use of a cardiac pacemaker

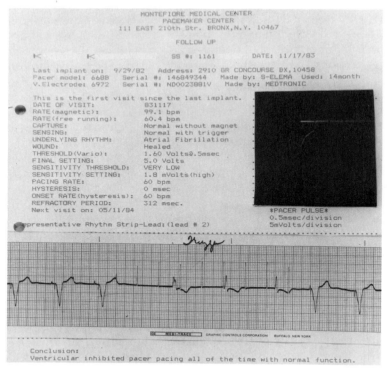

Figure 17. *The computer-generated clinic report designates historical data (top), the characteristics of the oscilloscopic artifact (center), and the data derived at the time of the visit. This includes mode of operation, rate, atrial and ventricular sensing thresholds, and final outputs. A summary of function is at the bottom. All data is retained in computer memory.*

requires improvements in hardware and personnel to improve the result. One measure of such improvement is the time to the first intervention after pacemaker implant. This has been calculated for the years 1965, 1970, 1975, 1977, 1980, 1982. The earlier pacemaker eras were less technologically stable and secondary intervention occurred much earlier. The time by which 10% of patients and then 50% of patients had the first reintervention was calculated in months (Figure 19).

Despite the increasing complexity of cardiac pacing involving multiprogrammability, dual-chamber pacing, and rate responsiveness, the overall result has been a stability of therapy, which means that, for pacemakers implanted during 1980, only 10% of devices will have undergone reintervention four years later. For those implanted during 1982 only 2.8% have undergone reintervention two years later. The

AUTOMATED PACEMAKER FOLLOW-UP (CLINICAL)
1. COMPUTER ASSISTED

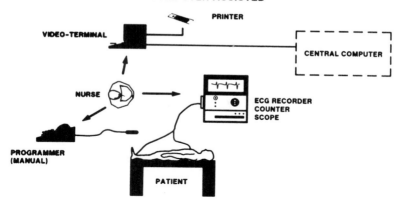

Figure 18. *Follow-up is computer-assisted at Montefiore Medical Center. The central computer contains data on all patients, records of their previous visits, and instructions and guidance on programming each of the pacemakers in use. The patient is attached to a counter, ECG, and oscilloscope. The nurse operates the program, derives data in cooperation with directions from the computer, and enters data into the computer. At the conclusion of the test procedure, all data has been entered into the computer, verified, and is in permanent memory. A printout, immediately available from a printer in the examination room, is provided for the chart and transmission to the referring physician.*

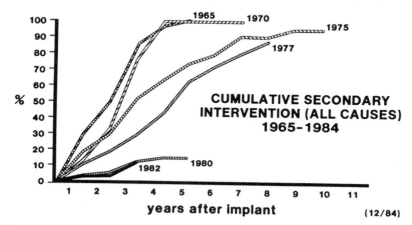

Figure 19. *The interval from implant to the first reintervention has prolonged over the years. Ten percent of patients implanted during 1965 had a secondary procedure by the end of three months, 50% by the end of twenty-four months, and all had a secondary procedure by the end of sixty months. Those implanted during 1982 had 2.8% secondary interventions by the end of the two years and fewer than 10% by the end of three years. The increased rate of reintervention was caused by exhaustion of short duration dual-chamber pulse generators and polyurethane lead failures.*

dramatic improvement of stability and durability of implanted pacing is remarkable.

BIBLIOGRAPHY

Benedek M, Furman S: Semiautomatic computer follow up for transtelephone patients. *PACE* 1983; 6:316.

Bilitch M, Hauser R, Goldman B, et al: Performance of cardiac pacemaker pulse generators. *PACE* 1985; 8:276–282.

Brevik K, Ohm OJ: Myopotential inhibition of unipolar QRS-inhibited (VVI) pacemakers assessed by ambulatory holter monitoring of the electrocardiogram. *PACE* 1980; 3:470–478.

Byrd CL, McArthur W, Stokes K, et al: Implant experience with unipolar polyurethane pacing leads. *Pace* 1983; 6:868–882.

Chardack WM, Gage AA, Federico AJ, et al: Five years' clinical experience with an implanted pacemaker: An appraisal. *Surgery* 1965; 58:915–922.

Choo MH, Holmes DR JR, Gersh BJ, et al: Permanent pacemaker infections: Characterization and management. *Am J Cardiol* 1981; 48:559–564.

Davies G, Siddons H: Prediction of battery depletion in implanted pacemakers. *THORAX* 1973; 28:180.

Dreifus LS, Pennock RS, Feldman M, et al: Experience with 3835 pacemakers utilizing transtelephonic surveillance. *Am J Cardiol* 1975; 35:133.

Edhag O, Elmqvist H, Vallin HO: An implantable pulse generator indicating asystole or extreme bradycardia. *PACE* 1983; 6:166–170.

Erbel R: Pacemaker syndrome. *Am J Cardiol* 1979; 44:771–772.

Escher DJW, Furman S: Oscilloscopic and recent other methods of implantable pacemaker follow-up. *Ann Cardiol Angeiol* 1971; 20:503.

Fisher JD, Escher DJW, Hurzeler P, et al: Recurrent syncope or dizziness after pacemaker implantation. *Clin Res* 1978; 26:231A.

Furman S: Cardiac pacing and pacemakers: V. Analysis of pacemaker malfunction. *Am J Cardiol* 1977; 94:378–379.

Furman S: Cardiac pacing and pacemakers VIII. The pacemaker follow-up clinic. *Am Heart J* 1977; 94:795–804.

Furman S: Transtelephone pacemaker monitoring. In EK Chung (Ed): *Artificial Cardiac Pacing: Practical Approach.* 2nd ed. Williams & Wilkins, Baltimore 1984, pp 345–358.

Furman S, Escher DJW: Transtelephone pacemaker monitoring. Five years later. *Ann Thorac Surg* 1975; 20:326–338.

Furman S, Parker B, Escher DJW: Transtelephone pacemaker clinic. *J Thorac Cardiovasc Surg* 1971; 61:827–834.

Goldman B, MacGregor D: Management of infected pacemaker systems. *CPPE* 1984; 2:220–235.

Greatbatch W, Lee JH, Mathias W, et al: The solid-state lithium battery; A new improved chemical power source for implantable cardiac pacemakers. *IEEE Trans Biomed Eng* 1971; 18:317.

Gribbin B, Abson CP, Clarke LM: Inhibition of external demand pacemakers during muscular activity. *Br Heart J* 1974; 36:1210–1212.

Hanson J: Sixteen failures in a single model of bipolar polyurethane-insulted ventricular pacing lead. *PACE* 1984; 7:389–394.

Hellend J: Pacemaker lead complications: Clinical significance and patient management. *Medtronic News* 1983; 13:8–14.

Hoffmann A, Jost M, Pfisterer M, et al: Persisting symptoms despite permanent pacing. Incidence, causes and follow-up. *Chest* 1984; 85:207–210.

Jacobs LJ, Kerzner JS, Diamond MA, et al: Myopotential inhibition of demand pacemakers: Detection by ambulatory electrocardiography. *Am Heart J* 1981; 101:346–347.

Judson P, Holmes DR, Baker WP: Evaluation of outpatient arrhythmias utilizing transtelephonic monitoring. *Am Heart J* 1979; 97:759–761.

Katzenberg CA, Marcus F, Heusinkveld R, et al: Pacemaker failure due to radiation therapy. *PACE* 1982; 5:156–159.

Laurens P: Nuclear-powered pacemakers: An eight-year clinical experience. *PACE* 1979; 2:356–360.

Lewis KB, Criley JM, Nelson RJ, et al: Early clinical experience with the rechargeable cardiac pacemaker. *Ann Thorac Surg* 1974; 18:490–493.

Lillehei RC, Romero LH, Beckman CB, et al: A new solid-state, long-life, lithium-powered pulse generator. *Ann Thorac Surg* 1974; 18:479–489.

MacGregor DC, Covvey HD, Noble EJ, et al: Computer-assisted reporting system for the follow-up of patients with cardiac pacemakers. *PACE* 1980; 3:568–588.

MacGregor DC, Noble EJ, Morrow JD, et al: Management of a pacemaker recall. *J Thorac Cardiovasc Surg* 1977; 74:657.

Mantini EI, Majors RK, Kennedy Jr, et al: A recommended protocol for pacemaker follow-up: An analysis of 1,705 implanted pacemakers. *Ann Thorac Surg* 1977; 24:62–67.

Mitsui T, Mizuno A, Hrsegawa T, et al: Atrial rate as an indicator for optimal pacing rate and the pacemaking syndrome. *Ann Cardiol Angeiol* 1971; 20:371.

Morse D, Fernandez J, Lemole G: A four year study of 123 programmable pacemakers. *Chest* 1976; 70:436.

Morse DP, Tesler UF, Lemole GM: The actual lifespan of pacemakers. *Chest* 1973; 64:454.

Mymin D, Cuddy TE, Sinha SN, et al: Inhibition of demand pacemakers by skeletal muscle potentials. *JAMA* 1973; 223:527.

Parsonnet V: Cardiac pacing and pacemakers VII. Power sources for implantable pacemakers Part 1. *Am Heart J* 1977; 94:517–528.

Parsonnet V, Myers GH: Residual function of explanted pulse generators. *AAMI* 1973; 7:203–207.

Parsonnet V, Myers GH, Gilbert L, et al: Prediction of impending pacemaker failure in a pacemaker clinic. Am J Cardiol 1970; 25:311–319.

Pennock RS, Dreifus LS, Morse DP, et al: Cardiac pacemaker function. *JAMA* 1972; 222:1379.

Rosenqvist M, Edhag O: Pacemaker dependance in transient high-grade atrioventricular block. *PACE* 1984; 7:63–70.

Ruben S: Sealed zinc-mercuric oxide cells for implantable cardiac pacemakers. *Ann NY Acad Sci* 1969; 167:627.

Rubenstein JJ, Laforet EG: Pacemakers runaway following intermittent output failure. *PACE* 1983; 6:645–647.

Schneider AA, Kulp JW: Lithium-iodine batteries for cardiac pacemakers. *Med Electron* 1978; 9:50–54.

Shaw GB, Evans A, Brewster GM, et al: Telephone monitoring of patients with pacemakers in the west of Scotland. *Br Med J* 1981; 283:127–129.

Sholder J, Levine PA, Mann BM, et al: Bidirectional telemetry and interrogation in cardiac pacing. In SS Barold, J Mugica (Eds): *The Third Decade of Cardiac Pacing*. Futura, Mount Kisco, 1982, pp 145–166.

Smyth NPD, Purdy DL, Sager D, et al: A new multiprogrammable isotopic powered cardiac pacemaker. *PACE* 1982; 5:761–767.

Smyth NPD, Millette M: The isotopic cardiac pacer: A ten year experience. *PACE* 1984; 7:82–89.

Steiner RM, Morse D: The radiology of cardiac pacemakers. *JAMA* 1978; 240: 2574–2576.

Stone JM, Bhakta RD, Lutgen J: Dual chamber sequential pacing management of sinus node dysfunction: Advantages over single-chamber pacing. *Am Heart J* 1982; 104:1319–1327.

Tyers GF, Foresman RA JR, Brownlee RR, et al: An automated tester for evaluation of pacemaker battery performance and reliability. *J Surg Res* 1974; 16:262–267.

Tyers GFO, Brownlee RR: The non-hermetically sealed pacemaker myth. Or, Navy-Ribicoff 22,000-FDA-Weinberger. *J Thorac Cardiovas Surg* 1976; 71:253.

van Gelder LM, El Gamal MI: False inhibition of an atrial demand pacemaker caused by an insulation defect in a polyurethane lead. *PACE* 1983; 6:834–839.

Venkataraman K, Bilitch M: Clinical experience with a programmable pacemaker. *PACE* 1980; 3:605–611.

Ward DE, Camm AJ, Spurrell RAJ: Ambulatory monitoring of the electrocardiogram: An important aspect of pacemaker surveillance. *Biotelemetry* 1977; 4:109–114.

Welti JJ: Pacemaker surveillance "A La Francaise": An attempt to detect faulty series of permanent pacemakers at an early stage. *PACE* 1978; 1:342–344.

Chapter 16

TELEMETRY

Seymour Furman

Telemetry is the transmission of data from an implanted pulse generator to an extracorporeal receiver. Unidirectional telemetry, i.e., from the pulse generator to the programmer is being supplanted by bidirectional telemetry in which commands are transmitted from the programmer to the pulse generator and responses are transmitted from the generator to the programmer. Telemetry is of great value in routine analysis of pacemaker function, especially during interpretation of complex electrocardiograms and especially troubleshooting of malfunction. Transmission is of two broad varieties, that of hardware and of physiological data. It is broken down further into five categories:

1. Hardware identification;
2. The electrogram (EGM);
3. ECG interpretation channels;
4. Memory contents including information placed into memory by the physician and memory of pacemaker function;
5. Combinations of the above (Table I).

It is also important to recognize that not all that is printed from a programmer is telemetered. Because of the complexity of modern programming, programmers commonly deliver a tape with the programmed details printed out. Some printouts show only what the operator has selected and the programmer transmitted, there is no implication that the signals have been received and that pacemaker function has been changed. In that instance, independent verification, such as on an ECG and an oscilloscope or other instrument, is required to ascertain that programming has indeed occurred. In other instances both the programmed commands and a telemetered confirmation will be printed. The operator must be aware of which data is simply a repetition of what has been entered into the programmer and what is actually telemetered from the implanted pacing system (Figure 1) (Table II).

Table I
Pacemaker Telemetry

I. Programmed pacemaker settings
II. Measured pacemaker stimulation parameters
III. Pulse generator and electrode hardware data
IV. Real-time pace sense events (ECG interpretation channel)
V. Electrogram (EGM)
VI. Memory Contents

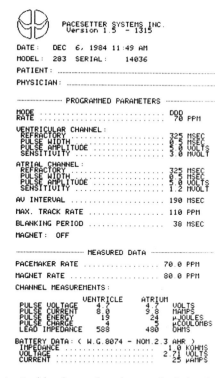

Figure 1. *A printout of hardware data from a dual-chamber pacemaker lists the output, sensitivity, and interval settings that have been programmed. These are not actually telemetered, rather they repeat the programmed settings. The telemetered data is indicated as "measured" data.*

Table II
Programmed Pacemaker Settings

1. Mode	5. Refractory period
2. Rate	6. Hysteresis
3. Pulse amplitude, duration, voltage	7. AV delay
4. Sensitivity	8. Upper and lower rates

HARDWARE IDENTIFICATION

Hardware identification may include battery status, battery voltage and impedance and lead impedance, the model and serial number of the pulse generator, its date of manufacture, and the date of implant (if placed into memory).

Hardware telemetry can be useful in determining the cause of malfunction. Several manufacturers allow telemetry of lead impedance during analysis of pacemaker function so that diagnosis of lead malfunction can be made noninvasively. If records of lead impedance, measured intraoperatively at implant or via telemetry early after implant, are available, then telemetric interpretation of impedance increase, indicating lead fracture, or decrease, indicating insulation disruption, can be accomplished preoperatively (Figure 2). Battery depletion can be indicated by a decrease in the magnetic pacer rate on ECG or by an increase in the impedance of a lithium battery measured telemetrically (Table III).

ELECTROGRAM

The electrogram is an especially important aspect of data transmission as it indicates the quality of the signal the pacemaker senses and upon which the generator's software decisions are based. The intrinsic deflection may be readily visible and indicate the time of sensing of antegrade and retrograde events and allow a decision concerning the quality of sensing and pacing function (Figure 3). The two major defects of EGM data transmission are the restricted response of the radio frequency link limited to approximately 300 Hz and the electrocardiograph upon which the data is printed, which may be further limited to 100 Hz (Figure 4). Both limitations reduce the quality of data.

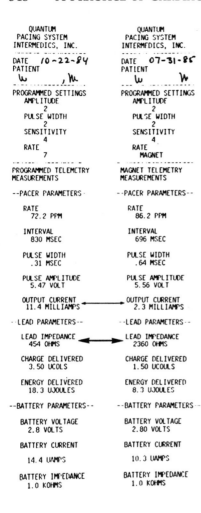

Figure 2. A telemetric diagnosis of lead fracture can be made when the lead impedance increases greatly from its stable value. In this instance, the lead impedance on 10-22-84 was 454 Ohms, on 7-31-85 it was 2,360 Ohms. Lead fracture was confirmed on x-ray. Note that the impedance reduced output current, battery current drain, and the energy delivered. The changes in rate, interval, and pulse width were not relevant.

Table III
Pulse Generator and
Electrode Hardware Data

1. Battery voltage
2. Battery current drain
3. Battery impedance
4. Electrode impedance

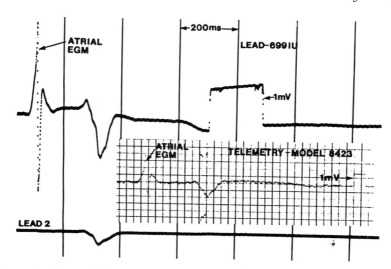

Figure 3. *The atrial electrogram, telemetered from a single-chamber unipolar pacemaker is illustrated and compared to the electrogram derived directly from the lead at a band width of 0.1−2,000 Hz. Despite the restricted telemetry frequency response, the overall quality and timing of the atrial EGM can be determined.*

Only a few systems can telemeter both atrial and ventricular electrogram channels simultaneously (Figure 5). Often this is accomplished by splitting the frequency response in such a way that the transmission frequency for each channel is no more than 100−150 Hz, which severely limits the quality of the electrogram. For systems that cannot transmit atrial and ventricular electrograms simultaneously, important relationships between atrial and ventricular function are not readily discernible via telemetry except as a far-field signal. ECG interpretation channels, therefore, may have an even greater capacity for troubleshooting, as the activity of both atrial and ventricular channels is indicated. While the transmission of the electrogram is an important capability and will assume greater importance in the future, its usefulness now is limited (Figure 6A, 6B).

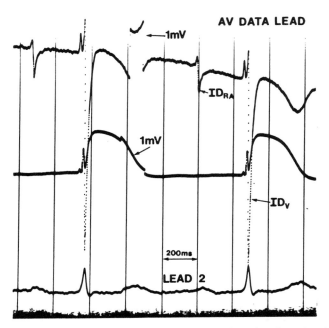

Figure 4. *An AV data lead has terminals in the ventricle and in the atrium in a single lead and is able to record atrial and ventricular events simultaneously on the same channel. As there is also a ventricular electrode for conventional sensing and stimulation, three electrogram channels are possible.* **ABOVE:** *The AV data channel with atrial and ventricular electrograms.* **MIDDLE:** *The ventricular electrogram from the lead tip.* **BELOW:** *Lead 2.*

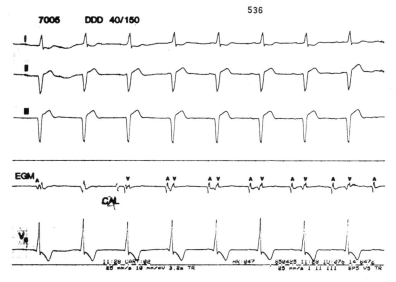

Figure 5.

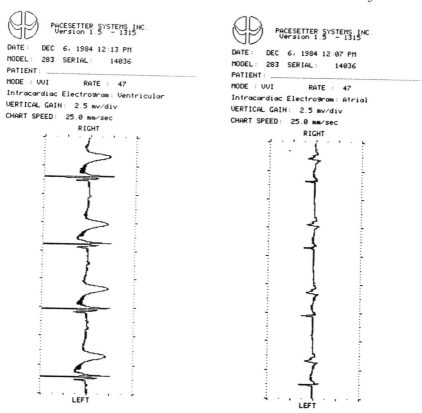

PACESETTER SYSTEMS INC.
Version 1.5 - 1315

DATE: DEC 6, 1984 12:13 PM
MODEL: 283 SERIAL: 14036
PATIENT: ....
MODE : UVI   RATE : 47
Intracardiac Electrogram: Ventricular
VERTICAL GAIN: 2.5 mv/div
CHART SPEED: 25.0 mm/sec
              RIGHT

              LEFT

6A.

PACESETTER SYSTEMS INC.
Version 1.5 - 1315

DATE: DEC 6, 1984 12:07 PM
MODEL: 283 SERIAL: 14036
PATIENT: ....
MODE : UVI   RATE : 47
Intracardiac Electrogram: Atrial
VERTICAL GAIN: 2.5 mv/div
CHART SPEED: 25.0 mm/sec
              RIGHT

              LEFT

6B.

Figure 6A. *An electrogram telemetered via the ventricular channel. The quality of the signal can be interpreted as can its amplitude, in this instance about 7.5 mV. The P wave can be discerned as a small distant signal.*

Figure 6B. *The electrogram telemetered via the atrial channel. The atrial intrinsic deflection is followed by a far-field QRS complex approximately 250 ms later. The amplitude of the atrial electrogram is approximately 2.5 mV.*

Figure 5. *(Opposite) Electrogram telemetry of the atrial channel with the far-field ventricular EGM recorded simultaneously. The surface leads give the impression that AV conduction with first degree AV block is present. The atrial EGM clearly demonstrates the lack of relationship between atrial and ventricular events, i.e., complete AV block.*

ECG INTERPRETATION CHANNEL

ECG interpretation channels are designed to indicate the pacing and sensing function of single- and dual-chamber pacemakers (Table IV). In each, the instant of sensing or pacing is indicated with associated events such as the onset of alert, and refractory and safety pacing intervals by a mark on the programmer printout. As sensing occurs at the intrinsic deflection, the mark indicates the timing of those events (Figure 7). ECG interpretation channels (which do not telemeter the electrogram) can indicate the relationship between atrial and ventricular sensing and stimulus emission (Figure 8). As the mark is an artifact of the pacemaker sensing and output circuits, an indicator of pacemaker response to cardiac function exists. In some telemetry, an artifactual ECG will have marks on it giving the impression of an actual ECG. A ladder diagram has also been developed in conjunction with an artifactual ECG, which indicates, much as a conventional ladder, the relationship between atrial and ventricular events, adding the appropriate alert, refractory, and blanking intervals (Figure 9).

A variety of different ECG interpretation channels, some wholly artifactual, others with telemetered EGMs or ECGs exist. It is important, in each instance to distinguish whether the apparent signal (ECG or EGM) is artifactual or real.

The atrial mark can indicate a sensed atrial event that starts a pacemaker cycle or one that occurs too early or too late in the timing cycle to begin a timing event. It can also indicate a stimulus emission from either ventricular or atrial channel, which, if not reflected on the ECG, can suggest a lead fracture (Figure 10). As sense and pace markers exist for both channels, the exact relationship between the two is shown, and, in some systems, can be recorded simultaneously with the ECG and clarify the ECG and pacemaker involvement. ECG interpretation channels clearly indicate which electrocardiographic events are being sensed properly and which start a timing cycle (Figure 11). The mark indicates which events do not begin such a cycle and which

---

Table IV
Real-time Pace and Sense Events
(ECG interpretation channel)

1. Sensing
2. Pacing

At atrial and/or ventricular levels

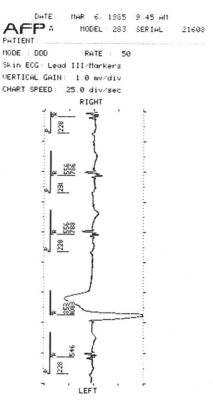

DATE: MAR 6, 1985 9:45 AM
AFP ж   MODEL: 283 SERIAL: 21608
PATIENT: ....
MODE : DDD   RATE :   50
Skin ECG: Lead III/Markers
VERTICAL GAIN: 1.0 mv/div
CHART SPEED: 25.0 div/sec

Figure 7.   *Timing intervals can be superimposed on a surface ECG, in this instance lead III simultaneously with the various intervals. The first P wave is sensed 228 ms before the QRS complex. The first conducted QRS is sensed near its beginning on the surface, but the VPC is sensed later within the deflection. The escape intervals between events and the refractory intervals are clearly indicated.*

are unsensed. The persistence of retrograde conduction can be recognized and quantified, and data used to determine the appropriate duration of a programmed atrial refractory interval. Most of the EGM and ECG interpretation channels print out on programmer paper tape. This defect will be corrected as printers and multichannel electrocardiographs become available that will allow input from the programmers either via a computer link or by direct input. In some systems the electrogram can be printed out on a multichannel recorder while the ECG interpretation channel can only be printed on programmer tape (Figure 12).

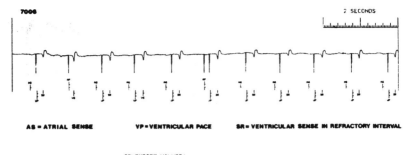

TELEMETRY VALUES:

	TEMP	PERM	
MODE :	DDD	DDD	
LOWER RATE :		60	PPM
A-V DELAY :		150	MS
UPPER RATE :		125	PPM
PULSE WIDTH:			
ATRIAL		0.5	MS
VENTRICULAR		0.05	MS
SENSITIVITY:			
ATRIAL		1.25	MV
VENTRICULAR		2.5	MV
AMPLITUDE:			
ATRIAL		2.5	V
VENTRICULAR		2.5	V
REFRACTORY :			
ATRIAL		325	MS
TACHY DETECTED:		NO	
SAFETY PACING :		ON	
BATTERY:		OK, ABOVE 2.5V	

Figure 8. *ECG interpretation channels can indicate what it is that the pacemaker senses when pacing occurs and the relationships between the various sensed and paced events. In this illustration, atrial sensing and ventricular sensing are normal, ventricular pulse duration is below threshold of capture. QRS complexes result from conduction following a spontaneous P wave that is normally sensed. The QRS complexes fall into the ventricular refractory period after the ventricular stimulus. They are unsensed and do not begin a timing cycle.*

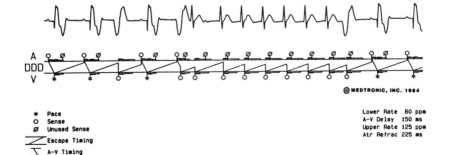

Figure 9. *An automatic, programmer drawn, ladder diagram is a useful telemetric indication of pacemaker function in which pace and sense events, and atrial and ventricular refractories can be indicated much as in a hand-drawn ladder diagram. This is a simulated ECG and does not represent actual cardiac events. A real ECG must be available to correlate with the ladder diagram findings.*

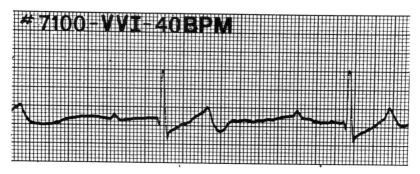

Figure 10. *A patient with complete heart block and an implanted VDD (atrial synchronous, ventricular inhibited) was seen without pacemaker stimuli on the electrocardiogram.* **A.** *The ECG is in the VVI mode programmed to a rate of 40 bpm. There is no evidence of pacemaker activity.*

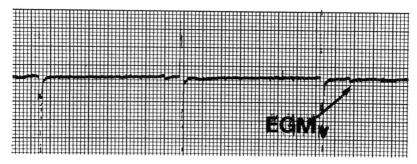

Figure 10B. *Telemetry of the ventricular EGM shows only a small deflection and ventricular stimuli, not seen on the ECG at a rate of 40 bpm.*

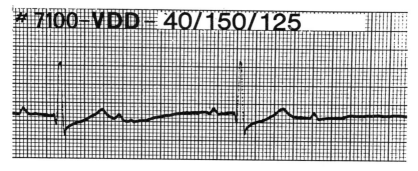

Figure 10C. *Programming to the VDD mode with an AV interval of 150 ms, a lower rate limit of 40 bpm, and an upper rate limit of 125 bpm again shows no evidence of pacemaker activity.*

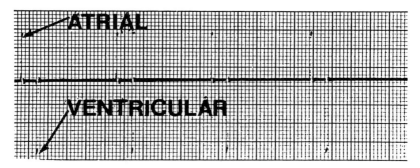

Figure 10D. *ECG interpretation channel telemetry shows normal sensing of atrial events, the absence of sensing of ventricular events, emission of ventricular stimuli at the programmed AV interval without visibility on the ECG, and the absence of ventricular capture. The most likely fit for these findings was ventricular lead fracture, which was subsequently radiographically confirmed.*

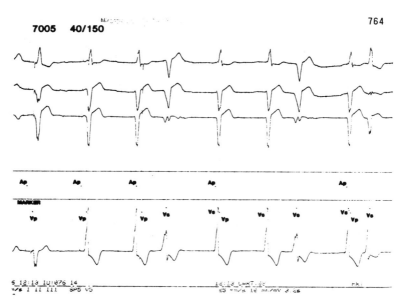

Figure 11. *Intermittent failure of atrial sensing and ineffective atrial stimuli are clearly indicated on the ECG interpretation channel. Three spontaneous ventricular events V_s are properly sensed. Ventricular complexes five and eight are sensed after the atrial stimulus during the safety pacing interval. Two ventricular marks occur, the first V_s for ventricular sensing, the second V_P for the "safety" stimulus. No ventricular stimulus V_p clearly captures the ventricle.*

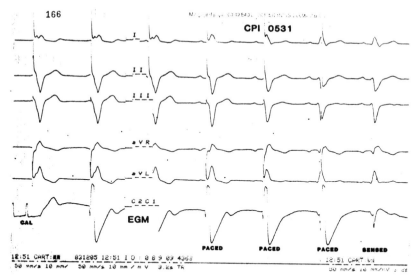

Figure 12. *Telemetry of the single-chamber electrogram is best printed simultaneously with several other electrocardiographic channels. In this display of five surface leads and the electrogram only, the last is an unpaced EGM. The CAL is 5 mV and the spontaneous EGM is, therefore, approximately 5 mV in amplitude and occurs late in the simultaneously recorded surface leads. The preceding EGM is a fusion beat with the stimulus occurring earlier than the intrinsic deflection of the ventricular depolarization.*

MEMORY CONTENTS

Memory contents fall into two subcategories, data placed into memory by the physician and that which results from pacemaker activity. The latter category can be further subdivided into activity generated by stimulation and that of sensed events (Table V):

1. Data placed into memory—Several pulse generators have a memory into which coded data can be entered. This data includes lead model and threshold, electrogram amplitude, and pacemaker settings at implant, medications the patient is consuming, and the indication for pacemaker implant. If the system is used, all of this data is entered by a coding arrangement provided by the manufacturer and can be read later from the pulse generator by the programmer. As there is no commonly accepted coding for different conditions, this data may be

Table V
Measured Impulse
Stimulation Parameters
1. Interval (rate)
2. Duration
3. Current
4. Voltage
5. Charge and energy

useful for the physician with the appropriate programmer, but less valuable should the patient visit another physician.

2. Data derived during pacemaker operation—Several pacemakers can store information concerning pacemaker activity. Categories can be made of: (a) atrial paced beats; (b) ventricular paced beats; (c) atrial and/or ventricular sensed beats; (d) ventricular premature contractions, which are defined as spontaneous ventricular events not preceded by a sensed or paced atrial event, and atrial premature contractions defined as atrial events that are sensed at specific times of the cardiac cycle during which atrial activity is not anticipated (Figure 13) (Table VI).

This data can be valuable if implantation is accomplished with less than absolute evidence of AV block or of sinus arrest or if atrial or ventricular ectopic activity occurs. Once the pacemaker is implanted it can be set at a rate sufficiently low so that, if a stimulus is emitted, it can be assumed that pacing is necessary. Coupled beats and runs of sensed tachycardia can be counted both as individual events and runs of tachycardia. All of the data now recorded is numeric. P waves and QRS complexes are not recorded individually. The compromises made in diagnosis of various arrhythmias do not allow the actual recording of the QRS complexes or P waves. This is a major defect as the reading of the actual ECG or EGM is of great value. This Holter capability will be very useful when it exists, but as the digitized ECG consumes very large amounts of computer memory, such Holter recordings are unlikely to be available soon.

UTILITY OF TELEMETRY

Telemetry is a relatively new addition to pacemaker technology. As such, its capabilities have not been fully explored and innovations can be anticipated as its electronic base becomes more sophisticated.

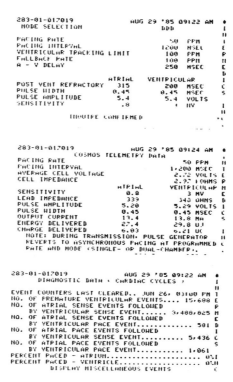

Figure 13. *Printout of telemetry from dual-chamber model 283-01. The top section consists of pacemaker settings determined by the INQUIRE command. The middle section is the telemetered hardware data. The lower section (Diagnostic data) is that of the pacemaker memory contents of data derived during pacer function. As the event counters are CLEARED and reset when read, it is possible to determine the number of events during the interval from the past clearing of the memory register. In this instance, the pacemaker was largely inhibited, but the atrium was stimulated 5,436 times with AV conduction inhibiting ventricular output. Other events are as indicated.*

Table VI
Memory Contents

A. Patient Data:
   1. I.D. Number
   2. Indication for pacing
   3. Medication, etc.

B. Pacemaker Data:
   1. Type and location of electrode
   2. Stimulation thresholds
   3. Model and serial Number
   4. Date of implant, etc.

C. Processed Data:
   1. Ratio of paced to sensed beats
   2. Absolute number of paced beats

Telemetry can be broken down into four broad areas, that of identification of the pulse generators and its functional setting; that of the output settings of the generator and such additional data as lead impedance, battery impedance, and battery voltage, indicating how much longevity remains in the unit. The third capability is memory for its own settings and its function so that a variety of Holter recordings can be interrogated from the device. The fourth capability is that of some variety of marker, either by telemetry of electrograms or of ECG interpretation channels to indicate its function.

The four functions are presently restrained because of the absence of a common means of transmitting and recording data. Each manufacturer uses a recording device of unique capability. Some are relatively easy to operate, the recording is rapid and readily interpretable, while others are arcane, the printers of hard copy are excruciatingly slow and present a barrier to use rather than providing assistance. Still, even single-chamber modern pulse generators are so complex and are programmable in so many different ways that automatic transmission of data for record keeping purposes is very useful. When programming a modern six function (a common number of functions for a multiprogrammable model) single-chamber pulse generator, a single printout of the new programmed setting is preferable to a two-person team, one to program and the other to transcribe.

The telemetry of battery impedance and voltage is useful, but the availability of a magnetic rate that is correlated with battery status (a technique widely used for two decades) is almost as good and has the advantage of being interpreted on an ECG alone and requiring only the use of the ubiquitously available magnet. In practical fact, it is easier to derive this data via transtelephonic monitoring with a magnet and a pulse generator magnetic rate than with telemetry of the data. An ECG interpretation channel indicating the instant of sensing, and refractory and alert intervals is useful in a single-chamber pulse generator.

The telemetry of memory function such as the number of times paced and the number of sensed events may be useful, but until there is a clear indication from the generator that a recorded paced event was indeed in response to need, the data will be of limited value. This "Holter" function will await the availability of adequate computer memory to allow the recording of an ECG of reasonable facsimile within the pulse generator and its telemetry to an external recorder. The widespread use of such telemetry will also probably await agreement on interfaces for the production of hard copy.

We are therefore left with the printing of programmed settings to allow the rapid knowledge of pulse generator function and the use of

ECG interpretation channels. While useful in single-chamber pulse generators, both are far more useful in dual-chamber pacing. While six programmable functions are common in single-chamber pulse generators, far more are needed in dual-chamber generators. The relationship between events on the electrocardiogram and the intervals between atrial and ventricular events, refractory and alert intervals, and upper and lower rate limits can only be recorded in a comprehensible fashion by a hard copy indication of the interplay between the pacemaker and the heart. It is in this area that telemetry of ECG interpretation channels is useful. With increasing complexity of the device, certainly when pacemakers are used more extensively for tachycardia management, telemetry will be more widely available and more widely used (Figure 14).

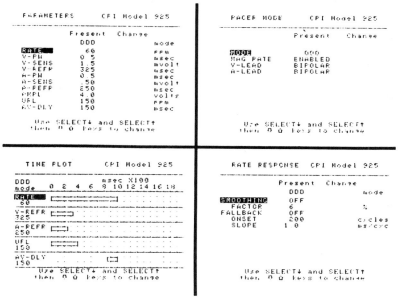

Figure 14.   *Data available from CPI Model 925 "DELTA" programmer pacemaker printout. The upper left corner of the figure displays the parameters at which the pacemaker is currently programmed. In the upper right corner is a screen indicating whether or not the magnet rate is enabled and if the leads are functioning in a unipolar or bipolar mode. In the lower left corner is a display of the rate, ventricular refractory period, atrial refractory period, upper rate limit, and AV delay plotted in a bar graph to allow the user a graphic display of the relationship of the various programmed intervals and how a change in one interval affects another programmed change. The lower right corner is the final screen of telemetered information and reflects whether or not smoothing and/or fallback is being utilized.*

BIBLIOGRAPHY

Byrd C, Schwartz S, Wettenstein E, et al: Computer-aided analysis of pacemaker function. *Comput Cardiol* 1984; 11:147.

Duffin EG: The marker channel: A telemetric diagnostic aid. *PACE* 1984; 7:1165–1169.

Halperin JL, Camunas JL, Stern EH, et al: Myopotential interference with DDD pacemakers: Endocardial electrographic telemetry in the diagnosis of pacemaker-related arrhythmias. *Am J Cardiol* 1984; 54:97–102.

Irnich W, Effert S: Telemetric control of pacemaker function. *Dtsche Med Wochenschr* 1971; 19:811–814.

Kruse I, Markowitz T, Ryden L: Timing markers showing pacemaker behavior to aid in the follow up of a physiological pacemaker. *PACE* 1983; 6:801–805.

Levine PA: Confirmation of atrial capture and determination of atrial capture thresholds in DDD pacing systems. *CPPE* 1984; 2:465–473.

Levine PA, Lindenberg B, Mace R: Analysis of AV universal (DDD) pacemaker rhythms. *CPPE* 1984; 2:54–73.

Levine PA, Sholder J, Duncan JL: Clinical benefits of telemetered electrograms in assessment of DDD function. *PACE* 1984; 7:1170–1177.

Olson WH, McConnell MV, Sah RL, et al: Pacemaker diagnostic diagrams. *PACE* 1985; 8:691–700.

Sholder J, Levine PA, Mann BM, et al: Bidirectional telemetry and interrogation in cardiac pacing. In SS Barold, J Mugica (Eds): *The Third Decade Of Cardiac Pacing*. Futura, Mount Kisco, 1982, p. 145–166.

Sutton R, Citron P: Electrophysiological and hemodynamic basis for application of new pacemaker technology in sick sinus syndrome and AV block. *Br Heart J* 1979; 41:600–612.

Sutton R, Perrins EJ, Duffin E: Interpretation of dual chamber pacemaker electrocardiograms. *PACE* 1985; 8:6–16.

Taylor KD: An FM telemetry demodulator for telephone pacemaker clinics. *Biomed Eng* 1978; 25:87–90.

Uhley HN: An inexpensive receiver for ECG telemetry. *Am Heart J* 1976; 91:346–348.

Ward DE, Camm AJ, Spurrell RAJ: Ambulatory monitoring of the electrocardiogram: An important aspect of pacemaker surveillance. *Biotelemetry* 1977; 4:109–114.

Chapter 17

PROGRAMMABILITY

David L. Hayes

Programmability can be defined as the ability to make noninvasive, stable, but reversible changes in pacemaker function. The pulse generator contains predetermined circuits from which one or several features or functions can be selected for variation within a restricted range. Using a "pacemaker programmer," one can change some aspects of pacemaker function. It is not possible to produce a completely new program with available pacemakers. (Although investigational work is being carried out with "software", i.e., microprocessor-based pacemakers in which new programs, not part of the manufacturing process, can be written, there are no commercially available products at this time.)

The first modern programmable units were introduced in 1972. In this pacemaker, a magnetic code was introduced from an external programmer to manipulate four levels of output and six rates. Since 1972, numerous changes have evolved in pacemaker programming capabilities. Not only have a progressively greater number of programmable functions been developed, but there has been a gradual change from the use of the initial magnetic code to the use of radio frequency signals (the only American manufacturer continuing to use magnetic code programming will supplant that system in the next generation of pulse generators).

Development of the technology of pacemaker programming has been extremely rapid in recent years. It was estimated in 1978 that programmable pacemakers accounted for 36% of all pacemaker implants. Pacemakers at that time were programmable for rate or pulse width (or both). By 1984, all initial pacemaker implants at our institutions were programmable for two or more variables. Some dual chamber pacemakers are now capable of as many as 2.5×10^{23} programmable combinations. The North American Society of Pacing and Electrophysiology/British Pacing and Electrophysiology Group (NASPE/BPEG) code designates the degree of programmability in the fourth position. In the NASPE/BPEG code, "M" denotes simple programmability, i.e., rate and/or output, and "P" indicates multiprogrammability (see Chapter 6) (Table I).

Table I
Uses of Programmability

	Increase	Decrease
Rate	Optimizes cardiac output	Adjusts below angina threshold
	Overdrives arrhythmias	Decreases pacing frequency to preserve atrial transport
Output	Adapts to threshold	Conserves energy
		Reduces extracardiac stimulation
Sensitivity	Senses low endocardial signals	Senses T waves
		Detects extracardiac signals
Refractory period	Minimizes T-wave sensing	Detects early diastolic premature ventricular contractions
	Minimizes QRS sensing (AAI)	
Hysteresis	Delays onset of pacing to preserve atrial transport	
Polarity	Converts to unipolar to correct lead fracture and to amplify low endocardial signal	Converts to bipolar to decrease pacemaker artifact distortion of QRS and to decrease electromagnetic interference

Table II
Potential Programmable Values

Single chamber	Dual chamber
Mode	Mode
Rate	Lower rate
Pulse duration or voltage amplitude (or both)	Atrioventricular delay*
Sensitivity	Upper rate
Hysteresis	Sensitivity: atrial and ventricular
Refractory period	Refractory periods: atrial and ventricular
Polarity	Polarity
	Upper rate limit response
	Blanking period
	Magnet on and off†

*Is a function of rate in some units.
†Available in a limited number of models.

Pacemaker programmability varies widely, depending on the design of the individual pulse generator (Table II). The first and greatest variable is whether the pacemaker paces a single chamber or has dual-chamber capabilities. Features such as atrial refractory period, blanking periods, atrioventricular (AV) delays, and upper rate response deal with dual-chamber pacemakers. These variables are in large part related one to another in maintaining and optimizing AV synchronous performance. These variables are in Chapter 7, "Comprehension of Pacemaker Timing Cycles" and discussed in Chapter 11, "Pacemaker Electrocardiography."

Although there are fewer variables to program with single-chamber pacing, optimal programming with any pacemaker can have a profound effect on its longevity, patient well-being, and avoidance of further invasive procedures. The remainder of this chapter deals with the basic programmable variables pertinent to all pacemakers; programmable features associated with dual-chamber pacing are described in the chapters cited previously (Table III).

RATE PROGRAMMABILITY

Rate programmability is the most frequently used programmable feature. The range of rate programmability varies widely among units. The major use of rate programming is to allow a patient to remain in sinus rather than in paced rhythm when sinus bradycardia with intermittent sinus arrest or intermittent AV block exists. Programming a rate of 60 bpm or even as low as 40 to 50 bpm may allow the patient's intrinsic sinus rhythm to exist as much of the time as possible. Only in

Table III
Common Ranges of Programmability

Parameter	Common range
Basic pacing rates (low rate)	30–150 bpm
AV interval	25–250 ms
Upper rate (maximal rate)	100–175 bpm
Atrial pulse width (ms)	0.05–2.0 ms
Ventricular pulse width (ms)	0.05–2.0 ms
Atrial sensitivity	0.25–11 mV
Ventricular sensitivty	0.5–14 mV
Atrial refractory period	150–500 ms
Ventricular refractory period	200–500 ms
Atrial pulse amplitude	2.5–8.0 V
Ventricular pulse amplitude	2.5–8.0 V
Blanking period	12–50 ms

the event of a more profound sinus bradycardia or asystole will a pacemaker programmed at this rate support the heart. Slower pacing rates (slower than the nominal value of 70 bpm) are helpful in the following circumstances:

1. to allow dominance of the patient's intrinsic rhythm;
2. to prolong longevity of the pulse generator in patients with sinus brady-cardia and intermittent sinus arrest;
3. to provide pacemaker protection from an underlying rhythm disturbance in patients with coronary artery disease and significant angina in whom a nonprogrammable pacemaker with a fixed rate of 70 to 72 bpm would increase myocardial oxygen consumption and complicate the medical management of angina;
4. to avoid the consequences of ventriculoatrial (VA) conduction occurring with VVI pacing and not with sinus rhythm.

More rapid pacing rates. i.e., greater than 70 bpm, are used most commonly in pediatric patients. In a few patients, a rate faster than 70 bpm may improve cardiac function or suppress an atrial or ventricular arrhythmia. Many of the reasons for pacing at slow rates are eliminated by restoration of the normal AV sequence now possible with dual-chamber pacing.

More rapid pacing rates also are used at the time of pacemaker follow-up. If the patient's intrinsic rate is greater than the programmed rate, the imposed rate is increased in order to assess the threshold of stimulation (Figure 1).

HYSTERESIS PROGRAMMING

Programming of hysteresis permits prolongation of the first pace-maker escape interval after a sensed event. A pacemaker programmed at a cycle length of 1,000 ms (60 bpm) and at a hysteresis of 1,200 ms (50 bpm) allows 200 ms more for another sensed QRS complex. Should another QRS complex not be recognized, the pacemaker will stimulate continuously at the programmed rate of 60 bpm, an escape interval of 1,000 ms (Chapter 11, Figure 13) until a sensed event restarts the cycle. The advantage of hysteresis is in the ability to maintain spontaneous AV synchrony as long as possible (Figure 2). This may prevent symptomatic retrograde VA conduction. In most patients with symptomatic VA conduction, hysteresis provides reliable backup pac-ing and increases the potential for the patient's own rhythm. (The possibility exists of hysteresis with an abbreviation of the paced inter-

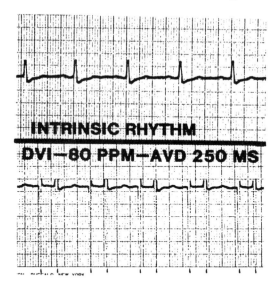

Figure 1. *ECGs during follow-up of a DVI (Medtronic Byrel 5993) pulse generator. The intrinsic sinus rhythm is at a rate of approximately 75 bpm. To ascertain stimulation threshold it is necessary to increase the pacing rate to greater than 75 bpm. In the lower panel the pacemaker is programmed to the DVI mode at a rate of 80 bpm to drive the atrium.*

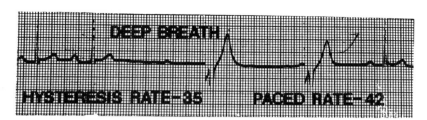

Figure 2. *ECG of a young man with episodic heart block upon deep inspiration. The hysteresis rate was set at 35 bpm (cycle length 1,714 ms) and the pacing rate at 42 bpm (cycle length 1,430 ms). With a deep breath, AV block occurs and a longer interval is allowed from the last spontaneous sensed event to between the two paced events. The episode is ended and recycled by a conducted ventricular event.*

val after the first sensed event. This capability is not present in any currently available pulse generator.)

PROGRAMMING OF OUTPUT (Pulse Width and Voltage Amplitude)

Although programming pulse generator output has been used less commonly than changing the rate, it may be more important. Programming output can be used to extend pulse generator life by output reduction or to solve the clinical problem of rising stimulation threshold. Presently available pulse generators have programmable output, from a minimum of approximately 2 or 3 μJ to a maximum of almost 200μJ. The customary pacemaker output of 5 V and 0.5 ms pulse duration, current limited to 10 mA (an output of approximately 25μJ) is an acceptable average, although some units are now delivered at 2.5 V output (i.e., $12-13$ μJ) as they are to be used with lower threshold leads than were available previously. In patients in whom stimulation thresholds are lower, decreasing output can result in significant prolongation of pulse generator life. Conversely, in a few patients, increasing thresholds develop after implantation. These high thresholds may be transient or permanent. The threshold may increase to an output requirement of 100 or more microjoules without obvious lead displacement. Output programmability is useful in transient and permanent situations. In patients with a transient elevation, maximal output can be used until thresholds return to a stable chronic level. In patients with chronic high thresholds, the pulse generator can be programmed to higher output to permit reliable pacing (albeit with shorter pulse generator longevity).

The rationale for output programming is illustrated by the three hypothetical patient stimulation threshold curves in Figure 3. At the time of implantation, patients A, B, and C had a similar threshold of approximately 0.75 V at 0.5 ms pulse duration. After implantation, stimulation threshold evolution for the three patients differed significantly. A more marked increase in the early threshold, exceeding 4 V, developed in patient A, but the threshold decreased thereafter to a stable long-term level. The threshold in patient B peaked at approximately 2.5 V two to three weeks after implantation. The longterm threshold was approximately twice the acute threshold. Patient C had a lower acute threshold of stimulation, approximately 0.4 V. During follow-up no increase in threshold was noted, and 6 months after implantation, threshold remained almost identical to that of the initial

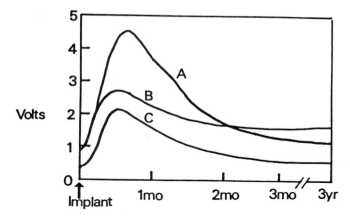

Figure 3.   *Three hypothetical patient stimulation threshold curves. (See text).*

value. This is the type of threshold evaluation seen in the modest number of patients with investigational steroid (dexamethasone)-tipped leads.

Not shown in Figure 3 is the very rare patient who has a late rise in threshold. In this patient, it is necessary to increase the pacemaker pulse duration or output voltage. For the individual patient, early and long-term threshold behavior cannot be predicted absolutely by the threshold value obtained at implantation. The value of output programmability to maintain the widest margin of patient safety is obvious.

The output function to be programmed for the most effective control of a rising threshold is still uncertain. Newer pulse generators allow programmability of pulse duration and output voltage. Of the options available, it is likely that pulse duration programming over the range 0.05 to 1.0 ms is more effective. Programming to a pulse duration greater than 1 ms approaches rheobase, does not provide much additional pacing margin of safety, and causes high current and energy drain. If pulse duration programmability defines a threshold greater than 1 ms in duration, then output voltage increase is the better option if it exists in the implanted pulse generator. If threshold is high, rheobase (the lowest voltage threshold at an infinitely long pulse duration) may be above a specific voltage setting no matter how long the programmed pulse duration. Output voltage programming is then required. As a general rule, if a proper pulse duration can be found between 0.5 to 1.0 ms, pulse duration programming is suitable, if pulse duration threshold is high, then output voltage is more useful. Conversely, if threshold is very low, i.e., in the range of 0.05–0.1 ms at a given output voltage, consider the reduction of voltage and the modest prolongation of pulse duration. The rationale for this approach is described in Chapter 3 "Basic Concepts." Indications for increasing the output of the pulse generator include:

1. maintaining cardiac pacing in a patient with poor electrode position or "microdislodgment";
2. use with an old, inefficient but still serviceable lead;
3. control of temporary high threshold evolution (Figure 4).

It should be pointed out that output programmability should not, at any time, be a substitute for proper lead placement (see Chapter 10, Troubleshooting).

Reduction of output from nominal (i.e., factory delivered) values is safe for most patients and translates into prolonged longevity of the pulse generator (Figure 5). Programming output to an efficient but safe level can increase the projected battery life by 50% or more. This is of

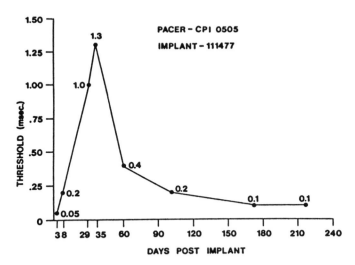

Figure 4.   *Occasional high threshold evolution following pacemaker implant can be managed with output programmability. In this instance, threshold at implant was 5.2 V and 0.05 ms pulse duration, the briefest pulse width that this pulse generator was capable of delivering. At 35 days threshold had risen to 1.3 ms pulse duration, an increase of 26 times. Threshold gradually decreased to stabilize at 0.1 ms, a normal level. Long-term threshold behaved normally, remaining stable at 0.1 ms pulse duration.*

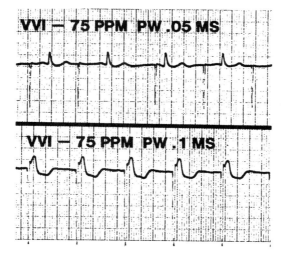

Figure 5. *Two ECGs from a patient with an implanted VVI pulse generator. Stimulation threshold had been determined noninvasively. At a programmed pacing rate of 75 bpm and pulse duration of 0.05 ms, ventricular capture does not occur. Note that the second QRS complex on the left is appropriately sensed to recycle the pulse generator. In the lower ECG, the pulse duration has been programmed to 0.1 ms and normal capture occurs.*

particular importance in patients with dual-chamber (therefore, potentially high current drain) pulse generators. Decrease in output can be used not only to increase pulse generator longevity but also to eliminate phrenic or diaphragmatic and local pectoral muscle stimulation. If extracardiac muscular or nerve stimulation occurs, reduction in output voltage is preferable to reduction in pulse duration. If a voltage can be found that is below the rheobase of the stimulation threshold of the organ being stimulated, the output pulse duration can be increased to provide consistent cardiac capture without extracardiac stimulation (Figure 6).

STIMULATION THRESHOLD

Determination of the stimulation threshold is an important consideration in setting pulse generator output. The process of determining stimulation threshold can be prolonged, tedious, and, if subthreshold output is reached and not promptly corrected, dangerous. Several pulse generator models have programmable features that allow auto-

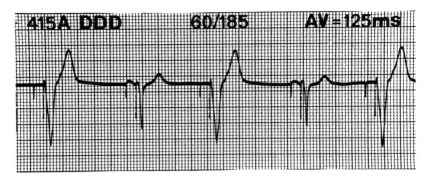

Figure 6.   *Output setting just below threshold causes intermittent capture. Increase in output can produce consistent capture. As atrial output is just below threshold, each alternate stimulus does not capture the atrium and the ventricular stimulus produces a paced ventricular QRS. Those atrial stimuli that cause an atrial contraction allow AV conduction with a fusion QRS.*

matic output testing. This can be done during programming in which the programming sequence reduces pulse duration through each step until the sequence is stopped manually (Figure 7). Another approach decreases output by 0.5 V in ten steps from full output when the magnet is applied when programmed to the threshold test mode (Figure 8). Still, a third approach is a proprietary mode called "Vario." It is a programmable option in several multiprogrammable pacemakers and is available for both atrium and ventricle in several models of dual-chamber pacemaker. In the Vario mode, magnet application reduces voltage output by $\frac{1}{15}$ progressively until zero output is reached. Removal of the magnet returns full output. The Vario mode can be activated for the test procedure only or allowed to be effective continuously.

SENSITIVITY PROGRAMMABILITY

All noncompetitive pulse generators sense and filter the intracardiac electrogram delivered through the electrode(s). For atrial and/or ventricular sensing, the R and P waves must have minimal amplitude (millivolts) and slew rate (dV/dt) for proper sensing to occur. The sensitivity of the pulse generator is the R (or P) wave of the lowest amplitude that the until will recognize as a ventricular (or atrial) depolarization (Figure 9). The pacemaker definition of whether it is an R or P wave depends on the channel through which it is sensed. Events

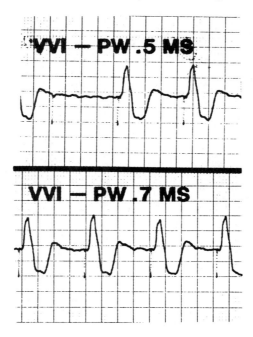

Figure 7. *ECGs from a patient with a Spectrax 5984 VVI,M pulse generator. Magnet application initiates three asynchronous pulses at a rate of 100 bpm. The first and second are of normal, i.e., programmed, pulse duration, and the third is at 75% of that duration. The pacing margin of safety can be assessed with magnet application if output is only slightly above threshold. In the upper panel, the first pacing artifact seen is the third of the three asynchronous pulses at 100 bpm and does not capture. A suprathreshold stimulus is at 0.5 ms, but at 75% of this output duration (equivalent to a pulse duration of 0.375 ms) failure to capture occurs. In the lower panel the programmed pulse duration is 0.7 ms. The first pacing artifact is again the third of the three asynchronous pulses and is therefore at 75% of programmed, or 0.525 ms. Capture is maintained.*

sensed through the atrial channel will be defined as P waves, those via the ventricular channel as R waves. For nonprogrammable models, the sensitivity is usually preset from 1.2 to 2.5 mV, and poor sensing will occur if the amplitude of the intracardiac R wave is too low. Although the amplitude of the intracardiac R wave may be adequate at the time of implantation, this amplitude may decrease for a variety of reasons, including metabolic and drug effects and lead dislodgment. Each electrogram decreases in amplitude and slew rate as chronicity occurs. Each ventricular focus is not sensed equally, and some ventricular foci (conducted or ectopic) may not reach an adequate level of amplitude or slew rate to be sensed. Some extrasystoles may be sensed, while

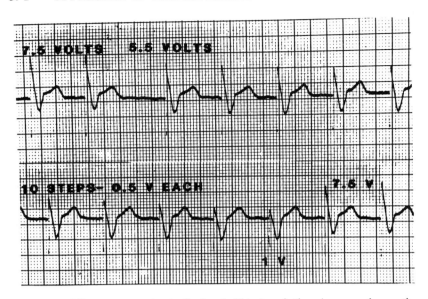

Figure 8.   *When programming to the threshold test mode there is a pause longer than the usual escape interval (between stimuli two and three), thereafter, from the nominal full output of 5.5 V, the output decreases by 0.5 V steps until 1 V is reached. The unit then returns to the programmed output. Should capture be lost, removal of the programmer from the pulse generator returns full output at the next stimulus. Pacing threshold can be readily calculated by counting the number of stimuli.*

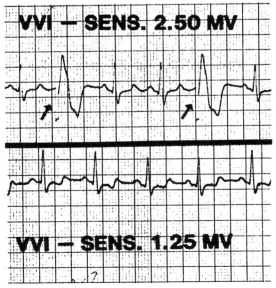

Figure 9.

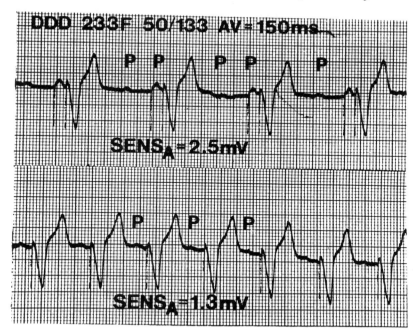

Figure 10. *Atrial sensitivity programming of a dual-chamber (DDD) pacemaker changes atrial sensing and mode of operation.* **ABOVE:** *Insensitivity to spontaneous P waves allows an atrial stimulus to produce an atrial contraction followed by a ventricular stimulus, both at the lower rate limit (50 bpm).* **BELOW:** *Increasing atrial sensitivity from 2.5 mV to 1.3 mV allows atrial sensing and the restoration of atrial synchrony.*

conducted beats may not be sensed and vice versa. If the pulse generator is used in the atrial position, the P wave must have a minimum amplitude and slew rate for proper sensing to occur, as described for ventricular pacing (Figure 10). Atrial and ventricular electrograms are similar, except that the atrial electrogram is of lower amplitude.

Sensitivity programming can be accomplished by an increase in the sensitivity of the amplifier, for example, decreasing the amplitude of the signal required to trigger the unit but maintaining the same frequency spectrum. Because poor QRS and P waves contain a pre-

---

Figure 9. *(Opposite) Two ECGs from a patient with a ventricular-inhibited pacemaker.* **ABOVE:** *A program ventricular sensitivity of 2.5 mV and a rate of 70 bpm (coupling interval 850 ms). On two occasions, pacing artifacts occur approximately 450 ms following a spontaneous QRS complex, equivalent to a pacing rate of 136 bpm, indicating failure to sense.* **BELOW:** *Sensitivity has been reprogrammed to 1.25 mV and returns sensing to normal.*

dominance of low-frequency signals, a program shift to lower frequencies and an increase in gain can be useful and is provided as a programmable option in some generators.

Sensitivity programmability to increase or decrease sensitivity has saved additional operative procedures. Increased sensitivity is especially useful in atrial pacing as the electrograms are usually far smaller than those obtained during ventricular pacing. Decreasing sensitivity is useful in eliminating oversensing of nonphysiological electromagnetic interference signals or such physiological signals as pectoral muscle artifacts (Figure 11).

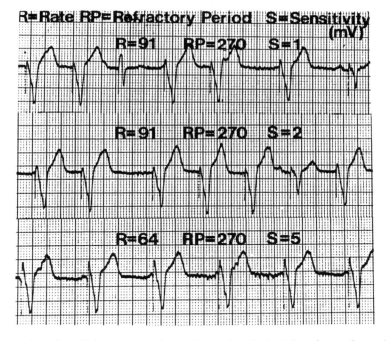

Figure 11.   *Sensitivity programming can be used to eliminate interference from a lead fixation mechanism. Because of interfering signals sensed by the pulse generator, the fifth interval is prolonged. At this time, the sensitivity level for ventricular pacing was 1 mV. Reprogramming and reduction of sensitivty to 2 mV did not eliminate artifact sensing, but further reduction to 5 mV produced consistent pacing without false inhibition.*

REFRACTORY PERIOD

Programming in Single-Chamber Pacemakers

Refractory period programming in single-chamber pacing is not commonly used. However, it can be advantageous in two situations. The first is in a pacemaker the refractory period of which is so long that it is prevented from sensing some ventricular electrograms. Should this occur, the subsequent pacemaker stimulus could fall on the T wave of the unsensed beat. Conversely, a refractory period too short can allow sensing of the T wave and inappropriate inhibition of the pulse generator. In the second situation, less commonly seen, some older pulse generators have sensed the afterpotential following a stimulus. The problem may be corrected by prolongation of the refractory period or, reduction of the pulse duration if an adequate pacing margin of safety still exists. If a single-chamber, unipolar, generator is used for atrial pacing, a longer refractory period is desirable to avoid sensing the QRS electrogram (Figure 12).

Programming Dual-Chamber Pacemakers

Refractory periods in dual-chamber dual-sensing units are much more complex than in single-chamber units because the events and timing cycles in one channel impact on the other. When programmed to a dual-chamber sensing mode (VDD, DDI, DDD), refractory periods exist for each sensing channel. The refractory period for the ventricular channel will behave as for single-chamber sensing. The operation of the refractory period on the atrial channel is quite different. Following an atrial stimulus or a sensed atrial event, the atrial sensing amplifier becomes refractory for the AV interval plus the programmed atrial refractory interval after the ventricular event. Immediately following a ventricular sensed event, an intrinsic QRS complex, or PVC, the atrial sensing amplifier will become refractory for the programmed refractory period.

Programmable flexibility of the atrial refractory period is especially important because of its role in preventing pacemaker-mediated tachycardia (Figure 13). Because pacemaker-mediated tachycardia can occur only when the atrial refractory period is shorter than the retrograde conduction time, this is an especially important interval (Figure 14).

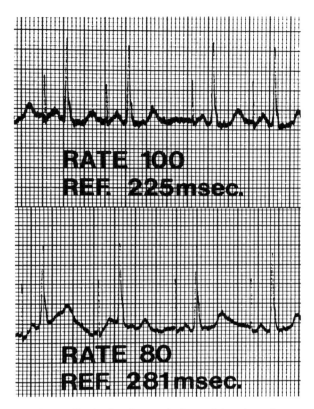

Figure 12. **ABOVE:** *Single-chamber, unipolar atrial pacing via a coronary sinus lead with sensing of the QRS complex, inhibition and recycle of the pacemaker. The duration of the refractory period in this pacemaker is a nonprogrammable function of the programmed rate, more rapid rates have a shorter refractory period.* **BELOW:** *The refractory period has been prolonged by reducing the programmed rate. Ventricular sensing no longer occurs.*

Figure 14. *(Opposite) Management of prolonged retrograde conduction requires prolongation of the atrial refractory interval (ARI) after the ventricular event.* **ABOVE:** *The ARI is briefer than the retrograde conduction time, 300 ms. Retrograde P waves are sensed and an endless loop tachycardia is sustained at a coupling interval of 640 ms (94 bpm) below the pacemaker upper rate limit.* **MIDDLE:** *The ARI is prolonged to 500 ms. Retrograde P waves cannot be sensed, and pacing and sensing occur at a coupling interval of 750 ms (80 bpm). The upper rate limit has been reduced to an interval of 675 ms(89 bpm).* **BELOW:** *The lower rate has been reduced to an interval of 1200 ms (50 bpm) and atrial sensing has been restored.*

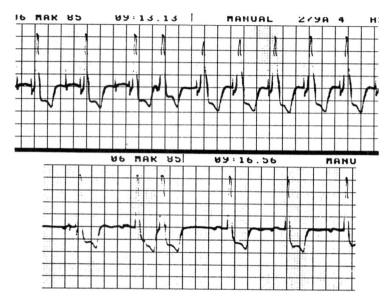

Figure 13. *ECGs from a patient with a DDD pulse generator.* **ABOVE:** *The fourth QRS complex is a premature ventricular contraction that produces a retrograde P wave and a pacemaker-mediated tachycardia at the programmed upper rate of 110 bpm.* **BELOW:** *The atrial refractory period has been programmed to 325 ms. The third complex is premature, but with a longer atrial refractory period, the retrograde P wave is unsensed and pacemaker-mediated tachycardia does not occur.*

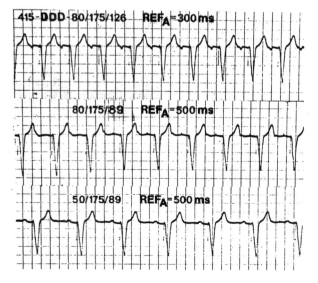

Figure 14.

Not all patients, however, have intact VA conduction; some have short retrograde conduction times. The effect of programming a long atrial refractory period on the upper rate and the possibility of endless loop tachycardia should be considered (Figures 14, 15, 16).

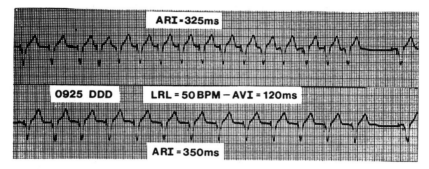

Figure 15.   *Programming of atrial refractoriness can allow endless loop tachycardia.* **ABOVE:** *An atrial refractory interval (ARI) of 325 ms allows sensing of retrograde P waves.* **BELOW:** *Prolongation of the ARI to 350 ms eliminates sensing of retrograde P waves and the possibility of endless loop tachycardia.*

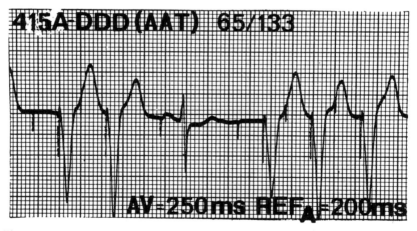

Figure 16.   *Evaluation of the possibility of endless loop tachycardia and the retrograde conduction time can be accomplished with some pulse generators in the DDD mode with atrial triggering, atrial output below capture threshold, a short atrial refractory period, and a long AV interval to encourage retrograde conduction. The fourth QRS complex is not preceded by a paced P wave (the atrial stimulus is ineffective), retrograde conduction occurs, and the retrograde P wave is marked by a triggered atrial stimulus. The fact of pacemaker-mediated tachycardia is demonstrated as well as the interval from the ventricular stimulus to the atrial intrinsic deflection.*

MODE PROGRAMMING

The combinations of available programmable stimulation modes have increased, as have all other programmable features. Most programmable single-chamber pacemakers can be programmed to the inhibited, triggered, or asynchronous mode. The inhibited mode is most commonly used for long-term pacing. The triggered (AAT, VVT) is helpful during follow-up to determine normal sensing (Figure 17). The triggered mode cannot be inhibited (this is only partially true in at

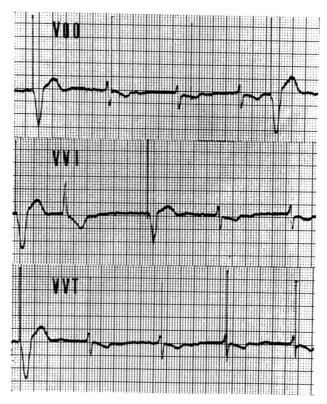

Figure 17. *Many single-chamber and some dual-chamber programmable pacemakers can be programmed to three different modes of ventricular pacing. In this example pacing is in the VOO (above), VVI (middle), and VVT (below) modes of operation.* **ABOVE:** *Spontaneous ventricular contractions are disregarded and stimuli continue at the programmed interval of 1,200 ms (rate of 50 bpm).* **MIDDLE:** *Spontaneous activity is sensed and pacemaker output is inhibited.* **BELOW:** *In the triggered mode, sensed ventricular events cause a stimulus to be placed onto the QRS complex.*

least one model) and is therefore useful when noncompetitive pacing is associated with EMI. The asynchronous mode is rarely used for long-term pacing because it is potentially competitive with spontaneous conducted or ectopic activity.

In dual-chamber pacemakers, multiple single- and dual-chamber modes usually are available. Newer dual-chamber pacemakers may have as many as 14 programmable pacing modes.

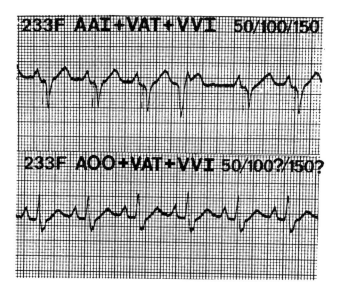

Figure 18.   *Restoration of atrial sensing changes the sequence of atrial and ventricular function.* **ABOVE:** *The function code is proprietary and is the equivalent of DDD pacing. As the sensed atrial event starts the AV interval, 100 ms later a ventricular stimulus is emitted.* **BELOW:** *This code is the equivalent of DVI pacing. As an AV interval is not started with a sensed atrial event, the ventricular rate which is above the lower rate limit of 50 bpm inhibits pacemaker output.*

A multimodal pacemaker pulse generator can be programmed to meet a variety of pacing modes and for troubleshooting (Chapter 10) and follow-up (Chapter 13).

PROGRAMMABLE PACING MODES

VOO—Ventricular pacing; no sensing.

AOO—Atrial pacing; no sensing.

VVT—Ventricular pacing; ventricular sensing and triggering.

AAT—Atrial pacing; atrial sensing and triggering.

VVI—Ventricular pacing; ventricular sensing and inhibited.

AAI—Atrial pacing; atrial sensing and inhibited.

VVIR—Ventricular pacing; ventricular sensing with inhibition; rate modulated pacing.

AAIR—Atrial pacing; atrial sensing with inhibition; rate modulated pacing.

DOO—Dual-chamber pacing; insensitive.

DVI—Dual-chamber pacing; ventricular sensing and inhibition; atrial insensitivity (Figure 18).

DDI—Dual-chamber pacing; dual-chamber sensing and inhibited; no tracking of the atrium.

DDD—Dual-chamber pacing; dual-chamber sensing; tracking of the atrium and ventricular inhibition. The dual-chamber sensing and pacing mode with atrial tracking can exist in four different versions, all of which have value in specific circumstances. If the atrium is sensed and a timing cycle started that will result in a ventricular stimulus in the absence of sensing in the ventricular channel during the AV interval, the sensed atrial event may result in inhibition of atrial output or may cause a stimulus to fall on the P wave as in the AAT mode of operation. Thus, there are two varieties of atrial operation in the DDD mode, neither can be specified on the code. Equally, the ventricular channel can be inhibited or triggered by a sensed ventricular event. If both atrium and ventricle are in the triggered mode of operation, the mode is DDT. The DDT mode is useful for antitachycardia overdrive using an external module. The atrial triggered mode is useful to determine the long-term duration of the retrograde conduction interval. The most commonly used is the mode of atrial and ventricular inhibition. Triggering in either atrium or ventricle is less commonly used.

DDDR—Dual-chamber pacing; dual-chamber sensing; tracking of the atrium and ventricular inhibition. Dual-chamber rate modulation.

DVIR—Dual-chamber rate-modulated pacing without atrial sensing or tracking. This mode will be available as part of the programmability of a DDDR pacemaker.

VDD—Ventricular pacing; dual-chamber sensing, tracking of atrium with ventricular inhibition.

OOO—In several models it is possible to program the device **OFF** to assess the underlying rhythm.

POLARITY

Recently polarity programmability has become available. This allows programming from unipolar to bipolar functions. The applicability of this technology is not fully known, but it appears to be most helpful in patients who have myopotential or electromagnetic inhibition in the unipolar mode but not in the bipolar mode. Unipolar and bipolar electrograms have distinctly different characteristics, and programming from one polarity to the other may result in superior sensing of an electrogram or the elimination of the sensing of an unwanted electrogram or interfering signal. For example, a retrograde P wave may be sensed in the unipolar mode but not the bipolar, or vice versa. Selective programming can then reduce or eliminate the possibility of endless loop tachycardia. At present, all polarity programmable pulse generators program the same polarity in both channels. Unipolar programmability in one channel and bipolar in the other is not an option at the present time (Figure 19).

DUAL-CHAMBER PROGRAMMABILITY

In complex dual-chamber pacing modes, programmable combinations are almost endless. With these pacing modes, programmability allows changes in output, rate, sensitivity, refractory period, and pacing cycle for each chamber. Inhibited or triggered modes, sensitive or insensitive modes, and pacing and sensing only in each chamber are all possible. Because of the number of options available from a given manufacturer, many possible combinations exist. Common ranges of programmability are given in Table III.

The importance and utility of noninvasive programmability is easily demonstrated in a series of electrocardiograms from a patient with a DDD pacemaker during routine Pacemaker Clinic follow-up.

PROGRAMMING SEQUENCE TO ESTABLISH NORMAL FUNCTION

1. Baseline (nonmagnet) electro-cardiogram (Figure 20);
2. Program to rate 30 ppm (or lowest available) to determine the underlying rhythm (Figure 21);
3. Program the ventricular-inhibited mode (VVI) at a rate greater than the intrinsic ventricular rate to determine the ventricular pacing threshold. Gradually decrease pulse width and voltage output until capture is lost and record the lowest values at which capture is maintained (Figure 22);
4. Determine the ventricular sensing threshold in either VVI or VVT modes by gradually making the ventricular channel less sensitive until failure to sense is noted (Figure 23);
5. Atrial pacing thresholds can be determined by programming AAI or DVI modes (depending on mode availability and underlying rhythm) and gradually decreasing atrial pulse duration and voltage amplitude (Figure 24) until failure to capture the atrium is noted;
6. Determine atrial sensing by gradually making the atrial channel less sensitive until failure to sense occurs (Figure 25);
7. Programming various AV intervals will help determine at what AV delay, if any, the patient will conduct through the AV node and result in an intrinsic QRS complex (Figures 26, 27, Chapter 3, Figure 18);
8. With the patient in any atrial sensing mode (AAI, AAT, VDD, DDD, or DDI), the patient can be assessed for potential over-sensing in the atrial channel while performing isometric exercises while programmed to various sensitivities (Figure 28);
9. The patient can be checked for the potential for pacemaker-mediated (endless loop) tachycardia by programming the atrial refractory period to its shortest programmable duration and observing the consequent rhythm. If a premature atrial or ventricular contraction occurs during the period of observation, this may be helpful in assessing the potential for developing pacemaker-mediated tachycardia. Because VA conduction is a dynamic state, a longer observation is required for a greater certainty that a pacemaker-mediated tachycardia will not occur. Magnet application and reduction of atrial output below threshold are useful in assessing the likelihood of retrograde conduction (Figures 13, 16);
10. The potential for crosstalk can be assessed by programming the atrial channel to its highest output and the ventricular output to its highest sensitivity value. These are the most likely settings under which crosstalk would occur and ventricular output would be inhibited. If, under these "worst case" condicitons, no crosstalk is observed, it is unlikely that it will occur at nominal or the usual programmed values.

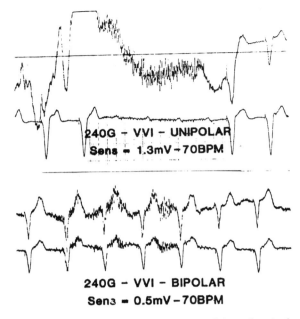

Figure 19. *A dual-chamber pacemaker programmed into the single-chamber VVI mode, into unipolar and then bipolar sensing to assess resistance to electromyographic interference.* **TOP:** *Programmed to a middle level of sensitivity, EMI causes inhibition of output and allows ventricular asystole.* **BOTTOM:** *In the bipolar mode at the highest sensitivity, EMI does not inhibit output.*

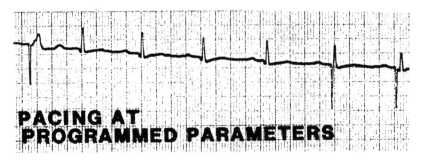

Figure 20. *ECGs obtained prior to any programming. The present settings are DDD mode, lower rate 60 bpm, upper rate 120 bpm. Atrial refractory period 220 ms, atrial and ventricular pulse durations of 0.45 ms, and atrial and ventricular voltage amplitudes of 5.4 V. The atrial sensitivity is 0.8 mV and the ventricular sensitivity 2.0 mV. There is one ventricular premature contraction at the left and two ventricular escapes at the conclusion of the AV interval that fuse with conducted QRS complexes at the right. There is the appearance of normal atrial and ventricular sensing and pacing.*

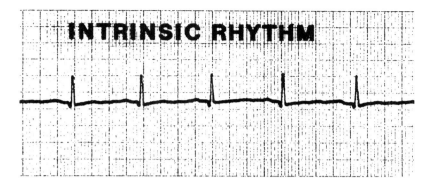

Figure 21. *Throughout this and the succeeding illustrative ECGs (through Figure 26) the spontaneous rate varies between 65–77 bpm. The pacemaker has been programmed to the ventricular inhibited (VVI) mode at 30 bpm. Observation of the underlying rhythm by programming the DDD pacemaker to a rate slower than the spontaneous rate is inadequate because the sensed P wave will start an AV interval that, if shorter than the AV conduction time, will end with a ventricular stimulus.*

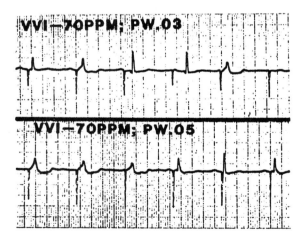

Figure 22. *In order to determine ventricular pacing thresholds, the ventricular pulse width can be decremented until capture is lost if the patient is known to have an adequate underlying rhythm. Once threshold has been determined, capture can be re-established by incrementing output or by the simple maneuver of programming standard or "Nominal" pacemaker output. In this example, ventricular capture was lost at a pulse duration of 0.03 ms, when intermittent capture occurred (ABOVE).* **BELOW:** *At a pulse duration of 0.05 ms normal ventricular capture occurs.*

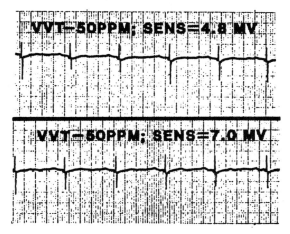

Figure 23.   *To determine ventricular sensing thresholds the patient should be pro-grammed either to the ventricular inhibited (VVI) or ventricular triggered (VVT) mode. In this example, the pacemaker has been programmed to the VVT mode which emits a stimulus in response to a sensed event. When programmed to a sensitivity of 4.8 mV, each QRS complex has a superimposed pacemaker stimulus. Programming to the lowest sensitivity level of 7 mV (Intermedics 283-01) continues appropriate sensing. The specific sensing threshold cannot be determined, but it is known that normal sensing exists throughout the programmable range.*

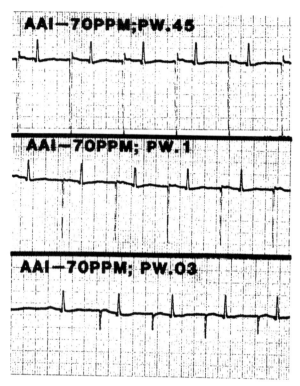

Figure 24. *Atrial pacing thresholds can be determined by programming to the AAI or DVI modes. The mode selected will depend on availability of the pulse generator and the patient's underlying rhythm. Several dual-chamber models do not have the AAI mode available. In this example, durations of 0.45 ms and 0.1 ms at a paced rate of 70 per minute showed normal atrial capture with antegrade conduction. While programming to a pulse duration of 0.03 ms, the spontaneous atrial rate had increased and stimuli had fused with the P wave. Two P waves, on the middle and the lower ECGs, inhibit atrial channel output. As 0.03 ms is the least programmable pulse duration, it can be stated that consistent capture occurs at a pulse duration of 0.1 ms and that the threshold is uncertain at shorter pulse durations.*

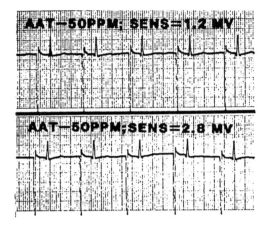

Figure 25.   *Atrial sensing can be assessed in the AAI or AAT modes. In this example, the AAT mode is used and pacing is at sensitivities of 1.2 and 2.8 mV. Normal AAT sensing is found at the minimum atrial channel sensitivity (2.8 mV). Pacemaker artifacts are superimposed and caused by the spontaneous P waves. As the automatic pacemaker rate is 50 per minute a more rapid stimulus rate is an indication of response to spontaneous atrial events.*

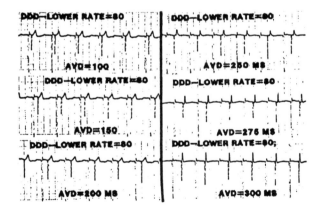

Figure 26.   *During the programming sequence, it is useful to program various AV delays (AVD) to determine at what duration, if any, conduction through the AV mode will produce a QRS complex from a paced atrial beat. In this example, AV delays have been programmed at 100, 150, 200, 250, 275, and 300 ms. The morphology of the QRS complex is wholly paced at 100, 150, and 200 ms. Thereafter, the morphology changes as the AV delay is prolonged. At 250 and 275 ms, fusion complexes appear, while at 300 ms, ventricular channel stimuli still occur but the complex seems to be wholly conducted. This may be considered a pseudo-fusion complex. In this patient, no degree of prolongation of the AV interval possible with this device will result in conducted ventricular activity and inhibition of ventricular output.*

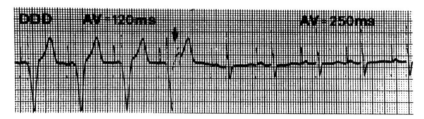

Figure 27. Programming of the AV interval may produce consistent ventricular capture or allow spontaneous ventricular depolarization—in this instance, with continuous fusion with conducted ventricular activity. A DDD pacemaker set at a lower rate limit of 750 ms (80 bpm) and an AV interval of 120 ms paces both atrium and ventricle. Reprogramming (arrow) to an AV interval of 250 ms allows AV conduction, but because the conduction time is prolonged, ventricular channel stimuli fuse with the conducted ventricular complexes.

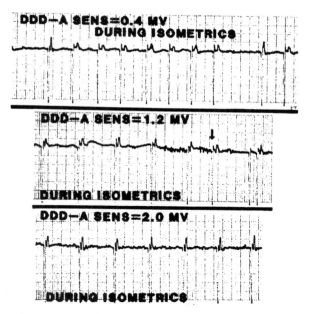

Figure 28. The possibility of sensing electromyographic interference via the atrial channel can be assessed by programming different atrial channel sensitivities while the patient is performing isometric exercises. In this example, atrial channel sensitivity has been programmed to 0.4, 1.2, and 2.0 mV. At an atrial sensitivity of .4 mV, isometric activity is sensed in the atrial channel to drive the ventricular channel at a rate of approximately 120 bpm (the upper rate limit of the pacemaker) for 8 consecutive beats. The relative absence of muscle artifacts on the ECG indicates that relatively light exercise was detected at this sensitivity. At an atrial channel sensitivity of 1.2 mV, the sixth beat occurs early (arrow), most likely as the result of the sensing of muscle activity. At an atrial channel sensitivity of 2.0 mV, no oversensing is detected.

PHANTOM PROGRAMMING

Programming signal transmission is via radio frequency signals or magnetic signals, which rapidly move a magnetic switch contained within the pulse generator. Radio frequency transmission of programming commands has become dominant and is used by almost all manufacturers. Magnetic reed switch programming sends very long duration signals for complex commands (Figure 29). Interruption of the signal during transmission can lead to false programming or failure of programming (Figure 30). In these pacemakers, magnet application itself rarely causes reprogramming (Figure 31).

Several categories of phantom or false programming have been defined, including misprogramming from faulty program emission signals, dysprogramming from anomalous sources, and, commonly, purposeful programming by a physician who fails to inform the patient or record the fact of this programming for future reference.

There are three major categories of phantom programming that occur or are detected in a hospital setting. The first is exposure to cold. The pulse generator may be exposed to severe cold in the cargo hold of an aircraft or the trunk of an automobile during delivery. New microprocessor-based pulse generators will revert, following exposure to severe cold, to a backup mode which is different for each generator but may be, for example, 52 bpm in the VOO mode. Cardioversion may cause reversion to the backup mode. A common cause of reversion to backup is the use of electrocautery, such as during open heart surgery. If the possibility of such reversion is not anticipated in each of these instances, pacemaker malfunction may be thought to be present.

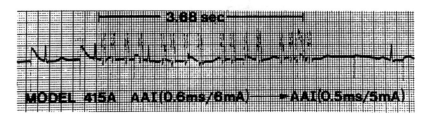

Figure 29. *Magnetic reed switch programming used in several models of single-and dual-chamber pulse generators requires a prolonged transmission time. Programming this dual-chamber pulse generator in the single-chamber atrial inhibited mode (AAI) from one output to another uses a pulse code 3.68 seconds in duration. If the programmer is decoupled (i.e., moved away from proper position in relation to the implanted pulse generator) during code transmission, a false code can be transmitted or programming will be unsuccessful.*

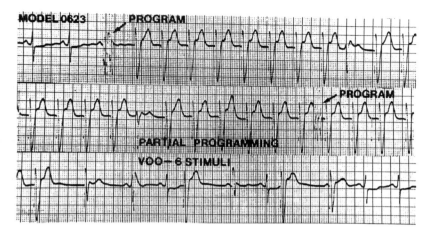

Figure 30. *A simple pulse generator with magnetic programming. Each programming effort begins with a five stimulus sequence at a coupling interval of 600 ms (100 bpm). Thereafter, six asynchronous stimuli are emitted at the newly programmed coupling interval. Inhibited pacing is then resumed. A programming attempt caused the 100 bpm rate, but because only partial programming had occurred, the newly programmed rate of 60 bpm did not begin until reprogramming (middle) completed the programming process.*

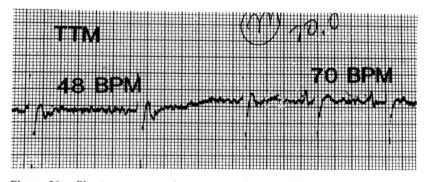

Figure 31. *Phantom programming may occur because of the unusual programming response to a stimulus that should not program the pacemaker. In this instance, recorded during transtelephonic monitoring, the rate had been programmed to 48 bpm. Magnet application programmed the rate to 70 bpm. Active programming to return to the original rate was required.*

When phantom programming occurs outside of the hospital setting, a detailed analysis of possible sources of reprogramming should be discussed with the patient in an attempt to determine (and avoid) the cause and ascertain that pacemaker malfunction does not exist.

CAUSES OF FALSE PROGRAMMING

1. medical equipment/hospital environment, i.e., electrocautery and nuclear magnetic resonance;
2. reprogramming by another physician without notification of the pacemaker center;
3. exposure to large industrial motors;
4. exposure to welding equipment;
5. exposure to large internal combustion engines;
6. farm equipment;
7. home appliances (rarely) (Figure 32).

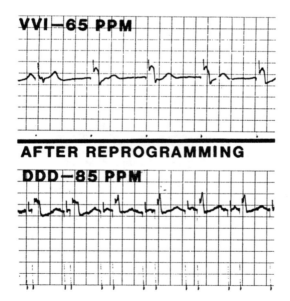

Figure 32.   *Two ECGs from a patient who had experienced reprogramming of an implanted pacemaker by a faulty kitchen appliance. The upper strip was obtained during transtelephonic monitoring and shows the pacemaker in the ventricular inhibited (VVI) mode at a rate of 65 bpm, the fallback mode for this pulse generator model. The patient had been previously programmed to the DVI mode. After reprogramming, the magnet application ECG was obtained showing a continuous paced rate of 85 bpm.*

BIBLIOGRAPHY

Barold SS: Clinical significance of pacemaker refractory periods. *Am J Cardiol* 1971; 28:237–239 (editorial).

Barold SS, Falkoff MD, Ong LS, et al: Programmability in DDD pacing. *PACE* 1984; 7:1159–1164.

Barold SS, Falkoff MD, Ong LS, et al: The third decade of cardiac pacing. Multiprogrammable pulse generators. *Br Heart J* 1981; 45:357–364.

Belott PH, Sands S, Warren J: Resetting of DDD pacemakers due to EMI. *PACE* 1984; 7:169–172.

Berman ND: T wave sensing with a programmable pacemaker. *PACE* 1980; 3:656–659.

Berman ND, Lipton IH, Dickson SE: The role of programmable pacemaker and assessment based on 264 implants. In *Cardiac Pacing—State of the Art* (Proceedings of the VIth World Symposium on Cardiac Pacing, Montreal, October, 1979). Montreal: Pacesymp, 1979.

Billhardt RA, Rosenbush SW, Hauser RG: Successful management of pacing system malfunction without surgery: The role of programmable pulse generators. *PACE* 1982; 5:675–682.

Curtis JJ, Walls JT, Madigan NP, et al: Effect of varying atrioventricular contraction intervals on cardiac output in man. *Surg Forum* 1982; 33:285–287.

Djordjevic M, Milosevic U, Velimirovic D: Programmable pacemakers to selected patients or to all patients. *PACE* 1983; 6:A-101 (abstract).

Fieldman A, Dobrow RJ: Phantom pacemaker programming. *PACE* 1978; 1:166–171.

Furman S: Pacemaker programmability. *Contemp Surg* 1982; 20:35–48.

Furman S: Pacemaker programmability. *PACE* 1978; 1:161–162.

Furman S: Spurious pacemaker programming. *PACE* 1980; 3:517–518.

Furman S, Pannizzo F: Output programmability and reduction of secondary intervention after pacemaker implantation. *J Thorac Cardiovasc Surg* 1981; 81:713–717.

Gabry MD, Behrens M, Andrews C, Wanliss M, Klementowicz PT, Furman S: Comparison of myopotential interference in unipolar-bipolar programmable DDD pacemakers. *PACE* 1987; 10(6):1322–30.

Goldschlager N, Thomas AM: Successful electrode catheter repositioning accomplished by determination of pacing system function using noninvasive programming. *PACE* 1982; 5:937–939.

Griffin JS, Quitman JA: Pacemaker programmability: The role of noninvasive pacing system revision. In *Cardiac Pacing-State of the Art* (Proceedings of the VIth World Symposium on Cardiac Pacing, Montreal, October, 1979). Montreal: Pacesymp, 1979.

Harthorne JW: Programmable pacemakers: Technical features and clinical applications. *Cardiovasc Clin* 1983; 14(2):135–147.

Hauser RG: Multiprogrammable cardiac pacemakers: Applications, results, and follow-up. *Am J Surg* 1983; 145:740–745.

Hauser RG, Susmano A: After-potential oversensing by a programmable pulse generator. *PACE* 1981; 4:391–395.

Hehrlein FW, Mulch J, Pahutan P, et al: Programmable cardiac pacemakers. First experiences with the Omnicor System. *J Cardiovasc Surg* 1974; 15:522–527.

Hollins WJ, Leman RB, Kratz JM, Gillette PC: Limitations of the long-term clinical application of rate hysteresis. *PACE* 1987; 10(2):302–4.

Levine PA: Proceedings of the policy conference of the North American Society of Pacing and Electrophysiology on programmability and pacemaker follow-up programs. *Clin Prog Pacing Electrophysiol* 1984; 2:145–191.

Luceri RM, Hayes DL: Follow-up of DDD pacemakers. *PACE* 1984; 7:1187–1194.

MacGregor DC, Furman S, Dreifus LS, et al: The utility of the programmable pacemaker. *PACE* 1978; 1:254–259.

Morse D, Samuel A, Fernandez J, et al: Preliminary experience with the use of a programmable pacemaker. *Chest* 1975; 67:544–548.

Morse D, Spagna P, Lemole GM: Charge levels in programmable pacemakers. *PACE* 1980; 3:38–43.

O'Keefe JH Jr, Hayes DL, Holmes DR Jr, et al: Importance and long-term utility of a multiparameter programmable pulse generator. *Mayo Clin Proc* 1984; 59:239–242.

Parsonnet V, Rodgers T: The present status of programmable pacemakers. *Prog Cardiovasc Dis* 1981; 23:401–420.

Pless P, Simonsen E, Arnsbo P, Fabricius J: Superiority of multiprogrammable to nonprogrammable VVI pacing: a comparative study with special reference to management of pacing system malfunctions. *PACE* 1986; 9(5):739–44.

Preston TA, Preston AW Jr: The automatic rate adjustment pacemaker. The possibilities of rate hysteresis. *PACE* 1978; 1:178–185.

Rosenqvist M, Vallin HO, Edhag KO: Rate hysteresis pacing: How valuable is it? A comparison of the stimulation rates of 70 and 50 beats per minute and rate hysteresis in patients with sinus node disease. *PACE* 1984; 7(Part I):332–340.

Sinnaeve A, Piret J, Stroobandt R: Potential causes of spurious programming: Report of a case. *PACE* 1980; 3:541–547.

Smyth NPD, Sager D: A multiprogrammable pacemaker with unipolar or bipolar option. *Am Heart J* 1983; 106:412–414.

Smyth NPD, Sager D, Keshishian JM: A programmable pulse generator with high output option. *PACE* 1981; 4:566–570.

Starke ID: Long-term follow up of cardiac pacing threshold using a noninvasive method of measurement. *Br Heart J* 1978; 40:530–533.

Thompson ME, Shaver JA: Undesirable cardiac arrhythmias associated with rate hysteresis pacemakers. *Am J Cardiol* 1976; 38:685–688.

Tyers GFO, Williams EH, Larrieu AJ, et al: Multiprogrammable pacemakers. *Can J Surg* 1981; 24:252–256.

Venkataraman K, Bilitch M: Clinical experience with a programmable pacemaker. *PACE* 1980; 3:605–611.

Vera Z, Janzen D, Mason DT: Longevity of programmable energy output pacemakers. Early results and experiences. *Br Heart J* 1977; 39:1364–1373.

Vera Z, Klein RC, Mason DT: Recent advances in programmable pacemakers: Consideration of advantages, longevity and future expectations. *Am J Med* 1979; 66:473–483.

Chapter 18

PRACTICAL CONSIDERATIONS

David L. Hayes

Patients with pacemakers have practical concerns after implantation. These are related to activity, environmental effect on the pacemaker, the effects of the surgical procedure and the responsibilities of long-term care of the foreign body. Some concerns about the environmental effect on a pacemaker stem from experience with early-generation pacemakers and electrical equipment and are no longer valid. They still must be addressed, and the anxieties of the patient must be allayed.

The optimal time for instruction is before hospital discharge after pacemaker implantation. Patients can be instructed in postoperative care of the incision, restrictions, techniques of taking and interpreting the pulse, basic principles and techniques of cardiac pacing, and details of pacemaker follow-up.

PHYSICIAN-PATIENT INTERACTION

Patient

Some patients become psychologically dependent on the implanted pacemaker. They date many life, other cardiac, and certainly medical events to the implant and existence of the pacemaker. Some even presume that the existence of the pacemaker cures a variety of unrelated cardiac conditions. An occasional patient, often a younger man, will deny the existence of any illness and consider the management of a cardiac arrhythmia by an implanted pacemaker to be equivalent to a "cure." The physician should attempt to emphasize that the pacemaker effectively manages a specific cardiac condition but does not cure all illnesses.

A young patient with atrioventricular block or sinus node dysfunction and an implanted pacemaker may want to return to the extremes of cardiac activity. If a dual-chamber pacemaker is implanted in such a patient who also has retrograde conduction, upper rate limit settings may not allow the patient to exercise to a high atrial rate, and activity may be limited. The patient must understand and accept this limitation. The patient must be aware that this implanted device is not a cure and has not restored absolutely normal health. Some limitations remain, and customary precautions about one's health are still required.

The patient must be encouraged to adopt the attitude that an illness is being managed and that cooperation in its management is required. The patient should recognize that prudent steps should be taken to protect the device and to maintain its correct function. The patient should also recognize that health may deteriorate, and the device may undergo progressive, routine, or even sudden failure. A prudent attitude devoid of apprehension and denial of disease is helpful.

Physician

A physician who implants a pacemaker or one who follows a patient with an implanted pacemaker should recognize the prolonged responsibility entailed. Electrical, electronic, or physiological malfunctions may occur, and the lead system or the pulse generator may be recalled or behave less well than expected.

Communications may be received from the manufacturer about a patient with an implanted pacemaker, and it may be desirable to notify the patient about the event. The physician should keep accurate records of the patient's location and if the patient moves from the physician's area of responsibility, should insist that pacemaker follow-up be continued elsewhere.

The physician should recognize, as should the patient, that the existence of a pacemaker does not protect against a variety of intercurrent illnesses. The physician should not blame each unrelated ache or pain on the implanted device. Pain in the shoulder adjacent to a pacemaker may be pacemaker-related or may be bursitis; precordial distress may be pacemaker syndrome or angina pectoris. Only careful evaluation can make the distinction.

POSTOPERATIVE CARE

Patients should be told to examine the pacemaker pocket and incision for unusual signs of puffiness, drainage, or erythema. If these develop, they are to contact the physician. They are instructed to watch for and document the recurrence of symptoms similar to those experienced before pacemaker implantation, new symptoms, any drop in the pulse rate below the programmed lower rate limit, or, for patients with dual-chamber pacemakers, a pulse increase above the programmed upper limit. Patients should be cautioned not to depend excessively on counting the pulse rate. The pulse normally varies in most patients with implanted pacemakers, especially in those with dual-chamber devices. The count of the pulse at the wrist is commonly incorrect, since its accuracy depends on accurate palpation, accurate timing, and the absence of "dropped" beats. For many patients, an accurate count is beyond their technical capacity.

FOLLOW-UP

Before hospital discharge, pacemaker follow-up schedules are arranged. In some centers, patients and their families are instructed in the use of the transtelephonic monitoring system. In other centers, a follow-up visit to the pacemaker clinic is arranged. Irrespective of approach, the importance of follow-up transmissions or visits to the pacemaker clinic should be stressed.

ELECTROMAGNETIC AND ELECTROMYOGRAPHIC INTERFERENCE

Electromygraphic interference is generated by somatic musculature adjacent to the pulse generator and is physiologic in origin. It is almost impossible to eliminate electromyographic interference in a unipolar pacemaker. Electromagnetic interference is derived from artificial electronic sources. Electromyographic interference is far more common and disturbing than electromagnetic interference. A patient who has a single-chamber, unipolar pacemaker and suffers recurrent dizziness may be having episodic inhibition of the pulse generator. Dual-chamber pacemakers can have triggering via the atrial channel and simultaneous inhibition via the ventricular channel. The net effect will depend on whether inhibition or triggering dominates. Ambulatory monitoring is the most effective means of detecting such inhibition. Electromyographic interference is, in fact, a common cause of recurrent symptoms. It can be almost completely eliminated by bipolar lead systems.

COMMON QUESTIONS

Travel

Patients who have cardiac pacemakers should carry an identification card that lists the type of pacemaker, type of lead system, patient's physician, and personal identification. For travel, a list of local physicians conversant with pacemakers aids in proper care if trouble develops. Travel should not be limited. The only requirement is that the patient carry the transmitter, if one is in use, and be in a part of the world where reliable telephone service exists and responsible medical attention is available. Neither commercial air travel nor the metal detector used in airports is a problem. A pacemaker may activate the metal detector, and having the identification card available should help avoid any confusion.

Medications

Although many cardiac medications and electrolyte solutions can have minor effects on the pacing threshold, therapy should not be withheld in a patient with a normally functioning pacemaker system. The change in threshold that can occur is so small that any system with an adequate pacing margin of safety will not be affected by such minor changes in threshold. Sympathomimetic amines that increase cardiac irritability should be avoided.

Work

A patient should be able to return to their previous occupation and recreational activity with few exceptions (See below). All patients, especially those who are pacemaker-dependent, should be warned to refrain from driving for two to three weeks after implantation to be certain to avoid problems related to lead dislodgment. Questions that arise about electromagnetic interference at work can usually be referred to the manufacturer, who can send a field engineer to investigate the workplace.

Sports

For many persons, contact sports must be restricted. There should be no limitations on other activities. For patients who insist on being involved in contact sports, it should be made clear that direct trauma can result in damage to the unit itself or fracture of the lead. Contact sports in which there is little risk of direct trauma to the placement site are reasonable if the patient wears a protective garment or dressing over the unit. Movements which stress the point of entry of a lead into the venous system should be limited. Strenuous activity that protects the shoulder can be undertaken, subject to cardiac reserve and tolerance.

Patients frequently inquire about several activities. One is golfing, which is not restricted after the first two to three weeks after implantation. Patients also ask about the use of a rifle or shotgun. This should be discussed before implantation. If this activity is important to the patient, the unit should be placed on the side opposite the shooting arm to avoid damage due to recoil. Patients also often ask about swimming. Swimming can be done after the incision has healed. Patients should be reassured that there is no danger of water causing problems with the pacemaker circuit.

Sexual Activity

Sexual activity is permitted as tolerated and is limited only by the cardiac reserve. Patients tend to be reluctant to ask questions about sexual activity. This topic is included in the literature and audiovisual material provided for the patient's instruction.

Clothing

Clothing usually has little impact on the implanted cardiac pacemaker. Patients with epicardial implants who have the pulse generator in the abdominal position should not wear a tight belt crossing the lead system because the belt can become a fulcrum about which the leads may bend or break. A woman may ask whether her brassiere will affect the pacemaker or lead. A brassiere will not damage the pacemaker lead, but the very thin patient or the patient in whom the pacemaker is poorly positioned may have some discomfort. A soft sponge or rubber pad may alleviate pressure on the leads or pulse generator. In some patients, a brassiere may support the breast and decrease discomfort related to the pacemaker itself. In occasional patients with pendulous breasts, a brassiere may be worn at night to alleviate discomfort.

In more recent years, patients have asked whether seat belts, especially shoulder straps, cause any problems with the pacemaker. They should be reassured that with transvenous systems in which the pacemaker has been placed in the anterior chest wall, there is no problem with seat belts or shoulder restraints. Patients who have epicardial systems should follow the same precautions as those noted above for wearing a tight belt. On balance, the seat belt is probably a more important safety measure than a cause of pacemaker difficulty. Certain state legislatures have required the use of seat belts but have realized the potential problem of discomfort or pressure on a pacemaker and have exempted pacemaker patients from that mandate. If the question arises, one should be aware of the law in the individual state.

EFFECT OF THE ENVIRONMENT ON THE PACEMAKER SYSTEM

Permanent damage to implanted pacemakers by electrical equipment normally encountered at home or at work has not been reported and is unlikely. The most frequent occurrence is temporary interference with pacemaker activity while the patient is in the presence of sustained electrical interference. Interpreted by the pacemaker as cardiac electrical activity, this electrical interference may inhibit pacemaker function episodically. With home appliances, interference is not a problem. Electrical interference may cause pacemaker inhibition but does not cause pacemaker damage.

There are potentially significant restrictions for some patients. Each circumstance is different and involves the individual decision of the implanting physician and the patient. In patients who work in close proximity to heavy motors, such as internal combustion engines, or arc welding, temporary interference with pacemaker activity can result in pacemaker inhibition. This problem involves a small percentage of the patient population and is quite infrequent. In these situations, patients may be required to change occupations or at least to avoid specific equipment. If the potential for such EMI is known before implant the use of bipolar leads can ameliorate or eliminate the problem.

Patients invariably inquire whether a microwave oven or radar of the type used in airports interfere with pacemaker function. With present-day pulse generators, these devices should not cause any interference.

ELECTROCAUTERIZATION, CARDIOVERSION, AND ELECTROSHOCK THERAPY

Interference with pacemaker function by electrocauterization, cardioversion, defibrillation, or electroconvulsive or electroshock therapy is possible and should be considered before the procedure.

In all instances, the electrocautery or paddles for cardioversion/ defibrillation should be kept at least 4–6 inches away from the pacemaker itself. For cardioversion, the pads should optimally be placed in an anteroposterior position rather than to the left and right of the anterior portion of the chest. This positioning minimizes the chance of placing the paddle over the pulse generator or having the current path go directly to the lead system.

After any electrical intervention, i.e., electrocautery during surgery, cardioversion, or electric shock therapy, the pacemaker should be rechecked because the pacing function may have been changed. Potential changes are pacemaker reversion to the noise mode, reprogramming, circuit damage, and myocardial damage caused by current transmission via the electrode, yielding so high a current density at the electrode-myocardial interface that tissue destruction occurs.

The most common problem is pacemaker inhibition. As long as the electrical intervention is only brief, it is not of concern in most patients. If prolonged electrocauterization occurs, the pacemaker may revert to the noise mode and pace the heart asynchronously, a change that rarely leads to difficulty. If the patient is to undergo a surgical procedure in which electrocauterization is to be fairly constant, the anesthesiologist should be consulted, and consideration given to reprogramming the pacemaker to an asynchronous mode to avoid intermittent inhibition or, in nonprogrammable units, to taping a magnet over the unit to convert it to an asynchronous mode. This course of action should be definitely considered in patients who are pacemaker-dependent. The cautery electrode should be at least 12 inches from the pacemaker, as it is possible to directly destroy the pacemaker if it is closer. As cautery will interfere with the ECG so much that it cannot be interpreted, palpation of a peripheral pulse is desirable.

Additional problems are the reprogramming of a generator to its "backup" mode of operation. Electrocautery is a sufficiently powerful electrical interference that the implanted generator may be reprogrammed rather than only inhibited. For example, if a DDD generator is in place and is operating at a fixed rate in the asynchronous single-chamber mode (VOO) after electromagnetic interference, the most likely occurrence has been reprogramming to its protected (backup) mode. It can be readily programmed to its former function. Other pacemakers may require access to special codes before such reprogramming can be performed.

If cardioversion is performed, the pads should be kept 4–6 inches away from the pulse generator and damage to the pacemaker should not occur. Cases have been reported in which, despite adherence to these guidelines, the angle of the electrical shock to the lead or pacemaker was sufficient to cause pacemaker damage. In this situation, the pacemaker should always be checked after an electrical intervention to ascertain that it is still programmed correctly and functioning normally.

The electrode-myocardial interface should be considered. Although rare, an electrical impulse delivered at the appropriate angle to the pacemaker lead can be transmitted through the electrode directly to the endocardium or myocardium where it can produce arrhythmia or local cardiac necrosis with high threshold and poor sensing.

ILLNESS, SURGERY, AND PREGNANCY

The patient with a cardiac pacemaker is subject to other illnesses and medical conditions. Tolerance to the stress of illness and surgery is a function of the patient's intrinsic cardiac reserve. A limiting factor of varying significance is the lessened ability of a patient with a single-rate pacemaker to increase the cardiac output in response to fever or stress. Nevertheless, the patient with a single-rate pacemaker and preserved left ventricular function can increase stroke volume and thus maintain cardiac output. If left ventricular function is poor and cardiac output is rate-dependent, the patient will do less well.

A patient with an activity sensing pacemaker (by far the most popular variety of rate-modulated devices now implanted) will not respond to a fever or other non-activity stress by increasing cardiac rate. The responses of other rate-modulated pacemakers to prolonged stress remain unclear. For example, during sustained fever, temperature sensitive devices return to the lower rate setting.

EFFECT OF OTHER MEDICAL
PROCEDURES AND TREATMENTS

Diathermy

Some types of diathermy equipment can cause pacemaker inhibition. Patients who are to receive such therapy should be alerted to notify the treating physician. Diathermy in close proximity to a pulse generator (such as for treatment of shoulder bursitis) can damage its circuit. Diathermy should not be used so close to a pulse generator that damage can occur.

Transcutaneous Nerve Stimulation

Transcutaneous nerve stimulation has been used with increasing frequency for a number of neurological and musculoskeletal problems. It appears to be safe in the patient with a permanent pacemaker and rarely causes inhibition, interference, or reprogranming, though an occasional patient with interference with pacemaker function has been reported. It is not known how close to the pacemaker the transcutaneous nerve stimulator can be placed and it is best to avoid applying the stimulator to a vector or path that would be parallel to the pacing lead until more information is available. Pacemaker dependent patients should be monitored during initial transcutaneous nerve stimulation to be certain no inhibition occurs. Most of the information regarding transcutaneous nerve stimulation in patients with permanent pacemakers has been obtained with relatively modern pacemakers. It is possible that some older pacemakers with less sophisticated filtering capabilities may be more susceptible to interference (Figure 1).

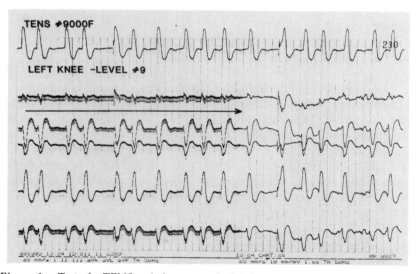

Figure 1. *Test of a TENS unit for use on the left knee. Normal pacemaker function persisted during TENS operation and thereafter. The TENS signals overly the ECG on the left.*

Radiation

Diagnostic X-ray does not interfere with pacemaker function. Therapeutic radiation levels can have a damaging effect on pacemaker function. The newer multiprogrammable pacemakers contain complementary metal oxide semiconductors (CMOS) for their integrated circuits, while older generators had discrete components. CMOS circuits are more readily damaged by therapeutic radiation than were discrete components. Specifically, when metal oxide semiconductor transistors are exposed to ionizing radiation, damage occurs to the silicone and silicone oxide insulators within the transistors. Therapeutic radiation may result in complete failure or random damage to circuit components. Sudden no output or runaway may occur. As the damage to the circuit is random and the radiation dose cumulative (i.e., from one therapeutic exposure to the next), no specific prediction relative to dose can be made. There have been some reports of pacemaker damage in CMOS devices from as small a radiation dose as 1,000 rads. In others, 3,000–15,000 rads have been reported to cause damage.

This effect is of particular importance in patients undergoing radiation for thoracic or chest wall malignancies. In these patients, the pulse generator should be shielded and the field of radiation limited as much as possible to avoid damage. In patients in whom the pacemaker is within the field of radiation, for example, those with carcinoma of the breast, a change in the position of the pulse generator may be required.

Magnet Application

For conventional pacemakers, application of a magnet results in asynchronous pacing. Because of the increased interest in pacing tachycardias with magnet-induced underdrive, this mode may be used with increasing frequency. Magnet application should be done by physicians experienced with the treatment of arrhythmias and only with electrocardiographic monitoring to document the arrhythmia and identify adverse consequences. The physician must understand the effect of magnet application on each individual pacemaker, particularly implantable defibrillators, which may be inactivated.

Magnetic Resonance Imaging

Magnetic resonance imaging (MRI) has developed as an important diagnostic tool. The MRI system, with its powerful static, time-varying magnetic, and radio frequency fields, can affect normal pace-maker operation and function. At the very least, exposure to MRI causes all pacemakers to revert to an asynchronous mode because of reed switch closure. This effect can be avoided only in those newer pulse generators in which the magnet mode can be programmed *off*. Limited investigation has been done with MRI and pulse generators at this time, but has already shown that MRI does not damage the reed switch or other pulse generator components. The radio fre-quency artifacts do not alter the acutely programmed variables, change the normal magnet rate, or induce pacing in most pacemakers tested. Certain single- and dual-chamber pacemakers implanted in animals and exposed to MRI do pace at the radio frequency pulse period used during radio frequency scanning. Because the radio fre-quency pulse period may be set at extremely short intervals for some diangostic procedures (20–2,000 ms), patients with those pulse gen-erators could be paced at rates as high as 3,000 bpm.

At this time, no generalizations can be made concerning which pacemaker patients can safely be exposed to magnetic resonance scanning, and until such recommendations can be made, magnetic resonance imaging should be avoided in a patient with an implanted pacemaker.

Extracorporeal Shock Wave Lithotripsy

Extracorporeal shock wave lithotripsy is being used with increas-ing frequency for the treatment of nephrolithiasis. This device can potentially cause multiple problems with permanent pacemakers. The shock waves produced by the lithotripsy device are usually syn-chronized to the patient's ventricular depolarization or to the output stimulus of the pacemaker. Early experience based on limited testing of devices in-vitro and anecdotal patient experience suggests that lithotripsy does not interfere with fixed rate VVI pacing as long as the focal point of the device is at least 6 inches from the pacemaker. Irregularities in the pacing rate of dual-chamber pacemakers have been reported. Sensing of the shock waves resulting in increased pacing rates and sensor damage has been reported when activity sensing rate-modulated pacemakers were exposed to lithotripsy.

If extracorporeal shock wave lithotripsy is necessary in the pa-tient with a permanent pacemaker, the pacemaker should be pro-grammed to the VVI or VOO mode, the focal point of the device should be greater than 6 inches from the pacemaker, and the patient should have cardiac monitoring throughout the procedure.

Care and attention to the device and its interaction with the host is a lifelong affair but need not be especially burdensome. Modern devices function for long periods, usually without any intervention. While some become troublesome, this is the exception rather than the rule. Understanding of what the device can accomplish, how it is to be observed and how to protect it and the patient from harm will lead to prolonged satisfactory function. The personal physician should have some broad knowledge of pacemaker function and where to seek consultation. The patient should not fix all illnesses on the pacemaker and equally should not assume that its presence is a guard against all cardiac disease.

BIBLIOGRAPHY

Adamec R, Haefliger JM, Killisch JP, Niedeuer J, Jaquet P: Damaging effect of therapeutic radiation on programmable pacemakers. *PACE* 1982; 5:146–150.

Blacher RS, Basch SH: Psychological aspects of pacemaker implantation. *Arch Gen Psychiat* 1970; 22:319–323.

Blamires NG, Myatt J: X-ray effects on pacemaker type circuits. *PACE* 1982; 5:151–155.

Calfee RV: Therapeutic radiation and pacemakers. *PACE* 1982; 5:160–161 (editorial).

Cooper D, Wilkoff B, Masterson M, et al: Effects of extracorporeal shock wave lithotripsy on cardiac pacemakers and its safety in patients with implanted cardiac pacemakers. *PACE* 1988; 11:1607–1616.

Domino KB, Smith TC: Electrocautery-induced reprogramming of a pacemaker using a precordial magnet. *Anesth Analg* 1983; 62:609–612.

Erlebacher JA, Cahill PT, Pannizzo F, Knowles RJR: Effect of magnetic resonance imaging on DDD pacemakers. *Am J Cardiol* 1986; 57:437–440.

Escher DJW, Parker B, Furman S, Mehra R: The effect of magnetic fields on cardiac pacemakers. *JAAMI* 1972; 6:165 (abstract).

Feldman RM: The use of diathermy in the presence of metal implants and cardiac pacemakers (ltr to ed). *Can Med Assoc J* 1980; 123:16–17.

Fetter J, Aram G, Holmes DR Jr, Gray J, Hayes DL: The effects of nuclear magnetic resonance imagers on external and implantable pulse generators. *PACE* 1984; 7:720–727.

Furman S: Radiation effects on implanted pacemakers. *PACE* 1982; 5:145 (editorial).

Hayes DL, Holmes DR Jr, Gray JE: Effect of 1.5 tesla nuclear magnetic resonance imaging scanner on implanted permanent pacemakers. *JACC* 1987; 10:782–786.

Holmes DR Jr, Hayes DL, Gray JE, Merideth J: The effects of magnetic resonance imaging on implantable pulse generators. *PACE* 1986; 9:360–370.

Irnich W, DeBakker JMT, Bisping HJ: Electromagnetic interference in implantable pacemakers. *PACE* 1978; 1:52–61.

Irnich W: Interference in pacemakers. PACE 1984; 7:1021–1048.

Jones SL: Electromagnetic field interference and cardiac pacemakers. *Phys Ther* 1976; 56:1013–1018.

Katzenberg CA, Marcus FI, Heusinkveld RS, Mammana RB: Pacemaker failure due to radiation therapy. *PACE* 1982; 5:156–159.

Levine PA, Barold SS, Fletcher RD, et al: Adverse, acute and chronic effects of electrical defibrillation and cardioversion on implanted unipolar cardiac pacing systems. *JACC* 1983; 1:1413–1422.

Manwaring M: What patients need to know about pacemakers. *Am J Nurs* 1977; 77:825–828.

Marbach JR, Meoz-Mendez RT, Huffman JK, Hudgins PT, Almond PR: The effects on cardiac pacemakers of ionizing radiation and electromagnetic interference from radiotherapy machines. *Int J Radiat Biol* 1978; 4:1044–1058.

O'Brien E: Environmental dangers for the patient with a pacemaker. *Br Med J* 1982; 285:1677–1678 (editorial).

Pannizzo F, Furman S: Pacemaker and patient response to the "point of sale" terminal as an actual and simulated electromagnetic interference source. *PACE* 1980; 3:461–469.

Pavlicek W, Geisinger M, Castle L, Borkowski GP, Meaney TF, Bream BL, Gallagher JH: The effects of nuclear magnetic resonance on patients with cardiac pacemakers. *Radiology* 1983; 147:149–153.

Pohost GM, Ratner AV: Nuclear magnetic resonance. *JAMA* 1984; 251:1304.

Rasmussen MJ, Hayes DL, Vlietstra RE, Thorsteinsson G: Can transcutaneous electrical nerve stimulation be safely used in patients with permanent cardiac pacemakers? *Mayo Clin Proc* 1988; 63:443–445.

Slusarczyk SM, Hicks FD: Helping your patient to live with a permanent pacemaker. *Nursing* 1983; 83:58–63.

Smyth NPD, Keshishian JM, Hood OC, Hoffman AA, Baker NR, Podolak E: Effect of an active magnetometer on permanently implanted pacemakers. *JAMA* 1972; 221:162–166.

Smyth NPD, Parsonnet V, Escher DJW, Furman S: The pacemaker patient and the electromagnetic environment. *JAMA* 1974; 227:1412.

Sowton E: Environmental hazards for pacemaker patients. *J R Coll Phys* Lond 1982; 16:159–164.

Sylven C, Levander-Lindgren M: Case report. Normally functioning inhibited pacemaker concomitant with vertebral nerve stimulation. *PACE* 1979; 2:645–647.

Venselaar JL: The effects of ionizing radiation on eight cardiac pacemakers and the influence of electromagnetic interference from two linear accelerators. *Radiother Oncol* 1985; 3:81–87.

Warnowicz MA: The pacemaker patient and the electromagnetic environment. *CPPE* 1983; 1:166–176.

Chapter 19

TROUBLESHOOTING

Seymour Furman

Implantable pacemakers will have occasional deficiencies with pacing and/or sensing, and pacemaker patients require periodic management of pacing defects. Complex modern devices must be carefully analyzed to understand the significance of pacing defects. Analysis must be undertaken in a logical and rational manner. Troubleshooting can occur during two different circumstances, nonoperatively (or preoperatively) and intraoperatively. During preoperative (or nonoperative) evaluation, direct access to the generator does not exist. Modern pulse generators have both programmability and telemetry which, added to X-ray and ECG findings, can often determine the nature of a specific malfunction. This chapter will deal with pacemaker hardware rather than physiological malfunction. Data from each of the other chapters, especially electrocardiography and radiology, has a bearing on this chapter and should be reviewed as this text is read.

Noninvasive evaluation will often allow management of difficulties by nonoperative change of pacemaker function. If nonoperative correction of pacemaker malfunction is impossible, then operative intervention will be required and will follow a second set of procedures to be described later. As in every medical discipline, preoperative diagnosis is preferable to intraoperative diagnosis. Management of problems must be undertaken in a rational and sequential manner (Table I).

Table I
Management of Complications
of Pacing

I. A. Knowledge of Hardware Function
   B. Careful Records
   C. Knowledge of Possible Difficulties
     1. Surgical
     2. Physiological
     3. Specific hardware
     4. Interference or radiation damage
II. Careful Preoperative Analysis
III. Careful Intraoperative Analysis
IV. Rational Repair

Identify The Symptomatic Nature of The Malfunction

Unless infection or local pain exist, malfunction usually will be manifest by return of symptoms that required pacemaker implant initially, i.e., fatigue, syncope or mental confusion. Malfunction may be noted by palpitations resulting from coupled beats, episodes of tachycardia or from the pounding in the neck and chest, which are associated with pacemaker syndrome. A careful history to define the nature of the malfunction may be less necessary if syncope recurs, though it must be remembered that syncope, especially in the elderly, may be caused by bradycardia, tachycardia or events unrelated to an implanted pacemaker or cardiac rate and rhythm. Alternatively, approximately one-third of patients will have significant but asymptomatic pacemaker malfunction.

Electrocardiographic Determination of Malfunction

A number of findings on ECG should be sought (Table II):

a) Is capture satisfactory in the sensitive period of the cardiac cycle for atrium, ventricle or both?
b) Is sensing normal?
c) Is there any evidence of pacemaker function, if so, is it at a "normal" rate, is it very slow, is it rapid or is it so rapid that it is impossible or unlikely that any pacemaker during normal operation could function in that manner; is it at a runaway rate, i.e., faster than 140 stimuli per minute; does cardiac capture occur at any rate?
d) Runaway pacemaker: rapid pacing rates that result from electronic malfunction have been referred to as "pacemaker runaway." Runaway has been the most lethal variety of pacemaker malfunction because of the rapid rates that can occur and because of instability of the pacemaker cicruit. Runaway almost always occurs without warning of any other preliminary malfunction. In some, stimulation rates were sufficiently slow so that a patient with a relatively healthy myocardium could survive a short episode of ventricular pacing runaway.

In others, the rapid rate was coupled with a decrease in pacemaker output for each stimulus, occasionally below pacing threshold. Some older pacemakers capable of high-rate runaway remain in service. Modern pacemakers are carefully designed to reduce the possibility of stimulation rates in excess of about 140 bpm. Many are also designed to reduce the incidence of runaway by requiring two separate and unrelated electronic failures before runaway can occur. Though it is still possible for more rapid rates to occur, pacemaker runaway has become extremely unusual. If runaway rate is seen, the pacemaker should be

Table II
Troubleshooting DDD Pacemakers—I

Free-Running ECG

1. Is the pacing rate as programmed?
2. Is the AV delay as programmed?
3. Is the atrium
   a. sensed properly?
   b. paced properly?
4. Is the ventricle
   a. sensed properly?
   b. paced properly?

5. Are the pulse durations as programmed?
6. Are both channels operating
   a. individually?
   b. together?

removed as an emergency under sterile conditions if time permits, or if necessary, in the emergency department under unsterile conditions. If sterile, a new generator can be attached to the lead system immediately; if unsterile, the implanted lead can be used for temporary pacing. The pulse generator that has demonstrated runaway should not be left in situ for observation. Normal function may alternate with runaway at a lethal level without warning. Once runaway has occurred, the unit must be deemed unreliable and potentially disastrous, even should it appear to return to normal function (Figure 1).

Distinction between runaway and a ventricular or atrial triggered (VVT/AAT) pacemaker tracking a native tachycardia must be made. Magnet application with cessation of sensing of spontaneous cardiac activity will assist in the distinction. Magnet application will, almost always, have no effect on a generator during runaway.

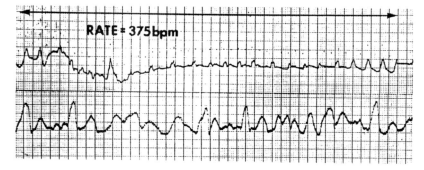

Figure 1. *Runaway pacemaker, the most potentially lethal of all pacemaker complications, still occurs. This runaway, seen during March 1985 in an external pacemaker, stimulated the ventricle at about 350 per minute and caused ventricular fibrillation and death.*

e) No Output: sudden "no output" is a common mode of electronic failure. (Though electronic failure of modern pulse generators is, itself, very uncommon, it is much less common than in former discrete component generators.) In this instance, no pacemaker activity will be found either during free running or magnet application. Despite the impression that the sudden absence of pacemaker function leaves the patient unprotected, and that pacemaker dependent patients will suffer severely, even having recurrent syncope, this situation is less dangerous than runaway. Possibly 30% of patients are sufficiently pacemaker-dependent as to have five seconds or more of asystole following sudden pacemaker failure.

f) Is the pacemaker single- or dual-chamber? If dual-chamber, is there evidence of atrial and ventricular pacing? Does all recycle occur from ventricular sensing only? Does escape after a sinus pause occur via an atrial escape, i.e., is the pacemaker DVI or DDD, or does escape occur only by a ventricular stimulus, i.e., VDD? Is each P wave tracked with a ventricular stimulus following each P wave? The answer to each of these questions will assist in determining the mode of pacemaker operation and whether operation is normal (Table III) (Figure 2).

Identify The Pacemaker

All pacemaker function is defined by the design of the individual pacing device, and unusual function may appear to be present when, in fact, it is normal operation of an unexpected variety. One possibility is the unusual atrial and ventricular recycle during normal function of a committed AV sequential pacemaker.

X-Ray The Pacing System

All pulse generators can be radiographically identified. Some are clear with a manufacturer's logo and model number while others

---

Table III
Troubleshooting DDD Pacemakers—II

Magnet ECG

1. Is the pacing rate as programmed?
2. Is the AV delay as programmed?
3. Are the outputs as in the magnet mode?
4. Have the timing cycles become those of the magnet mode?

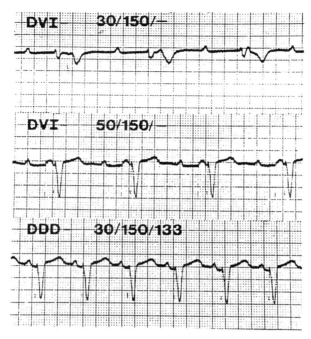

Figure 2. When interpreting a dual-chamber electrogram (ECG) it is important to recognize which chamber(s) are sensed and which are paced. Timing cycles are started and ended by sensed and paced events. **TOP:** The DVI mode senses only ventricular activity. The unsensed atrial event does not initiate a timing cycle. As the ventricular rate is more rapid than the automatic pacemaker rate of 30 bpm, both atrial and ventricular channels are inhibited. **MIDDLE:** The spontaneous ventricular rate is slower than the pacemaker rate so that continuous ventricular pacing occurs, always preceded by an atrial stimulus, in this instance competitive with unsensed atrial activity. **BELOW:** In the DDD mode, atrial sensing exists, and each sensed event starts an AV interval—in this instance, of 150 ms duration. Each sensed P wave is thus followed by a ventricular stimulus.

have a letter designation. Most can be identified by the X-ray configuration of the battery and circuit. All manufacturers provide tables and charts of identifying material, and a number of pacing books tabulate the data under one cover. If identification demonstrates that the pacemaker is one for which the physician has the appropriate programming hardware, s/he should proceed with diagnosing the malfunction. If not, the manufacturer can be asked to provide the appropriate programmer and a technical consultant. The lead system can be identified as unipolar or bipolar, whether a bipolar lead has been unipolarized and whether the electrode tip is in the atrium or ventricle, or leads are in both for a dual-chamber system. X-ray can identify fracture or lead displacement or inadequate connection and consequent intermittent pacing (Figure 3). X-ray and ECG are the two basic approaches for evaluating a pacing system. In more modern pacemakers, telemetry of pacemaker function is an important addition (Table IV).

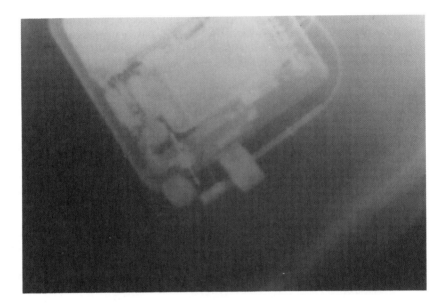

Figure 3.   *Intermittent sensing and pacing was caused by inadequate placement of the lead pin connector into the receptacle of the pulse generator. Contact between the generator and the lead was, therefore, intermittent. Correction was by resetting the pin and the set screw. The defect is readily visible on X-ray.*

Table IV
Troubleshooting DDD
Pacemakers—III

Chest X-ray—PA and Lateral

Is the atrial lead in RA appendage?
Is the ventricular lead in RV apex?
Is either lead fractured?
Are connections to PG secure?

LEAD DESTRUCTION

Pacemaker implantation is commonly and widely achieved via subclavian puncture. In order that introduction of the needle and introducer be safely accomplished, the vein that is entered traverses the costoclavicular space, as do the leads. This space may be narrow so that one, and especially two leads may bind and be subjected to continual pressure and local friction. In the event of continual friction, insulation deterioration, especially of a polyurethane lead will be rapid. Early failure of leads after such implantation can be detected radiologically, and as in other polyurethane deterioration, will be initially manifest by oversensing and possibly pacemaker inhibition (Figure 4).

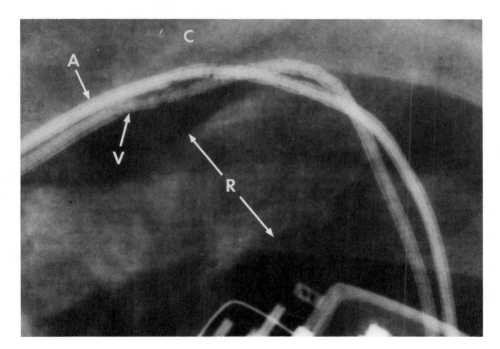

Figure 4. *Pressure caused destruction of atrial and ventricular leads in the costo-clavicular space. The insulation of both leads is extensively notched with the conductor exposed. No ligatures have been placed in this region. A = atrial lead, V = ventricular lead, C = clavicle, R = first rib. (Courtesy of F. Earl Fyke III, M.D.)*

PULSE GENERATOR MANIPULATION

Pulse generators generally lie in the subcutaneous tissue, usually in the right or left pectoral region. The well sited pulse generator will be well medial of the anterior axillary fold, and will be sufficiently below the clavicle so that body movement, especially of the arm will not cause the generator to impinge on the axilla or the clavicle. The pulse generator should be comfortable while the patient is at rest, and pain free during body and especially arm movement. The skin overlying the generator should be non-tender, of normal color and without local heat. The pulse generator should not be adherent to the skin, subcutaneous tissue or the underlying fascia. If any of these circumstances exist, the unit may be malpositioned or infected.

A lead fracture or the rare fracture of the header (connector) on the pulse generator, or a loose set screw holding the lead may be demonstrated by manipulating the pulse generator and lead. With the ECG running, the pulse generator is grasped through the skin and moved superiorly, inferiorly and medially and laterally. A lead fracture may be detected by distraction of the fragments. With the patient in the standing position, holding a weight in the arm on the side of the pacemaker is also useful to distract lead fragments. X-ray with a weight can also be helpful in demonstrating fracture.

If infection of the pacemaker site is suspected because of local erythema, swelling, fluid collection, pain or adherence of the pulse generator to surrounding tissue, wound culture is wise. As bacteria can be introduced, extreme care to avoid contamination should be exercised. The pulse generator site should be carefully shaved (if necessary) and washed as if for an operative procedure. It should then be painted with antiseptic solution and draped with sterile towels. The person performing the wound culture should wear sterile gloves and a sterile gown over clothing. Anesthetic solution, saline for intravenous use or for irrigation should be available as should sterile syringes and aerobic and anaerobic culture media. Saline for parenteral injection often contains an antibacterial preservative, and cultures diluted with it will be sterilized. An antibiotic solution for subsequent irrigation is useful. If the site appears to be infected it can be irrigated after the culture is taken, and provide short-term symptomatic relief while awaiting culture growth and determining the future course.

A dependent portion of the wound is then infiltrated with local anesthetic. A #14 or #16 Angiocath can then be introduced through the anesthetized site. This relatively large needle size is useful because purulent fluid is thicker and more viscous than either serous fluid or blood, and a larger lumen will be useful in aspirating it. The needle is directed toward the device and should strike it. The sensation of hitting a hard metallic object is unmistakable. As much as possible is withdrawn from the cavity made by the fluid accumulation. If the fluid is too viscid, or if little has accumulated, saline can be introduced and then aspirated. The fluid removed is sent for culture. As much as possible of the accumulated fluid is removed; then, if the assessment is that the wound has become infected, the antibiotic solution can be instilled and removed several times until the return is relatively clear. This process may provide brief symptomatic relief, but should not be confused as being curative.

RADIATION DAMAGE

Implanted pulse generators are not damaged by diagnostic levels of radiation. However, the thousands of RADs that are used for therapeutic radiation can damage and destroy an implanted generator. Older generators, which were constructed with discrete resistors, condensers and transistors are far less sensitive to radiation damage than are newer generators with CMOS circuits. The difference between the two pacemaker designs is striking and older concepts of pacemaker resistance are not relevant to modern multiprogrammable single- or dual-chamber pacemakers.

If radiation therapy is required, the generator should be carefully shielded from scatter. If shielding is impossible, for example, in the case of breast or lung cancer in which the pulse generator lies directly in the field of radiation, the generator should be moved to another site. Radiation dose is cumulative and the mode of failure is random. The generator may lose sensing or output function, may suddenly stop or may suddenly runaway. Leads can be radiated without risk.

SUPERFAST RECHARGE

An occasional patient with unipolar dual-chamber pulse generator model #7005 implanted will complain of episodic or continuous stimulation at the site of pulse generator implantation. Evaluation will demonstrate that this occurs only when the atrium is being stimulated and not during ventricular stimulation alone or with atrial sensing and ventricular stimulation. Analysis of the atrial stimulus artifact will show it to be normal. Other evidence of lead insulation failure   the most common cause of local pectoral muscle stimulation—will be absent. The muscle stimulation during atrial pacing is likely to persist despite reduction in atrial channel output, even if it is below the stimulation capture threshold.

The event occurs because of a superfast recharge circuit placed into the atrial channel output and is intended to reduce the necessary duration of the ventricular blanking period, which begins with the atrial stimulus. Reduction in duration of the recharge time allows a shorter blanking period, but produces a greater amplitude recharge spike, though of shorter duration. This stimulus may, in a few patients, be suprathreshold for stimulation of the local pectoral musculature.

As there is no certain means of stimulating the atrium and avoiding local musculature stimulation, the best means of management is the reduction of the incidence of atrial pacing. Model #7005 has no VDD mode, i.e., with atrial sensing but without pacing. Should atrial pacing be required to maintain synchrony, then local muscle stimulation cannot be avoided. If atrial activity is normal, then the lower rate limit should be reduced below the anticipated slowest atrial rate (this may be a problem for sleeping atrial rates), so that only sensing will occur. As atrial stimulation may occur during upper rate operation, especially should fixed ratio AV block occur, it is wise to increase the upper rate limit as high as is reasonable.

Should all other means of management fail, pulse generator replacement may be required. As this mechanism is part of normal operation of model #7005, replacement of one unit by another of the same model is not likely to help. Another model pulse generator will be required.

PULSE GENERATOR INSULATION DEFECT

Insulation defect, which is known to exist and be extremely troublesome in lead systems, can also exist on a pulse generator. Unipolar pulse generators are insulated on one side, generally that opposite to the side engraved with the pulse generator identification. The insulated side should be placed toward the muscle, and the uninsulated side toward the subcutaneous tissue. The insulation material can be removed or rubbed from the pulse generator. Should that occur, two circumstances may follow. The first is that electromyographic interference (EMI) may occur and inappropriately inhibit the pulse generator. Alternatively, a small area of defect may shunt a relatively high current density to the muscle, causing a local twitch with each stimulus. This is especially true in the case of the atrial stimulus in a pulse generator with a superfast recharge circuit. It may not then be possible to program an atrial channel output sufficiently low to avoid local muscle stimulation. This may be especially true in a patient with chronotropic incompetence who requires continued atrial stimulation.

If the pacemaker can operate in the effective VDD mode, in which there is no atrial stimulation, this effect can be avoided. If there is no possibility of ending atrial channel stimulation, operative intervention will be required. Once the insulation defect is found, an accessory silicone rubber boot may be placed on the generator. Alternatively, the pulse generator may be replaced. This condition is unusual, but has been seen by the author on several occasions. It should be suspected when local muscle stimulation occurs in model #7005, and when atrial stimulation causes local muscle stimulation, and ventricular stimulation does not. No detectable defect may be present during preoperative evaluation, as the current leak is extremely close to that which occurs during normal unipolar DDD pulse generator function.

PACING SYSTEM ANALYZER

The Pacing System Analyzer (PSA) is the basic device for determination of threshold of pacing and sensing. Equally important, it allows testing the function of an implanted pulse generator and lead system during pacemaker implant and during intraoperative analysis of pacemaker malfunction. As with any other device, knowledge of its proper operation is essential to derivation of useful data. This is especially true for the PSA, because these devices are not universally compatible with all implanted pacemaking systems, either for the lead system or for the pulse generator. For this reason, it is a wise policy to use the same make PSA as the generator to be tested and implanted. As each PSA operates somewhat differently, its manual should be carefully read and understood. There are two major differences that affect the method of interpretation of data derived from a PSA.

Measurement of Output Voltage

Two different means of pulse generator output are in widespread use. One is constant voltage in which output current is largely determined (within limits) by the impedance of the lead system. If the output voltage is 5 V and the impedance is the relative standard of 500 Ohms, the current flow will be 10 mA. If however, a short circuit exists, and the impedance is only 250 Ohms, then the current flow may be 20 mA. A PSA that measures constant voltage output will read both voltage outputs similarly and calculate current output at the higher level.

The second mode of output is constant current. In this mode, output current is largely independent (within limits) of lead impedance. The PSA that reads constant voltage output will not read accurately the constant current output of a pulse generator. The voltage reading will be falsely low. Determination of the output characteristics of a specific pulse generator may not match the nominal because of differences in measurement criteria. Only one manufacturer provides constant current pulse generators and a PSA reading constant current output.

The sensing circuits of different pacing system analyzers use different criteria. Each manufacturer's standard differs from a natural intrinsic deflection depolarization; all are artificial. The sensing circuit of a pulse generator will test differently on each PSA and therefore, the specific response of each generator must be known for each specific PSA. As the volume of detail involved will probably exceed the management capability of most laboratories, and as manufacturers are unwilling to provide data concerning test results of generators not of their manufacture, it is best to use the PSA provided by the manufacturer of the pulse generator being tested.

At the conclusion of noninvasive evaluation of pacemaker function, the nature of the malfunction is usually known. If unknown, it is likely that all possible diagnostic modalities have not been exhausted.

DIAGNOSTIC MODALITIES

1. Passive ECG
2. X-ray
3. ECG–free running and in the magnet mode
4. Ambulatory ECG
5. Programming
6. Manipulation of the pulse generator (to accentuate lead fracture or insulation defect)
7. Telemetry

Table V
Programmability for Lead Malfunction

OPERATIVE REPAIR	INCREASE SENSITIVITY
1. Fracture	1. Poor electrogram
DECREASE OUTPUT	REDUCE SENSITIVITY
1. Diaphragmatic stimulation	1. Electromagnetic interference
2. Phrenic nerve stimulation	2. Electromyographic interference
INCREASE OUTPUT	CHANGE MODE
1. Insulation failure	1. Electromagnetic interference
2. Poor position	2. Electromyographic interference
3. Displacement	3. "Noisy lead"
4. High threshold	
5. Threshold evolution	

Most often, these maneuvers will give sufficient information to allow preoperative diagnosis of pacemaker malfunction. It is as important to begin surgical intervention well informed (concerning pacemaker malfunction) as in any other surgical approach. Because of the limited causes of malfunction, the cause usually can be ascertained preoperatively. Each approach, preoperative evaluation and operative assessment, offers the possibility of diagnostic procedures unavailable to the other; each should be used. For example, a hairline lead fracture may be visible on X-ray, but invisible to the unaided eye following exposure of the pacemaker hardware but, once again, present as a high impedance on telemetry or at operation. A summary of the procedure for troubleshooting dual-chamber pacemakers is contained in Tables II, III, IV and V.

TELEMETRY

Telemetric data transmission which includes hardware, stimulation, physiology, and electrogram data is becoming increasingly more available and important in troubleshooting pacemaker defects and analyzing the intricacies of normal pacemaker function. See the chapter on telemetry for delineation of this capability.

OPERATIVE ASSESSMENT OF PACEMAKER MALFUNCTION

If noninvasive assessment of pacemaker malfunction has been unsuccessful in determining the nature of the problem, or if the programmability available has not been adequate for resolution of the problem, then operative intervention is undertaken (Table V).

The Incision

If it has been determined with a reasonable degree of certainty that the pulse generator only is at fault, then it alone should be approached, and the incision can be made over the center of the implanted generator, which can then be lifted from the subcutaneous or submuscular pocket, detached from the lead(s), which can then be tested for contact with the chamber of placement, and for electrical and mechanical integrity. This is usually the case if pulse generator battery depletion has occurred.

If the leads have been determined preoperatively to require replacement or reposition, then the incision should be made via the original implant incision that had been placed to approach the venous system. If the leads need not be manipulated, an incision over them risks damage, as they are difficult to palpate in the subcutaneous tissue, and can readily be cut with scapel or scissors. If the revision does not require dissection of leads, they should not be approached.

The Wound

When the wound is opened it should be inspected and reviewed for infection. An infected wound should be abandoned (see infection). A clean wound is free of purulence, erythema and tenderness. Upon opening the wound, if the lining of the pacer site is reddened or purulent, or if there is other than a small volume (1–2 cc) of clear light yellow fluid, then the wound should be cultured and not reused as a pacer site.

Pulse Generator and Leads

The Leads are Exposed

Measurement should be made of the impedance of each lead separately. If the lead is bipolar, then the impedance measurement should be of the bipolar pair. Measurement should be with any of the pacing system analyzers commercially available. The impedance is a measurement determined at a specific pulse duration and at a specific output, usually 10 mA (constant current) or 5 V (constant voltage). Lead impedance is very important data and varies with the method of measurement; it is, therefore, important that measurement be undertaken so that readings at the time of implant and later, at secondary intervention, are comparable.

Low Impedance

Late evolution of impedance after implantation is modest, i.e., several years after implantation, impedance will not be more than 20% greater than the impedance at the time of implantation (again measured by similar techniques). Virtually all electrode impedances will approximate 500 Ohms, as all are designed to that general specification. Some will be as low as 400 Ohms and others will be as high as 750 Ohms. Any significant deviation outside of these limits should suggest strongly the possibility of electrode defect.

If the impedance is lower than the given range, an insulation defect can be anticipated with current leak into the tissue before reaching the electrode. In the presence of a bipolar lead system, the possibility exists that the short circuit is between the two conductors. If low impedance is present, current is escaping either to the surrounding tissue in a unipolar or bipolar lead system, or between the two conductors in a bipolar system (Figure 5). If an insulation disruption is visible (in a unipolar system) in the exposed tissue it can probably be repaired. If it is at the connector, repair is readily possible with equipment provided by all manufacturers. If the disruption is

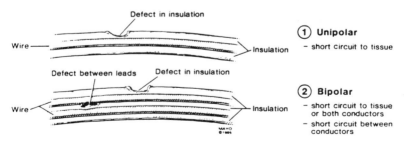

Figure 5. Short circuit of a pacer lead follows insulation deterioration. In the unipolar system, short circuit allows escape of current to the surrounding tissue. In the bipolar lead, the defect may be to the surrounding tissue of one conductor, of both conductors or between the two.

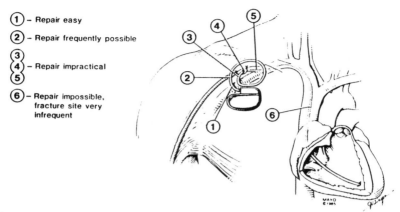

(1) – Repair easy

(2) – Repair frequently possible

(3)
(4) – Repair impractical
(5)

(6) – Repair impossible,
fracture site very
infrequent

Figure 6. *Lead fracture still occurs as a constant, ongoing phenomenon following implant. For a unipolar lead, attempt at repair depends on the site of fracture. If fracture is well beyond (i.e., outside) entry to the vein, repair may be easy; if adjacent to entry to the vein, it is impractical; and if within the vein, the fracture site is unapproachable.*

somewhere within the venous system, repair will be difficult (if possible at all), or practically impossible. If one limb of a bipolar system is intact, the resolution may be by unipolarization of the lead system but only if the lead to the tip is intact, not the lead to the electrode ring (Figure 6).

While a lead fracture protects an implanted pacemaker from depletion, an insulation disruption can cause rapid depletion. Even at short circuit, a constant current device will deliver approximately its rated output. A constant voltage pacemaker also will deliver a current at short circuit that will be limited only by the low internal resistance of the output circuit. Consequently, a constant voltage unit can deliver large currents and deplete itself rapidly and prematurely. If revision is undertaken for lead insulation failure, the generator should be investigated carefully for evidence of depletion before it is reused. This is especially true for insulation defects of polyurethane leads in which the defect is commonly associated with short circuit to the subcutaneous tissue, or between the two conductors of a biopolar lead.

High Impedance

If lead impedance is high it is important to check the measurement. Calibrate the PSA. If the PSA is satisfactory, short circuit the test cables used to measure the lead impedance, one to the other. The impedance on the PSA should now approximate zero or the minimum reading of the PSA. Separate the two clips, the impedance should be infinite. If these findings are consistent, the PSA is probably operating satisfactorily and the cables are intact. Most PSA impedance measurements range from 250–2,000 Ohms and so these will be the measurement limits. If the impedance exceeds the presumed upper limit or if it is higher by 50% or more than that at implant, lead fracture has probably occurred. Such a fracture may not be visible on x-ray. Negative x-ray findings do not eliminate the possibility of fracture. Elevated lead impedance is a more sensitive indicator of fracture than x-ray. If the impedance reading is above 1,000 Ohms, fracture is almost certain; if it is above 2,000 Ohms, i.e., reading at infinity, lead fracture is certain. If the break is within the venous system, repair is impossible; if the break is outside the venous system and in the subcutaneous tissue, repair depends on whether an adequate length is present to repair without stress. If repair cannot be accomplished either with low or high impedance conditions, the connector pin should be insulated and the lead abandoned.

A lead that is clean (uninfected) and has been chronically in place may be difficult to remove. If it is fractured within the venous system, i.e., distal to the point at which it can be grasped, it may not be possible to remove it without an invasive procedure. Abandonment of an uninfected lead may be preferable to an attempt at removal. Occasionally, total removal of a lead will be unsuccessful, leaving fragments of the lead in situ. Such fragments may cause more difficulty than an intact, inactive lead. Removal of an inactive lead should be performed only after carefully considering the consequences of leaving the lead in place or removing it destructively. If the high impedance is felt to be caused by lead failure, several options exist— abandonment, partial removal or complete removal.

Threshold of Pacing

Each lead should be tested for pacing threshold and whether the threshold is within the output capability of the pulse generator. If the threshold is low (compared to the output capability of the pulse generator), then, all is well. If the threshold is in the general middle range of output, the generator can be programmed to accommodate threshold. If threshold is near or above maximum pulse generator output, the lead requires revision. The distinction between high threshold and lead defect lies in the impedance. High or low impedance associated with lack of capture indicates lead defect. Normal impedance with high threshold implies defect of the electrode myocardial interface.

It is generally easy to decide when threshold is well within the output capability of the pulse generator intended for implant. It is equally easy to determine when threshold is excessively high. The major difficulty occurs when threshold is high but margin still exists. The following rules may be useful:

1. Determine that the lead impedance is normal, i.e., that high threshold is not a result of a lead defect;
2. Determine that the voltage and current thresholds are proportional. If the voltage threshold is high, the current threshold should be equally high. High voltage threshold and low current threshold indicate high impedance and lead fracture. Low voltage threshold and high current threshold indicate short circuit or lead defect. For virtually all pacing system analyzers the voltage is measured directly, just as the impedance, and the current flow is derived, i.e., calculated from the two. It should be recognized that voltage threshold and impedance are measured values, current is derived.
3. A stable, sharply defined threshold that is high may be useful, nevertheless. If threshold is high and varies as it is tested, it is unreliable and should not be used. High pulse generator output consumes the battery rapidly, and all estimates of prolonged pacemaker longevity are based on "normal" levels of output. If "normal" output cannot accommodate pacing and an adequate safety margin, lead revision should be undertaken. Special circumstances may, of course, dictate that prolonged longevity is less important than immediate and short-term restoration of pacing. "Normal" output can be considered to be a maximum output voltage of 5 V and a pulse duration of 0.5–1.0 ms.
4. 8–10 V outputs consume battery capacity rapidly. They should be used sparingly and only for good reason.

Once pulse duration threshold has been determined at 2.5 V, output should be set at 5 V and at least at the pulse duration threshold. This situation will work well if threshold pulse duration is briefer than 1.0 ms. If threshold pulse duration is determined at 5 V, output should be set at least three times the threshold pulse duration if that pulse duration does not exceed 1.2 ms. If pulse duration threshold at 5 V output is 0.5 ms or longer, careful consideration should be given to revision or replacement of the lead. Longer pulse durations or lesser safety margins can be used in special circumstances.

Sensing Threshold

As with the pacing threshold, the amplitude of the electrogram should be measured either directly on a physiological recorder or with a PSA. If the electrogram is of amplitude and slew rate (frequency content) adequate to be readily sensed, then no revision is required.

If not, the lead may require repositioning. The display of the electrogram on a physiological recorder has the additional virtue, not available on the PSA, of identifying the chamber in which the lead lies. Since erroneous placement of an atrial appendage lead in the outflow tract of the right ventricle can occur, display of the atrial EGM is especially valuable and will definitively identify the site of the lead; simple electrogram amplitude will not (Figure 7). If the signal (i.e., the EGM) is too small to be sensed by the maximum sensitivity of the pulse generator, lead revision is required. If the signal is adequate, attention can be turned to the pulse generator.

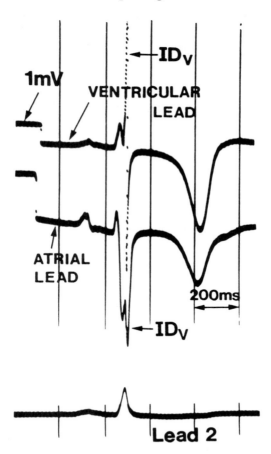

Figure 7. *Following displacement of an atrial lead to the right ventricular outflow tract, X-ray was reported as normal. Simultaneous electrogram recording from the atrial and ventricular leads demonstrated ventricular electrograms from both leads, simultaneous with the QRS complex on the surface.*

Electrogram

One of the best tests for lead integrity and placement is determination of the electrogram via the implanted lead. In a number of generators, the electrogram can be telemetered noninvasively and indicate by its quality whether the lead is intact. If this capability does not exist, or if there is doubt (even if there is little doubt), the electrogram derived from the implanted lead should be displayed during pacemaker revision. The appearance of the implanted lead electrogram should be similar to that shown elsewhere in this text. A carefully done electrogram   using cables now provided by various manufacturers and displayed on a physiological recorder   should be recorded at 0.1–2,000 Hz, and will be clean and well defined. An electrogram recorded on an electrocardiograph will be frequency-limited but will be readily recognizable and interpretable (Figures 8,9). Possible defects include:

1. Artifacts on the EGM indicating the reason for "false recycle" (Figure 10);
2. Sixty Hz interference, indicating a loss of lead continuity;
3. Intermittent loss of signal, i.e., intermittent lead contact;
4. Small EGM, below the level of sensing capability (Figure 11).

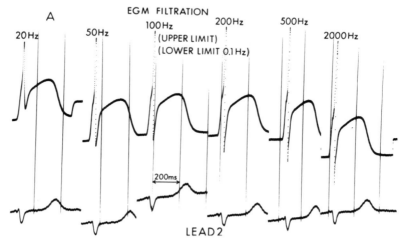

Figure 8.   *The quality of the electrogram (EGM) depends on the frequency response of the recorder. In each of these tracings, the lower frequency response is 0.1 Hz, the upper is as listed. Since much of the electrogram amplitude is at higher frequency levels, recording at a lower frequency limits the amplitude of the recording. The recording at 100 Hz will approximate that on an electrocardiograph. It is best to record the EGM at an upper frequency cutoff of 500 or more Hz.*

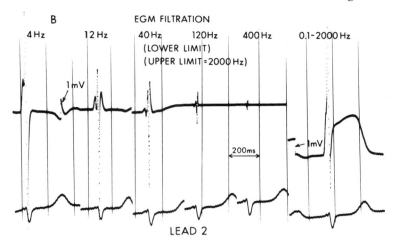

Figure 9. *The quality of the electrogram (EGM) depends on the frequency response of the recorder. In each of these tracings, the upper frequency response is 2,000 Hz, the lower is as listed. Since much of the electrogram amplitude is also at lower frequency levels, recording at a higher frequency only limits the amplitude of the recording. It is best to record the electrogram at a lower frequency response of 0.1 Hz, and an upper limit of at least 500 Hz.*

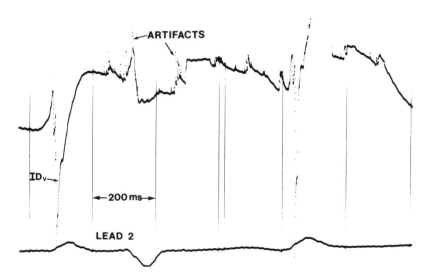

Figure 10. *An electrogram recorded with superimposed random artifacts. These artifacts may result from a poor connection between test lead and pacing lead, or lead fracture. The persistance of these artifacts after careful attention to the various connections is an indication of conductor deterioration, even if no fracture is visible on X-ray.*

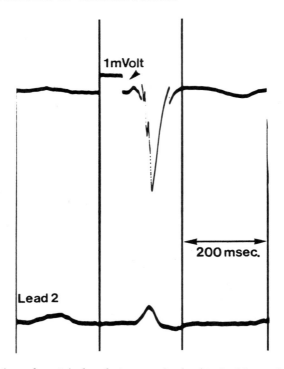

Figure 11. *A good ventricular electrogram is characterized by a sharply defined intrinsic deflection of adequate amplitude, with an intrinsic deflection that has minimal visible slope. A poor electrogram is characterized by visible slope, poor amplitude (in this instance no more than ¾ mV), and occasionally, a reversal of the intrinsic deflection, which makes each component too small to be sensed.*

In each instance it is very important to be certain that the connecting cables are intact, because defects in the cables can mimic each of these problems.

RETAINED LEAD

Occasionally, a lead will be damaged or will have deteriorated so that it cannot be continued in use. When such a lead is found to be present either because of high threshold, incorrectible sensing, or because of impending insulation deterioration or lead fracture, the lead should not be reused. Two additional circumstances exist: the lead may be infected or it may be clean. If it is infected it must be removed, otherwise cure of the infection and sterilization of the blood will be virtually impossible. While occasional reports of infection relief without removal of hardware have appeared, these should be looked at with suspicion. The only certain means of clearing the infection is lead removal with subsequent antibiotic management.

If the lead is clean it may be abandoned in situ. The connector pin should be insulated with a cap provided for that purpose. The lead should be carefully attached to the subcutaneous tissue with nonabsorbable ligature so that it cannot migrate.

LEAD REMOVAL

If the lead is infected it must be removed. The lead must be carefully mobilized, and a secure portion of the lead in the subcutaneous tissue grasped. Gentle traction under fluoroscopy should be exerted while watching the lead move from the right ventricular apex into the superior vena cava and out, via the site of insertion. If implantation is via thoracotomy, then repeat thoracotomy will be necessary. The incision is made to approach the electrode at the myocardial level. Once the electrode is carefully removed from the myocardium by unscrewing or by cutting the ligatures holding it, the electrode is cut from the lead and removed. The lead can then be removed by traction as it moves through the tract in the subcutaneous tissue. Removal of the electrode at the myocardial level is usually easily accomplished if infection is present, as it has already been lifted from the heart by the infectious process (Figure 12).

If the transvenous lead cannot be removed by gentle manual traction, weighted traction can be used. The lead is exposed, and a hemostat grasps the exposed end. A weight over a pulley at the end of the operating table or the bed then applies continuous traction until the lead falls from the heart. The process may occupy several hours. Once the pulley is in place, water is added to a plastic bag to serve as the weight until several ventricular premature contractions (VPC) are seen. Approximately 350 ml will be required to start. Water is then continually added until VPC occur as the traction removes the lead from the myocardium. This process contaminates the lead, which must be removed eventually, once this process has started. If the lead cannot be removed, a direct approach to the heart, via open heart surgery, if necessary, will be required (Figure 13).

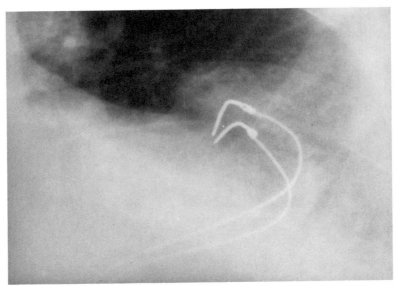

Figure 12.   *An infectious mass surrounds the two electrodes implanted by thoroco-tomy, which are no longer capable of stimulating the heart. At exploration, the electrodes lay free in a gelatinous infected mass.*

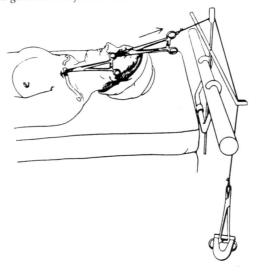

Figure 13.   *Removal of a chronically implanted ventricular lead can usually be accomplished by slow, progressive, and gentle traction. The lead must be surgically mobilized and then attached to a Buck's traction on which progressive weights are placed. The weight is increased progressively to the level at which an occasional ventricular premature contraction (VPC) occurs. As the lead moves from the ventricle, the weight can be increased.*

Atrial leads can also be removed, but since the atrium is fragile it may be lacerated by the procedures listed above. Only a few successful removals of a retained atrial lead have been reported, and the risk of removal of an atrial lead by traction is uncertain. If traction is deemed too risky, then thoracotomy may be used with amputation of the atrial appendage.

When traction is not successful for chronic lead removal, other techniques are available. Special lead extractors have been described that fit over the chronic lead and are passed along the lead to the endocardial surface, at which point a grasping mechanism is activated. While this concept is attractive, no such device is commercially available yet.

A chronically implanted lead can often be removed if tension can be applied to the lead near its tip. The technique used at the Mayo Clinic is as follows. If the tip of the lead cannot be removed by traction, a pigtail catheter is passed into the heart via the femoral vein. The pigtail portion of the catheter is positioned around the permanent pacing lead, as near to the tip as possible (Figure 14). Twisting the pigtail catheter multiple times in a clockwise direction will entwine the pacing lead in the pigtail catheter (Figure 15). Traction is then applied to the pigtail catheter. Traction applied to the pacing lead near its point of endocardial attachment will frequently free the lead (Figure 16A). If the lead tip is dislodged from the endocardial surface, continued traction is placed on the pigtail catheter, and the lead is pulled into the inferior vena cava. Because the entwined pacing lead and pigtail catheter are bulky, and because with traction the pigtail catheter may now slip off the free end of the pacing lead, the pigtail catheter is removed. This is done by twisting the pigtail catheter in a counterclockwise direction (Figure 16B). Once the pigtail catheter is removed, a Dotter retriever is then passed into the inferior vena cava via the femoral vein. The Dotter retriever consists of a retractable wire basket that is passed within a sheath. When the wire basket is extended beyond the sheath, the basket opens, and the operator attempts to catch a portion of the pacing lead in the wire basket. When the retractor is then pulled back, the pacing lead will be firmly entrapped in the Dotter retriever. Applying traction on the Dotter retriever, the lead can then be extracted via the femoral vein. Prior to attempting extraction, the connector portion at the proximal end of the pacing lead must be transsected (Figure 16C).

If initial traction on the entwined pigtail catheter fails to dislodge the tip of the pacing lead, any redundancy in the lead is pulled into

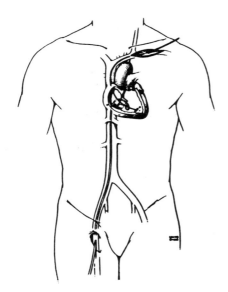

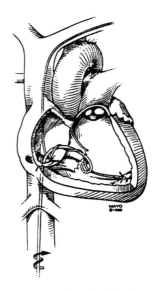

Figure 14. A pigtail catheter is passed via the right femoral vein into the right ventricle. The pigtail portion of the catheter is positioned around the permanent pacing lead as near to the tip of the lead as possible.

Figure 15. The pigtail catheter is then twisted in a clockwise fashion. This effectively entwines the pigtail catheter and the permanent pacing lead.

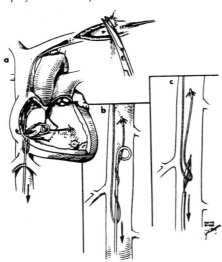

Figure 16. A. With the pigtail catheter and the permanent pacing lead firmly entwined, traction is then applied on the pigtail catheter in an attempt to free the lead tip from the endocardial surface. *B.* If traction is successful in freeing the tip of the lead, the lead is pulled into the inferior vena cava. The pigtail catheter is rotated in a counterclockwise direction to free the pigtail catheter and is then removed via the femoral vein. *C.* The pigtail catheter is replaced with a Dotter retriever. The wire basket is extended, and under fluoroscopy it's positioned so that a portion of the pacing lead is within the wire basket. The wire basket is then retracted around a portion of the pacing lead so that the pacing lead is firmly caught in the Dotter retriever. Traction is then applied to the Dotter retriever in an attempt to extract the whole lead via the femoral vein. The most proximal portion of the pacing lead (the lead connector) should be transected prior to extraction.

the inferior vena cava in an effort to form a small loop of pacing lead that can subsequently be grasped by the Dotter retriever (Figure 17A). Again, by turning the pigtail catheter in a counterclockwise direction, the pigtail catheter is freed from the pacing lead and removed. The Dotter retriever is then passed into the inferior vena cava and with the

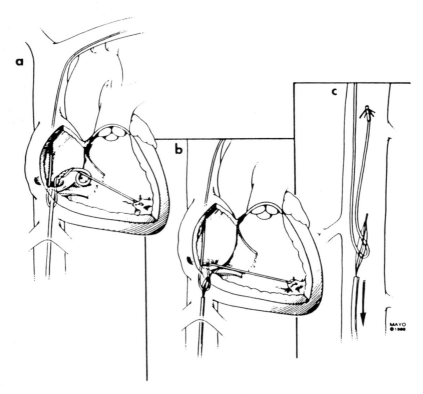

Figure 17. A. *With the pigtail catheter firmly entwined with the permanent pacing lead, traction is applied, but the lead tip cannot be dislodged from the endocardial surface. Traction is applied on the pigtail catheter and the still attached lead in an effort to position a small loop of the pacing catheter within the inferior vena cava. The pigtail catheter is then rotated in a counterclockwise direction in an effort to separate the pigtail catheter from the pacing lead. The pigtail catheter is then removed. **B.** The Dotter retriever is passed into the inferior vena cava. With the Dotter retriever extended, an attempt is made to snare the loop of the pacing lead in the Dotter retriever. Once this is accomplished, the basket portion of the Dotter retriever is retracted, firmly securing a portion of the pacing lead in the Dotter retriever. Traction is then applied on the Dotter retriever to free the tip of the pacing lead from the endocardial surface. **C.** If the tip of the pacing lead is successfully dislodged from the endocardial surface, the lead is extracted via the femoral vein.*

basket extended, an attempt is made to capture the loop of pacing lead within the inferior vena cava in the Dotter retriever. Once the pacing lead has been entrapped in the wire basket, the retractor is pulled back and with the pacing lead firmly snared, traction is placed on the Dotter retriever in an effort to dislodge the tip of the lead (Figure 17B). The Dotter retriever is successful sometimes in dislodging the lead tip when the pigtail catheter has failed, because better traction can be applied with the pacing lead securely snared in the Dotter retriever. If the lead tip is successfully dislodged, continued traction is placed on the Dotter retriever, and the lead is extracted via the femoral vein (Figure 17C). Extracting the lead via the femoral vein, while it is still entangled in the Dotter retriever, can potentially damage the femoral vein because of the bulk of the catheters being extracted. In our experience, no significant hematomas have resulted from the extraction, nor has venous repair ever been required. However, a pressure dressing should be placed over the puncture site, and the site must be carefully observed.

Although the procedure can be time-consuming and technically difficult, it may prevent the need for thoractomy.

LEAD REMOVAL BY OPEN HEART SURGERY

If all other approaches for removal of an infected lead(s) have failed, removal is still mandatory if cure of endocarditis is to occur. If the lead cannot be safely removed, and this may be especially so for atrial leads, a direct approach by thoracotomy must be made.

If a ventricular lead has been removed and only the atrial lead remains, it may be attached at the atrial appendage. With median sternotomy, the superior and inferior vena cava are dissected and looped with tapes, and the azygous vein is also occluded. The attachment of the atrial lead to the atrial appendage can be palpated, and with inflow occlusion, the tip of the atrial appendage can be amputated, freeing the lead. The amputated atrium is then reclosed with a partially occluding clamp and subsequently repaired. Separately, the site of insertion of the lead, probably at the pectoral area, is opened, the lead mobilized and withdrawn from the venous system. This approach obviously does not involve cardiopulmonary bypass and can be accomplished briefly (with one to two minutes of inflow occlusion, or none at all).

If the atrial lead cannot be removed, as above, or if a ventricular lead is adherent to the ventricular apex, or if a lead has deteriorated and traction only causes it to unravel, leaving portions of the lead within the ventricle, then an open heart surgical approach is required for its removal. The chest is opened via median sternotomy, and cardiopulmonary bypass is established. The right atrium is opened and the ventricular lead is grasped as it traverses the tricuspid valve. The lead is detached from the valve, and the traction on it pulls the point of attachment in the ventricle to the tricuspid valve. The site of attachment may be encased in infected thrombus, which can now be removed along with any vegetations on the tricuspid valve. As much infected tissue as possible should be debrided. The fibrous tissue holding the lead in place can be readily identified and cut with a scalpel. The lead can then be readily removed from the ventricle. The fibrous mass should be debrided, but need not be entirely resected.

Having freed the lead from within the heart, the site of attachment to the pulse generator in the pectoral region can be approached, and the lead withdrawn. A chronically implanted lead may have become adherent to the subclavian vein, which may be lacerated by traction. Bleeding may then be virtually uncontrollable.

Once the lead and vegetations have been removed from the heart, the atriotomy can be reclosed in routine fashion, and cardiopulmonary bypass ended. If the patient has been on prolonged antibiotic management, and the blood stream has been sterilized, thoracotomy implantation of new myocardial leads may be accomplished at this time. Antibiotic administration should be continued for the full course of management of bacterial endocarditis.

The Pulse Generator

The pulse generator should be tested to determine whether it is operating properly. Most of the available PSA systems will allow the determination of pulse generator output, sensitivity and pulse duration. The pulse generator should be programmed to several of its capabilites and then checked with the PSA. If the generator has been, in fact, programmed to the outputs displayed on the programmer, then it is probably functioning normally and may be reused. Sterile programming heads and cables are readily available. If the pulse generator is contaminated during testing, it should not be returned to the original pacer site but be resterilized with ethylene oxide, and then reused in the same patient. Directions for resterilization with ethylene oxide are beyond the capability of this text; temperature limits should not be exceeded, the device should be allowed to wait, and should be adequately washed with saline to remove residual gas before reimplantation. The generator should be carefully inspected for mechanical defects, especially at the connector. If the unit is sterile and intact mechanically and electrically, it can be reused, but most warranties will be voided. Each manufacturer may have a different policy and this should be checked. If in doubt, use a new generator suitable for the patient.

Pulse Generator Reuse

Reuse of a previously implanted pulse generator is an issue fraught with legal and ethical problems. During October 1988, the FDA approved refurbishment of used pulse generators for export. Refurbished units are not reimplanted in the United States, as of this writing. Reuse of a generator that has been removed from the wound and is to be replaced during the same procedure, into the same patient is commonly performed and is appropriate. Reuse of a pulse generator removed from a patient, cleansed sterilized and reused in the same patient at a later date, is appropriate. Nevertheless, subjecting the pulse generator to that process will usually void the manufacturer's warranty and if incorrectly done, may destroy the generator. The generator, if it is to be reused, should be carefully cleaned with antiseptic solution such as quaternary ammonium, carefully rinsed in isotonic saline to remove residual antiseptic and then tested. If it is still functioning normally, it can be sterilized with ethylene oxide gas. Sterilization by steam autoclave will destroy the generator. It should be retested, after sterilization, at the operating table, to ascertain that it has not been destroyed during processing.

Pulse Generator Eccentricity

Pacemaker eccentricity is an apparent deviation from presumed normal function, but is normal pacemaker function for that model. Eccentricities should be distinguished from unexpected function, which has been designed to be normal pulse generator function. There are many such eccentricities of both single- and dual-chamber pulse generators. All represent normal rather than abnormal function and when found, should not lead to a conclusion of malfunction.

Single-chamber pulse generator eccentricities include:

1. Prolonged periods of asystole during programming of models #5984/5. Depending on the rate from which the device is programmed to the rate at which it is programmed, a period of almost four seconds of asystole may occur (Figure 18).
2. Partial programming during programming of devices using magnetic reed switch manipulation. Partial rate programming may result in an intermediate rate. For example, the #0505 generator rate moves during rate programming from the previous rate to 100 bpm, and finally to the new rate. It may remain at 100 bpm and can be returned to the normal function by repeating the programming sequence (Figure 19).

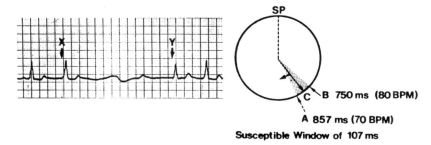

Figure 18. *Asystole can occur during programming from a lower to a higher rate in one make of multiprogrammable pacemaker. The timing "clock" has a 2,000 ms cycle (lowest rate 30 bpm) starting from "SP." The programmed rate acts as a release point (A). When the moving cursor (the diagrammatic arrow C) reaches A the stimulus is released. If, after the cycle has started and the cursor (C) has passed the higher rate (which it reaches first) but not reached the lower rate, the lower rate stop (A) can be moved (by rate programming) behind the advancing cursor. No "stop" exists, and no stimulus is emitted until that stop is reached. Depending on the rates programmed, the maximum duration of asystole can be almost 4 seconds.*

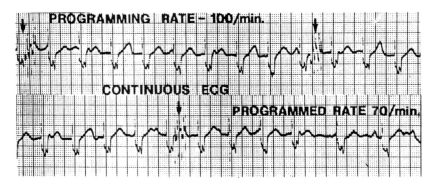

Figure 19. *Partial programming can occur, especially in pulse generators that are programmed by magnetic reed "dithering" and that move through an intermediate step before reaching the programmed value. In this unit, model #0505, the intermediate rate during rate or output programming is 100 bpm for four stimuli. Each programming episode is indicated by an arrow. Only the last completes the programming cycle. Partial programming results from incomplete transmission of the signal caused either by distance from the pulse generator, or by removing the programming head before the programming transmission has been completed. Note, that the programming signal is about 0.3 seconds in duration. Thousands of these generators remain in service.*

3. Several models of unipolar dual-chamber pacemaker can use the opposite leads (atrial and ventricular) as the ground for sensing and pacing. A unipolar pacemaker requires the pacemaker case in contact with the tissue to complete the circuit. In this instance, the pulse generator can be lifted from the wound and continue to pace and sense well.
4. At least one model dual-chamber pacemaker (#283-01) will stimulate the ventricle if threshold is in the low normal range during pacing in the AAI mode, due to current leak via the ventricular lead. This effect is not subject to correction by reduction of ventricular output, but only by reduction of atrial output.
5. Crosstalk is the sensing of the atrial stimulus in the ventricular channel with consequent inhibition of output in that channel. It occurs more often during high atrial output, and reduction of output can often reduce or eliminate crosstalk. Other methods of management include increase of the duration of the ventricular blanking period, programming to the triggered mode in the ventricular channel, and reducing ventricular sensitivity.
6. The single-chamber pacemaker may sense the repolarization effect following a high output stimulus. Reduction of stimulus amplitude or increase in duration of the ventricular refractory period may resolve the problem.

Many other eccentricities will be manifest as devices proliferate and become more complex. It is most important that these be distinguished from truly abnormal function.

INTERPRETATION OF DATA

The interpretation of data is of utmost importance in the decision concerning the variety of revision to be undertaken. The PSA can only provide numerical data for such interpretation. In the end, all interpretations are made because of the operator's knowledge of pacing hardware and physiology. Some guides are valuable; four measurements are useful:

1. voltage threshold;
2. current threshold;
3. impedance;
4. electrogram.

Based on intraoperative data derived from these four factors, diagnosis and resolution can be made (Table VI). Troubleshooting of implanted hardware problems may be extremely difficult or relatively simple since the number of problems and resolutions are limited.

Table VI
Lead and Electrode Test Data

	Fracture	*Insulation Failure*	*Dis-placement*	*High Threshold*	*Poor Sensing*	*Poor Position*
Voltage	High	Low	High	High	Normal	High
Current	Variable May be normal	High	High	High	Normal	High
Impedance	High	Low	Normal	Normal	Normal	Normal
Electrogram	Variable	Variable	Low	May be normal	Low	Low
Resolution	Repair	Repair	Reposition	Higher output or reposition	High sensitivity	Reposition

DIAGNOSIS OF MALFUNCTION

The failure of different components of the pacing system should be analyzed to assist in making a rational choice concerning revision. It is important to define the part of the system at fault before attempting revision. There are characteristic deficiencies that would lead to the conclusion that the electrode, lead, pulse generator circuit or power source is at fault.

The prevalence of polyurethane leads at risk, models #6972, #6990U, and #6991U implanted in over 100,000 patients, makes it likely that defects will be widely seen. Failure rates of up to 20% occur and as the failures are time dependent, more are likely to be seen. If unusual pacemaker failure circumstances are observed with one of these urethane leads, the possibility of lead failure should be considered promptly (Figure 20).

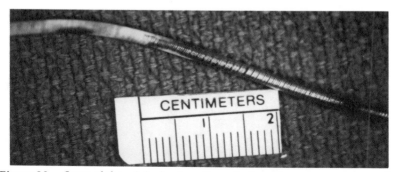

Figure 20. Some of the original polyurethane leads underwent spontaneous deterioration during contact with body fluids. Pressure of a ligature could also destroy the underlying polyurethane. Milky opacification of the clear polyurethane, cracking and insulation loss with short circuit all occurred.

DIAGNOSIS OF MALFUNCTION

POWER SOURCE
1. Rate decline in the magnet mode;
2. Loss of capture in a high threshold lead system;
3. Loss of sensing as a late manifestation;
4. Erratic stimulation rate as a late manifestation.

CIRCUIT
1. Erratic stimulation rate and erratic magnet rate;
2. Erratic or absent sensing of cardiac signals and absent sensing of chest wall stimuli;
3. Programming defect;
4. Telemetry defect;
5. Absent or erratic magnetic mode;
6. Sudden "no output," lead intact on x-ray.

ELECTRODE
1. High threshold, apparently normal pulse generator function;
2. Poor sensing, apparently normal pulse generator function;
3. High threshold with poor sensing;

4. Oversensing, i.e., false recycle from inapparent events is frequently electrode in origin.

LEAD
1. Absent sensing and pacing usually is caused by a lead fracture;
2. False sensing may result from insulation defect;
3. Polyurethane lead deterioration causes the following complex of:
   a) low lead impedance;
   b) early battery depletion (caused by large output drain in a constant voltage pacemaker);
   c) false sensing and recycle from artifacts;
   d) high threshold;
   e) stimulation of the pectoral musculature caused by subcutaneous insulation defect;
   f) stimulation of the right phrenic nerve caused by local insulation defect;
   g) undersensing of spontaneous cardiac activity.

REVISION AND REPAIR

High Threshold Electrode.   Program to high pacemaker output but if the threshold persists, operatively revise the electrode position.

Malposition of the Lead.   Revise the position.

Ventricular Lead Perforation.   Withdraw the lead into the main right ventricular cavity. Note for pericardial bleeding, which however, rarely occurs.

Lead Fracture.

(a) Repair if the fracture site is accessible, and a new connector can be placed without repair of the lead itself;
(b) abandon the lead if the fracture is intravascular or if the stump remaining in the subcutaneous tissue is too short to repair securely;
(c) remove the lead if it is infected.

Insulation Failure.

(a) Repair if accessible, but not if the insulation failure is caused by general deterioration of the material;
(b) if a recalled urethane lead, remove or abandon;
(c) abandon and insulate the connector.

Pulse Generator Depletion. Replace the generator.

Pulse Generator Electronic Failure. Replace the generator if failure is of the pulse forming or sensing circuits. Other circuits such as telemetry, can malfunction without affecting vital pacemaker function. Consult the manufacturer, as many malfunctions are generic to a design rather than unique to a single unit, and the manufacturer may be willing to provide valuable advice of expectation concerning function.

SUMMARY

Troubleshooting of implanted cardiac pacemakers involves knowledge of the hemodynamics, electrophysiology, radiography and electrocardiography of pacing. If the findings on x-ray or ECG are clearcut and straightforward, then diagnosis of the problem and its resolution may be straightforward. If the findings are subtle or confusing, the diagnosis and consequent resolution can be very difficult. Diagnosis can, in the end, be made from the perspective of maximum information concerning pacemaker function and interaction with the patient.

BIBLIOGRAPHY

Alicandri C, Fouad FM, Tarazi RC, et al., Three cases of hypotension and syncope with ventricular pacing: Possible role of atrial reflexes. *Am J Cardiol* 1978; 42:137–142.

Aulenbacher CE: Hydrothorax from subclavian vein catheterization. *JAMA* 1970; 214:372 (letter to editor).

Ausubel K, Furman S: The pacemaker syndrome. *Ann Int Med* 1985; 103:420–429.

Ausubel K, Gabry MD, Klementowicz PT, Furman S: Pacemaker-mediated endless loop tachycardia at rates below the upper rate limit. *Am J Cardiol* 1988; 61:465–467.

Barber K, Amikam S, Furman S: Atrial lead malposition in a dual chamber (DDD,M) pacemaker. *Chest* 1984; 84:766.

Barold SS, Gaidula JJ: Failure of demand pacemaker from low-voltage bipolar ventricular electrograms. *JAMA* 1971; 215:923.

Barold SS, Levine PA: Autointerference of demand pulse generators. *PACE* 1981; 4:274–280.

Bernard RW, Stahl WM: Mediastinal hematoma: Complication of subclavian vein catheterization. *NY State J* Med 1974; 74:83–84.

Calfee RF: Therapeutic radiation and pacemakers. *PACE* 1982; 5:160–161.

Campo I, Garfield GJ, Escher DJW, et al: Complications of pacing by pervenous subclavian semifloating electrodes including two extra-luminal insertions. *Am J Cardiol* 1970; 26:627.

Carter R, Dickerson SC, Berry R: Axillary-subclavian vein thrombosis as a complication of permanent transvenous cardiac pacing. *Va Med* 1978; 105:515–518.

Chatterjee K, Sutton R, Davies JG: Low intracardiac potentials in myocardial infarction as a cause of failure of inhibition of demand pacemakers. *Lancet* 1968; 1:511.

Chauvin M, Brechenmacher C: Muscle stimulation caused by a pacemaker current leakage: The role of the insulation failure of a polyurethane coating. *J Electrophysiol* 1987; 1:326–29.

Christensen KH, Nerstrom B, Baden H: Complications of percutaneous catheterization of subclavian vein in 129 cases. *Acta Chir Scand* 1967; 133:615–620.

Collins DWK, Black JL, Sinclair IN: Predicted early failure of cardiac pacemakers. *PACE* 1985; 8:544–548.

Coumel P, Mugica J, Barold SS: Demand pacemaker arrhythmias caused by intermittent incomplete electrode fracture. Diagnosis with testing magnet. *Am J Cardiol* 1975; 36:105–109.

Crook, BRM, Gishen P, Robinson CR, et al.: Occlusion of the subclavian vein pacemaker electrodes. *Br J Surg* 1977; 64:329–331.

Daly JE, Whitte AA: Non-invasive analysis of simulated pacemaker failure available in multiprogrammable pulse generators. *PACE* 1982; 5:4–9.

Danielson GK, Shabetai R, Bryant LR: Failure of endocardial pacemaker due to late myocardial perforation. Successful restoration of cardiac pacing by conversion to an epicardial system. *J Thorac Cardiovasc Surg* 1967; 54:42–48.

Davies JG, Siddons H: The detection of impending failure in implanted pacemakers. *Thorax* 1969; 24:74–77.

Dekker E, Buller J, Schuilenburg RM: Aids to electrical diagnosis for pacemaker failure. *Am Heart J* 1965; 70:739.

Epstein E, Quereshi MSA, Wright JS: Diaphragmatic paralysis after supraclavicular puncture of subclavian vein. *Br Med J* 1976; 1:693–694.

Falkoff M, Ong LS, Heinle RA, Barold SS: The noise sampling period: A new cause of apparent sensing malfunction of demand pacemakers. *PACE* 1978; 1:250–253.

Farhat K, Nakhjavan FK, Cope C, et al: Iatrogenic arteriovenous fistula: A complication of percutaneous subclavian vein puncture. *Chest* 1975; 67:480.

Fisher JD, Furman S, Parker B, et al: Pacemaker failures characterized by continuous direct current leakage. *Am J Cardiol* 1976; 37:1019–1023.

Flanagan JP, Gradisar IA, Gross RJ, et al: Air embolus: A lethal complication of subclavian venipuncture. *N Engl J Med* 1969; 281:488–489.

Frick MH: Efficiency of a pacemaker clinic to prevent sudden pacing failures. *Br Heart J* 1973; 35:1280–1284.

Frumin H, Furman S: Endless loop tachycardia started by an atrial premature complex in a patient with a dual chamber pacemaker. *JACC* 1985; 5:707–710.

Fulkerson PK, Leier CV, Vasko JS, et al: Use of chest wall stimulation to localize and treat pacemaker sensing failure. *J Electrocardiol* 1980; 13:283–284.

Furman S, Escher DJW, Lister J, et al: A comprehensive scheme for management of pacemaker malfunction. *Ann Surg* 1966; 163:611.

Furman S, Escher DJW, Parker B, et al: Electronic analysis for pacemaker failure. *Ann Thorac Surg* 1969; 8:57.

Fyke FE III: Simultaneous insulation deterioration associated with side-by-side subclavian placement of two polyurethane leads. *PACE* 1988; 11:1571–1574.

Gabry MD, Behrens M, Andrews C, Wanliss M, Klementowicz PT, Furman S: Comparison of myopotential interference in unipolar-bipolar programmable DDD pacemakers. *PACE* 1987; 10:1322–1330.

Gerst PH, Bowman FO, Fleming WH, et al: An evaluation of function and failure of cardiac pacemakers. *J Thorac Cardiovasc Surg* 1967; 54:92–102.

Giedwoyn JO: Pacemaker failure following external defibrillation. *Circulation* 1971; 44:293.

Goldman BS, MacGregor D: Management of infected pacemaker systems. *CPPE* 1984; 2:220–235.

Goldman BS, Noble EJ, MacGregor DC: Pacemaker panic. *Am J Cardiol* 1972; 30:705 (letter to editor).

Goldman LI, Mailer WP, Drezner AD, et al: Another complication of subclavian puncture: Arterial laceration. *JAMA* 1971; 217:78.

Gould L, Maghazeh P, Reddy CVR: Subclavian vein thrombosis following cardiac pacemaker implantation. *Vasc Surg* 1978; 12:262–268.

Gould L, Patel S, Gomes GI, et al: Pacemaker failure following external defibrillation. *PACE* 1981; 4:575–577.

Griepp RB, Daily PO, Shumway NE: Subclavian-axillary vein thrombosis following implantation of a pacemaker catheter in the internal jugular vein. *J Thorac Cardiovasc Surg* 1970; 60:889.

Gschnitzer F: Thrombose der Vena subclavia and axillaris nach Herzschrittmacher Implantation. *Wien Klin Wschr* 1972; 84:393.

Haas JM, Strait GB: Pacemaker-induced cardiovascular failure hemodynamic and angiographic observations. *Am J Cardiol* 1974; 33:295–299.

Hanson J: Sixteen failures in a single model of bipolar polyurethane-insulated ventricular pacing lead. *PACE* 1984; 7:389–394.

Hauser RG: Bipolar leads for cardiac pacing in the 1980's: A reappraisal provoked by skeletal muscle interference. *PACE* 1982; 5:34–37.

Hauser RG, Edwards LM, Giuffre VW: Limitations of pacemaker system analyzers for the evaluation of implantable pulse generators. *PACE* 1981; 4:650–657.

Hauser RG, Giuffre VW: Clinical assessment of cardiac pacemaker performance. *J Cont Ed Cardiol* 1979; 14:19–35.

Hayes D, Holmes D Jr, Merideth J, et al: Apparent pacemaker failure due to reversion circuitry within the programming device. *PACE* 1984; 7:237–239.

Hearne SF, Maloney JD: Pacemaker system failure secondary to air entrapment within the pulse generator pocket. A complication of subclavian venipuncture for lead placement. *Chest* 1982; 82:651.

Heilbrunn A: Fatal subdural hematoma: An unusual complication of pacemaker failure. *Chest* 1970; 57:283–285.

Hepburn F: Discriminating between types of pacemaker lead failure. *J Med Eng Tech* 1978; 2:130–135.

Katzenberg CA, Marcus FI, Heusinkveld RS, et al: Pacemaker failure due to radiation therapy, *PACE* 1982; 5:156–159.

Klein B, Mittelman M, Katz R, et al: Osteomyelitis of both clavicles as a complication of subclavian venipuncture. *Chest* 1983; 83:143.

Kohler F, Schmitt CG, Ellringmann U: Extraction of tricuspid valve tissue and myocardium, as a complication of transvenous cardiac pacing. *Thoraxchirurgie* 1977; 25:97–100.

Kukral JC: Transvenous pacemaker failure due to anomalous venous return to the heart. *Chest* 1971; 59:458–461.

Lasky II: Pacemaker failure from automobile accident. *JAMA* 1970; 211:1700 (letter to editor).

Levick C, Mizgala H, Kerr C: Failure to pace following high dose antiarrhythmic therapy—reversal with isoproterenol. *PACE* 1984; 7:252–256.

Levine PA: Confirmation of atrial capture and determination of artrial capture thresholds in DDD pacing systems. *CPPE* 1984; 2:465–73.

Levine PA: Pacemaker pseudomalfunction. *PACE* 1981;4:563–565.

Levine PA, Barold SS, Fletcher RD, et al: Adverse, acute and chronic effects of electrical defibrillation and cardioversion on implanted unipolar cardiac pacing systems. *JACC* 1983; 1:1413–1422.

Levine PA, Klein MD: Myopotential inhibition of unipolar pacemakers: A disease of technologic progress. *Ann Int Med* 1983; 98:101–103 (editorial).

Levine PA, Seltzer JP: Magnet rates and recommended replacement time indicators of lithium pacemakers. (Part 2). *CPPE* 1983; 1:287–292.

Lewin AA, Serago CF, Schwade JG, et al: Radiation induced failures of complementary metal oxide semiconductor containing pacemakers: A potentially lethal complication. *Int J Radiat Oncol Biol Phys* 1984; 10:1967–69.

Lister JW, Escher DJW, Furman S, et al: Heart block: A method for rapid determination of causes of pacing failure in artificial pacemaking systems. *Am J Cardiol* 1966; 18:64–72.

Lister JW, Furman S, Stein E, et al: A rapid determination of pacemaking defects in patients with artificial pacemakers. *Bull NY Acad Med* 1964; 40:982.

MacGregor DC, Noble EJ, Morrow JD, et al: Management of a pacemaker recall. *J Thorac Cardiovasc Surg* 1977; 74:657.

Martin CM, Klein JJ: Pseudofusion beats masquerading as pacemaker failure. *J Electrocardiol* 1974; 7:179.

McGuire LB, Breit RA, Steinberg S, et al: Reflections on an epidemic of premature pacemaker failures. *PACE* 1981; 4:335–338 (editorial).

McGuire LB, Nolan ST: The care of patients at increased risk of premature pacemaker failure. *JAMA* 1979; 24:701–703.

McWilliams E, Buchalter M, O'Neill C: An unusual form of pacemaker failure *PACE* 1984; 7:765–766.

Misaki T, Iwa T, Mastunaga Y: Atrial amplitude mapping to avoid P wave sensing failure. *PACE* 1983; 6:A–3. (abstract)

Nathan DA, Lister JW, Keller JW, et al: Percutaneous access to implanted electrodes. *Am J Cardiol* 1971; 27:397.

Nevins MA, Landau S, Lyon LJ: Failure of demand pacemaker sensing due to electrode fracture. *Chest* 1971; 59:110–113.

Obel IWP: Transient phrenic nerve paralysis following subclavian venipuncture. *Anaesthesiology* 1970; 33:369–370.

Ong LS, Barold SS, Craver WL, Falkoff MD, Heinle RA: Partial avulsion of the tricuspid valve by tined pacing electrode. *Am Heart J* 1981; 102:798–799.

O'Reilly MV, Murnaghan DP, Williams MB: Transvenous pacemaker failure induced by hyperkalemia. *JAMA* 1974; 228:336–337.

Oseran D, Ausubel K, Klementowicz PT, Furman S: Spontaneous endless loop tachycardia. *PACE* 1986; 9:379–386.

Pappas G, Shoultz Ch A Jr, Blount SG Jr: Fractured intracardiac transvenous pacemaker catheter. An unusual cause of pacemaker failure. *Am Heart J* 1969; 78:807.

Parsonnet V, Myers GH, Manhardt M: A pacemaker follow up clinic: An analysis of detection of signs of impending pacemaker failure. In P Samet, N El-Sherif (eds): *Cardiac Pacing.* Grune & Stratton, New York, 1980, p. 257.

Parsonnet V, Myers GH, Gilbert L, et al: Prediction of impending pacemaker failure in a pacemaker clinic. *Am J Cardiol* 1970; 25:311–319.

Pourhamidi AH: Radiation effect on implanted pacemakers. *Chest* 1983; 84:499–500.

Preston TA, Fletcher RD, Lucchesi BR, Judge RD: Changes in myocardial threshold. Physiological and pharmacologic factors in patients with implanted pacemakers. *Am Heart J* 1967; 74:235–242.

Quertermonus T, Megahy SM, DasGupta DS, et al: Pacemaker failure resulting from radiation damage. *Radiology* 1983; 148:257–258.

Raymond R, Nanian K: Insultaion failure with bipolar polyurethane leads. *PACE* 1984; 7:378–380.

Reinhart S, McAnulty JH, Dobbs J: Type and timing of permanent pacemaker failure. *Chest* 1982, 82:433–435.

Rockland R, Parsonnet V, Myers GH: Failure modes of American pacemakers: In vitro analysis. *Am Heart J* 1972; 83:481.

Rowley BA: Electrolysis: A factor in cardiac pacemaker electrode failure. *IEEE Trans Biomed Eng* 1963; 10:176.

Rubenstein JJ, Laforet EG: Pacemaker runaway following intermittent output failure. *PACE* 1983; 6:645–647.

Rubin IL, Arbeit SR, Gross H: The electrocardiographic recognition of pacemaker failure and function. *Ann Intern Med* 1969; 71:603.

Ryden L, Hedstrom P, Leijonhufvud S: A new apparatus for detection of impending pacemaker failure in patients treated with implanted pacemakers. *Cardiovasc Res* 1970; 4:242.

Seltzer JP, Levine P: Magnet rates and recommended replacement time indicators of the available implanted pulse generators in North America (part I). *CPPE* 1983; 1:81–84.

Seltzer JP, Levine PA, Watson WS: Patient-initiated autonomous pacemaker tachycardia. *PACE* 1984; 7:961–969.

Sheridan DJ, Reid DS, Williams DO, et al: Mechanical failure causing leakage with unipolar pacemakers. Significance and detection. *Eur J Cardiol* 1978; 8:1–8.

Slepian M, Levine JH, Watkins L Jr, Brinker J, Guarnieri T: Automatic implantable cardioverter defibrillator/permanent pacemaker interaction: Loss of pacemaker capture following AICD discharge. *PACE* 1987; 10:1194–1197.

Sowton E: Detection of impending pacemaker failure. *Isr J Med Sci* 1967; 3:260.

Stanford W, Coyle FL, Dooley BN, et al: Transvenous pacemaker failure; migration of catheter lead by patient manipulation. *Ann Thorac Surg* 1968; 5:162.

Stroobandt R, Willems R, Depuydt P, Holvoet G, Sinnaeve A: The superfast atrial recharge pulse: A cause of pectoral muscle stimulation in patients equipped with a unipolar DDD pacemaker. *PACE* 1989; 12:451–455.

Tegtmeyer CJ, Bezirdjian DR, Irani FA, et al: Cardiac pacemaker failure: A complication of trauma. *South Med J* 1981; 74:378–379.

Tulgan H: Electrocardiographic misrepresentation of impending pacemaker failure. *Ann Intern Med* 1970; 72:251.

Warnowicz MA, Goldschlager N: Apparent failure to sense (undersensing) caused by oversensing: Diagnostic use of noninvasively obtained intracardiac electrogram. *PACE* 1983; 6:1341–1343.

Weinman J: Comments. Electrolysis. A factor in cardiac pacemaker electrode failure. *IEEE Trans Biomed Eng* 1964; 11:114–115.

Yarnoz MD, Attai LA, Furman S: Infection of pacemaker electrode and removal with cardiopulmonary bypass. *J Thorac Cardiovasc Surg* 1974; 68:43–46.

Yatteau RF: Medical Intelligence: Brief recordings. Radar-induced failure of a demand pacemaker. *N Engl J Med* 1970; 283: 1447–1448.

GLOSSARY

AICD™:   Abbreviation for the automatic internal cardioverter defibrillator. A permanently implanted device with the function of sensing ventricular tachycardia and/or ventricular fibrillation and delivering an electrical shock when such a rhythm has been detected. The term AICD is a trademark.

ALERT PERIOD: That part of the ventricular or atrial cycle during which the pacemaker is sensitive, i.e., "alert" to incoming signals.

AMPERE (A):   The basic unit of electrical current. Pacemaker systems require small amounts of current, measured in thousandths of an ampere (milliampere, abbreviated mA) or in the millionths of an ampere (microampere, abbreviated μA). The fluid equivalent is a measure of flow, i.e., quarts or gallons of water/sec.

AMPERE HOUR: The basic unit of battery capacity. All batteries are rated in ampere-hours and output voltage. The voltage is specific for any one battery, the overall capacity depends on the size of the cell, i.e., greater or lesser ampere-hour capacity. The implication is that under standardized conditions the battery will deliver a given number of amperes for a stated number of hours. The equivalent might be the capacity to deliver a specific number of gallons of water for a specific number of hours.

ANODE: The positive terminal of a pacemaker or electrode. In a battery, the terminal that receives electrons.

ASYNCHRONOUS: A mode of operation in which the pacemaker is insensitive to incoming signals from the chamber being paced. The antonym of asynchronous in pacing terms is not synchronous, rather it is responsive.

A-V BLOCK: The mode of approach to the upper rate interval by maintaining the AV interval constant until a P wave is unsensed or blocked.

A-V CONDUCTION: A description of the conduction of atrial impulses from the atrium through the AV node and the His-Purkinje system to the ventricle. The term in also applied to the conduction of paced beats from the atrium to the ventricle via the pacemaker.

A-V INTERVAL: (Atrio-ventricular interval, A-V delay) The interval between the sensed or paced atrial event and the next sensed or paced ventricular event.

A-V SYNCHRONY: The relationship between atrial and ventricular systole. This relationship is lost in patients with AV block. It is also lost in some patients with ventricular pacing.

AUTOMATICITY: An electrophysiological mechanism of arrhythmia in

651

which there is abnormal impulse formation. Automatic arrhythmias can usually not be reliably induced or terminated by electrical stimulation.

AUTONOMOUS PACEMAKER TACHYCARDIA (APT):   A tachycardia of a dual-chamber pacemaker in which the arrhythmia is begun by a combination of pacemaker and sensed cardiac events, but once begun is sustained without regard to cardiac interaction. No electronic malfunction exists.

BATTERY: The power source of the pulse generator. Strictly speaking, a battery consists of more than one cell. Each cell of a battery is of a specific chemistry and develops a specific voltage. In a cell or battery of cells power is evolved from a chemical reaction.

BEGINNING OF LIFE (BOL):   The electronic characteristics of a pulse generator when it has been freshly manufactured. These are usually maintained until the approach of end of life. This term relates to the operation of the pulse generator battery.

BIPOLAR: Both pacemaker electrical terminals, anode and cathode, are in contact with stimulatable tissue.

BLANKING PERIOD: The time during and after a pacemaker stimulus during which the opposite channel of a dual channel pacemaker is insensitive. The intent is to avoid sensing the electronic event of one channel in the opposite channel.

CAPACITOR (Condenser):   A device that can store an electrical charge. It is made of two conductors separated by an insulator, or by an electrolyte or air.

CARDIAC OUTPUT: The volume of blood ejected per unit of time, measured in liters per minute. This may be adjusted to account for body surface to yield the cardiac index, i.e., liters per minute per meter^2.

CAROTID SINUS SYNCOPE (CSS):   Attacks of syncope and related symptoms that usually occur with the patient in the upright position and that can be reproduced regularly by means of mechanical stimulation of the carotid sinus.

CATHODE: The negative terminal of a pacemaker or electrode. In a battery, the terminal that emits electrons.

CELL: See Battery.

CHRONAXIE TIME: See Strength Duration Curve.

CMOS: Complementary metal oxide semiconductor. Modern low power semiconductor.

COMMITTED: A dual-chamber pacemaker in which the delivery of an atrial stimulus forces the delivery of a ventricular stimulus. Either both stimuli are emitted or neither.

CONDUCTOR: A material that allows the passage of electrical current. As all materials will allow the passage of current at a sufficiently high voltage, a conductor is one which will allow the passage of current at a low voltage.

CONNECTOR: The mechanism that connects the output of the pulse generator to the lead. There are two parts, one on the generator, the other on the lead.

CONSTANT CURRENT: A pacemaker that maintains its constancy of current output over a wide range of impedance. The output voltage is as required to maintain the current output constant.

COULOMB (C): The measure of charge. It is equivalent to the term gallons. As pacemaker outputs are small, the common measurement would be in the micro terms, i.e., 1/1,000,000 of a coulomb (μC).

CROSSTALK: Sensing of electronic events generated in one channel in the other channel. Sensing an atrial stimulus in ventricular channel with consequent recycle is an example.

CYCLE LENGTH: The interval in milliseconds from one event to the next. The term is used in measuring cardiac rate or a pacemaker stimulation rate.

DEFIBRILLATION THRESHOLD (DFT): The energy in Joules that consistently terminates ventricular fibrillation.

DEMAND (Standby): A noncompetitive pacemaker, this term now is almost obsolete.

DISCRIMINANT P-WAVE SENSING: The ability of the pacemaker to discriminate between an antegrade and a retrograde P wave. Such discrimination may be helpful in preventing endless loop tachycardia.

dP/dt: An abbreviation denoting the change in pressure that occurs over a given amount of time. When applied to cardiac hemodynamics, this refers to contractility. dP/dt measurements may serve as a possible biological sensor for rate modulation.

dV/dt: See slew rate.

DUAL CHAMBER: A pulse generator that can stimulate and/or sense atrium and/or ventricle.

DUAL DEMAND: A pacemaker that paces to support the cardiac rate during bradycardia and will begin pacing (usually asynchronously) during tachycardia.

ECCENTRICITY: An apparent deviation from presumed normal function but which is normal function for that model.

EJECTION FRACTION: The relationship between the volume of blood ejected and the end-systolic (ES) X end-diastolic (ED) volume. ED volume−ES volume/ED volume.

ELECTROCARDIOGRAM (ECG, EKG): The electrical signal emitted by active cardiac tissue recorded from the body surface.

ELECTRODE: The interface with living tissue across which the stimulus is transmitted. It is usually metal but may be carbon or, potentially, other material.

ELECTROGRAM (EGM): The electrical signal emitted by active cardiac tissue recorded from within or upon the heart.

ELECTROMAGNETIC INTERFERENCE (EMI):   Electrical signals of nonphysiological origin that affect pacemaker function.

ELECTROMYOGRAPHIC INTERFERENCE (EMI):   Electrical signals of muscular origin that affect pacemaker function.

ELECTROPHYSIOLOGIC TESTING: An invasive study with placement of a variable number of catheters in the heart for stimulation and recording. During this study the basic properties of conduction and refractoriness are assessed. The mechanism of tachycardia is assessed by analyzing conduction and termination sequences.

ENDLESS LOOP TACHYCARDIA (ELT):   (Pacemaker Mediated Tachycardia; Pacemaker Mediated Re-entry Tachycardia; Pacemaker Circus Movement Tachycardia). A re-entry arrhythmia in which the dual-chamber pacemaker acts as the antegrade limb of the tachycardia and the natural pathway as the retrograde limb.

END OF LIFE (EOL):   The electronic characteristics of a pulse generator when it should be electively removed from service. This term relates to the operation of the pulse generator battery.

EPICARDIAL LEAD: A lead stimulating the heart by onlay upon the epicardial surface of the atrium or ventricle.

EPIMYOCARDIAL LEAD: A lead placed into the myocardium from the epicardial surface of the heart. All modern leads implanted by thoracotomy are myocardial, colloquially referred to as "epimyocardial."

ESCAPE INTERVAL: The interval between a sensed or paced event to the next paced event. (See hysteresis)

EVOKED RESPONSE: The response of the myocardium to a pacemaker stimulus. The response may be modified by the activity state of the cardiac tissue.

FIXATION: The means of attachment of an endocardial electrode to the endocardium once it is introduced. Two modes exist:
Active: The electrode actively grasps the endocardium via fine metal pins, a jaw-like device, or a screw.
Passive: The lead proximal to the electrode is irregular with a conical "shoulder" fins or tines. Local tissue reaction places enough fibrous tissue about the lead irregularity to hold it in place.

FUSION BEAT: A ventricular or atrial depolarization which starts from two foci (one spontaneous, the other, a pacemaker stimulus) and has characteristics of each.

HEADER: The portion of a pulse generator that contains the receptacle(s), which receive the lead connector pins.

HERMETIC: The ability to seal a device so that neither water vapor nor any other gas can enter or leave the "hermetic seal." The standard measurement technique is in leakage of helium molecules.

HERTZ (Hz):   Frequency of a signal in cycles per second.

HYSTERESIS: A difference in the duration of the pacemaker escape interval depending on whether it is started by a sensed or paced event. The interval may be shorter or longer than the escape interval and will be referred to as "positive or negative," although in the context, the terms are undefined.

IMPEDANCE: The total impediment to the flow of electrical current in a conductor. It is a more complex function than resistance alone and accounts for all impediments to the flow of current.

INHIBITED (INHIBITORY): A pacemaker response in which a stimulus is withheld in response to a sensed event.

INTERVAL: The elapsed time between pacemaker and/or cardiac events. A more useful concept than rate.

INTRINSIC DEFLECTION: The portion of the electrogram that represents the depolarization wave moving past the sensing electrode. It is the part of the electrogram that is sensed because of adequate amplitude and slew rate (frequency content).

JOULE (J): The unit of energy. It is the product of current volts and time. In pacemakers, microJoules (μJ) would be used; in defibrillators Joules.

LEAD: The insulated wire that connects the output of the pulse generator to the electrode.

LOWER RATE INTERVAL: Also referred to as the "lower rate limit," etc. It is the maximum interval the pacemaker will allow between two pacemaker ventricular stimuli or between a sensed ventricular event and the next ventricular paced event.

MAGNET MODE: The response of a pacemaker to the closure of its magnetic switch. Many different magnetic modes exist so that the mode of operation for a specific pacemaker must be known.

MAXIMUM SENSOR RATE: The programmed value for a rate modulated pacemaker that determines the maximum rate that can be achieved with the artificial sensor. In a rate modulated dual-chamber pacemaker the maximum sensor rate may be the same, higher, or lower than the maximum atrial trigger (tracking) rate.

MAXIMUM TRACKING RATE: The maximum rate (or minimum coupling interval) at which an atrial sensing pacemaker will respond to atrial events. In a rate modulated dual-chamber pacemaker the maximum tracking rate may be the same, higher, or lower than the maximum sensor rate.

MINUTE VENTILATION: Respiratory rate X tidal volume = minute ventilation. This parameter is used as a biological indicator for rate modulated pacing.

MYOCARDIAL ELECTRODE: An electrode which penetrates the myocardium and is held in place by a suture, or by a plastic, fabric, or rubber plate.

NOISE MODE: The pacemaker operation when it receives signals defined as being electrical noise. For example, the asynchronous (VOO) operation of a ventricular inhibited pacemaker during sensing of 60 Hz current.

NONCOMPETITIVE: A pacemaker that senses cardiac function and avoids a stimulus during the sensitive portion of a spontaneous depolarization.

OVERDRIVE PACING: Pacing at a more rapid rate than a tachycardia in order to interrupt and terminate a re-entrant arrhythmia.

OVERVOLTAGE: A reverse voltage developed by a reactive metal in a biological solution, i.e., a non-noble metal electrode, e.g., Elgiloy (a steel alloy) in contact with myocardium. The more noble (i.e., nonreactive) the metal, the lower the overvoltage. Overvoltage is part of the impedance measurement.

PACEMAKER: The entire cardiac stimulating system, it includes power source (battery) and circuit, which are always one package, lead, and electrode.

PACEMAKER-INDUCED ARRHYTHMIA (PIA):   An arrhythmia caused by a pacemaker stimulus or stimuli that once begun continues without further pacemaker function, e.g., ventricular fibrillation.

PACEMAKER-MEDIATED ARRHYTHMIA (PMA):   An arrhythmia that requires a pacemaker to start and be sustained, e.g., atrial fibrillation or flutter sensed by the pacemaker to drive the ventricle, endless loop tachycardia.

PACEMAKER SENSOR: A sensor incorporated into an implantable pulse generator for the purpose of detecting a physiological or nonphysiological function in order to modulate its rate, and possibly, other characteristics.
Closed Loop: A pacemaker sensor that responds to a physiological stimulus such as respiration, evoked response, or central venous temperature.
Open Loop: A pacemaker sensor that responds to a nonphysiological stimulus such as motion or activity.

PACEMAKER SYNDROME: A syndrome of pounding in the chest and neck and waves of weakness during cardiac pacing that results from loss of AV synchrony and retrograde activation of the atrium. Other causes include restricted cardiac output, because of the absence of rate increase with exercise.

PACING FOR TACHYCARDIA AUTOMATIC DEVICES: Pulse generators capable of automatic tachycardia detection and treatment.

PACING FOR TACHYCARDIA INTERACTION DEVICES: Pacemakers that require that the patient detect tachycardia, manually interact (operate) with the pulse generator, and recognize return to sinus rhythm.

POLARIZATION: Resistance to the flow of current because of the accumulation of electrons about an electrode. These act as an insulator until diffused. Polarization is measured as part of the impedance.

PRE-EJECTION INTERVAL: The interval from the beginning of ventricular depolarization to the beginning of ventricular ejection. The pre-ejection interval is made up of the electrical mechanical interval plus the isovolumetric contraction time. When used as an indicator for rate modulation, timing starts with a pacemaker stimulus.

PROBABILITY DENSITY FUNCTION: A technique that determines the diagnosis of ventricular fibrillation by the time the electrogram spends at the isoelectric line, more during sinus or ventricular tachycardia, and less with ventricular fibrillation.

PROGRAMMING: The ability to alter a pacemaker setting noninvasively. A variety of selections exist each with its own designation. If inadvertent or undetected, it is phantom programming.

PSEUDOFUSION BEAT: A spontaneous cardiac depolarization with a superimposed stimulus. The depolarization is of unpaced origin only.

PULSE DURATION: The duration of the pacemaker stimulus from its beginning to the return to the zero line. Some pulse shapes require measurement from the beginning to some other point. This is specified by the manufacturer.

PULSE GENERATOR: The metal enclosed power source and electronic circuit with its attached lead connector. The pulse generator is often mistakenly referred to as the pacemaker.

RATE: The reciprocal of the sustained pacemaker stimulation interval. The number of beats per minute, spontaneous or paced.

RATE MODULATED: A pacemaker that is able to adjust its stimulation interval (rate) based on input from a biological sensor. It is sometimes considered synonymous with rate responsive, adaptive rate, and sensor driven.

RATE RESPONSIVE: The change in pacemaker stimulation interval caused by sensing a physiological function other than the atrium. The physiological functions sensed may be stimulus-T interval, activity, right ventricular temperature, etc.

RATE SMOOTHING: Capability to avoid marked R-R cycle variations by placing limits on how much a subsequent R-R cycle length can vary from the preceding cycle length. In general, this is programmable in values of percent, i.e., 3, 6, 12 percent. When rate smoothing is utilized in a DDD device, it will result in AV dissociation.

REED SWITCH: A magnetically activated switch sealed (usually in glass) and contained within a pulse generator. Open (electricity does not flow), the generator functions in one way, closed (current flows) by placement of a magnet, in another manner, referred to as the magnet mode. Unless a magnet is placed, the resting position of the switch is "open."

REENTRY: The most common mechanism of tachycardia. It requires two pathways with differential conduction and unidirectional block. Re-entrant arrhythmias can usually be induced and terminated by electrical stimulation.

REFRACTORINESS: A measure of the recovery of excitability of the cardiac tissue under electrophysiological investigation.

REFRACTORY PERIOD: A time after a sensed or paced event during which the pacemaker is insensitive.

REFRACTORY PERIOD (ATRIAL): The time after a sensed or paced event during which the atrial pacemaker or channel of a dual-chamber pacemaker is insensitive. The intent is to avoid sensing a physiological event.

REFRACTORY PERIOD (VENTRICULAR):   The time after a sensed or paced event during which the ventricular pacemaker or channel of a dual-chamber pacemaker is insensitive. The intent is to avoid sensing a physiological event.

RESISTANCE: The impediment to the flow of electrical current in a conductor. All conductors present some degree of resistance to the flow of current. It is the ratio of the voltage to current of an electrical circuit connected to a direct current source. The measurement of resistance is in Ohms.

RESISTANCE, INTERNAL: The resistance to the flow of current within a battery. This limits the ability to deliver current flow. A high internal resistance battery may have the overall capacity to deliver a large amount of electrical capacity, but only at a slow rate. The lithium iodine battery fails by increase of internal resistance rather than depletion of the iodine or the lithium. At a sufficiently high internal resistance (approximately 50,000 Ohms), the ability of current to flow out of the battery is reduced below the needs of the pulse generator circuit.

RHEOBASE: See Strength Duration Curve

SAFETY PACING: A mechanism in which an event sensed during an interval after the end of the ventricular blanking period causes emission of a ventricular stimulus. It is designed to eliminate crosstalk or EMI inhibition of the ventricular channel.

SCANNING PACEMAKER: An underdrive pacemaker which progressively scans diastole in an attempt to stimulate during the critical time window during which tachycardia can be terminated.

SENSOR DRIVEN: A pacemaker that is capable of rate modulation via a sensor. Sensor driven may be used as a synonym for rate modulation, adaptive rate, and rate responsive pacemakers.

SINGLE-CHAMBER: A pulse generator that can stimulate and sense one cardiac chamber only. Often the same generator can be used for either atrium or ventricle.

SLEW RATE: The rate of movement of an electrical field, measured in volts/second. It is characteristic of a biological signal such as an electrogram. By a complex mathematical process known as the Fourier transform it can be converted into a series of signals of different frequencies.

STANDBY (DEMAND):   A noncompetitive pacemaker.

STRENGTH DURATION CURVE: The quantity of charge, current, voltage, or energy required to stimulate the heart at a series of pulse durations. The *RHEOBASE* is the lowest point on such a curve at an infinitely long pulse duration. *CHRONAXIE TIME* is the pulse duration twice the rheobase value.

STROKE VOLUME: The volume of blood ejected per heart beat. It equals end-diastolic volume minus end-systolic volume.

STYLET: The thin flexible wire that can be shaped and inserted in the lumen of the pacing lead to allow its manipulation.

SUTURELESS LEAD: A myocardial lead in which the means of its introduction is the means of its fastening. One example is the "corkscrew-" like electrode, which once screwed into the myocardium is fixed in position and stimulates the heart.

SYNCHRONIZED: A stimulus emitted simultaneously with a sensed atrial or ventricular event so that the pacemaker stimulus falls into the absolute refractory interval of spontaneous depolarization.

SYNCHRONOUS: A pacemaker stimulus that is emitted in response to a sensed event after an appropriate delay, as in atrial synchronous.

TACHYCARDIA: A ventricular rate more rapid than 100 bpm. It may be entirely normal as in sinus tachycardia, a response to exercise, emotion, fever, etc.
Malignant: A tachycardia that accelerates and may result in ventricular fibrillation.
Monomorphic: A tachycardia that originates from one ventricular focus.
Polymorphic: A tachycardia that originates from more than one ventricular focus.
Supraventricular: A tachycardia that originates above the ventricle, i.e., sinus, atrial fibrillation, or flutter, etc.

THRESHOLD: The threshold of cardiac stimulation is the least cathodal electrical stimulus which, when delivered in diastole after the absolute, relative refractory and the hypersensitive periods, is able to maintain consistent capture of the heart.
Acute: The threshold immediately after implantation of the lead-electrode system.
Chronic: The threshold after stability has been reached.

TIME WINDOW: Range of critical coupling intervals during which extrastimuli can initiate and terminate tachycardia.

TOTAL ATRIAL REFRACTORY PERIOD: The time in which the atrial pacemaker channel is insensitive. It usually consists of the AV interval and the atrial refractory interval after the ventricular event.

TRIGGERED: (See Synchronized.) A pacemaker response in which a stimulus is emitted in response to a sensed event.

UNDERDRIVE PACING: Pacing at a slower rate than a tachycardia which can interrupt and terminate a re-entrant arrhythmia.

UNIPOLAR: All pacemaker systems have two electrical terminals for each channel, one anodal, the other cathodal. If one (always the cathode) is in contact with sensitive tissue while the other is remote, i.e., away from the heart, the system is termed unipolar.

UPPER RATE INTERVAL: Also referred to as the "upper rate limit," "maximum tracking rate," etc. It is the minimum interval of response of the pacemaker ventricular channel to signals received via the atrial channel. It is the shortest interval the pacer will allow between two ventricular stimuli, or between a sensed ventricular event and a ventricular stimulus. The concept of interval is much more useful than that of rate.

VA CONDUCTION (ventriculo-atrial):   The conduction of a ventricular impulse retrograde to the atrium via the AV node.

VA INTERVAL (ventriculo-atrial):   The interval between the sensed or paced ventricular event and the next sensed or paced atrial event.

VOLT (V):   The force with which current is driven. The proper term is electromotive force which is measured in volts. Pacemaker output is indicated in volts. Biological signals, such as electrogram amplitudes, are indicated in millivolts (mV).

VULNERABLE PERIOD: That portion of the electrical complex, either atrial or ventricular, during which stimulation may induce arrhythmia.

WENCKEBACH: AV conduction at progressively greater intervals until one P wave is unsensed. The cycle then restarts.

WENCKEBACH UPPER RATE LIMIT: A mode of approach to the upper rate interval by automatically prolonging the interval between the sensed or paced ventricular event.

INDEX

Electrolyte balance, 24–25
Electromagnetic interference, 599
Electromyographic interference, 599
Electroshock therapy, 603–604
Endless loop tachycardia, 68–72, 143–156
  balanced, 151–156
  caused by atrial premature complex,
    146
  differentiation from primary supraven-
    tricular tachycardia, 146, 148–149
  spontaneous, 149–151
Endocardial evoked potential, 389–392
Endocardial systems, 431, 434, 436, 438
Endocardial thickening, 24
Energy, 44, 54, 55–56, 469–471
Environment, 602–603
Epicardial systems, 229–230
Epimyocardial systems, 271–273, 434, 436, 438
Exercise, 180–188
  and atrial pacing, 181
  and atrial synchronous pacing, 181–182
  and AV sequential pacing, 182–184
  byproducts emitted during, 374–375
  complete heart block with, 372
  and DDD systems, 184–186
  physiological changes during, 373
  and rate modulated pacing, 404–411
  and rate responsive pacemakers, 186–188
  testing after pacemaker implant, 404–
    411
External pulse generators, 218–219
External transcutaneous pacing, 231
Extracorporeal shock wave lithotripsy,
  607–608

Fibrosis, 23–24
First-degree heart block, 8
Follow-up, patient. See Patient follow-up

Heart block, 8–10, 370, 372
Heart rate, 168–169, 180, 430
Heart surgery, 638–642
Hematoma, 488–489
Hemodynamics, 167–188
His bundle, 211–213
Holter monitoring, 536
Hysteresis, 160, 312, 566–568

Illness, 604. See also specific illnesses
Impedance, 47, 49, 54, 60, 624–627
Implantation, permanent pacemaker, 239–285
  anatomic approach, 240–248
  anesthesia, 239–240
  atrial lead placement, 255–260
  after cardiac transplantation, 285
  cephalic approach, 245–246
  complications, 268–271
  connectors, 274–277
  dual-chamber, 253–260
  epimyocardial systems, 271–273
  facility for, 239
  hardware adaptations, 274–277
  jugular approach, 246–248
  measurement of pacing and sensing
    thresholds, 261–265
  pacemaker pocket, 265–268, 271
  pediatric patients, 278–284
  securing lead, 252
  subclavian approach, 240–245
  venous access and entry, 269
  ventricular lead placement, 248–252
Incision, 624
Infection, 236, 503
Interatrial conduction, 107–110

Jugular implantation approach, 246–248

Leads
  active fixation, 39
  anatomical variations, 324, 326–327
  arterial puncture, 489–490
  atrial, 255–260, 324, 339
  and automatic implantable cardioverter
    defibrillator, 430–438
  bipolar, 401–402
  damage, 493
  destruction, 617
  dislodgment, 231–234, 497–498
  endocardial fixation, 37–39
  impedance, 624–627
  insulation, 32–34
  integrity, 348
  intracardiac dislodgment, 231–234
  multiple, 349
  myocardial and epicardial, 37, 339, 341
  orthogonal, 94–107
  perforation, 490–492
  placement for permanent pacemaker im-
    plantation, 248–252, 255–260, 270–271
  polarity, 341, 344
  positioning, 348–350
  and radiography, 338–350
  removal, 633–642
  retained, 632–633
  retained fragments, 503, 505
  securing, 252
  specialized, 402–403
  steroid, 35–37
  systems for rate modulated pacing,
    401–403
  transvenous, 338, 434
  type, 344, 346
  unipolar, 401–402
  ventricular, 248–252, 324, 338–339
  See also Electrodes
Lithium, 55, 56, 58
Local muscle stimulation, 501–502
Lower rate behavior, 160
Lyme disease, 19–21

Magnet, 291–296, 606
Magnetic resonance imaging (MRI), 606–607
Medicare regulation, 3–8
Medication. See Drugs
MRI. See Magnetic resonance imaging
Multiple sensing channels, 163
Muscle stimulation, 501–502
Myocardial infarction
  anterior, 13
  inferior, 12
  local, 23–24
  permanent pacing after acute, 12–13
  and temporary pacing, 212, 213

Nuclear pacemakers, 55–56, 58
Nursing care, 228–229

Open heart surgery, 638–642
Overdrive suppression, 459–460
Oxygen saturation, 399

Pacemaker allergy, 505
Pacemaker clinic, 512, 536–539
Pacemaker codes, 193–204
  ICHD, 193, 194
  NASPE specific, 200–204
  NBG, 193, 195–200
Pacemaker electrocardiography. See Electrocar-
  diography
Pacemaker implantation, permanent. See Im-
  plantation, permanent pacemaker
Pacemaker malfunction. See Troubleshooting
Pacemaker pocket, 265–268, 271